AF834702

CLINICAL PSYCHIATRY: ASSESSMENT AND TREATMENT

Levan Maglakelidze

ALLIED HEALTH PRESS

Clinical Psychiatry: Assessment and Treatment

Author: **Levan Maglakelidze**

Allied Health Press
4164 Lakeshore Road
Burlington ON L7L 1A4
Canada
www.alliedhealthpress.com
Email: orders@arclereducation.com

ISBN: 978-1-77956-841-0

ABOUT THE AUTHOR

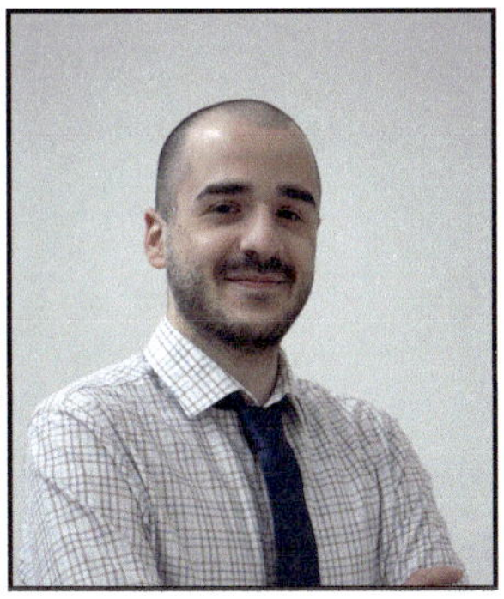

Levan Maglakelidze holds an M.D. from David Tvildiani Medical University, Tbilisi, with a clinical background in intensive care, cardiac and neurosurgical assistance, and psychiatry. He is currently working as a Research Study Coordinator at Evexi Clinic, Tbilisi, contributing to international clinical trials with organizations including ICON, Merck, and PPD. He also serves as an invited lecturer in American medical programs at the University of Georgia. His research interests include psychiatry, precision medicine, and medical data analysis. He holds a Good Clinical Practice (GCP) certificate obtained through his research work, and has previous experience as an ICU junior doctor, surgical assistant, and junior psychiatrist.

Brief Table of Contents

Getting Started with This Book

Chapter Openers

A list of Chapter Outline is presented providing a brief Introduction to what will be covered in the chapter.

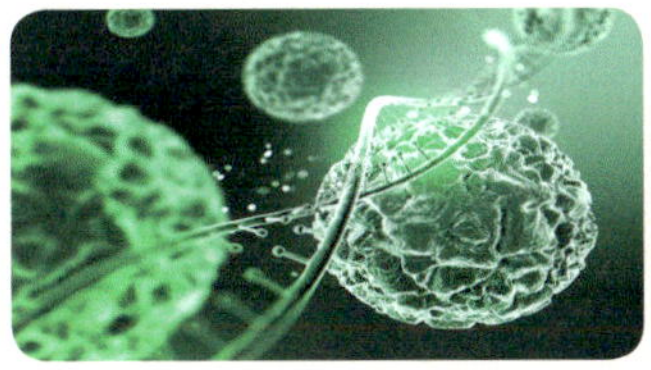

Introduction

Often referred to as the science of life, biology is a broad field of study aimed at comprehending the several kinds of life on Earth, from tiny creatures to sophisticated multicellular entities. Comprising several subfields, including molecular biology, ecology, and evolutionary biology, each of which advances our knowledge of living systems, this field clarifies the mechanisms controlling life events, including development, reproduction, and interaction with the surroundings, which is the central goal of biology. Moreover, biology fills in the void between the natural sciences and medicine by offering a necessary understanding of health, illness, and the interactions between organisms and their environments. Dealing with urgent global issues such as climate change, biodiversity loss, and new diseases depends on an awareness of these complex biological interactions, therefore highlighting the critical part biology plays in modern civilization. Fundamentally, biology explores and tests ideas about the living world using the scientific method. Through methodical observation and experimentation,

LEARNING OBJECTIVES

After studying this chapter, you will be able to:

1. Discuss the scientific method in biology;
2. Explain the cell theory;
3. Discuss the genetics and heredity;
4. Evolution and natural selection;
5. Focus on ecology and ecosystems;
6. Learn about human biology;
7. Evaluate the plant biology;
8. Explain the microbiology;
9. Focus on current trends in biology.

1.1. The Scientific Method in Biology

Learning Outcome

1. Describe the steps of the scientific method;
2. Focus on hypothesis formation;
3. Learn about experimental design.

Learning Outcomes

The beginning of each section of every chapter contains a set of Learning Outcomes that inform students of concepts they should understand. These outcomes help students understand what they should be able to do if they have mastered the material in that section.

Test Your Knowledge

Throughout each chapter, Test Your Knowledge cues you to note which topics have been covered and to self-test your understanding of the material presented.

Test Your Knowledge

1. Explain why correlation does not imply causation in scientific experiments.
2. How does the scientific method help reduce the influence of personal opinions in research?

Chapter Summary

The Summary Section appear at the end of each chapter and summarize main concepts covered throughout the chapter. These points provide key concepts in an engaging and meaningful way.

Summary

The investigation of biological principles highlights the importance of a comprehensive view of life by reflecting the intricate interactions that occur within living systems. The complexity of biology goes beyond individual species or systems, as this essay highlights; it also includes the interactions that mold ecosystems and affect biodiversity. Researchers can conduct in-depth analyses of metabolomic data using sophisticated technologies like MetaboAnalyst, which offer insights into the molecular mechanisms underlying these interactions. As demonstrated by the developments in MetaboAnalyst, for example, the integration of diverse omics data promotes a thorough understanding of metabolic pathways and helps identify important biological markers necessary for research on development and disease (Chong et al., 2018). Additionally, the phenomenon of ecological invasions is a key component of biological research and a vital field of study. The introduction of non-native species into unfamiliar habitats has significant ramifications and calls for multidisciplinary management strategies. Examining the origins and effects of these biological incursions, invasion science has become a crucial field that highlights the need to comprehend ecological dynamics and community interactions. As interest in biological invasions increases, new findings are emerging that put conventional ecological theories and practices to the test. The importance of incorporating various scientific viewpoints is shown by this developing discipline, which also highlights how invasive species shape ecosystems and advances our knowledge of ecological resilience (David et al., 2013). When taken as a whole, these discoveries from invasion science and metabolomics highlight the value of multidisciplinary biology research. Fostering cross-disciplinary collaboration and utilizing technological breakthroughs to improve our comprehension of intricate biological interactions are crucial as we look to the future of biological research. In addition to deepening our understanding of the complexities of life, this method lays the groundwork for tackling urgent environmental issues. Future studies can ensure the continued relevance of biology in a world that is constantly changing by acknowledging the interconnection of biological systems and opening the door to creative solutions that support sustainability and biodiversity conservation. We might imagine a thorough comprehension of life that serves both academia and society at large through ongoing investigation and integration of scientific knowledge.

Knowledge Assessment

The chapter includes material designed to review and reinforce each content. It includes Critical Thinking Questions to help test of your understanding of information presented in the chapter and Short answer Questions to review your understanding of the key concepts presented in the chapter.

Critical Thinking Questions

1. **Who is known as the "Father of Modern Biology"?**
   a. Aristotle
   b. Charles Darwin
   c. Gregor Mendel
   d. Louis Pasteur
2. **What is the basic unit of life?**
   a. Atom
   b. Molecule
   c. Cell
   d. Organism
3. **Which branch of biology studies the interaction of organisms with their environment?**
   a. Genetics
   b. Ecology
   c. Physiology
   d. Botany
4. **Which macromolecule is the main source of energy for living organisms?**
   a. Proteins
   b. Lipids
   c. Carbohydrates
   d. Nucleic acids
5. **DNA is primarily responsible for which function in living organisms?**
   a. Energy production
   b. Protein synthesis
   c. Storing genetic information
   d. Regulating body temperature

Short Answer Questions

1. What is biology, and why is it important to study biology?
2. What are the three main domains of life, and how are they different from one another?
3. Define homeostasis and give an example of how it works in living organisms.
4. What is the cell theory, and why is it fundamental to biology?
5. How do autotrophs and heterotrophs differ in the way they obtain energy?
6. What is the scientific method, and how is it applied in biological research?
7. Discuss how biology helps address global challenges such as climate change, disease, and food security.
8. Explain the levels of biological organization from the smallest unit to the largest. Provide examples at each level.
9. Describe the relationship between structure and function in biology, giving specific examples from cells or organs.
10. How has the discovery of genetics shaped our understanding of inheritance and variation among organisms?

Supplementary Materials

Key Terms: A list of key terms is given for quick reference

KEY TERMS FROM THIS CHAPTER

Annotation enrichment analysis	Biological structure	Cell
Cell theory	Cellular structure	Ecology
Ecosystems	Genetics	Human biology
Microbiology	Natural selection	Organism
Plant biology		

Further Resources: Recommendations for additional readings, websites, and multimedia resources.

References

1. Argelaguet, R., Velten, B., Arnol, D., Dietrich, S., Zenz, T., Marioni, J. C., Buettner, F., et al. (2018). Multi-omics factor analysis—A framework for unsupervised integration of multi-omics data sets. *Molecular Systems Biology, 14.* https://doi.org/10.15252/msb.20178124.
2. Bacher, S., Blackburn, T. M., Essl, F., & Genovesi, P. (2017). *Socio-Economic Impact Classification of Alien Taxa (SEICAT).* https://core.ac.uk/download/286567949.pdf (accessed on 8th March 2025).
3. Barnett, R., Brace, S., Cucchi, T., & Dobney, K. (2013). *Divergent Evolutionary Processes Associated with Colonization of Offshore Islands.* https://core.ac.uk/download/20664364.pdf (accessed on 8th March 2025).

Detailed Table of Contents

CHAPTER 3

Diagnosis and Case Formulation 67

CHAPTER 4

Schizophrenia and Psychotic Disorders 101

CHAPTER 5

Mood Disorders 137

CHAPTER 6

Anxiety Disorders 177

CHAPTER 7

Obsessive-Compulsive and Related Disorders 207

CHAPTER 8

Trauma- and Stressor-Related Disorders 243

CHAPTER 9

Personality Disorders 277

CHAPTER 13

Somatic Symptom and Related Disorders 409

CHAPTER 14

Psychiatric Emergencies 441

CHAPTER 15

Treatment Modalities in Psychiatry 475

LIST OF FIGURES

PREFACE

Understanding human behavior, emotions, and mental functioning has been one of the most challenging and vital aspects of modern medicine. The mind influences every facet of human life—from decision-making and relationships to physical well-being. When mental health is disrupted, the effects can be far-reaching and debilitating. Unlike many other medical conditions that present with clear biological markers, mental health disorders often require nuanced clinical judgment, careful observation, and a comprehensive understanding of individual experiences. Professionals working in this field must combine empathy with analytical skill to address these complex issues and improve patient's quality of life.

The practice of psychiatry stands at the intersection of science and clinical care. It encompasses an extensive range of disorders, each with distinct symptom patterns, diagnostic criteria, and therapeutic strategies. Ranging from acute psychotic decompensation and debilitating mood attacks to chronic personality disorder and the mental health problems of the child and older person, the psychiatric field demands a well-structured and complete methodology. With each advancement in diagnostic models and emerging treatment strategies, mental health workers are required to keep current on the knowledge base required to provide competent, ethical practice.

Clinical Psychiatry: Assessment and Treatment is designed to be an expansive textbook for students beginning or professionals established in the mental health field. It covers fundamental principles such as clinical interviewing and diagnosis and proceeds into detailed coverage of specific psychiatric disorders. The text is structured to provide utility for academic education, applied practice, and board preparation. The book emphasizes clarity, clinical relevance, and cutting-edge standards of care, and each chapter is written to address the needs of psychiatric training programs and clinical guidelines. The text is designed throughout academic programs, residency programs, and psychiatric inpatient units to be a trusted companion for education and clinical utility.

Chapter 1 presents a general overview of psychiatry, offering a broad history, scope, and application of the specialty. It offers brief overviews of broad classification systems, the need for biopsychosocial methods, and the ethical issues that are most prominent in psychiatric treatment.

Chapter 2 focuses on the psychiatric interview and mental status examination, two pillars of psychiatric practice evaluation. Chapter 2 outlines the structure of a clinical interview, communication competencies, and interpretive skill for understanding patients' verbal and nonverbal communication. The mental status examination is illustrated in a systematic manner with regards to factors such as appearance, mood, perception, and cognition.

Chapter 3 addresses psychiatric diagnosis and case formulation. It explains the use of classification systems like DSM and ICD, and the instruction on individualized construction of case formulations. Comorbidities, differential diagnosis, and contextual factors are emphasized to promote critical assessment.

Chapter 4 deals with schizophrenia and other psychoses. It outlines symptom clusters such as delusions, hallucinations, and disorganized behavior and has a section on course, prognosis, and treatment strategy , including pharmacologic and psychosocial interventions.

Chapter 5 covers the mood disorders such as major depression, bipolar disorder, and related conditions, in turn reviewing symptom presentation, functional impairment, differential diagnostic issues, and the array of therapeutic options , including medication, psychotherapy, and lifestyle modifications.

Chapter 6 is about the anxiety disorders. It covers generalized anxiety disorder, panic disorder, social anxiety, phobias, and other anxiety disorders. Both the biological and psychological underpinnings and the therapeutic approaches with medications and cognitive-behavioral techniques are discussed.

Chapter 7 presents obsessive-compulsive and related disorders, and their distinction from obsessive thinking, compulsive action, and their variations. The chapter includes disorders like body dysmorphic disorder and hoarding, and their clinical presentation and evidence-based treatments.

Chapter 8 presents trauma- and stressor-related disorders, with post-traumatic stress disorder (PTSD) and acute stress disorder being the main features. It highlights diagnostic characteristics, neurobiological models, and models of treatment such as trauma-focused treatments and medication.

Chapter 9 is devoted to personality disorders. It describes the main clusters of personality pathology, maladaptive trait causation in development, and diagnostic and treatment obstacles of these disorders. Treatment resistance, therapeutic boundaries, and long-term management strategies are widely covered.

Chapter 10 discusses substance use and addiction disorders. It presents diagnostic features, substance abuse patterns, withdrawal syndromes, and dual diagnoses. Treatment models like detoxification, maintenance therapies, relapse prevention, and psychosocial support systems are discussed.

Chapter 11 addresses child and adolescent psychiatry. It addresses developmental, emotional, and behavioral disorders that are prevalent in young age groups , such as ADHD, autism spectrum disorders, and mood dysregulation. The chapter is an age-based assessment and family-based treatment.

Chapter 12 covers geriatric psychiatry. It introduces the psychiatric disorders of older adults, including dementia, late-life depression, anxiety, and medication problems. Special features of assessment and intervention among the elderly are discussed, keeping in mind cognitive impairment and comorbid medical illnesses.

Chapter 13 covers somatic symptoms and related disorders. These are the disorders where psychological distress is expressed in physical symptoms, such as somatic symptom disorder, illness anxiety disorder, and conversion disorder. Diagnosis, conversation with the patient, and the avoidance of unnecessary medical treatment are highlighted.

Chapter 14 addresses psychiatric emergencies. Topics addressed include suicide potential, violent behavior, acute agitation, and severe psychotic crises that need immediate correction. The chapter describes assessment methods and emergency management techniques within the outpatient and hospital setting.

Chapter 15 is a comprehensive review of psychiatric treatment modalities. It discusses pharmacotherapy, including the categories of psychotropic drugs and their indications, side effects, and monitoring. Psychotherapeutic modalities , such as cognitive-behavioral therapy, psychodynamic therapy, and supportive therapy are addressed. Other modalities , such as electroconvulsive therapy (ECT), transcranial magnetic stimulation (TMS), and new neuromodulation techniques, are included.

This book is intended for the broad spectrum of mental health professionals. It will be particularly valuable for medical students, psychiatric residents, postgraduate clinical psychologists, psychiatric nurses, and social work trainees. Clinicians in practice who want to brush up or solidify their knowledge may also benefit. Educators and training programs can also use this book as a reference text or guide to direct programs.

INTRODUCTION TO PSYCHIATRY

1

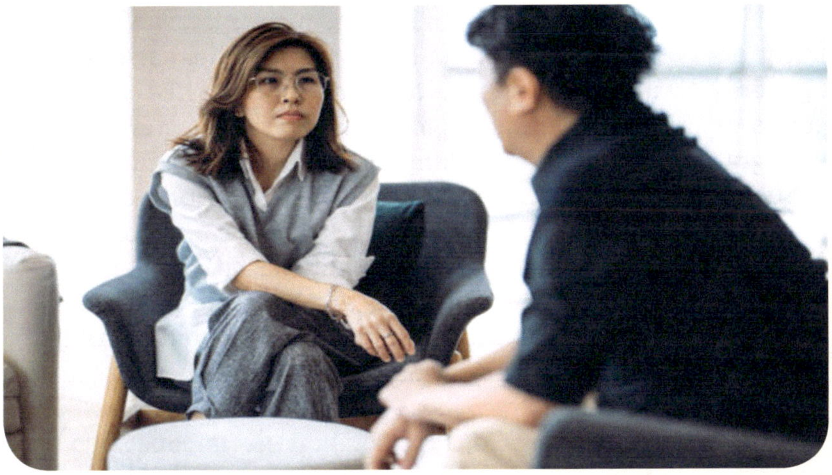

LEARNING OBJECTIVES

After studying this chapter, you will be able to:

1. Describe major theoretical approaches;
2. Explore the diagnostic criteria and classification;
3. Identify the treatment modalities;
4. Define the role of the psychiatrist;
5. List the current trends in psychiatry;
6. Focus on the challenges in the field.

Definition and Scope of Psychiatry

The definition and scope of psychiatry have shifted broadly since its founding, as there is an increased understanding of mental illness and the fact that it is intimately associated with physical health. Psychiatry has been defined as the medical specialty that treats, prevents, and diagnoses mental illness, which encompasses a broad array of psychological disorders from mild symptoms like depression and anxiety to grave mental illnesses like schizophrenia. Psychiatry as a medical specialty holds elements of psychology, neuroscience, and pharmacology and applies various interventions to treat, including psychotherapy and psychotropic medication. Furthermore, the integration of behavioral science and psychiatry has seen practitioners consider the interplay between body and mind, a perspective that recognizes bidirectional influences between soma and psyche (Gautam et al., 2022). The field of psychiatry is increasingly broadened beyond the traditional limits, with an interdisciplinary approach that encompasses collaboration with other specialties. This is evident especially in the expanding field of consultation-liaison psychiatry, where psychiatrists are engaged in providing comorbid psychiatric treatment within general medical treatment. This way, psychological aspects of physical conditions are addressed in a proper fashion, resulting in improved patient outcomes overall. As nearly one-fifth of global disease burden is attributed to neuropsychiatric disorders, the demand for such psychiatrists as are capable of addressing complex cases together with other healthcare professionals is in a persistent increase. The demand for collaboration and communication between mental health practitioners, general practitioners, and medical specialists points to the growing role of psychiatry as an integral component of patient care (Mark et al., 2019).

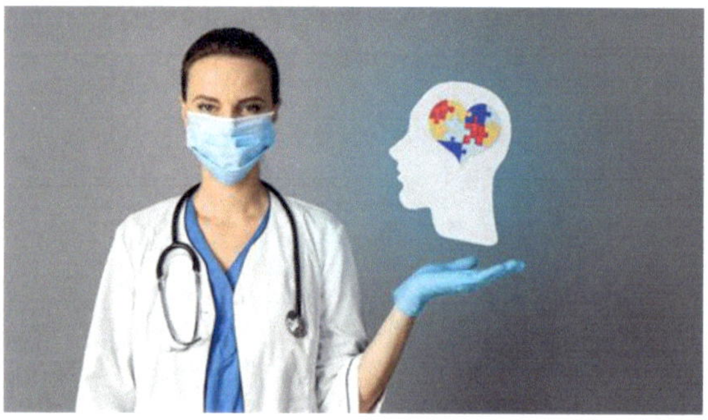

Figure 1.1. Psychiatry.

Source: https://external-content.duckduckgo.com/iu/?u=https%3A%2F%2Ftse3.mm.bing.net%2Fth%2Fid%2FOIP.KtAiXxqXquHa0VXUUqu6agHaEK%3Fpid%3 DApi&f=1&ipt=3905a6de02239d5fbf795e1467247faa6483a632ed9fcda630fce27b3d8278cc.

Historical Background of Psychiatry

The history of psychiatry in the background reflects an evolving understanding of mental illness and health on the basis of cultural, social, and scientific factors across centuries. It is possible to follow a line of evolution of modern psychiatry from ancient cultures where early medical practitioners sought to describe aberrations of the mind on a supernatural or religious basis. Ancient Egyptian, Greek, and Persian writings indicate that mental diseases were most commonly attributed to demonic possession or the anger of god. But during the Renaissance, explanations became more humanistic and logical. This transition period set the stage for the establishment of psychiatry as a distinct field, based on the belief that mental illness could be diagnosed, treated, and explained like physical illness. During the late 19th and early 20th centuries, the field started to become more systematic on the basis of developments in medical science and psychology. Key individuals like Emil Kraepelin and Sigmund Freud played a crucial role in establishing more refined diagnostic classifications and treatment approaches, respectively. Kraepelin's psychiatric nosology laid the groundwork that classified mental disorders according to symptomatic patterns, which significantly contributed to contemporary classification systems. At the same time, Freud's psychoanalytic ideas brought with them new models for conceptualizing the unconscious mind and the influence of early experience on adult psychopathology. These initial advances highlighted an increasing concern with mental health as a key component of overall wellness, further entrenching psychiatry's place in the medical world at large. Over the last several decades, the educational context of psychiatry has undergone alterations designed to improve the training of future doctors. Such evolutions are consistent with social changes and increased acknowledgment of the complexity involved in mental health treatment. For instance, the competency-based education framework proposed by the National Medical Commission has transformed the manner in which psychiatric training is taught, with increased emphasis on applied skills and professional conduct compared to theoretical concepts. In India, several of the significant advances in training in psychiatry have resulted from initiatives undertaken by the Indian Psychiatric Society, with a focus on the need for robust faculty development programs to produce future leaders. This constant evolution points to the importance of psychiatry evolving in tandem with what society needs and with scientific progress to maintain the discipline sensitive and responsive to the constantly changing world of health care (Romão et al., 2022; Narasimha et al., 2024).

Key Concepts and Terminology

In psychiatry, fundamental concepts , such as mental disorders, diagnosis, and treatment modalities are fundamental elements that underpin clinical practice. Mental disorders present a wide range of psychological disorders that significantly impair an individual's functioning and quality of life. The Diagnostic and Statistical Manual of Mental Disorders (DSM) is the primary tool employed by clinicians to classify these disorders according to a standard set of criteria. Accurate diagnosis is critical since it has a direct influence on the modality of treatment that is selected for the patient. Understanding the variance between various mental health conditions not only adds to effective treatment planning but also enhances the ability of clinicians to communicate findings and approaches to patients and other healthcare providers, thus providing an interprofessional therapeutic setting. Another basic term in psychiatry is "neuropsychiatric presentation," or the confluence of neurological and psychiatric symptoms observed during the clinical interviews. Neuropsychiatric presentations are particularly important to grasp, because most medical disorders, including infectious illnesses, can have profound psychiatric impact. For instance, in SARS, MERS, and COVID-19 epidemics, patients developed a range of psychiatric syndromes, from anxiety, depression, and confusion states (Rogers et al., 2020). Such findings pressure clinicians to have an integrated view of the health of patients beyond traditional psychiatric horizons; clinicians are forced to consider potential neuropsychiatric impacts stemming from acute and chronic diseases of medicine, thereby pointing to a holistic treatment method of psychiatric disorders. Furthermore, the argument between technology's impact on mental health, in this case smartphone addiction, has contributed to psychiatric knowledge, new mechanisms and definitions. With popular assertions of smartphone addiction, existing literature questioning the classification term smartphone addiction suggests that excessive phone use would better be described as problematic, not necessarily being addictive (Panova & Carbonell, 2018). This ongoing theoretical discussion highlights the importance of scrutinizing new behaviors mimicking past addiction patterns for mental health practitioners and psychiatrists. It also demands more study of the use of technology in its sociocultural context and its effects on mental illness, challenging the field to look into more complex terminology that most appropriately explains the complexity of modern psychological processes.

Distinction Between Psychiatry and Psychology

The distinction between psychiatry and psychology ultimately resides in their conceptual models and clinical treatment. Psychiatry is a branch of medicine concerned with the diagnosis, treatment, and prevention of mental illness. Psychiatrists are physicians capable of prescribing medicine and employing biological interventions, and therefore practicing a medical model in treatment. Psychology concerns itself with the more specific focus on explaining behavior and mental functioning through therapy. Psychologists most often employ a range of psychotherapeutic techniques, examining thought and feeling patterns separate from pharmacological treatment. The key here is that it indicates the difference in methodologies between each field and how their different approaches can complement one another when treating mental illness. There is a great deal of overlap that occurs in psychology and psychiatry, particularly in diagnosis and treatment planning. Both disciplines emphasize the importance of comprehensive evaluations in order to be familiar with a patient's state in depth. The character of these evaluations differs, nevertheless; psychiatry is more inclined to implement a medical examination with psychological testing, whereas psychology utilizes behavioral assessment and talking about it during therapy. This becomes even more complicated when referring to idiographic and narrative judgments, as emphasized by the World Psychiatric Association.

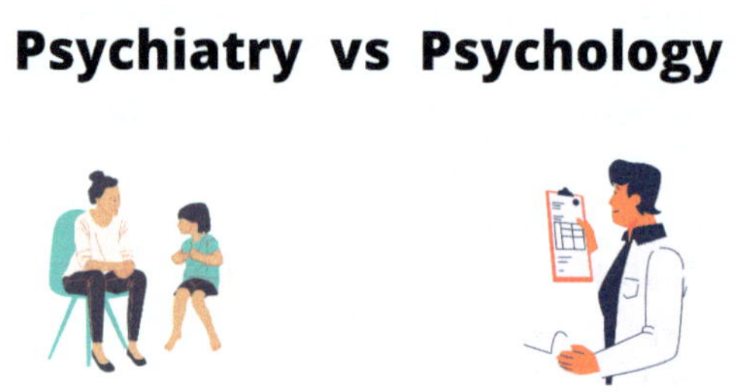

Figure 1.2. Distinction between psychiatry and psychology.

Source: https://external-content.duckduckgo.com/iu/?u=https%3A%2F%2Fcordialpsychiatry.com%2Fwp-content%2Fuploads%2F2023%2F12%2F1_20220806_003809_0000.png&f=1&nofb=1&ipt=514fca04312454fa28d8686d450a6b51583cc787a25f6a2d2e2380ac54d8eb4f.

While idiographic judgments are with individual differences that may invalidate psychiatric diagnoses, narrative judgments have the potential to enable rich contextual understanding of patients' experiences so that clinicians can incorporate personal histories into their treatment models and improve patient care (Thornton, 2008). Moreover, the ethical and philosophical issues in both fields guide their practice and identity, as is evident in accounts of mad identity from the perspective of mental health advocacy movements, such as accounts given by Gail Hornstein. In bringing into account the complexities of mental illness, psychology can provide a wider sense of personal experience that psychiatric models are unable to perceive. This dialogue illustrates a pivotal tension between the two professions: the biological emphasis of psychiatry and the social and cultural interests of psychology. As a result, the distinct identities of psychiatry and psychology coexist in a broader discourse surrounding mental health, forcing clinicians to adopt an integrative position that recognizes the biopsychosocial model as an efficacious approach to the multifaceted nature of mental illness (Huxley et al., 2018) (Figure 1.2).

1.1. Major Theoretical Approaches

Learning Outcome

1. Biological perspective.
2. Psychological theories.
3. Sociocultural influences.

The field of psychiatry is marked by an array of theoretical models that seek to explain and treat mental illness disorders. One of the prevailing theoretical models is the biological perspective, which focuses on the role of neurobiological factors in psychiatric disorders. The biological perspective believes that genetic factors, imbalance of neurotransmitter activity, and irregularities in brain structure are important causes of mental illness. For instance, our understanding of the biochemical mechanisms of depression or anxiety has led to the development of drugs that target these imbalances directly. Yet while the biological model yields such insights, it may omit the complex interplay of psychological and environmental factors, so that the full picture of the complexities of mental illness requires a more integrated approach. A second crucial psychiatry framework is the psychosocial one, emphasizing social, emotional, and cognitive factors in shaping mental health. This one is particularly useful in accounting for the effects of experiences during youth and adolescence on individuals' mental health trajectories. Early intervention and the incorporation of social support systems are key elements of this perspective, as evidenced by recent studies that emphasize the success of school-based mental health interventions. Research supports an immediate necessity for consensus in the operationalization of constructs addressing school mental health, revealing that promotion of mental health in schools can serve to create resilience and social-emotional learning among children (Cavioni et al., 2020). Thus, the psychosocial view complements the biological perspective by highlighting the environment within which the development of mental health disorders takes place. The coordination of various theoretical approaches may lead to an extended, enlarged understanding of psychiatric illness with the possibility of interdisciplinary collaboration in practice. For example, developments in emotion and affective science would mean that integration with psychiatric research can enhance treatment efficacy and diagnostic sensitivity (Larsen & Hastings, 2018). Through the rationalization of the interdependence between affective entities and psychiatric illness, these multidisciplinary efforts establish a path for sharpening diagnostic categories as well as clinical information systems. Ultimately, this operational framework can give the driving force to innovative interventions that take advantage of the individual strengths of both biological and psychosocial models, such that patients receive holistic care able to cope with the multi-dimensional nature of mental illness disorders.

1.1.1. Biological Perspective

The biological approach in psychiatry involves an integrated view of mental illness, assuming that bodily functions play a major role in influencing psychological well-being. It combines neurobiological mechanisms with manifestations of behavior, demarcating how genetic factors, neuroanatomy, and chemical imbalances in neurotransmitters are responsible for psychiatric illness. For instance, research has indicated that genetic susceptibility variations can dramatically influence disorders , such as schizophrenia and bipolar disorder, further supporting the necessity of considering biological underpinnings in diagnosis and treatment strategies. Additionally, developments in neuroimaging technology have illuminated structural and functional brain abnormalities in regions of the brain associated with mood control, further cementing the necessity for a biological approach to psychiatry. This perspective not only enhances our comprehension of mental illness but also guides the development of biologically-driven treatments, which indicate that empirical evidence needs to drive psychiatric practice. Biological concepts are also useful in the treatment of psychiatric disease, where pharmacologic treatments are a cornerstone of modern psychiatry. These treatments are generally directed at distinct neurotransmitter systems to remedy chemical imbalances that cause mental illness. For example, selective serotonin reuptake inhibitors (SSRIs) have revolutionized the treatment of depression by increasing serotonin levels in the synaptic spaces and thereby improving mood and functionality. Furthermore, the investigation of stress disorders , such as post-traumatic stress disorder (PTSD) has been facilitated by biological knowledge, employing the neurobiology and cognitive neuroscience models to understand the cognitive impairments of these disorders. Contemporary hypotheses, such as active inference, present a unifying model explaining how biological processes impact cognitive function and responses to stress, exemplifying the importance of a stringent biological paradigm in establishing well-timed therapeutic interventions (Linson & Friston, 2019). Apart from pharmacotherapies, the biological approach permits new therapeutic modalities that cure mental illness through physiological means. New studies emphasize the interface of neurobiology and treatment methods with investigations into how brain functioning, as well as the processes of the environment, can be controlled to promote mental health.

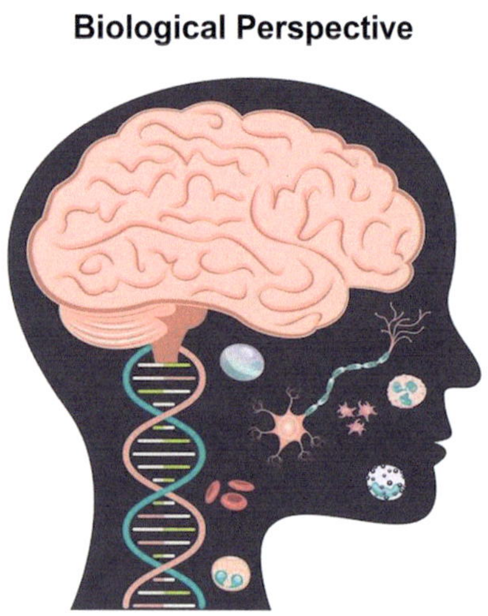

Figure 1.3. Biological perspective.

Source: https://external-content.duckduckgo.com/iu/?u=https%3A%2F%2Fimg.freepik.com%2Fpremium-vector%2Fbiological-perspective-psychology-education-vector-illustration-design_683773-768.jpg&f=1&nofb=1&ipt=4db798ffab2f250e9c0d25ee2a6d6997d105c6d672254ae33596d7bb9b5ba637.

Examples include therapies , such as electroconvulsive therapy (ECT) and transcranial magnetic stimulation (TMS), as the biological method's capacity to control neural functioning and treat severe depression symptoms and other psychiatric illnesses. Furthermore, the integration of social and biological models, as highlighted by Kępiński, underlines the complex relationships among biological processes, psychosocial factors, and therapeutic outcomes. Acknowledging these multifaceted interactions aligns contemporary psychiatric practice with Kępiński's reflections on the relevance of biological considerations while advocating for comprehensive treatment protocols that also include psychosocial determinants (Zawiła-Niedźwiecki et al., 2016) (Figure 1.3).

1.1.2. Psychological Theories

Psychological theories are part of the arsenal employed to comprehend psychiatric illnesses, blending schools of thought in analyzing the interaction between biological, cognitive, and sociocultural factors. From psychoanalytic models with intense reliance on unconscious processes to cognitive-behavioral models with reliance on present thoughts and behaviors, these models provide clinicians with several frameworks through which to assess and treat mental illness. The emergence of cognitive theories, for instance, brought the cognitive distortions and dysfunctional thought processes to center stage in disorders , such as depression and anxiety, emphasizing the cognitive restructuring aspect of therapy interventions. Moreover, psychological theories have evolved to include the role of vicissitudes of emotions and physical states, as indicated by recent studies on interoception, opening up how internal bodily information can influence emotional experience and mental health outcomes (Camilla et al., 2022). These complexity theories demand that psychiatric practice follow a dimensional approach, ensuring that treatment modalities vary and are patient-centered. Complementing traditional psychological theory, modern scholarship increasingly intersects with social and environmental environments to address issues of mental health. The recognition of the profound impact of one's social and physical environments on psychological health has created the disciplines of social psychiatry and health geography. This conceptual framework presupposes that psychological distress most often stems from environmental forces, that is, socioeconomic conditions, interpersonal relationships in the community, and accessibility to healthcare amenities. By studying the way social space and relations impact mental health, researchers have a deeper insight into the nature of conditions , such as anxiety and depression. These studies highlight the need for an integrative approach that recognizes social determinants of health and not just psychological ones, giving a more accurate representation of mental illnesses (Curtis, 2016). This shift to conceptualizing the environment not only enhances theoretical models but also informs public health policy toward improved mental health outcomes at the population level.

Finally, the integration of psychological theory and environmental thinking demands a multidisciplinary approach in psychiatry. Treatment modalities more and more draw from other disciplines, such as neuroscience, sociology, and behavioral science, in an attempt to develop comprehensive therapeutic approaches. As an example, neurobiological developments of the relation between physical health and emotional life have placed emphasis on the importance of bodily regulation in the treatment of mental illness (Camilla et al., 2022). Through the realization of the dynamic interaction among emotional regulation, cognition, and social components, clinicians are able to deliver interventions that are more functional and relevant to the patient's daily life. Moreover, this multidisciplinary model facilitates ongoing dialogue between clinicians and academics and, as a consequence, creative research and practice, which could lead to better therapies. Hence, psychological theories, founded upon other disciplines' knowledge, continue to develop in response to the sophistication of mental health and deepen the importance of multidisciplinary treatment modalities in psychiatry (Figure 1.4).

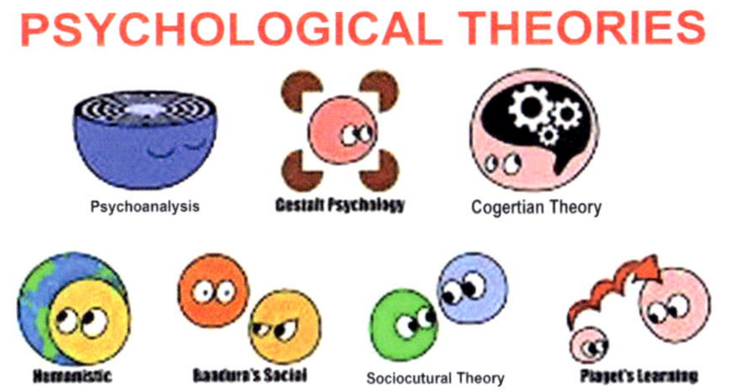

Figure 1.4. Psychological theories in psychiatry.

Source: https://i.ytimg.com/vi/kzRIXpFlMVc/mqdefault.jpg.

1.1.3. Sociocultural Influences

It is crucial to know about sociocultural influences in the field of psychiatry since human beings do not live their lives in isolation but within complex social frameworks that affect their mental well-being. These include cultural practices, socioeconomic status, to communal dynamics and they all bear some influence on how and what is perceived and treated in terms of mental illness. For instance, mental illness might be defined differently by cultures and thus psychiatric conditions are dealt with differently. In societies in which mental illness is extremely stigmatized, patients may forgo treatment, leading to continued. The forming of such dynamics requires that practitioners of mental health become culturally competent, something that will enable them to understand the multifaceted processes sociocultural settings use to mold patients' behaviors and conceptualizations of their own mental health. As such, awareness of such factors enhances the efficacy of psychiatric practice since interventions are aligned with patients' cultural environments and social realities. Second, the interplay between resource availability and social class intensely depicts the sociocultural determinants of mental health. Socioeconomic standing might ascertain the availability of mental health care services, perceived quality of care, and even awareness of mental illness.

Individuals with lower socioeconomic status experience less access to healthcare, less education about mental illness, and higher exposure to stressors , such as violence and instability. Not only does this inequality affect a person's mental health outcome, but it also challenges psychiatric professionals to develop interventions that are protective against these disparities. Attending to sociocultural concerns necessitates sensitivity to broader systemic issues to allow psychiatrists to address fair mental health treatment. Understanding the interaction of social class and mental health serves to clarify that good care in psychiatry needs to engage with patients' lived realities and social circumstances. The integration of sociocultural articulations into psychiatric models is needed to advance the field. The biopsychosocial model, which synthesizes biological, psychological, and social elements, has been one of the major paradigms to address the expanding challenges in psychiatric therapy. The model allows mental health practitioners to gain a greater understanding of how psychological processes of individuals are intricately embedded in sociocultural contexts. As noted by the literature, the traditional employment of a combination of different theoretical orientations has been found to lead to disagreement and inconsistency. But adopting a biopsychosocial perspective might unite practitioners in the sharing of a particular viewpoint that emphasizes the impact of sociocultural determinants on psychological practice and research. Its use can enhance educational practices in professional psychology as well as overall mental health treatment effectiveness, thereby aligning psychiatry with contemporary social needs (Holtzman, 1979; Melchert, 2007).

Test Your Knowledge

1. What are the core principles of the biological, psychological, and sociocultural approaches in understanding mental disorders?
2. How do cognitive-behavioral and psychodynamic theories differ in explaining the development and maintenance of psychiatric conditions?

1.2. Diagnostic Criteria and Classification

Learning Outcome

1. Overview of the DSM-5.
2. Common psychiatric disorders.
3. Importance of accurate diagnosis.

Diagnostic classification and mental disorder criteria are the foundation stones in the science of psychiatry, with an influence on clinical work as well as research. Central to this system is reliance on systematic classification systems , such as the International Classification of Diseases (ICD) and the Diagnostic and Statistical Manual of Mental Disorders (DSM). The ICD, following merely witnessed massive revisions in its 11th version, emphasizes universal usage and clinical utility and therefore aims to develop a comprehensive approach to the diagnosis of mental illnesses. Such changes are decided upon by professionals to align the diagnostic guidelines closer to modern practice, thereby eventually being able to capture better involvement of the diverse healthcare settings.

The implications of these developments extend beyond theoretical controversy, impacting the way practitioners diagnose, formulate treatment plans, and deliver overall mental health treatment (Berk et al., 2020). In mental illness, the necessity for classification cannot be overstated. Regular diagnostic criteria facilitate greater understanding and transmission of mental disorders among clinicians, researchers, and patients. They notify the organization of treatment strategies and can influence policy decisions for resource allocation and planning of health effects. Moreover, powerful classification systems play an important role in the possibility of more research, as they create exact parameters for data gathering and analysis. The cyclical process present within these classification systems reflects continuous refinements in our knowledge of mental health, with new knowledge necessitating adjustments to diagnostic criteria. The interactive dialectics between classification systems and clinical practice highlight the imperative for continuous evolution in the practice of psychiatry, as it moves towards the integration of new evidence and cultural considerations into existing frameworks (Bebbington et al., 2016). The recent developments in the diagnostic classification of mental disorders are such that they highlight the increasing emphasis upon the biopsychosocial model. This paradigm believes that the mental illnesses cannot be explained by biological or psychological factors alone but require a coming together of social factors. Diagnostic criteria have now begun to incorporate features related to social determinants of health, including environmental influences and life stressors. This multi-factorial process benefits not only the comprehensive assessment of patients but also encourages a humane approach towards understanding their condition. As the science progresses, the issue will be one of balancing the scientific caution of diagnosis with the nuanced complexities of individual patients. This ongoing dialogue in psychiatric communities will be crucial in ensuring the continued validity and efficacy of diagnostic criteria and classifications in the future (Berk et al., 2020) (Figure 1.5).

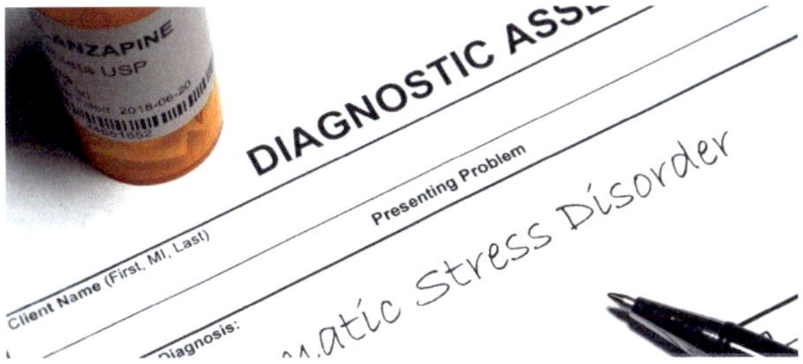

Figure 1.5. Diagnostic criteria and classification in psychiatry.

Source: https://media.licdn.com/dms/image/v2/C4D12AQHdhsshT7dMUw/article-cover_image-shrink_600_2000/article-cover_image-shrink_600_2000/0/1644499666529?e=2147483647&v=beta&t=xqtiM5utIxMXbH0XzNmURe796R4B6MWND2KeVudSzfY.

1.2.1. Overview of the DSM-5

The Diagnostic and Statistical Manual of Mental Disorders, Fifth Edition, or DSM-5, represents a milestone in the evolution of psychiatry that provides a comprehensive system for the classification and diagnosis of mental disorders. Ever since its release in 2013 by the American Psychiatric Association, the DSM-5 has become a go-to reference book for clinicians, researchers, and policymakers dealing with mental health conditions on a day-to-day basis. This volume not only provides definitive diagnostic criteria but also encompasses the wide range of disorders that embody contemporary views of mental health, both common and rare. Drawing on new research and clinical developments, the DSM-5 aims to increase diagnostic precision and the effectiveness of treatment for patients with mental health disorders. One of the most important features of the DSM-5 is its focus on dimensional rating, the acknowledgment of the spectrum of symptom severity and the complexities of human experience. This is opposed to the categorical division of disorders, realizing that mental health issues come in a continuum format rather than as compactly defined discrete entities. This revision allows clinicians to offer interventions more specifically tailored to individual patients' needs, with potentially greater success. The DSM-5 also includes new categories, including trauma- and stressor-related disorders, which reflect the evolving nature of psychiatric diagnoses to be consistent with current understanding of mental health. This flexibility is the DSM-5's commitment to applying ongoing research and clinical feedback to its format, ultimately making it more practical in day-to-day applications. Furthermore, the DSM-5 has also been extensively criticized and argued regarding the inclusion and definition of various disorders.

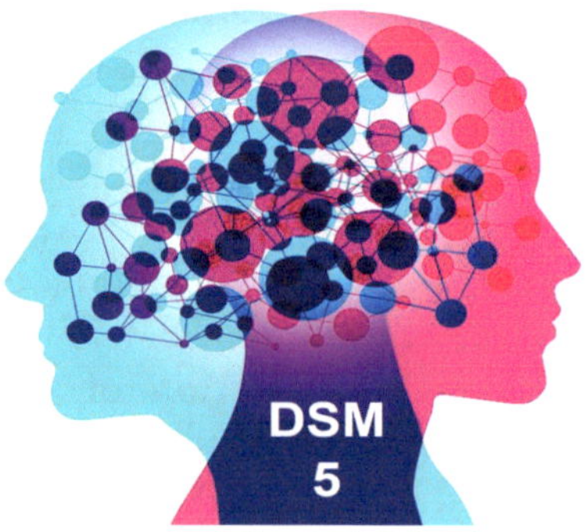

Figure 1.6. DSM-5.

Source: https://external-content.duckduckgo.com/iu/?u=https%3A%2F%2Fceu.uky.edu%2Fwp-content%2Fuploads%2F2020%2F06%2Fdms5.jpg&f=1&nofb=1&ipt=6c10f9fdd36c8c36db19646151e0f7a1d49434e5f52b9446618c10a29595f6cd.

As a case in point, there have been recent controversies about the classification of disorders like posttraumatic stress disorder (PTSD), which includes complicated symptoms that have a tendency to disrupt day-to-day functioning. The development of innovations , such as therapy progress indicators (TPI) is an indication of an ongoing quest to measure treatment outcomes best for disorders , such as PTSD, showing an evolution of treating and managing such disorders (Cohn et al., 2009). New conditions , such as gaming disorder (GD) have also called for the application of standardized diagnostic tools that are in line with DSM-5 and ICD-11 standards (King et al., 2020). This ongoing exchange reflects the dynamic nature of psychiatric classification systems and the imperative to keep abreast with changing trends within the field for the betterment of patient care for individuals wrestling with mental challenges (Figure 1.6).

1.2.2. Common Psychiatric Disorders

In psychiatry, common psychiatric disorders are a wide range of disorders that have a huge impact on the individual's mental health and function. Anxiety, depression, and bipolar disorder are a few of the most common ones and may be found in populations across the board. Anxiety disorders, as constituted by excessive worry, fear, and apprehension, are one of the most common mental illnesses, affecting millions of individuals globally. These disorders typically manifest in varied forms, either as social anxiety disorder or generalized anxiety disorder, in which individuals experience varied degrees of impairment within their everyday lives. These disorders result from genetic, environmental, and psychological factors, highlighting the nature of the mental health problems experienced by individuals in contemporary society. The second general category of psychiatric diseases includes the mood disorders, and the most prevalent disease on the planet is depression. Major depressive disorder, which can be described as low-grade episodes of unhappiness, disinterest in activities, and other cognitive symptoms, has been determined to significantly affect an individual's performance at school and work. Additionally, bipolar disorder, in which there are fluctuating cycles of depression and mania, further muddies the clinical picture. Above all, mood disorder patients often report comorbid conditions that complicate their symptoms. For example, studies indicate that 32% of clients being treated for mood disorders also report substance abuse issues, a dual diagnosis problem. Identification and treatment of the interface between mood disorders and substance abuse are of critical concern for effective treatment and care intervention in psychiatric care (Berry et al., 2008). Comorbidity is a recurring pattern within the backdrop of psychiatric disorders, illustrating how varied disorders may coexist and have an effect on one another.

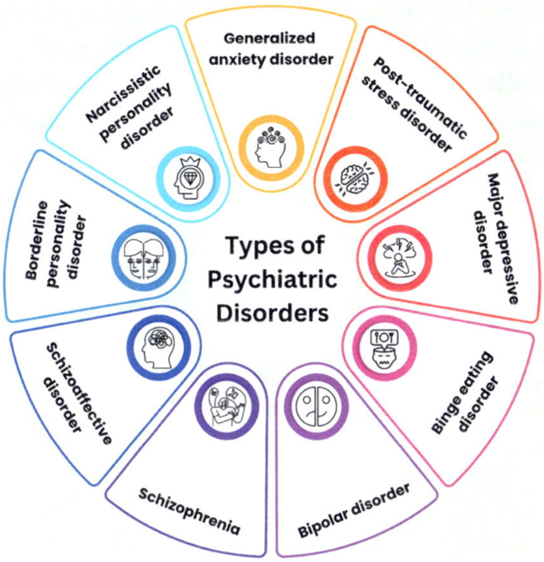

Figure 1.7. Common psychiatric disorders.

Source: https://www.onlinepsychiatrists.com/wp-content/uploads/2023/08/Types-of-Psychiatric-Disorders.jpg.

A good illustration consists of literacy problems in childhood and how they correlate with psychiatric disorders , such as attention deficit hyperactivity disorder (ADHD) and anxiety disorders. Current studies suggest that children with literacy problems are at greater risk for both externalizing and internalizing psychiatric illness and will require an integrated treatment plan addressing academic and mental health concerns (Angold et al., 2006). With respect to these observations, mental health professionals must adopt comprehensive models of treatment that consider the relationship between multiple psychiatric disorders to ensure the highest possible impact of interventions and the general outcome among affected persons. This is not only a mirror to the focus on intensive assessment but also a clarion call for interdisciplinary services among sectors , including education and healthcare, to adequately intervene among people with co-occurring psychiatric disorders (Figure 1.7).

1.2.3. Importance of Accurate Diagnosis

Accurate diagnosis is a foundation underlying psychiatry that is of significance to the process of treatment as well as overall therapy response in patients. Misdiagnosis leads to ineffective or even injurious treatment because the treatment provided is not directly addressing the actual condition of the patients. DSM-5 Field Trials illustrate this relevance by verifying the various levels of reliability in psychiatric diagnosis; the majority of diagnoses fell within the good to very good range of inter-rater reliability, thus reassuring clinicians concerning their validity of diagnosis in practice. Such a reliability is significant not only for establishing a solid ground for treatment plans but also to ensure that patients are offered adequate treatment that is tailor-made to their respective issues. Therefore, accurate and consistent diagnoses are at the heart of best health facilitation and optimization of the effectiveness of psychiatric treatment in general. Moreover, accurate diagnosis is essential to an understanding of the majority of psychiatric illnesses, which all present with comorbid symptoms. Comorbid symptoms can pose diagnostic problems for clinicians, who must sort through disorders , such as anxiety, depression, and ADHD. For instance, ADHD, the most common childhood neurobehavioral disorder, can seriously interfere with a child's educational and social life unless it is correctly diagnosed and treated. The American Academy of Pediatrics clinical guidelines for diagnosing ADHD emphasize the need to have an advanced understanding of the disorder's symptomatology and the requirement of evaluating broad information from multiple sources. Without proper diagnosis, it is possible that significant factors affecting the performance and behavior of a child and, by extension, future well-being may be missed. In addition, the implications of accurate diagnosis extend beyond the care of the individual patient to public health programs and utilization of resources in the healthcare system. Specific criteria for diagnosis guarantee uniformity in clinical practice, allowing the collection of reliable epidemiological data that are essential in estimating the prevalence and impact of psychiatric disorders in different groups. The DSM-5 Field Trials placed great emphasis on the establishment of accurate definitions of diagnostic reliability, demonstrating that the majority of the diagnoses accurately depicted the examined clinical populations, but some continued to be questionable or unacceptable. This heterogeneity calls for ongoing research to further refine diagnostic tools and improve the overall accuracy of psychiatric assessment. Hence, the continuous refinement of diagnostic criteria by virtue of new discoveries accentuates the indispensable role of accurate diagnosis in the direction of meaningful treatments, policy-making, and ultimately, maximizing mental health outcomes for society at large.

Test Your Knowledge

1. What are the key differences between DSM-5-TR and ICD-11 in classifying mental disorders?
2. How are diagnostic criteria operationalized to improve reliability and validity in psychiatric assessment?

1.3. Treatment Modalities

Learning Outcome

1. Psychopharmacology.
2. Psychotherapy techniques.
3. Alternative and complementary therapies.

The efficacy of treatment modalities in psychiatry relies on a diversified, individualized process to address the diverse needs of patients. Psychotherapy, pharmacological interventions, and other treatments are some of the therapeutic modalities that become part of the overall treatment weave of mental health care. An understanding of such complexities is crucial for clinicians who aim to deliver global and effective treatment. For instance, psychotherapy can incorporate cognitive-behavioral therapy, psychodynamic treatment, and others that enable patients to introspect themselves and rebuild their cognition. These therapies commonly lead to improved coping strategies among patients with anxiety, depression, and other psychiatric illnesses, pointing to the incorporation of diverse treatment methods (Hoque, 2016). Pharmacotherapy is another mainstay in treating psychiatric disorders, primarily in combination with psychotherapeutic interventions. Drugs , such as antidepressants, antipsychotics, and anxiolytics are valuable tools in symptom management that can thwart the ability of a patient to respond to therapy. Knowledge of the pharmacokinetics and pharmacodynamics of such medications is critical for clinicians to tailor treatment regimens, minimizing side effects while maximizing therapeutic effect. Furthermore, the evolving setting of psychiatric treatment requires clinicians to regularly keep themselves informed of emerging pharmacologic therapy to keep treatment modalities evidence-based and patient-focused (Masiriri, 2008). These constant adjustments and integrations of updated information encapsulate the dynamic nature of psychiatric treatment. Within recent years, new treatment modalities , such as sensory integration therapy have been widely reported for their capacity to treat a broad spectrum of psychiatric symptoms.

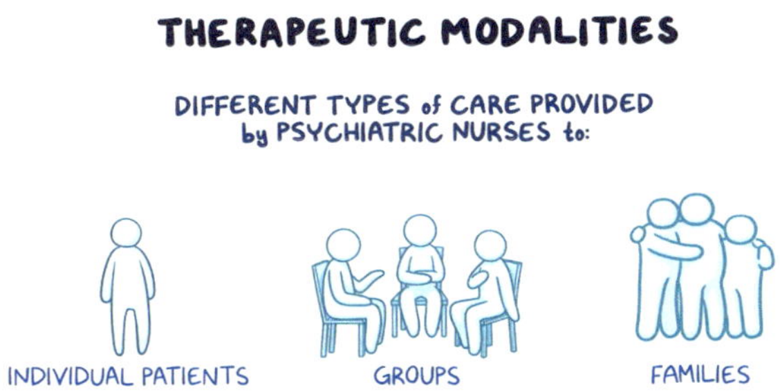
THERAPEUTIC MODALITIES
DIFFERENT TYPES of CARE PROVIDED by PSYCHIATRIC NURSES to:
INDIVIDUAL PATIENTS
GROUPS
FAMILIES

Figure 1.8. Treatment modalities for psychiatric disorders.

Source: https://www.osmosis.org/_next/image?url=https%3A%2F%2Fd16qt3wv6xm098.cloudfront.net%2FuoiCV6xcTD28hXGJDofMtiqTTcaGAVXh%2F_.jpg&w=3840&q=75.

According to Dr. Ayres' Sensory Integration Theory, clinical applications of sensory modulation have been shown to reduce distress, anxiety, and agitation in patients. Research indicates that the implementation of sensory-based approaches in mental healthcare settings can be used as a substitute for more coercive treatments like seclusion and restraint. This modality empowers staff and patients alike, promoting a symbiotic partnership that optimizes therapeutic relationships and improves outcomes. The study evidence pertaining to sensory modulated approaches reflects a stringent need for additional research aimed at determining their role in clinical practice, ultimately to cultivate the field of psychiatry and improve patient outcomes (Hoque, 2016) (Figure 1.8).

1.3.1. Psychopharmacology

The field of psychopharmacology is at the core of managing psychiatric disease, examining how medications affect mood, cognition, and behavior. With its nature as a cross-disciplinary science, it brings together ideas in psychology, neuroscience, and pharmaceutical science to understand the complex mechanisms of drugs acting on the central nervous system. The field is particularly critical given the global prevalence of mental illness, where an effective treatment choice is required. Notwithstanding the major progress within psychopharmacology, for example, the creation of selective serotonin reuptake inhibitors (SSRIs) like fluoxetine, many patients are not sufficiently treated. The study shows that although SSRIs have transformed depression treatment by augmenting monoaminergic transmission, a substantial percentage of patients are still symptomatic, reflecting the challenges involved in psychiatric pharmacotherapy (Bel et al., 2014). Hence, the phenomenon of treatment resistance emerges as a critical psychopharmacology challenge. The majority of patients diagnosed as "treatment resistant" experience minimal responses to conventional pharmacological interventions, entailing tremendous social, economic, and psychological impacts. The lack of direct consensus on what constitutes treatment resistance provides a hindrance in estimates of prevalence and highlights the value of detailed definitions within clinic contexts (Jakovljevi, 2015). This environment necessitates that treatment strategies be reevaluated, fostering a move away from traditional, mechanistic notions of psychopharmacology towards an integrated, individualized model. Through an emphasis on the need for individualized treatment plans, practitioners can better address the diverse spectrum of needs presented by those who do not respond favorably to usual care, maximizing overall treatment efficacy in the process. Moreover, the defeat of drug resistance would likely demand a complete understanding of drug mechanisms and their effect on neuroplasticity. For instance, fluoxetine's action is not merely serotonin reuptake blockade, but it also triggers neuroplasticity and adult neurogenesis, which play a major role in regulating mood and thinking (Bel et al., 2014). Speaking this knowledge into clinical practice would bring into being the possibility of the creation of novel therapies consisting of the marriage of more than one modality of treatment. An integrative strategy that combines pharmacologic intervention with psychotherapy and lifestyle change could enhance outcomes in patients struggling with refractory symptoms. Lastly, a paradigm shift in psychopharmacology would provide more functional, contextually relevant treatment decisions and, thereby, elevate the quality of care for patients with chronic psychiatric illness (Jakovljevi, 2015) (Figure 1.9).

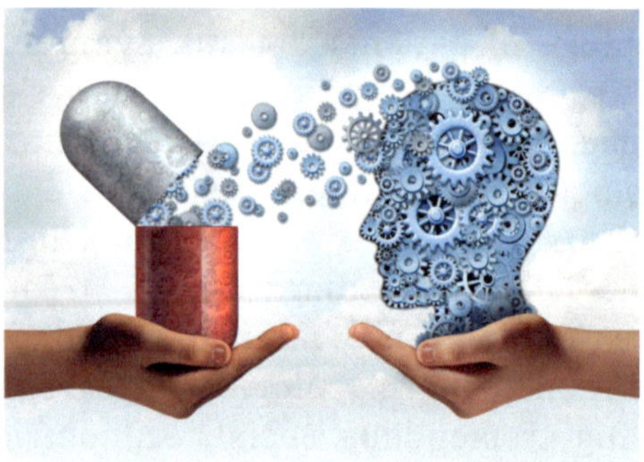

Figure 1.9. Psychopharmacology.

Source: https://medworksmedia.com/wp-content/uploads/2017/04/shutterstock_235393648.jpg.

1.3.2. Psychotherapy Techniques

Psychotherapy is a series of techniques applied to alleviate mental anguish and improve mental well-being. Essentially, this form of therapy capitalizes on the interaction between patient and psychotherapist to explore emotional difficulties and behavioral patterns. Techniques may include cognitive behavioral therapy (CBT), which addresses the identification and reversal of distorted thinking, or psychodynamic therapy, which analyzes unconscious forces from experiences in early life. Both models emphasize the importance of knowing the client's personal history in facilitating healing. Of special interest is the application of evidence-based practices, as applied in Project Reach, which aims to provide quality mental health care through innovative treatment and assessment. In its provision of integrated care within the school and primary settings, Project Reach depicts the ways psychotherapy techniques can be adapted to meet the unique demands of individuals who have experienced specific traumatic events, such as Hurricane Harvey (Cepeda et al., 2019). In the process of therapy, different modalities are likely to be employed to counteract the intricate level of issues of mental health. For instance, narrative therapy allows clients to reinterpret their narratives in a way that they are able to feel a sense of empowerment and agency. Such a practice assists individuals in reframing negative narratives, which can hinder personal growth and recovery. In like manner, art and film therapies have become valuable tools in psychotherapy, such that clients are able to express emotion, which is difficult to verbalize. Such strategies allow a window of reflection and dialogue, facilitating a better understanding of complex emotions. As maintained, utilizing films as starters in educational contexts emphasizes the therapeutic potential of artistic portrayal in therapy, allowing clients to work through their concerns through an indirect medium (Amann, 2010). Greater emphasis on models of integrated therapy highlights the importance of integrating the clients' overall needs during psychotherapy. Integrating mainstream psychotherapy practice with programs at the community level is likely to enhance accessibility and effectiveness of mental health interventions. Initiatives like Project Reach illustrate the potential of long-term mental health treatment through collaboration with schools and primary healthcare providers. This integration not only improves the delivery of services but also strives to remove stigma from seeking help, thus promoting healthier communities. With the evolution of psychotherapy, it will likely address a broader range of techniques and methods, solidifying the idea that mental health care must be adaptable to meet the ever-changing wave of societal demand and individual experience (Cepeda et al., 2019) (Figure 1.10).

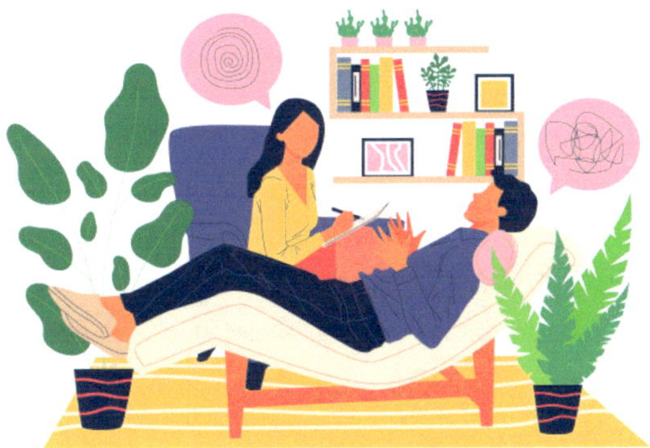

Figure 1.10. Psychotherapy techniques.

Source: https://mozartcultures.com/en/wp-content/uploads/2021/06/patient-counseling-with-psychologist-illustration_179970-799.jpeg.

1.3.3. Alternative and Complementary Therapies

The application of complementary and alternative therapy presents a significant trend in the area of psychiatry, synthesizing conventional healing mechanisms with contemporary mental health strategies. Interventions , such as massage and aromatherapy have garnered attention over time as vehicles to enhance psychological health. Research confirms that modern therapeutic massage, once a symbol of the ancient world, has become an integral part of complementary and alternative medicine (CAM) in the present day. The effectiveness of massage therapy has been established by research conducted on its physical, physiological, and psychological impact, which shows that the therapy has minimal side effects and supports mental health, thus acting as an alternative for psychiatric treatment (Cavaye, 2012). With psychiatric professionals increasingly recognizing the limitations of conventional pharmacologic treatments, the normalization of such unconventional interventions heralds a growing sensitivity to mental health care. Another cutting-edge approach within varied therapeutic models is the integration of sensory experiences into treatment.

The examination of olfactory input, particularly through advancements in perfumery technology, highlights the profound influence of odors on psychological states. Current multidisciplinary works, such as the JENTIL® Collection, explore the relationship between fashion and mental health and suggest that garments can be designed to react sensitively to the subject's emotional state, thereby constituting a healing space. This is manifest in the potential of marrying multisensory design with therapies where the subject can receive emotional nurturing through personalized scent bubbles that can exert a positive influence on mood and self-worth (Tillotson et al., 2008). These advancements reveal the multifaceted interaction between mental illness and sensory experience, adding richness to the psychiatric field in terms of new, promising intervention methods that address emotional and psychological needs. Furthermore, the rising popularity of complementary therapies suggests a shift towards holism in psychiatric treatment. As patients become increasingly adamant about seeking therapies that resonate with personal experiences, the demand for integrative approaches increases. Alternative therapies, including yoga, meditation, and herbal treatments, allow patients to have numerous means of dealing with stress, anxiety, and depression. The focus on the interaction of mind and body allows these therapies to complement other traditional psychiatric care and give patients active roles in their recovery. Psychiatric clinicians are now being called upon to examine a more integrated model that honors the patients' preferences for alternative therapies, ultimately leading to a more holistic and supportive model of mental health care. The integration of these therapies not only signifies a new cultural shift toward holistic care but also is another sign of ongoing innovation in psychiatric care in the 21st century (Figure 1.11).

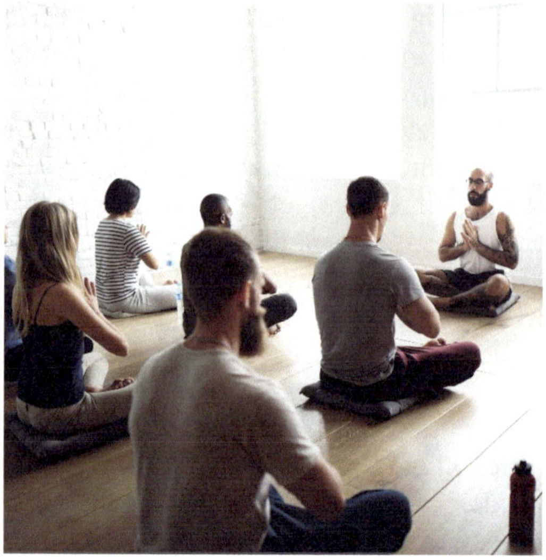

Figure 1.11. Alternative and complementary therapies.

Source: https://files.nccih.nih.gov/files/yoga-class-meditation-ThinkstockPhotos-637955386-square.jpg.

Test Your Knowledge

1. What are the main pharmacological and psychotherapeutic treatment options for common psychiatric disorders?
2. How do biological treatments such as ECT, TMS, and neurostimulation compare in terms of indications and effectiveness?

1.4. Role of the Psychiatrist

Learning Outcome

1. Education and training requirements.
2. Responsibilities and duties.
3. Ethical considerations in practice.

The psychiatrist's function in modern mental illness treatment is more than the classical role of diagnosis and treatment. Psychiatrists are uniquely trained to examine, diagnose, and treat a wide spectrum of mental illnesses, ranging from mood disorders to severe psychiatric illnesses. Their combined treatment model frequently utilizes biological, psychological, and social aspects in treatment plans, satisfying the multidimensionality of mental illness needs. For acute crises, psychiatrists are skilled at emergency interventions that create a sense of immediate relief and support to ensure that individuals affected by extreme mental distress receive timely intervention that matters. Through the utilization of evidence-based practices and research, psychiatrists help improve mental health outcomes by creating fundamental care platforms that address the needs of varied patients (Akbarzadeh et al., 2017). Furthermore, implementation of emerging models of care, such as Crisis Resolution Teams (CRTs), illustrates how the role of psychiatrists is evolving in community practice. The teams work towards diversion of hospitalization in mental health emergencies through early assessment and home interventions. Psychiatrists play a central role in these teams to provide proper interventions in the comfort of familiarity, thereby designing a supportive environment for recovery. Research indicates that CRTs can reduce hospitalization demand and simultaneously enhance patient satisfaction with psychiatric treatment. Psychiatrists are thus essential in optimizing the effectiveness of these teams by concentrating on particular characteristics, which further enhance crisis intervention and treatment quality, a sign of expanding psychiatric practice environments beyond clinics (Churchard et al., 2015). Apart from direct patient care, psychiatrists are also highly engaged with public health education and advocacy on mental health issues. They frequently participate in stigma reduction of mental illness and mental health resource awareness within communities. This aspect of their practice plays a great role in facilitating early intervention and encouraging people to access help before issues escalate. Psychiatrists work with multidisciplinary teams, including psychologists, social workers, and other health care professionals, to treat the broader social factors that cause mental illness. In their advocacy work, they influence public policy and educational initiatives that aim to increase access to mental health services and increase the overall level of mental illness awareness within the population. Therefore, the role of a psychiatrist is thus diversified, focusing on integral care, creative delivery of services, and community outreach, all of which are necessary to further the cause of psychiatry (Akbarzadeh et al., 2017) (Figure 1.12).

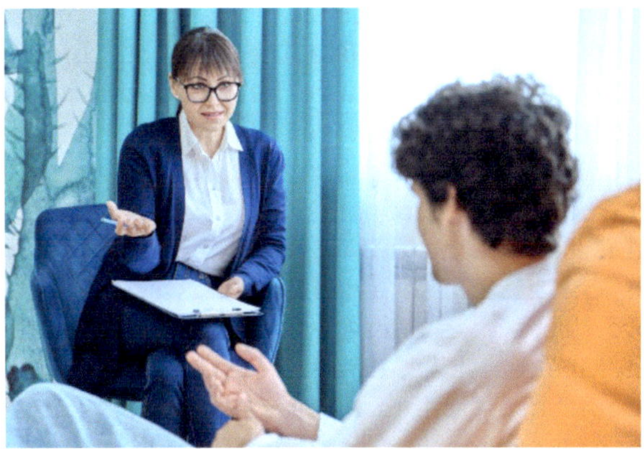

Figure 1.12. Role of the psychiatrist.

Source: https://www.merylwalmsley.top/wp-content/uploads/2025/06/female-psychologist-talking-to-young-male-individ-2024-12-08-02-08-42-utc-min-scaled.jpg.

1.4.1. Education and Training Requirements

The education and training required for psychiatric professionals are at the heart of quality and effectiveness in mental health care. Individuals who want to become professionals in this field typically begin with a bachelor's degree in psychology, social work, or a related field. This initial learning provides fundamental information about human behavior and mental processes. Then, a future psychiatrist must attend medical school and obtain a Doctor of Medicine (MD) or Doctor of Osteopathic Medicine (DO) degree. Medical school involves a lot of education in overall medicine, which is crucial in learning about the biological aspects of mental illness and treatment. This heavy training equips future psychiatrists with the necessary competence to handle complex mental illnesses, ultimately enhancing the quality of care they offer to patients. It follows that the initial years of training are the groundwork for a successful career in psychiatry. Following medical school, training continues with residency training for specialists. Typically lasting four years, a psychiatry residency provides extended experience with subspecialties like geriatric psychiatry, child and adolescent psychiatry, and addiction psychiatry. Residents can apply theoretical principles to real-world scenarios and acquire practical experience in the assessment and management of patients with various mental illnesses during this period of core training. Psychiatrists also acquire supervised clinical practice, which enhances their diagnostic and therapeutic skills, through residency. Besides, the training emphasizes the importance of interprofessional collaboration with other health professionals and an understanding of the way in which interdisciplinary practice brings value to patient care. Through such skills, psychiatric workers can address the multifaceted needs of their patients more effectively and contribute positively to the mental health workforce. The preparation of the mental health workforce also heavily relies on the existing policies for education and training. As suggested, quality mental health care also hinges not only on providers' competence but also on their availability, which has direct connections with education access and policies of the workforce (Bagalman et al., 2013). Moreover, mental health care expenses always correspond to providers' required salaries, which affect whether psychiatry is an appealing career (Heisler, 2018). Enhancing training opportunities and strengthening educational programs can lead to solutions for workforce deficiencies and improved access to high-quality care. These could include steps like loan forgiveness for psychiatric specialty-track students who are medical students or greater funding for residency positions. With these considerations of policy, stakeholders can work towards a more resilient and better-prepared mental health workforce that is capable of addressing the psychiatric requirements of society.

1.4.2. Duties and Responsibilities

In psychiatry, the responsibilities and obligations of psychiatric practitioners extend beyond clinical practice to involve a wide array of ethical responsibilities and regulatory requirements. Practitioners are required to ensure that they are providing competent care, adhering to professional guidelines, and being current with evolving practice. For instance, monitoring and regulation of Approved Mental Health Professional (AMHP) training schemes are a necessary framework for guaranteeing quality across the profession. The General Social Care Council (GSCC) inspected AMHP schemes to ensure adherence to mandatory standards and correct variations in training quality, as per the reports. This highlights the importance of regulation and monitoring in safeguarding public health as well as ensuring that practitioners possess the skills required to function within their capacities, thereby leading to more authentic care for patients. Moreover, the ethical concerns of the psychiatrist's role include balancing patient confidentiality, informed consent, and the requirement of proper assessments. These psychologists are charged with the mandate of evaluating their patients' mental well-being while maintaining respectful and transparent therapeutic relationships. This is particularly so in cases where psychological evaluations are mandated for work purposes. These evaluations influence employment and licensing practices, which mandate that psychologists adhere to stringent standards that promote ethical practice. By adhering to these standards, professionals can not only determine their observations correctly but also fairly, thereby upholding the dignity of the psychiatric profession and gaining the confidence of patients and the public at large.

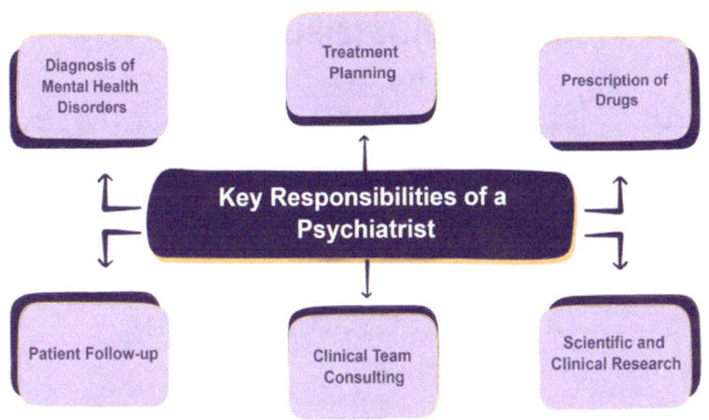
Diagnosis of Mental Health Disorders
Treatment Planning
Prescription of Drugs
Key Responsibilities of a Psychiatrist
Patient Follow-up
Clinical Team Consulting
Scientific and Clinical Research

Figure 1.13. Responsibilities and duties of the psychiatrist.

Source: https://www.theknowledgeacademy.com/_files/images/Key_Responsibilities_of_a_Psychiatrist.png.

Additionally, the administrative and collaborative roles of psychiatrists are fundamental elements of their professional practice. Accepting leadership roles in interdisciplinary teams, psychiatrists have a responsibility to themselves and others to make treatment plans clearly communicated and executed across all healthcare stakeholders. Such collaboration can involve working with other mental health professionals, including psychologists, social workers, and general practitioners, in the provision of comprehensive care to patients. The ethical consideration of such collaborative approaches is being responsible and transparent regarding all contact. Such responsibility is even more emergent in work settings, where psychological tests also need to follow established guidelines to ensure a fair and equitable working environment. Involvement in these cooperative duties not only enhances patient treatment but also enhances the role of the psychiatrist in enhancing mental health consciousness in the broader societal context (Figure 1.13).

1.4.3. Ethical Considerations in Practice

Ethics in psychiatric practice entailed a complex interplay of values, professional standards, and patients' rights. The most significant feature of this is the appreciation of the subjective character of mental illness, which contradicts traditional diagnostic models that strive to portray mental disorders as purely factual phenomena. Ethical values must rise above seeing diagnosis as a fixed classification in order to embrace a more dynamic conception of mental health through values-based practice (VBP). This encourages the importance of knowing the individual patients' experiences and the societal context that informs their mental well-being. This process enables practitioners to avoid reductionist tendencies that would neglect the profound moral implications of their therapeutic decisions, thereby building a therapeutic community that appreciates patient autonomy and promotes customized care (Thornton, 2014). The ethical implications are reflected in practical applications in psychiatry, particularly in areas related to informed consent and the responsibility model attributed to patients. Current models responding to mental illness must critically examine their capacity to embrace normative values, hence influencing diagnostic and treatment protocols.

This is raised while determining the moral responsibilities of patients. Utilizing a normative framework in psychiatric diagnosis, not only can professionals classify mental health conditions more precisely, but they can also establish the capabilities needed by individuals to perform their responsibilities. This educated awareness enables a deeper conversation between patients and clinicians regarding available options for treatment, encouraging decision-making that balances therapeutic goals with the patient's values and circumstances (Seely, 2019). Further, the ethical framework of psychiatry is provided by case studies that illustrate the complexity surrounding the treatment of mental diseases. For instance, examining cases like Alcohol Dependence Disorder can illustrate how principles of morality intersect with clinical practice. Under these circumstances, a detailed understanding of responsibility, the gravity of the disorder, and patient consent becomes critical. Ethical demands require that an equipoise be maintained between clinical judgment and patient welfare, particularly while clinicians attempt to develop individualized treatment plans that respect both medical prudence and patient values. This integration is not merely an ethical practice in conformity but promotes patient-centered care that is centered on healing and wellness, such that the therapy process is fair and righteous for all presenting (Seely, 2019) (Figure 1.14).

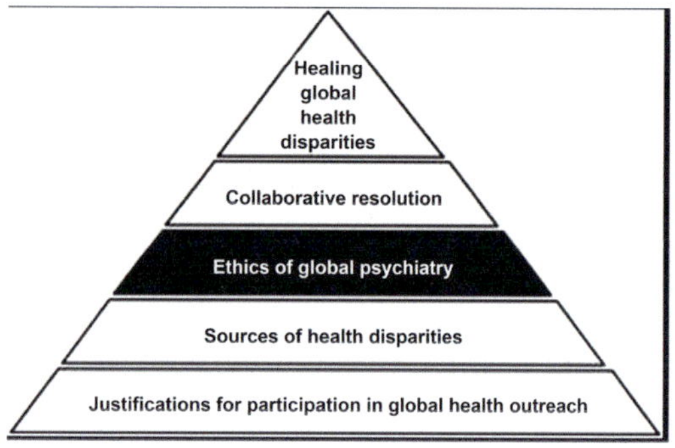

Figure 1.14. Ethical considerations in the practice of the psychiatrist.

Source: https://www.researchgate.net/publication/263514604/figure/fig1/AS:267457659142148@1440778283893/The-ethical-practice-of-global-psychiatry-requires-understanding-of-motivators-for.png.

Test Your Knowledge

1. What responsibilities does a psychiatrist have in the diagnosis, treatment, and long-term management of mental disorders?
2. How does a psychiatrist collaborate with psychologists, social workers, and other professionals in multidisciplinary mental health care?

1.5. Current Trends in Psychiatry

Learning Outcome

1. Advances in neuroimaging and genetics.
2. Integration of technology in treatment.
3. Focus on mental health awareness and stigma reduction.

Current trends in psychiatry recognize a salient shift toward evidence on the age patterns of onset of mental disorders, with significant consequences for prevention and treatment. Recent systematic reviews have established that the median age of onset of most mental disorders is generally in childhood or early adolescence. For instance, neurodevelopmental disorders , such as autism spectrum disorder and attention-deficit/hyperactivity disorder have a median age at onset of approximately 5.5 years, underlining the importance of interventions among early stages of population. Furthermore, the trends indicate that by the age of 25, up to 62.5% of individuals may be experiencing some form of mental disorder. This knowledge contradicts normative treatment models that compartmentalize mental health services for children and adults, but instead demands a more integrated approach to the promotion of mental health and preventive interventions throughout the life course that bridges the developmental gap (Solmi et al., 2021). Growing awareness of mental health issues among university students is still another new trend in contemporary psychiatry. The COVID-19 pandemic has compounded existing vulnerabilities in this population, causing increased stress, anxiety, and depressive symptoms. Acknowledging this change, many schools are starting to make mental health services a top priority, thus creating a nourishing environment for both academic and emotional health. Besides, the pandemic has sped up a broader conversation around mental health, encouraging colleges to implement whole-of-population outreach programs and mental health services tailored to the specific needs of students. Such progressive change demonstrates growing awareness that stresses of education can have a significant impact on mental health, hence the need to have integrative systems of care enabling students to access required psychiatric treatment (Son et al., 2020). Lastly, the incorporation of telepsychiatry and technology is a signature trend that will shape the future of psychiatric practice.

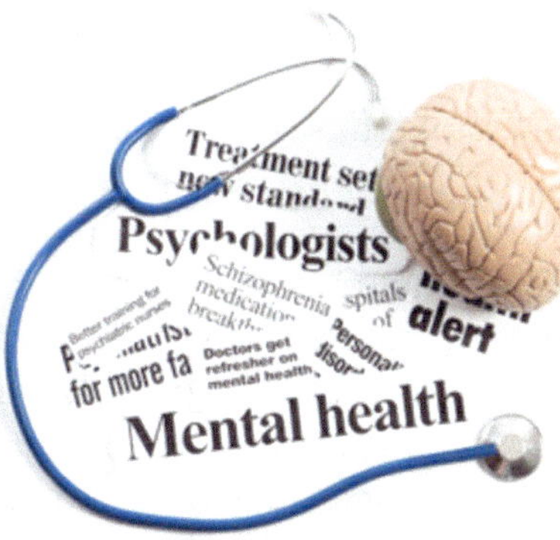

Figure 1.15. Current trends in psychiatry.

Source: https://blogger.googleusercontent.com/img/b/R29vZ2xl/AVvXsEjegRRR1w8NJYYG4KxoBm1IeVdRi_hM0CO5kUo8bZabfYretWDCzft-TzSaX-Pi2QNUqHmPyq1q4Yuzc1V3fLB9mLKn5AwmZgni5LPKR8vS4H33yPQBaE_KJhbjhy6wSsbT4ZsD0CSPpxew96tadsQ7qridsaTRxL-fbf3wDOZQOmINh__qTZgRa-Go6Q/s380/mental%20health.jpg.

The trend has gained momentum with the crisis caused by the pandemic, enabling psychiatrists to remotely perform consultation and therapy sessions. Telehealth emerges as a viable option, particularly in rural areas where mental health professionals are scarce. Moreover, utilization of electronic platforms offers the potential for enhanced patient involvement with self-assessment tools, web forums, and mobile mental health apps. However, the concern of confidentiality of patients and efficacy of these computerized interventions remains. With continued advancement in telepsychiatry, it is important to formulate guidelines that maintain quality of care but enhance access and, therefore, enhance the overall mental health climate in psychiatry (Solmi et al., 2021) (Figure 1.15).

1.5.1. Advances in Neuroimaging and Genetics

The rapidity of the evolution of intelligence in neuroimaging devices has significantly contributed to our understanding of the neural basis of psychiatric disorders. Advanced modalities , such as functional magnetic resonance imaging (fMRI) and positron emission tomography (PET) allow researchers to create images of brain activity in real time, providing insight into the neurobiological underpinnings of complex behaviors and emotional processes. These imaging technologies have been valuable in the identification of dysfunctional brain networks involved in disorders like schizophrenia and major depression. More particularly, neuroimaging research has pointed to disrupted patterns of connectivity in areas implicated in cognition and emotion regulation, demonstrating the complexity of these disorders at a biological level. Furthermore, the integration of neuroimaging data and genetic data has unlocked the potential for personalized therapy in psychiatry, matching specific neural changes with genetic vulnerabilities and eventually guiding more tailored therapeutic interventions (Wilke et al., 2020). Along with these advances in neuroimaging are monumental advances in genetics that have elucidated the complex heritability of psychiatric disorders. Through genome-wide association studies (GWAS), researchers have identified numerous genetic variants with a higher risk for several mental illnesses. These findings have enhanced the understanding of the biological processes that contribute to mental illnesses and reinforced the importance of polygenic risk factors. Identification of some genes associated with diseases like bipolar disorder, schizophrenia, and autism spectrum disorders increases the potential for developing new genetic screening devices. Such technologies have the potential to provide insightful knowledge of early diagnosis, assessment of risks, and quantification of treatment efficacy, leading to more effective individualized treatment approaches. However, the ethical considerations of genetic testing and genetic discrimination are some of the long-standing issues that will need to be addressed as this technology advances (Michael et al., 2019). Moreover, the marriage of genetics and neuroimaging has propagated a more convergent understanding of psychiatric illness. By linking neuroimaging results to genetic information, researchers are beginning to create a more comprehensive picture of psychiatric illness incorporating biological as well as environmental factors. This convergence gives a better picture of how genetic risk can manifest as observable alterations in brain structure and function that translate into specific psychiatric symptoms. For example, increased levels of neurofilament proteins in the blood may serve as biomarkers of neuronal damage, as agreed with neuroimaging findings and genetic predisposition factors in conditions , such as spinocerebellar ataxia type 3 (Wilke et al., 2020). As further research illuminates our understanding of these relationships, the potential for developing targeted treatments that consider an individual's neurobiological and genetic profiles could revolutionize the practice of psychiatry, leading to more effective treatments tailored to each patient.

1.5.2. Integration of Technology in Treatment

Inclusion of technology in treatment planning in the field of psychiatry is transforming care delivery paradigms. Telemedicine, mobile health applications, and electronic health records (EHRs) have revolutionized access and control of mental health care. Telehealth services, in particular, have become more and more vital, providing ease of use for patients who otherwise would have been constrained by limitations in accessing customary face-to-face consultations. Such a shift not only subverts geographical constraints but also benefits patients with mobility or anxiety conditions, thus ensuring that quality care is not undermined due to accessibility concerns. Moreover, the use of EHRs enhances continuity of care through facilitating better information exchange among medical professionals, thus a more uniform treatment approach. With these technologies advancing, the potential of individualized, patient-centered interventions becomes increasingly clear, an important development in the history of psychiatric treatment strategies. Furthermore, co-operative models , such as the research-practice integration (RPI) model underscore the pivotal role that technology is playing in bridging the research-practice gap. This model supports collaboration between stakeholders like researchers, clinicians, and health plan administrators to establish a solid platform for taking empirical evidence to practice. This model not only uses technology for conveying research results effectively, but also tries to improve the quality of treatment through evidence-based practices. For instance, the application of technology in treating teen alcohol and other drug (AOD) use illustrates such integration to a tee, how research findings can practically be utilized to inform service delivery in actual contexts. Such a partnership is key in developing an innovative mental health environment where the implementation of innovations is accelerated, which consequently results in better patient outcomes as well as optimized utilization of resources (Sterling et al., 2006). In the integration setting, the development of learning collaboratives , such as those in New Hampshire, signifies the collaborative effort of alignment of primary care and behavioral health. These types of programs establish a sense of value on mutual learning as well as transparency of data among multiple stakeholders, thereby promoting a more unified treatment approach. The NH Behavioral Health Integration Learning Collaborative, for instance, stems from the necessity of behavioral health service integration into primary care as a way to address the complex nature of co-occurring disorders. By using health information technology in enabling communication and data sharing, such programs not only improve patient care but also advance sustainable payment models for service effectiveness. This integrated model ultimately aims to create a health setting where behavioral health is dynamically intertwined with physical health, providing integrated care for patients with complicated health issues (Bartels et al., 2016).

1.5.3. Focus on Mental Health Awareness and Stigma Reduction

The growing awareness of mental health has become increasingly important in today's world, particularly in psychiatry. This is a testament that there is a greater awareness that mental health is as important as physical health, and that a lack thereof would have severe repercussions on individuals and communities. By this, campaigns and education contribute to de-stigmatization of mental illnesses and promoting open talk about such issues. Awareness-raising campaigns try to counter existing myths and stigmas and urge individuals to obtain help without fear of being judged. Furthermore, incorporating mental health education into coursework encourages less stigmatizing environments for young adults who all too frequently struggle with depression and anxiety as they seek to plow through academic pressure and personal development. Mental illness stigma is most often the cause of impediments to treatment, deterring individuals from accessing the treatment that they need. Most people perceive mental illness as a weakness that provokes shame or withdrawal. Stigma is particularly prevalent in work and academic settings, where pressure to wear a mask of competence can be intense. Healthcare workers, for instance, during the COVID-19 pandemic reported high rates of anxiety, depression, and sleep disturbances but isolated themselves from support networks to which they had access (Muller et al., 2020). These disparities bring into relief the necessity of programs that not only provide necessary mental health care but also work to address the issues of challenging and transforming stigma about mental illness, encouraging exposure and candor in communication regarding mental health. The issues related to awareness on the topic of mental health are particularly critical in higher education students, who possess unique pressures that can magnify underlying mental health issues. The COVID-19 pandemic brought the spotlight to this population with reports of staggering rates of anxiety and depressive symptoms among university students (Son et al., 2020). With schools and universities working to build resilience and foster well-being, stigma reduction strategies become essential. This includes the incorporation of peer support groups and mental health workshops that create safe spaces where individuals can speak freely. Additionally, learning institutions can promote the availability of mental health services, with students knowing where to turn for help. Lastly, addressing stigma and creating an open atmosphere in academically oriented environments not only enhances the well-being of individuals but also strengthens the overall resilience of the student community, paving the way for a healthier environment towards mental health in the context of psychiatry (Figure 1.16).

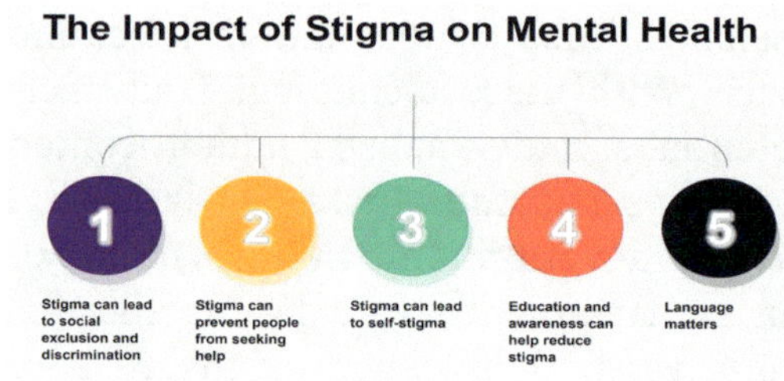

Figure 1.16. Focus on mental health awareness and stigma reduction.

Source: https://fastercapital.co/i/Mental-health--Shattering-Stigmas--Embracing-Mental-Health-and-Distressale--The-Impact-of-Stigma-on-Mental-Health.webp.

Test Your Knowledge

1. How are digital mental health tools, such as telepsychiatry and AI-based assessment platforms, transforming psychiatric practice?
2. What role do advances in genetics, neuroimaging, and precision medicine play in shaping the future of psychiatric diagnosis and treatment?

1.6. Challenges in the Field

Learning Outcome

1. Access to mental health care.
2. Misconceptions and stigma.
3. The impact of socioeconomic factors.

The field of psychiatry is faced with a broad array of challenges that may significantly impede successful intervention and the promotion of mental well-being among different groups. Stigma about mental illness is among the greatest impediments. It discourages individuals from going for health care and enables underdiagnosis and undertreatment, thereby increasing cycles of mental suffering as well as social isolation. Moreover, the culturally variable understanding of mental illness provides an impediment to devising universally successful psychiatric treatment. Patients within varying cultures and ethnicities may have assumptions contrary to conventional psychiatric practice, and communication and establishing trust with mental health workers becomes problematic. Merging mental health care into the overall health sector is the other essential challenge within the psychiatric business. Despite growing concern over mental ill health, even in elite sport, funds allocated to psychiatric care are generally inadequate. Paralympic athletes are but one case in point, wherein their cases reveal enormous gaps in mental health care even as the demand for the same continues to grow. Experience has indicated that sporting success can not only enhance mental well-being but also heighten psychological stress inherent in competitive sport. This dualism highlights the necessity of an effective healthcare plan for the prevention and management of mental disorders, as mentioned in the study highlighting the role required for the promotion of the utilization of sports psychiatry and psychotherapy services (Heiniger et al., 2023).

Lastly, the new face of mental health diagnosis and treatment is accompanied by a list of challenges for the practitioner. Advances in neuroscience and psychology have yielded a more nuanced understanding of mental disorders, yet they must be continually learned and adapted to by mental health professionals. The sheer pace of these advances is enough to make some professionals feel unready or overwhelmed and unable to effectively impart new methods. Further, the interface of technology advances , such as telepsychiatry, facilitates both challenges and opportunities regarding how to ensure accessibility without compromising the quality of care. Addressing these challenges requires a psychiatric community dedication towards lifelong learning as well as interprofessional collaboration to dismantle barriers to present more effectiveness in mental health treatment across different settings (Heiniger et al., 2024).

1.6.1. Access to Mental Health Care

Mental health access remains a chronic issue, often compounded by societal stigma and system-related issues. Mental health patients are usually confronted with issues hindering them from receiving appropriate care. For instance, sufferers of Functional Somatic Syndromes (FSS) have experienced high stigma levels, which may discourage them from seeking care. The emotional identification with public and professional views further complicates access because these patients are susceptible to internalizing stigmatizing beliefs and, thus, shun services they require. The condition underlines the need for mental health systems to address stigma openly, establishing an environment that enables people to access help without stigma or judgment (Cox, 2011). Such measures not only enhance access but also the overall effectiveness of mental health care. Teenagers have particular challenges with accessing mental health care. Research has indicated that approximately 20% of teens have mental health and addiction disorders, but timely evidence-based services are scarce. The traditional mental health system is strained to provide for this group, and therefore treatment wait times are longer. Contributing to this is low awareness, lack of proper resources, and a not youth-friendly enough setting. As a response, innovative models like the Integrated Collaborative Care Team (ICCT) model have been developed, with the aim of providing rapid, need-based access to services in a treatment setting. This model is designed not just to reduce wait times but also to include youth and families in the treatment continuum, ultimately developing a more responsive mental health care system (Chaim et al., 2017). Moreover, the effect of increased access to mental health care on public health outcomes as a whole must be taken into consideration. Greater access can lead to enhanced functioning in individuals with mental illness, and this can pay substantial dividends to health care systems and to communities as well. Through collaborative and integrated care models, mental health treatment can more effectively address the diverse needs of patients. This shift not only addresses the short-term issues of the individual in crisis but also promotes long-term stability and recovery. With the progress in mental health care, stakeholders , such as policymakers and health care providers are critical in prioritizing accessibility, hence promoting equitable and inclusive mental health care for all segments (Cox, 2011; Chaim et al., 2017) (Figure 1.17).

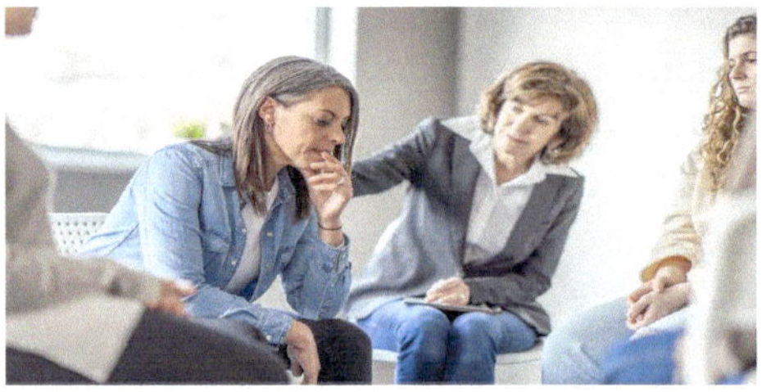

Figure 1.17. Access to mental health care.

Source: https://www.bonterratech.com/wp-content/uploads/2024/10/istock-1388265659.jpg-1.webp.

1.6.2. Misconceptions and Stigma

The field of psychiatry is often draped in myths that contribute significantly to mental illness stigma. The myths are likely to generate a social picture of mental illness as a failure or weakness and not as a tangible health condition warranting treatment. Negative attitudes are not only likely to deter individuals from seeking assistance but can also stimulate feelings of shame and isolation. As indicated in self-stigma studies, internalization of such stigmatizing assumptions is capable of profoundly affecting a person's mental self-esteem and overall well-being. Individuals bothered by such harmful beliefs tend to avoid seeking help from mental health care, ultimately impeding their recovery process and well-being, a basic issue in psychiatric practice (Lasalvia et al., 2025). Moreover, psychiatry is stigmatized and it not only falls on the mentally ill but also on professionals. Psychiatry residents, for example, even experience their own stigma, which makes them uncomfortable in declaring their specialty choice or discussing their experience with their own mental health. A survey of psychiatry residents revealed that a majority of them reported being exposed to negative stereotypes regarding mental health clinicians and individuals with severe mental illness. The high stigma scores indicate that not only are these residents battling against extrinsic stigma but also with an internalized version of it, one that can influence their employment satisfaction and professional identity (Masmoudi et al., 2024).

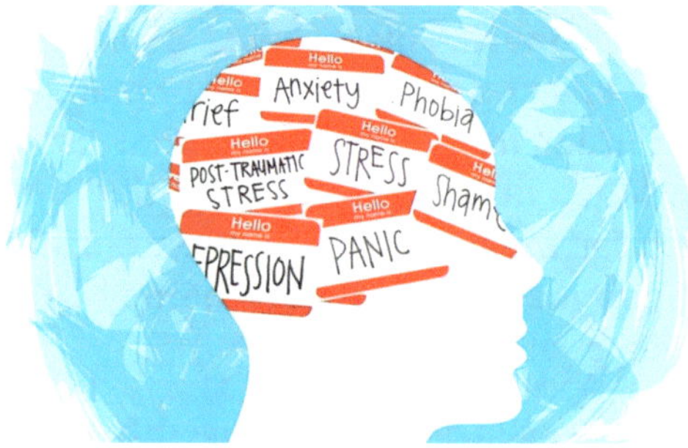

Figure 1.18. Misconceptions and stigma of psychiatry.

Source: https://www.fitpaa.com/wp-content/uploads/2023/10/Untitled-design-2023-10-31T184050.372-jpg.webp.

These processes underscore the intricacy of stigma in psychiatry and underscore the necessity of systemic change in mental health education and practice. Myth-busting and dispelling stigma are necessary to develop a society where mental health receives the same dignity and seriousness that physical health receives. Public education campaigns to create awareness about mental health diseases go a long way towards reducing stigma. For instance, therapies like Narrative Enhancement and Cognitive Therapy (NECT) have been used successfully to combat self-stigma among individuals with severe mental illnesses by promoting positive self-esteem and enabling individuals to embrace themselves despite societal prejudice. By integrating such interventions within public mental health systems, particularly stigmatized ones, treatment reach and effectiveness are made easier to enhance, thereby contributing to a more supportive society and eventually improved recovery outcomes for such persons dealing with mental illness (Lasalvia et al., 2025) (Figure 1.18).

1.6.3. The Impact of Socioeconomic Factors

Socioeconomic status is a major predictor of mental health status and access to psychiatric treatment. Individuals in lower socioeconomic groups are more likely to endure higher stressors, such as poverty, few educational years, and unstable housing, that serve to magnify mental illness. For instance, research has documented that impoverished individuals are more vulnerable to anxiety and depression caused by chronic financial stress and uncertainty. Secondly, such individuals may have limited access to mental health treatment due to financial limitations, stigma, or lack of available resources in their regions of residence. The compounding of these factors affects not only individuals on an individual level but is an even larger issue for public health since untreated mental illnesses are associated with greater morbidity and societal costs overall. The intersection of socioeconomic status with physical health issues also captures the intricate interaction of fiscal ability with mental health. Poor people have higher rates of comorbid conditions, like diabetes and cardiovascular disease, that contribute to mental health concurrently. As per research, mental illness sufferers are at greater risk of acquiring serious physical health conditions, illustrating how socioeconomic disadvantages may present themselves across a range of health areas (Demarin et al., 2021). The issue is further complicated by the reality that people with mental disorders might be less conscious of their physical health threats and less capable of effectively coping with them. This lack of awareness and control exacerbates existing mental health issues, creating a cycle of causation that is perpetuating rising rates of hospitalization and mortality among economically disadvantaged populations. In addition, the impact of socioeconomic determinants continues in certain aspects of health, like oral health, which has a staggering impact on quality of life. A study reveals the prevalence of high rates of dental issues among individuals with mental illness because it hypothesizes that poor oral health is largely due to socioeconomic factors, hence resulting in poor oral hygiene and related diseases (Borgamwar et al., 2024). Urban residents from lower socioeconomic backgrounds can be fairly deprived of dental care, and this further exacerbates the problem, mainly because individuals with mental illness have difficulty maintaining personal hygiene. This is particularly problematic in psychiatric populations, where compounding of poor self-care, restricted financial resources, and diminished access to healthcare represents a profound public health crisis. It serves particularly well to illustrate the necessity of closing socioeconomic disparities as a central strategy for improving overall health outcomes for individuals with mental illness.

Test Your Knowledge

1. What are the major barriers to accessing quality psychiatric care in low- and middle-income countries?
2. How do stigma, ethical dilemmas, and workforce shortages continue to hinder progress in global mental health?

Summary

The study of psychiatry calls for a mature intersection of several disciplines of study, in which mental health is perpetually constructed through clinical practice and scientific research. According to the description in recent studies, advancement of the field emphasizes the diverse impacts on people's lives. The conclusion of our exploration reveals that an integrated model, considering economic, social, and environmental factors, is central to policy-making and effective destination development in the psychiatric context (Vyas et al., 2025). This analysis thus not only directs attention to the multifaceted nature of psychiatric disorders but also emphasizes the importance of inter-provincial collaboration to achieve stronger paradigms that holistically address mental health issues. Also, psychiatric practice changes in the backdrop of significant alterations induced by precision psychiatry, which aims to provide personalised treatment modalities. Precision medicine is premised on a continuum of information across genetics, symptomatology, and psychosocial attributes, enabling clinicians to identify individual clinical phenotypes (JFżaryn et al., 2025). The ultimate goal is not a question of diagnosis but of working out individualized interventions that maximize patient benefit. As the field evolves, the incorporation of computational psychiatry into clinical practice can spur a paradigm change, promoting more precise diagnostic processes and response to treatment optimized to the specific circumstances of individual patients and thereby improving the overall strategy of mental healthcare. In short, as we navigate through the complexities of psychiatry, it is increasingly clear that interdisciplinarity and individualized treatment will shape the future of mental treatment. With emphasis placed on interdisciplinarity, the results of the current study highlight the need for organized investigations and the adoption of new approaches. The discipline is poised at the border of tradition and innovation, with a potential for such approaches as computational psychiatry to transform our understanding of mental health diseases. Lastly, final thoughts on this journey through psychiatric concepts and practices recognize that continued research, with policy support, is the highest priority to avoid the pressing mental illnesses of our time, thereby creating a more holistic vision of personal health (JFżaryn et al., 2025).

Psychiatry is a field of study that deals with a wide array of complex concepts and practices that are essential in the examination of mental health diseases. Among the key issues within the field is the intricate relationship between mental processes and behavior. This association illustrates the importance of learning why thoughts can impact emotions and behavior, already foreshadowed by the central observation that the association between possessing a mind and conforming to a rational model is still a valuable insight (Thornton, 2011). This approach underscores the need for an integrative approach to psychological therapy, which needs to encompass cognitive-behavioral therapies. Knowledge of such dynamics is crucial because it underlies evidence-based practice, which is capable of meeting the specific needs of diverse patients, suggesting that effective psychiatric treatment entails an integration of psychological theory and practice. Of equal significance in psychiatry is the application of various therapeutic modalities to minimize symptoms that are associated with mental illnesses. For instance, exposure and response prevention (ERP) has been recognized as a first-line behavior therapy for disorders , such as obsessive-compulsive disorder and Tourette syndrome (Black & Black, 2018). A recent modification, reward-enhanced exposure and response prevention (RE–ERP), illustrates how technology can enhance therapeutic interventions. RE–ERP uses a web-based platform, TicTrainer, where patients are taught tic suppression with the aid of an incentive system. This innovation marks a shift towards the application of digital technology for the augmentation of accessibility and effectiveness in treatment. Such advances in psychiatric interventions mark a continued change in the ways that practitioners can make use of new technology to benefit patients, particularly those in low-resource settings. Finally, understanding how psychiatric theories intersect with emerging practices further demonstrates the continued development of the field of psychiatry. The integration of behavior-based interventions, as seen in RE–ERP, into typical treatment models is a dedication to acting on the needs of patients in real-world contexts. The usability of interventions , such as TicTrainer not only enhances engagement but also maintains over time, demonstrating the potential of technology within mental health treatment. As the field grows, it is imperative that practitioners remain attuned to both the scientific underpinnings and real-world applications of emerging interventions. Focusing on holistic, evidence-based practice, psychiatry can continue to evolve, eventually leading to improved patient outcomes as well as the health of mental health knowledge overall (Vyas et al., 2025).

KEY TERMS FROM THIS CHAPTER

- Antidepressants
- Anxiety disorders
- Bipolar disorder
- Cognitive behavioral therapy
- Delusion
- Depression
- Electroconvulsive therapy
- Hallucination
- Mental illness
- Mental status examination
- Mood disorders
- Neurosis
- Obsessive-compulsive disorder
- Personality disorders

CRITICAL THINKING QUESTIONS

1. **Which of the following best defines psychiatry?**
   a. The study of childhood development
   b. The branch of medicine focused on diagnosing and treating mental disorders
   c. The study of the nervous system
   d. The practice of counseling for relationship issues
2. **Which professional is primarily responsible for prescribing medications for mental illness?**
   a. Psychologist
   b. Psychiatric nurse
   c. Psychiatrist
   d. Social worker
3. **The Diagnostic and Statistical Manual of Mental Disorders (DSM) is used to:**
   a. Measure intelligence
   b. Provide psychological counseling
   c. Classify and diagnose mental disorders
   d. Treat physical injuries
4. **A major depressive episode includes which of the following symptoms?**
   a. Elevated mood and energy
   b. Decreased need for sleep
   c. Persistent sadness and loss of interest
   d. Excessive talking and risky behaviors
5. **Which of the following is considered a psychotic disorder?**
   a. Panic disorder
   b. Schizophrenia
   c. Generalized anxiety disorder
   d. Obsessive-compulsive disorder

Short Answer Questions

1. Define psychiatry and explain how it differs from psychology.
2. What are the main categories of mental disorders commonly treated in psychiatry?
3. Who is considered the founder of psychoanalysis, and what is the main focus of this approach?
4. What is the DSM-5, and why is it important in psychiatric practice?
5. List three common symptoms that may indicate a psychiatric disorder.

Answer to Critical Thinking Questions

1. (b); 2. (c); 3. (c); 4. (c); 5. (b)

REFERENCES

1. King, D. L., Chamberlain, S. R., Carragher, N., Billieux, J., Stein, D., Mueller, K., Potenza, M. N., Rumpf, H. J., Saunders, J., Starcevic, V., Demetrovics, Z., Brand, M., Lee, H. K., Spada, M., Lindenberg, K., Wu, A. M. S., Lemenager, T., Pallesen, S., Achab, S., Kyrios, M., ... Delfabbro, P. H. (2020). Screening and assessment tools for gaming disorder: A comprehensive systematic review. *Clinical psychology review*, *77*, 101831. https://doi.org/10.1016/j.cpr.2020.101831 (accessed on 28th July 2025).
2. Akbarzadeh, F., Ebnehoseini, Z., Irajzade, M., et al. (2017). Designing the minimum data set of psychiatric emergency record. https://core.ac.uk/download/234708006.pdf (accessed on 28th July 2025).
3. Amann, C. (2010). *Cine-Therapie/Film-Therapie: Eine Erste Bibliographie.* https://core.ac.uk/download/14513746.pdf (accessed on 28th July 2025).
4. American Academy of Pediatrics. (2011). ADHD: Clinical practice guideline for the diagnosis, evaluation, and treatment of attention-deficit/hyperactivity disorder in children and adolescents. *Pediatrics, 128*, 1007–1022. https://doi.org/10.1542/peds.2011-2654 (accessed on 28th July 2025).
5. American Psychological Association. (2017, February 24). *Professional practice guidelines for occupationally mandated psychological evaluations.* https://www.apa.org/practice/guidelines/psychological-evaluations (accessed on 28th July 2025).
6. Angold, A., Banaschewski, B., Maughan, B., Byrne, C., et al. (2006). Literacy and mental disorders. https://core.ac.uk/download/49099.pdf (accessed on 28th July 2025).
7. Bagalman, E., & Heisler, E. J. (2013). The mental health workforce: A primer. https://core.ac.uk/download/18615793.pdf (accessed on 28th July 2025).
8. Bartels, S. J., Beaty, S., Blount, A., et al. (2016). Integrating behavioral health & primary care in New Hampshire: A path forward to sustainable practice & payment transformation. https://core.ac.uk/download/215540992.pdf (accessed on 28th July 2025).
9. Bauer, M. S., & Kirchner, J. (2019). Implementation science: What is it and why should I care? *Psychiatry Research, 283*, 112376. https://doi.org/10.1016/j.psychres.2019.04.025 (accessed on 28th July 2025).
10. Bayley, K., Christian, L., Hammond, N., et al. (2012). GSCC targeted inspections of Approved Mental Health Professionals (AMHP) courses in England (2011–12). https://core.ac.uk/download/30612948.pdf (accessed on 28th July 2025).
11. Bebbington, P. E., Brugha, T., Jenkins, R., et al. (2016). Mental health and wellbeing in England: The Adult Psychiatric Morbidity Survey 2014. https://core.ac.uk/download/286715532.pdf (accessed on 28th July 2025).
12. Bel, N., Bergstrom, R. F., Bravo, L., Bremner, J. D., Burrows, G. D., Chouinard, G., Datla, K. P., et al. (2014). Fluoxetine: A case history of its discovery and preclinical development. https://core.ac.uk/download/161360681.pdf (accessed on 28th July 2025).
13. Berk, M., Brewin, C., Briken, P., et al. (2020). Mental, behavioral and neurodevelopmental disorders in the ICD-11: An international perspective on key changes and controversies. https://core.ac.uk/download/287582535.pdf (accessed on 28th July 2025).

14. Berry, M., Meier, P. S., Schulte, S., et al. (2008). Treatment approaches for dual diagnosis clients in England. https://core.ac.uk/download/50706.pdf (accessed on 28th July 2025).

15. Black, J. K., & Black, K. J. (2018). Software for web-based tic suppression training [version 2; referees: 3 approved]. https://core.ac.uk/download/212866338.pdf (accessed on 28th July 2025).

16. Borgamwar, V., Kumar, P., P. C., M., et al. (2024). Dental conditions in patients with psychiatric disorders–A pilot study. https://core.ac.uk/download/613707967.pdf (accessed on 28th July 2025).

17. Cavaye, J. (2012). Does therapeutic massage support mental well-being? https://core.ac.uk/download/9720241.pdf (accessed on 28th July 2025).

18. Cavioni, V., Grazzani, I., & Ornaghi, V. (2020). Mental health promotion in schools: A comprehensive theoretical framework. https://core.ac.uk/download/322748597.pdf (accessed on 28th July 2025).

19. Cepeda, S. L., Christian, C. C., et al. (2019). Project Reach: Implementation of evidence-based psychotherapy within integrated healthcare for Hurricane Harvey affected individuals. https://core.ac.uk/download/228022778.pdf (accessed on 28th July 2025).

20. Chaim, G., Cheung, A., Cleverley, K., et al. (2017). Integrated collaborative care teams to enhance service delivery to youth with mental health and substance use challenges: Protocol for a pragmatic randomized controlled trial. https://core.ac.uk/download/275573011.pdf (accessed on 28th July 2025).

21. Churchard, A., Fitzgerald, C., Fullarton, K., et al. (2015). Implementation of the Crisis Resolution Team model in adult mental health settings: A systematic review. https://core.ac.uk/download/29414640.pdf (accessed on 28th July 2025).

22. Cohn, J., Dijkstra, T., Nijholt, A., et al. (2009). Therapy Progress Indicator (TPI): Combining speech parameters and the subjective unit of distress. https://core.ac.uk/download/pdf/11473070.pdf (accessed on 28th July 2025).

23. Cox, P. (2011). An examination of the psychiatric experiences of patients diagnosed with functional somatic syndrome within the National Health Service: A qualitative study. https://core.ac.uk/download/370473.pdf (accessed on 28th July 2025).

24. Curtis, S. (2016). *Space, Place and Mental Health*. Routledge eBooks. https://doi.org/10.4324/9781315610160 (accessed on 28th July 2025).

25. Demarin, V., & Morović, S. (2021). Comorbidity from a neuropsychiatric perspective. https://core.ac.uk/download/512503374.pdf (accessed on 28th July 2025).

26. Linson, A., & Friston, K. (2019). Reframing PTSD for computational psychiatry with the active inference framework. *Cognitive neuropsychiatry*, *24*(5), 347–368. https://doi.org/10.1080/13546805.2019.1665994 (accessed on 28th July 2025).

27. Gautam, S., Gautam, M., Jain, A., & Yadav, A. N. (2022). Overview of practice of consultation-liaison psychiatry. *Indian Journal of Psychiatry, 64*, S201–S210. https://doi.org/10.4103/indianjpsychiatry.indianjpsychiatry_1019_21 (accessed on 28th July 2025).

28. Green, M. F., Horan, W. P., & Lee, J. (2019). Nonsocial and social cognition in schizophrenia: Current evidence and future directions. *World Psychiatry, 18*, 146–161. https://doi.org/10.1002/wps.20624 (accessed on 28th July 2025).

29. Larsen RR and Hastings J (2018) From Affective Science to Psychiatric Disorder: Ontology as a Semantic Bridge. Front. Psychiatry 9:487. doi: 10.3389/fpsyt.2018.00487(accessed on 28th July 2025).

30. Heiniger, A., Imboden, C., Kiselev, N., et al. (2023). Perspectives on mental health and well-being. https://www.zora.uzh.ch/id/eprint/238077/1/ludi_et_al_2023_perspectives_on_mental_health_and_well_being.pdf (accessed on 28th July 2025).

31. Heiniger, A., Imboden, C., Kiselev, N., et al. (2024). Voices of Swiss Paralympic athletes: Perspectives on mental health and well-being. https://core.ac.uk/download/636780120.pdf (accessed on 28th July 2025).

32. Heisler, E. J. (2018). The mental health workforce: A primer. https://core.ac.uk/download/233839585.pdf (accessed on 28th July 2025).

33. Holtzman, W. (1979). Delivery of mental health services: Social, cultural, and family factors. https://core.ac.uk/download/211348844.pdf (accessed on 28th July 2025).

34. Hoque, S. (2016). Care team education on the use of sensory resources in inpatient psychiatry. https://core.ac.uk/download/79664899.pdf (accessed on 28th July 2025).

35. Huxley, A., Komaromi, A., Sinfield, A., Sweeney, A., Woods, A., Woods, A., Smith, A. D., et al. (2018). Madness decolonized? Madness as transnational identity in Gail Hornstein's *Agnes's Jacket*. https://core.ac.uk/download/42369304.pdf (accessed on 28th July 2025).

36. Jakovljević, M. (2015). Creative, person-centered and narrative psychopharmacotherapy or how to prevent and overcome treatment resistance in psychiatry. https://core.ac.uk/download/81389163.pdf (accessed on 28th July 2025).

37. Lasalvia, A., Bodini, L., Cristofalo, D., Fin, V., Yanos, P., & Bonetto, C. (2025). Assessing the effectiveness and the feasibility of a group-based treatment for self-stigma in people with mental disorders in routine mental health services in North-East Italy: Study protocol for a pragmatic multisite randomized controlled trial. *Trials, 26*. https://www.semanticscholar.org/paper/652518e9d3b4949942110575011607c4409cedf2 (accessed on 28th July 2025).

38. Masiriri, T. (2008). The effects of managed care on social work mental health practice. https://core.ac.uk/download/10685663.pdf (accessed on 28th July 2025).

39. Masmoudi, R., Ajmi, S., Guermazi, A., Cherif, F., Sallemi, R., & Masmoudi, J. (2024). Perceived stigma evaluation among residents in psychiatry. *European Psychiatry, 67*, S798. https://www.semanticscholar.org/paper/fd66df1770d1a15004a65aef29d9c8e8c75660b3 (accessed on 28th July 2025).

40. Melchert, T. (2007). Strengthening the scientific foundations of professional psychology: Time for the next steps. https://core.ac.uk/download/213077244.pdf (accessed on 28th July 2025).

41. Możaryn, J. F., & Szczegielniak, A. (2025). Computational psychiatry: A bridge between translation and precision. *International Journal of Neuropsychopharmacology, 28*, i276–i277. https://www.semanticscholar.org/paper/7caa74ecbd4a3530b3881e61185437046177f049 (accessed on 28th July 2025).

42. Muller, A. E., Hafstad, E., Himmels, J. P. W., Smedslund, G., Flottorp, S., Stensland, S. Ø., Stroobants, S., et al. (2020). The mental health impact of the COVID-19 pandemic on healthcare workers, and interventions to help them: A rapid systematic review. *Psychiatry Research, 293*, 113441. https://doi.org/10.1016/j.psychres.2020.113441 (accessed on 28th July 2025).

43. Narasimha, V., Suhas, S., Kishor, M., Dixit, A., & Murthy, P. (2024). Advances in psychiatry training and faculty development in India. *Indian Journal of Psychological Medicine, 46*, 391–399. https://www.semanticscholar.org/paper/5326b27eb838266dfdad0ddb7c536ce4207d15ba (accessed on 28th July 2025).

44. Nord, C. L., & Garfinkel, S. N. (2022). Interoceptive pathways to understand and treat mental health conditions. *Trends in Cognitive Sciences, 26*, 499–513. https://doi.org/10.1016/j.tics.2022.03.004 (accessed on 28th July 2025).

45. Panova, T., & Carbonell, X. (2018). Is smartphone addiction really an addiction? *Journal of Behavioral Addictions, 7*, 252–259. https://doi.org/10.1556/2006.7.2018.49 (accessed on 28th July 2025).

46. Regier, D. A., Narrow, W. E., Clarke, D. E., Kraemer, H. C., Kuramoto, S. J., Kuhl, E. A., & Kupfer, D. J. (2013). DSM-5 field trials in the United States and Canada, Part II: Test-retest reliability of selected categorical diagnoses. *American Journal of Psychiatry, 170*, 59–70. https://doi.org/10.1176/appi.ajp.2012.12070999 (accessed on 28th July 2025).

47. Rogers, J., Chesney, E., Oliver, D., Pollak, T. A., McGuire, P., Fusar-Poli, P., Zandi, M. S., et al. (2020). Psychiatric and neuropsychiatric presentations associated with severe coronavirus infections: A systematic review and meta-analysis with comparison to the COVID-19 pandemic. *The Lancet Psychiatry, 7*, 611–627. https://doi.org/10.1016/s2215-0366(20)30203-0 (accessed on 28th July 2025).

48. Romão, J., Gonçalves, M., André, R., Felix, F., Saraiva, R., & Abreu, M. (2022). From Akute Primäre Verrückheit to Bouffée Délirante: The background of acute transient psychosis. *European Psychiatry, 65*, S197, S198. https://www.semanticscholar.org/paper/e84978eb0ed10e41311bc3dfe23f83cc2724b516 (accessed on 28th July 2025).

49. Seely, M. (2019). Managing madness: The ethics of identifying and treating mental illness. https://core.ac.uk/download/215444329.pdf (accessed on 28th July 2025).

50. Solmi, M., Raduà, J., Olivola, M., Croce, E., Soardo, L., Salazar de Pablo, G., Shin, J. I., et al. (2021). Age at onset of mental disorders worldwide: Large-scale meta-analysis of 192 epidemiological studies. *Molecular Psychiatry, 27*, 281–295. https://doi.org/10.1038/s41380-021-01161-7 (accessed on 28th July 2025).

51. Son, C., Hegde, S., Smith, A., Wang, X., & Sasangohar, F. (2020). Effects of COVID-19 on college students' mental health in the United States: Interview survey study. *Journal of Medical Internet Research, 22*, e21279. https://doi.org/10.2196/21279 (accessed on 28th July 2025).

52. Sterling, S., & Weisner, C. (2006). Translating research findings into practice: Example of treatment services for adolescents in managed care. https://core.ac.uk/download/323072702.pdf (accessed on 28th July 2025).

53. Thornton, T. (2008). Should comprehensive diagnosis include idiographic understanding? https://core.ac.uk/download/341079.pdf (accessed on 28th July 2025).

54. Thornton, T. (2011). Recent developments for naturalizing the mind. https://core.ac.uk/download/341071.pdf (accessed on 28th July 2025).

55. Thornton, T. (2014). Values based practice and authoritarianism. https://core.ac.uk/download/42138025.pdf (accessed on 28th July 2025).

56. Tillotson, J. (2008). JENTIL: Responsive clothing that promotes a 'holistic approach to fashion as a new vehicle to treat psychological conditions. http://ualresearchonline.arts.ac.uk/4907/1/Tillotson_Scent_IFFTI2008_doc_.pdf (accessed on 28th July 2025).

57. Vyas, B., Patoliya, J., Doshi, R., Shah, P., Vijay, A., Gandhi, Z., et al. (2025). Socioeconomic and environmental impact of tourism: A review and future research agenda. *Journal of Information Systems Engineering and Management*. https://www.semanticscholar.org/paper/b43d29fe3a6f27f1d4a966b9da2dd19ee7020ce7 (accessed on 28th July 2025).

58. Wilke, C., Haas, E., Reetz, K., Faber, J., García-Moreno, H., Santana, M. M., van de Warrenburg, B., et al. (2020). Neurofilaments in spinocerebellar ataxia type 3: Blood biomarkers at the preataxic and ataxic stage in humans and mice. *EMBO Molecular Medicine, 12*. https://doi.org/10.15252/emmm.201911803 (accessed on 28th July 2025).

59. Zawiła-Niedźwiecki, J. (2016). Antoni Kępiński's philosophy of medicine–An alternative reading. https://core.ac.uk/download/83117222.pdf (accessed on 28th July 2025).

PSYCHIATRIC INTERVIEWING AND MENTAL STATUS EXAMINATION (MSE)

2

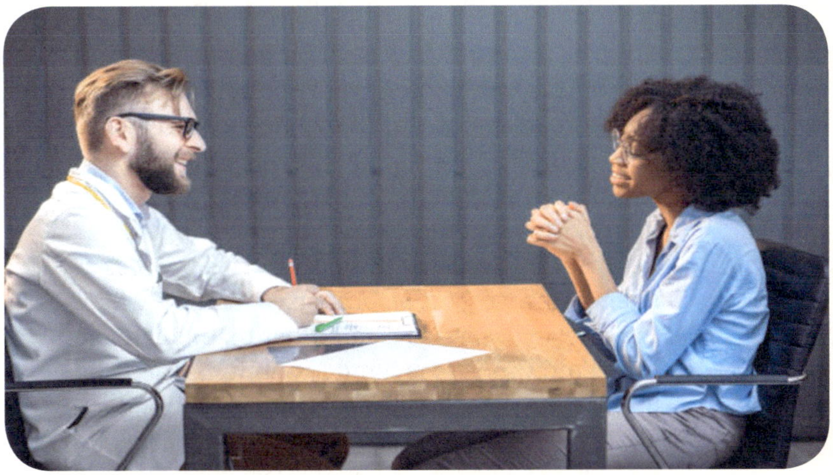

LEARNING OBJECTIVES

After studying this chapter, you will be able to:

1. Define the purpose of clinical interviewing;
2. List the types of clinical interviews;
3. Explain the key components of clinical interviewing;
4. Give an introduction to mental status examination (MSE);
5. Focus on the components of the mental status examination;
6. Explore the challenges in clinical interviewing and MSE.

Introduction

The practice of the clinical interview is a cornerstone in mental health, and it serves as the foundation upon which one can observe a client's state of mind. The process involves not only the gathering of information via the initial contact, but also the successful assessment of a client's state of mind. The importance of this skill cannot be overestimated since it can guide clinicians in forming a complete picture of the client's cognitive, emotional, and behavioral function. The mental status examination (MSE) bridges the gap in the clinical interview by providing a structured method of examining different facets of a client's mental well-being. As identified in literature, the MSE is an essential component of the psychiatric clinical interview, but there has been a stark deficiency in the use of evidence-based instructional design in order to adequately educate skills (Chivu et al., 2022). In teaching, future mental health professionals must have the tools required for conducting holistic interviews and conducting MSEs. The format of this learning project often includes lectures, case studies, and interactive experiences with students. These methods work to build the diagnostic skills and understanding of mental disorders, as presented in the Diagnostic and Statistical Manual of Mental Disorders, Fifth Edition (DSM-5) (Miyakuni et al., 2022). Through the focus on etiology and classification of mental illness, students come to realize the nuances involved in diagnosis as well as proper treatment planning. Moreover, through the employment of several instructional modalities, an interactive learning environment has been developed that not only enhances clinical skills but also promotes problem-solving by encouraging teamwork in dyadic and small group settings.

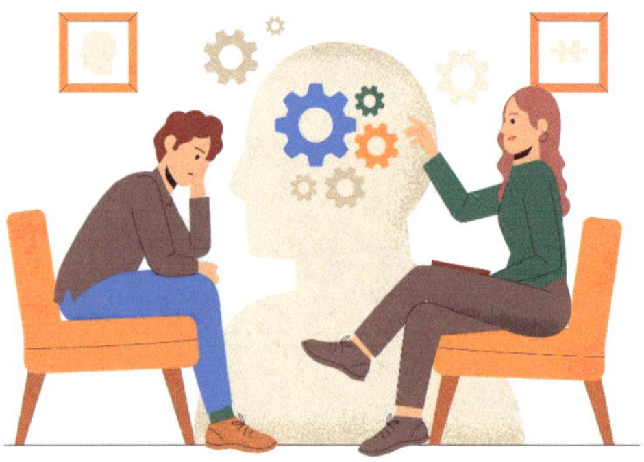

Figure 2.1. The mental state examination (MSE).

Source: https://www.psycourse.in/upload/shares/Course/Image/Other/Mental-State-Examination.jpg.

The integration of MSE and clinical interviewing skills in psychiatric training underscores the necessity of systematic education based on evidence. Despite the existence of educational case reports and teaching exercises, there remains a gap in studies to compare the effectiveness of different methods of instruction in this area (Chivu et al., 2022). To enhance the practice of clinical interviewing and the application of the MSE in the future, educational programs should stress empirical research and the application of diverse instructional design models. Through this means, mental health educators can ensure that practitioners are adequately trained to engage in effective clinical interviewing, thereby leading to improved client outcomes and quality mental health services. Consequently, creating training methods is required to close the already existing gaps and enhance the quality of care in psychiatric practice (Figure 2.1).

Definition of Clinical Interviewing

Clinical interviewing is an integral aspect of the field of psychology, particularly in mental health assessment. It is known to be a structured yet flexible interaction between a clinician and client, for the purpose of gathering relevant information on the emotional, psychological, and behavioral status of the client. The process is likely to incorporate an organized method, where the interviewer uses a combination of open and direct questions to facilitate communication and encourage the client to be open. Notably, good clinical interviewing not only requires a solid knowledge base of psychological theories and models but also empathetic interpersonal skills to establish rapport and a safety net for the revelation of the client. This conflict between structure and exploring detailed individual narratives is integral to proper assessment and treatment planning. A critical aspect of clinical interviewing is the inclusion of the Mental Status Examination (MSE) as part of the assessment process. The MSE provides a structured format for evaluating a client's cognitive and emotional status, including such areas as appearance, behavior, thought processes, mood, and insight. Clinical psychologists employ the MSE to identify mental disorder symptoms so that an exhaustive understanding of a client's general mental status is realized. As documented in psychological training research, such as tests conducted at the University of KwaZulu-Natal, student psychologists often encounter barriers as they transition from theoretical learning to practical application when administering the

MSE (Seshadri et al., 2019). This poses the importance of learning clinical skills that add to the effectiveness of the interview, as trainees must manage the complexities of clients to gain appropriate clinical information. Additionally, variables that influence clinical interviews cannot be overstated in terms of promoting good communication and understanding between different clients. Challenges to performing clinical interviews include discomfort with a particular kind of question and needing cultural competence in order to address the subtleties involved in client histories (Seshadri et al., 2019).

In addition, findings from research on child sexual abuse disclosures demonstrate that predictors of disclosure can dramatically differ across individual factors and social environments, indicating that clinicians must attain a sophisticated knowledge of these variables to be prepared for encounters with such difficulties. Eventually, the meaning and application of clinical interviewing must evolve in perpetuity to accommodate those complexities in order to allow for thorough evaluations and well-informed treatment interventions (Figure 2.2).

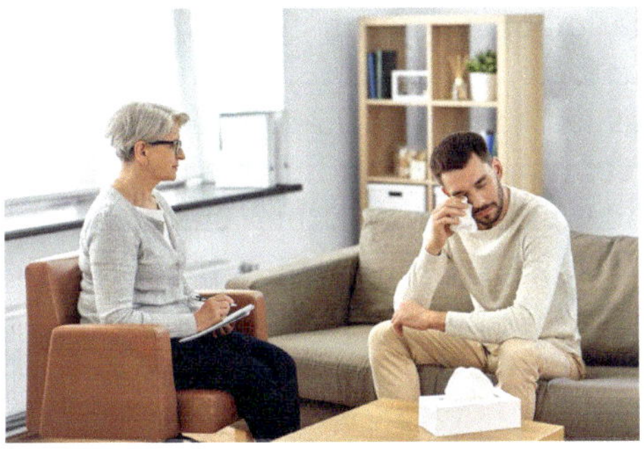

Figure 2.2. Clinical interviewing.

Source: https://external-content.duckduckgo.com/iu/?u=https%3A%2F%2Fwww.filepicker.io%2Fapi%2Ffile%2FMMXGBhTgeSXE5vqDUOQc&f=1&nofb=1& ipt=b2460c76fb8cba720e72f7bf121318d5454c90c2d17d64fb373aeec3beffb4fa.

Importance of Mental Status Examination

Mental Status Examination (MSE) is an important aspect of clinical interviewing, being a major component in the assessment of a patient's mental functioning. MSE is a systematic interview that allows clinicians to observe and record systematically different cognitive and emotional components, including appearance, behavior, mood, and thought. The total effect of such observation is a summary of the patient's mental state, allowing for accurate diagnosis and treatment planning. The MSE not only facilitates the identification of specific mental illness disorders but also facilitates monitoring progress over time, thus providing important feedback regarding treatment efficacy. Employed in its rightful use, the MSE can function simultaneously as both a diagnostic and a therapeutic intervention, and it assists in enhancing a greater clinician-patient understanding. Incorporating the MSE into practice enhances the clinician's capability for individualized care. Accurate mental status examination leads to tailored interventions, which are essential to improve the patient's outcome. As more focus and urgency for mental health are given in healthcare systems, the significance of a good MSE cannot be underscored any further. By thorough analysis of cognition and emotion, clinicians can offer tailored measures that align with the specific demands of unique patients, closing the gap between theory and practice of clinical practice. Furthermore, the incorporation of measures , such as the Patient Activation Measure (PAM) allows for a more nuanced understanding of a patient's ability to manage their healthcare, thus validating the value of the MSE in the broad framework of health management planning (Smith, 2016). The MSE is also critical beyond the individual assessment; it has an essential role in aggregating and assessing data in different populations. Through integration of findings from a series of assessments, researchers and clinicians can identify trends in mental health status, informing public health programs and resource allocation. Instruments , such as the Source Guide developed by Mathematica Policy Research shed light on best practice in data gathering and analysis, highlighting the importance of documenting systematically the mental status of diverse populations with disabilities (Bleeker et al., 2006). This collaborative data collection not only provides richness to knowledge of mental health phenomena but also encourages evidence-based practice, which can be disseminated across the healthcare continuum, thus fostering a culture of continual improvement in the provision of mental health care.

2.1. The Purpose of Clinical Interviewing

Learning Outcome

1. Establishing rapport with the patient.
2. Gathering a comprehensive patient history.
3. Identifying presenting problems and symptoms.

The clinical interviewing purpose extends beyond mere data collection; it is an anchoring process employed in setting the client-clinician therapeutic relationship. This relationship is crucial since it ensures a safe environment in which people feel free to expose themselves to personal information concerning their minds. Effective clinical interviewing abilities enable the probing of patient history and current problems and can assist in determining patterns that are most probably the underlying cause of psychological distress. Here, healthcare professionals learn to employ open-ended questioning, empathy, and active listening skills. These not only encourage rapport, but they also ensure an integrated understanding of the client's experience and improve the treatment plan, as well as increasing the likelihood of desired outcomes. Clinical interviewing is thus a significant element of mental health treatment, as it engages the patient constructively and helps in understanding their unique requirements. In addition, our clinical interviewing is an important diagnostic assessment method practiced in mental health centers. With formally structured or semi-structured interviews, clinicians gather elaborate information regarding symptoms, conduct, and psychosocial issues to establish proper diagnoses. The comprehensive assessment process is instrumental in the identification of underlying psychiatric disorders as well as co-occurring disorders. The understanding that arises from good-quality interviews can be used to guide clinical interventions such that they are tailored in a specific manner for the particular needs of the client. Furthermore, by placing symptoms in the broader picture of the patient's everyday living, clinicians can provide better referrals and set up evidence-based treatments into action. Clinical interviewing, thus, is not a curtain raiser; it is a part of the entire clinical assessment process that lends itself to effectiveness in treatment over the long term. In addition, the ability to adapt clinical interviewing approaches according to the personal client's situation and needs is the foundation of success in mental health practice. Various factors , such as cultural background, age, and issues presented necessitate interviewing to be conducted with a flexible orientation. For instance, children or other culturally diverse people might require other than the general strategies in order to communicate their thoughts and feelings effectively. In addition, the infusion of knowledge on the basis of contemporary controversies in the field can also enrich the interviewing practice. The takeaways from the Infectious Diseases Society of America Training Program Directors Committee, specifically about competencies for remediation, highlight the importance of formulating targeted communication strategies and continuous enhancement in interviewing skills to meet various types of issues in mental health (Escota et al., 2020). It is through these adaptive and knowledge-driven interviewing processes, then, that mental health professionals are ultimately able to develop a deeper understanding of their clients, resulting in improved treatment and care (Figure 2.3).

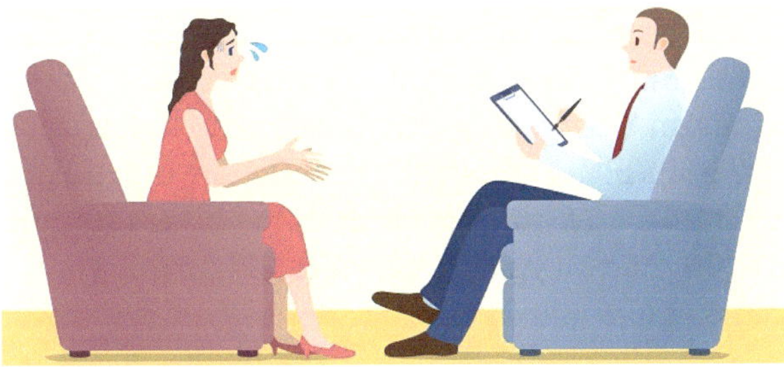

Figure 2.3. The purpose of clinical interviewing.

Source: https://external-content.duckduckgo.com/iu/?u=https%3A%2F%2Fwww.tutorix.com%2Farticles_assets%2Fimages%2F539016-1676283575.jpg&f=1&nofb=1&ipt=d7ff2dd39cf63c43737cea115b97f27816addb76e0bb294e441db90e442187b4.

2.1.1. Establishing Rapport with the Patient

Rapport building is a major component in clinical interviewing and mental status examination (MSE). An effective rapport establishes a therapeutic relationship wherein patients are able to share their experiences and concerns without reservation. When clinicians create an empathic and non-critical atmosphere, patients are likely to reveal sensitive information necessary for proper diagnosis and treatment planning. This early rapport is especially necessary when considering the intricacy of psychological assessments, where trust will be a critical factor in the validity of information received. A clinician's ability to engage with empathy, understanding, and attentive listening is the basis for a successful encounter, where patients sense their clinician is a partner in managing their mental well-being. Furthermore, building rapport is a dynamic process involving empathic listening and understanding of the patient's emotional process. By being specially interested and concerned in the patient's account, clinicians can respond more effectively in line with the patient's affective context. This is particularly pertinent given the complexity of arriving at insight into family patterns and historical forces that influence personal development, as revealed in the shifting conversation about these forces in psychotherapy.

Emotional validation is one method that can be used to enhance the patient's responsiveness to therapeutic intervention and ultimately lead to more successful interventions. Without having reached this comfort level, the clinician cannot obtain complete information, which is necessary to conduct a thorough mental status examination and to properly treat the patient. Furthermore, there not being sufficient mental health professionals specializing in child and adolescent psychology makes the utilization of effective rapport-building skills even more critical. As identified by more recent studies, however, there remains a huge variation in access and training of clinicians who work with the younger populations that can further consolidate already established mental health problems.

By equipping nascent clinicians with the tools and techniques of rapport building, including developmentally responsive communication and intervention, the field can work towards an overall improvement in the quality of care being dispensed. Resources , such as tip sheets and clinical reference guides are valuable resources to aid clinicians in effectively dealing with therapy-interfering behaviors and establishing effective therapeutic relationships, ultimately enhancing clinical outcomes for youth (McQueen et al., 2024).

2.1.2. Gathering Comprehensive Patient History

Patient history taking is a component of clinical interviewing with far-reaching consequences for the outcome of mental status examination (MSE). A good history not only provides information about a patient's state of mind at the time, but also contextualizes his or her behavior within a life history. This is a historical view from which clinicians can view potential causal psychological or social stressors and guide diagnosis and treatment planning. Research points out that the integration of patient history and MSE heightens the clinician's sensitivity to identifying symptoms of mental disorders and their severity and duration. Taking such information should be carried out with sensitivity and some flexibility, as personal concerns, such as discomfort with a few questions—may arise while conducting the interview, impacting the completeness of the attained history (Seshadri et al., 2019). Also, the subtleties surrounding cultural and demographic challenges bear significant influence on the taking of patient history. Professionals must be attuned to the influence that age, gender, and cultural background have on communication and patients willingness to reveal private data. For instance, cultural congruence enables more open communication in the MSE, and dissimilarity makes it difficult to interact and leads to misinterpretation or omission. Understanding these dynamics enables practitioners to tailor their interview styles to become more inclusive and effective. The significance of these aspects is also complemented by studies highlighting the extent of MSE application in relation to client histories and characteristics as a response to the necessity for adaptive techniques that ensure optimal rapport and trust between practitioner and patient (Seshadri et al., 2019). Lastly, the history constructed from the entire patient history is of utmost significance to the continuous evaluation and treatment of mental illness. This background history interweaves with the data obtained from the mental status examination to create an entire picture of the patient's mental state. The lack of standardized processes for recording and integrating patient histories in psychiatric practice can prove disastrous to the efficiency of diagnosis and to therapeutic intervention. As already mentioned in Brazilian psychiatry, variation in methodology and vocabulary among professionals can lead to differential interpretation of MSE results, underlining the need for a standardized training program addressing this matter. Such progress can help bring about more efficient diagnostic methods and improved results in treatment within mental health services (Figure 2.4).

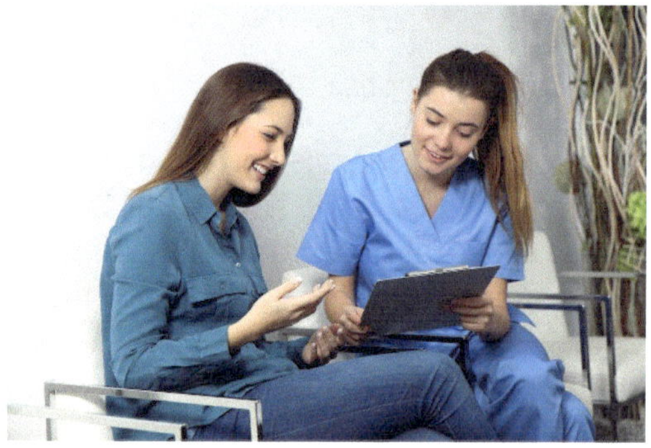

Figure 2.4. Gathering a comprehensive patient history.

Source: https://external-content.duckduckgo.com/iu/?u=https%3A%2F%2Fwww.richmondnursing.co.uk%2Fwp-content%2Fuploads%2F2018%2F07%2FPatient-history-what-you-need-to-ask.jpeg&f=1&nofb=1&ipt=0106a0651fe323777cc8c7f6ecbafe0463b86b29aeb8eb445301f6ad0da71086.

2.1.3. Identifying Presenting Problems and Symptoms

Identification of the presenting symptoms and problems is part of the clinical interview and the MSE. The initial part of assessment can be the taking of a clinical history, which captures the client's experience in their own words, and it helps to establish rapport and build trust. Patients must be prompted by clinicians to speak freely about their concerns so that there can be a better understanding of the presenting problems. Gathering detailed information on the onset, duration, and intensity of symptoms is important as it can distinguish episodic from chronic problems. In addition, information on the client's background, for instance, socio-economic status and support systems, might highlight the possible causes of distress. This integrated process of questioning serves to distinguish pertinent behavioral, emotional, or cognitive indicators that are not easily observed, thus serving as the basis for proper diagnosis and intervention. Throughout this process, a clinician must keep an eye out for linguistic and cultural differences that can influence how symptoms are presented. Different cultural backgrounds may dictate how individuals experience and convey their challenges, which may conceal important information if not well identified. For instance, differences in symptom presentation across cultures may lead to misplacement of the client's distress as a mere cultural idiosyncrasy rather than real mental health challenges. In cases where there is stigma of mental illness, clients are apt to be resistant to revealing symptoms entirely. As clinicians try to uncover presenting problems, they must employ assessment methods that are culturally conscious in conjunction with having good people skills so that they can establish a sense of safety and understanding, thereby ensuring symptom accuracy for correct treatment planning. In addition, the use of structured tools and questionnaires can be combined to enhance the qualitative data derived from interviews and yield a more complete account of a client's state. Although clinical interviews are precious, standardized assessments can help recognize specific symptoms and the extent of their severity, as baselines for tracking change across time. The employment of evidence-based assessment tools enables clinicians to draw on a rich treasure trove of investigation and clinical excellence and couple observations with tried-and-true diagnostic criteria. This systematic process accrues benefit to not only the enhancement of diagnosis but also the tailoring of intervention to individuals' unique presentations. In all, the synergy of clinical interviewing, cultural sensitivity practices, and standardized assessment materials creates a thorough description of presenting problems and symptoms, ultimately leading to improved outcomes in mental health services (Bleeker et al., 2006; Escota et al., 2020).

Test Your Knowledge

1. How does the clinical interview help clinicians develop an initial understanding of a patient's psychological functioning?
2. In what ways does clinical interviewing contribute to diagnosis, treatment planning, and rapport building?

2.2. Types of Clinical Interviews

Learning Outcome

1. Structured interviews.
2. Semi-structured interviews.
3. Unstructured interviews.

Clinical interviews are a central part of the clinical psychology assessment process, facilitating the clinician's ability to gather thorough data on a client's history, symptoms, and functioning. Structured interview is one of the principal subgroups of clinical interviews that consist of pre-defined questions read out by the clinician in a predetermined order. The format facilitates consistency across interviews, and this consequently improves the reliability of information collected. Structured interviews are best suited to assess specific disorders because they reflect diagnostic criteria. Unstructured interviews, on the other hand, have the opposite, offering more leeway in investigating questions in detail based on the client's answer. This can lead to richer descriptions and insight into the client's experience, but it brings variance into data collection that may affect comparability across cases. Generally, the clinical interview format used significantly affects how much information and what kind of information a clinician is able to obtain about a client's mental status. A second significant type of clinical interview is the semi-structured interview, which has characteristics of both the structured and unstructured interview types. In this approach, clinicians work from a script of questions but are still able to deviate from it to deliver follow-up questions tailored to the client's specific response. This tension can facilitate effective exploration of issues at hand while simultaneously offering some level of standardization across interviews. For instance, the semi-structured interview methodology is widely practiced in research settings and clinical practice, particularly with the employment of assessment tools , such as the Structured Clinical Interview for DSM Disorders. Semi-structured interviewing can be supportive of the flexibility of clinicians to reformulate questions based on the course of conversation and thereby enhance the client-clinician relationship and ensure that the assessment has meaningful implications. In this context, clinician flexibility and competence are critical to gain the maximum benefit of such interviews.

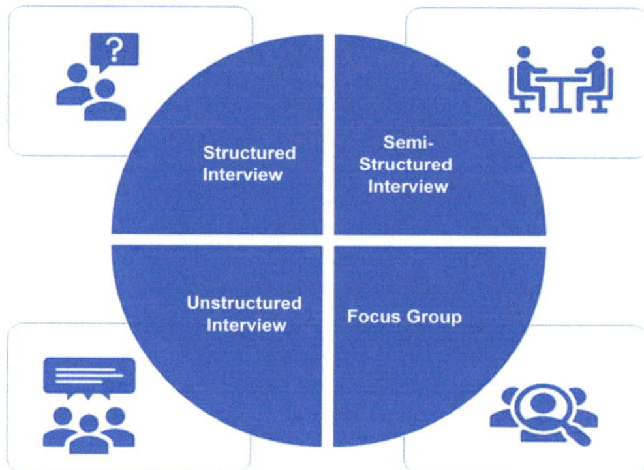

Figure 2.5. Types of clinical interviews.

Source: https://www.bachelorprint.com/wp-content/uploads/2023/07/Types-of-interviews-in-research.jpg.

Even the selection of an appropriate clinical interview format can influence the reliability of family history assessment, a factor which has gained increased recognition in clinical interviewing. As recent studies have shown, the complexity of family functioning requires a profound appreciation of an individual's developmental influences beyond symptom monitoring. Several tests have been created to measure family history, but their validity and reliability are not always consistent. The clinical interview process is able to somewhat counteract some of these issues through the ability of clinicians to delve further into patterns of generation and family relationships that play a major role in the understanding of the client's presenting concerns. By designing this interview, clinicians not only take an indispensable history but also use the therapeutic relationship to introduce clients to an exploration of their family lives. Clinical interview choice is thus key, as it predefines the narrative and influences subsequent interventions and treatment planning (Figure 2.5).

2.2.1. Structured Interviews

Increasing emphasis is laid on the use of structured interviews in clinical practice, which is a standardized way of gathering full information regarding a patient's mental health status. Compared to unstructured interviews that are susceptible to interviewer bias and variation, structured interviews follow a series of preset questions that ensure consistency in every evaluation. This standardization also becomes especially relevant while conducting a mental status examination (MSE) because it raises the validity and reliability of information gathered. With a structured format, clinicians can assess various areas, including mood, cognition, and behavior, in a systematic way that reduces the likelihood of misinterpreting answers. Structured interviews not only enhance the assessment process but also render comparison among patients easier, hence advancing the quality of clinical care in mental health organizations. Structured interviews also assist in providing a major solution to restricting the effect of extraneous variables that can distort the results of clinical interviews. This is particularly required when interviewing patients with varying backgrounds because biases during questioning may lead to misdiagnosis or misinterpretation of patient responses. The technique's structured nature ensures that clinicians avoid such biases by using standardized methods of questioning. Furthermore, evidence supports that structured methods of interviewing increase not only the validity of information gathered but also the engagement of the patient throughout the assessment process. When patients feel that the evaluation is being conducted in a clear and consistent framework, they will be more likely to feel respected and understood, creating an atmosphere that is conducive to open communication and effective diagnosis. Concerning investigating the application of structured interviews within the MSE, it is interesting to note its applicability across diverse populations, such as children and those with cognitive impairments. Studies indicate that different populations can elicit differential responses in accordance with cognitive capacity and development. Since the literature on children's testimony in forensic settings recommends a systematic approach must accounts for differences , such as these to facilitate accuracy and reliability of assessment. It is essential to understand the underdeveloped neurological state and contextual dependency determining children's response, as indicated in the studies. Thus, though systematic interviews can provide a good framework, clinicians need to adapt their strategy to the unique requirements of their clients so that the assessments can remain effective as well as ethically appropriate (Bleeker et al., 2006; Brubacher et al., 2014) (Figure 2.6).

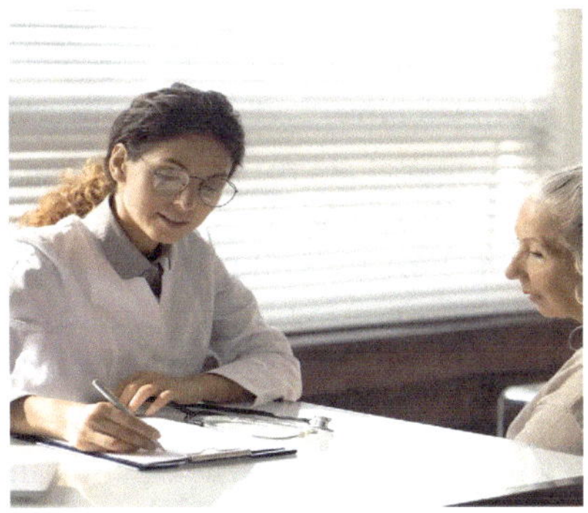

Figure 2.6. Structured interviews.

Source: https://lifesciences.transperfect.com/sites/default/files/styles/1000x1000_square/public/2023-07/shutterstock_1971115199.jpg.webp?itok=nlrU4Ihc.

2.2.2. Semi-Structured Interviews

Semi-structured interviews are the perfect method under the circumstances of clinical interviewing since they provide the benefits of both structured and unstructured interviews, allowing clinicians to adhere to a pre-decided list of questions but possess the flexibility necessary to explore appropriate themes arising during the process. This adaptability is particularly important in clinical settings, wherein patient narratives encompass complex emotional and psychological themes. By incorporating semi-structured interviews, professionals are better able to present a safe space for patients to articulate their sentiments and thoughts, leading to the possibility of richer data collection. Practitioners are also enabled to affirm their understanding of patients' particular contexts through this method, thus reinforcing rapport and catalytic listening throughout the process. Applying semi-structured interviewing can transform the conduct of Mental Status Examinations (MSE). Unlike rigid forms of questioning, semi-structured interviewing permits clinicians to probe those domains most relevant to a patient's mental status, such as mood disturbance or inconsistencies in cognition. By allowing the conversation to naturally develop, practitioners can uncover inherent trends or patterns within the patient's response, which can further indicate more complicated psychological pathology. Furthermore, it is possible with this technique to discuss a patient's history, present functioning, and future goals to have an overall perspective of their mental health. The aspect of flexibility in asking questions depending on the first response allows for the pertinent problems to be discussed comprehensively, and this can support the diagnosis and development of individually oriented therapeutic interventions. In specific studies of chronic illness, semi-structured interviewing revealed in-depth information about patient experience that would otherwise be masked with more structured approaches. For instance, when looking at health issues like Dupuytren's disease, semi-structured interviewing revealed four interrelated themes like awareness of the disease and living with its limitations, which enabled clinicians to better individualize treatment and patient education (Byrne et al., 2009). Similarly, findings based on participatory methodologies for child-centered research highlight the importance of this interview format. By asking children directly about their physical activity behaviors, researchers were able to gain significant results that might otherwise go unobserved by routine quantitative measures (Hayball et al., 2018). These examples illustrate how semi-structured interviews not only serve as information-providing tools in clinical interviewing but also as catalysts for better patient care and understanding (Figure 2.7).

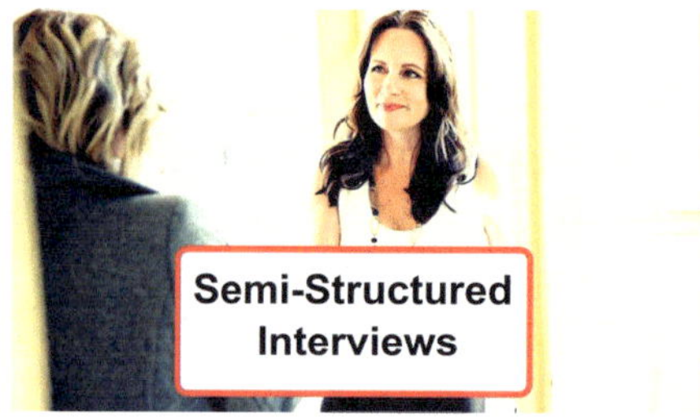

Figure 2.7. The semi-structured interviews.

Source: https://worlddanceheritage.org/wp-content/uploads/2023/07/interviews-min.jpg.

2.2.3. Unstructured Interviews

Unstructured interviews are an integral component of the Clinical Interviewing and Mental Status Examination (MSE) process and offer an evocative approach that captures the unique dynamics of the therapeutic dyad. As opposed to structured interviews, which incorporate a standard order of questions, unstructured interviews allow mental health professionals to engage with clients naturally. This process offers a more spontaneous dialogue, which encourages clients to express their feelings and ideas more authentically. The practitioners steer the discussion as they probe the emergent themes in real time, therefore potentially obtaining information lost in the strict format. The unstructured interview's criticality owes to its flexibility because it provides the practitioners with a chance to adapt questions according to the response of the client in exchange, resulting in a comprehensive comprehension of the mental status of the individual. The advantages of unstructured interviews are most pronounced when taking into consideration the evaluation of mental health. By creating a feeling of openness and trust, clinicians can develop rapport, which allows for deeper probing of clients' issues and experiences. The style is particularly suited to the purpose of the MSE, which allows for an overall understanding of the client's psychological function. Furthermore, unstructured interviews enable clinicians to keep tabs on non-verbal cues and emotional responses that can have a rich influence on their interpretation. Research at the University of KwaZulu-Natal involving trainee psychologists outlines the challenges and benefits of employing unstructured elements within the MSE process. Trainees were faced with difficulties in handling structured and unstructured components, which indicates that while flexibility is essential, it demands that practitioners possess a high level of proficiency and responsiveness (Seshadri et al., 2019). Despite the benefits, the use of unstructured interviews also involves some difficulties that need to be overcome by clinicians. Trainee psychologists, for instance, might have difficulty with personal bias and the anxiety involved in departing from an established style. This can lead to discomfort in handling a particular MSE question, which can be exacerbated by clinician-client cultural differences. These things are all important to recognize when further developing training for mental health professionals. These challenges can be learned from the trainee experiences to redesign the curriculum, promoting the acquisition of skills that integrate both unstructured and structured interviewing techniques. Overcoming these challenges, future clinicians will then be able to perform thorough and empathetic mental status exams, thereby improving accurate assessment and client outcomes (Leads et al., 2017) (Figure 2.8).

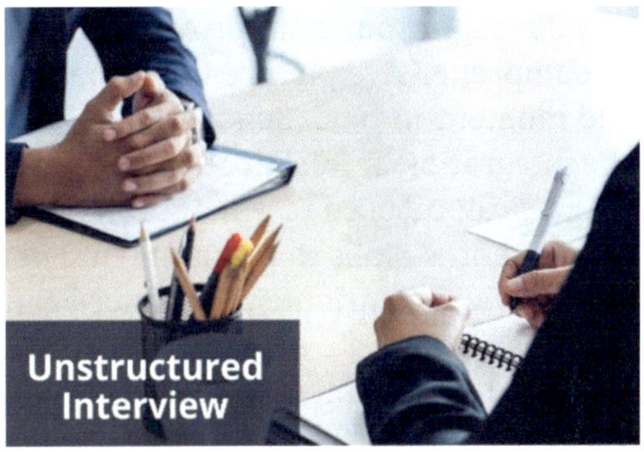

Figure 2.8. Unstructured interviews.

Source: https://www.totalassignment.com/blog/wp-content/uploads/2022/04/Unstructured-Interview.jpg.

Test Your Knowledge

1. What distinguishes structured, semi-structured, and unstructured clinical interviews from one another?
2. How do specialized interview types—such as crisis interviews and intake interviews—serve different clinical purposes?

2.3. Key Components of Clinical Interviewing

Learning Outcome

1. Verbal communication skills.
2. Non-verbal communication skills.
3. Active listening techniques.

Clinical interviewing is a crucial component of patient assessment and diagnosis in the practice of mental health. One of the key elements in this process is the Mental Status Examination (MSE), a standardized method of formalized structured interviewing of a patient's cognitive, emotional, and behavioral functioning by clinicians. The MSE addresses several areas of functioning , such as appearance, behavior, thought content, mood, and cognition, that provide clinicians with a comprehensive picture of the patient at any one moment in time. Scholarship indicates that the integration of fresh instructional design approaches can be used to enhance instruction on these essential skills to future mental health professionals and contribute to enhanced clinical interviews and accurate assessments (Chivu et al., 2022). Thus, a full understanding of the aspects of clinical interviewing and the MSE is a requirement for successful psychiatric practice. Clinical interviewing in the clinical environment is not just a process of gathering data, but also one of establishing a clinician-patient relationship. By this process, an atmosphere of trust is established that is necessary in gathering correct and informative information about the patient's experience. Issues , such as personal bias or discomfort with certain questions can get in the way of success with this interaction, and the transmission of the MSE will become more difficult (Seshadri et al., 2019). Trainee psychologists, for instance, often struggle to go from the theoretical aspects to practically applying things, particularly with handling the structured but flexible aspects of the MSE. To recognize these complexities is essential for clinicians and educators alike because it highlights the importance of having individually tailored training programs that equip future mental health professionals with the competencies and expertise necessary to conduct effective clinical interviews. Furthermore, cultural competence seems to be an essential element in the clinical interviewing process, impacting both interactional dynamics and the validity of the MSE findings. Age, gender, or racial differences may greatly affect communication and the ability of the clinician to effectively evaluate the mental state of the patient. For instance, shared cultural backgrounds may lead to improved understanding, while divergent background may result in misunderstanding or embarrassment in the interview (Seshadri et al., 2019). Therefore, clinicians must develop sensitivity to cultural factors that might influence their clinical judgment. Such awareness promotion not only enhances the therapeutic alliance but also enhances diagnostic accuracy, for it enables mental health professionals to view each patient as a unique individual in need of his or her own perspective, hence enhancing clinical interviewing and MSE that follows.

2.3.1. Verbal Communication Skills

Effective verbal communication skills are required in clinical interviewing practice and conducting a Mental Status Examination (MSE). Practitioners must balance language, tone, and nonverbal communication to gather information about patients. Effective responding and listening carefully foster a culture of trust, and patients are comfortable in providing sensitive information that will be utilized for appropriate evaluation and diagnosis. This aspect of communication is more than mere exchange of words; it is about empathy, listening to the views of the patient, and cultural factors that may impact the interaction. As communication is closely related to outcomes for patients, medical professionals must hone such skills to create effective interactions to the point that patients are heard and valued within the healthcare setting. In clinical education, experiential learning activities, such as the use of standardized patients (SPs), have been useful in enhancing oral communication skills of healthcare students. Through simulated interactions with SPs, students are provided with a unique setting to rehearse and enhance their interviewing skills. This method has proven to lead to significant increases in confidence and competence in communication, substantiating the value of experiential learning in their development. Studies indicate that students who go through guided interactions with SPs achieve greater self-efficacy and performance, particularly in communicating empathy and rapport, inherent components of effective verbal communication. Thus, incorporating such methodologies can significantly contribute to academic programs in clinical interviewing and MSE to equip future practitioners with the necessary skills. Furthermore, information on the scientific foundation of verbal communication in clinics can further render interviews and MSEs efficient. Research has confirmed a direct correlation between effective communication and positive patient outcomes, including improved satisfaction and better treatment compliance. As highlighted by recent research, significant gains in the level of communication skills were observed among students exposed to regular SP interactions compared to those who were not given such training (Cuchna et al., 2017). The findings highlight the relevance of the curriculum to prioritize making communication training a priority and reassess its impact on both the competence of the students and on the experiences of the patients. As medicine continues to evolve, the development of oral communication skills should remain the priority of professional development programs, recognizing their vital role in developing the therapeutic alliance and ultimately improving patient care (Figure 2.9).

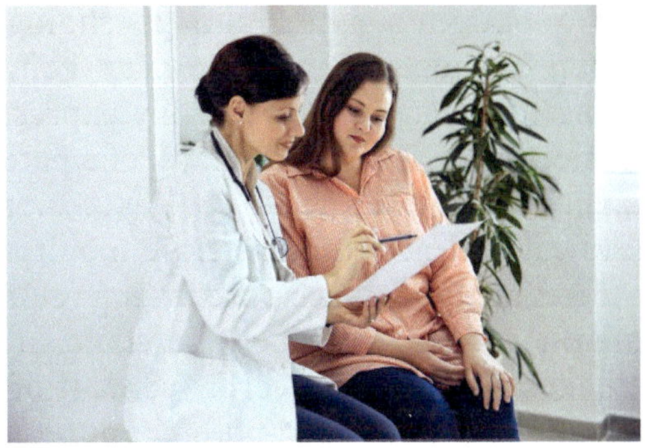

Figure 2.9. Verbal communication skills.

Source: https://publichealth.tulane.edu/wp-content/uploads/sites/3/2021/09/Strategies-for-Effective-Communication-in-Health-Care.jpg.

2.3.2. Non-Verbal Communication Skills

Non-verbal communication skills are a vital component of the clinical interviewing process and play a great deal in carrying out an effective Mental Status Examination (MSE). These skills include a range of non-verbal behaviors like body postures, facial expressions, and eye contact, which can play a substantial role in shaping the patient's responses and therapeutic relationship. For instance, the open body position of a clinician and sustained eye contact will assist in establishing trust and calmness, making it easier for patients to provide sensitive information. On the other hand, negative non-verbal messages , such as crossed body position or distracted behavior, may deter information gathering and even exacerbate a patient's feeling of anxiety. Because such interactions are of clinical importance, the acquisition of non-verbal communication skills constitutes a critical component of psychiatric training programs, as per the focus literature in instructional design in this respect (Chivu et al., 2022). Non-verbal communication skills are not merely employed in rapport-building; they are essential for accurately evaluating the patient's affect and emotional status while conducting MSE. Non-verbal answers usually mirror a patient's mood and psychological condition because they can convey genuine emotions that may not be verbally expressed. A flat affect or physical withdrawal of a patient, for example, can indicate severe depression or withdrawal and may require close monitoring from the clinician. Such an observation requires a systemic process, in which the clinician not only makes a note of the verbal content of the conversation but also takes note of the non-verbal signals, so that the mental status examination is comprehensive and advanced. This general grasp allows mental health clinicians to identify incongruities between the said and expressed non-verbally, thereby improving the assessment process (Seshadri et al., 2019).

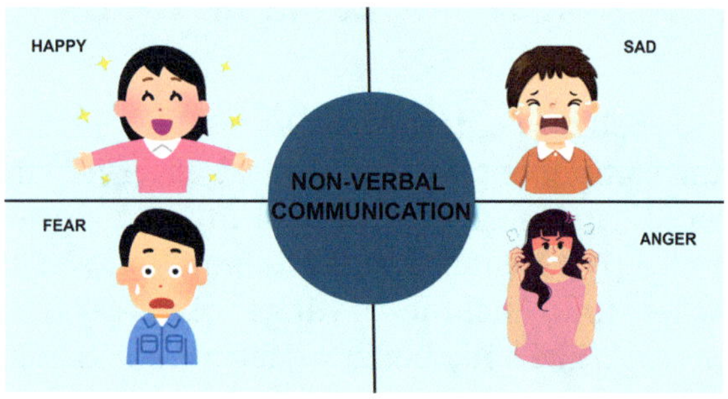

Figure 2.10. Non-verbal communication skills.

Source: https://engvarta.com/wp-content/uploads/2024/05/Cue-Cards-5-min.png.

Moreover, gaining practical skills in non-verbal communication is particularly useful in multicultural environments in which language is an obstacle to verbal communication. Student psychologists commonly refer to problems with conducting MSEs on culturally diverse clients, where variations in non-verbal behavior lead to misinterpretations or misunderstandings. For instance, cultural norms of eye contact, body space, and body contact can vary dramatically, affecting the process of the clinical interview. As discussed in research into trainee psychologists' experience, knowing such cultural nuances is indispensable for effective communication with clients and effective implementation of the MSE (Seshadri et al., 2019). Hence, cultural competence training should be introduced in the curriculum of training schools along with training for non-verbal communication skills so that future practitioners possess the power to handle these complexities in their evaluation (Figure 2.10).

2.3.3. Active Listening Techniques

The active listening skill is an integral part of clinical interviewing and the mental status examination (MSE). Active listening is to attend closely to the speaker, more than simply hearing what is said. Clinicians need to create a safe environment for open discussion where patients can freely give their opinions and feelings without worry of attack. Reflecting, summarizing, and clarifying skills guarantee not only comprehension of the verbal data by the interviewer but also comprehension of the underlying emotion and intent. Such interaction builds rapport and trust and is essential to effective diagnosis and treatment planning. By utilizing active listening techniques, clinicians are able to more effectively gather important information that enables them to determine potential psychological disturbances which may impact the patient's mental health status and overall well-being. Active listening is particularly critical in the clinical environment when dealing with sensitive matters, such as the emotional issues or situation of a patient. Vulnerable populations, including those struggling financially or with severe mental illnesses, may struggle specifically to pursue access to care services since they feel alienated. Active listening is useful in countering such barriers by allowing the patients to be understood and heard, thus raising their motivation for sharing personal fears and difficulties. By using positive listening skills as demonstrated in the (Deale et al., 2006), therapists are able to adopt a non-judgmental attitude that exudes empathy and understanding. This becomes critical for encouraging patients to verbalize their challenges, thus leading to an effective therapeutic partnership and better outcomes. In addition, integrating active listening skills into clinical interviewing makes room for best practices in mental illness therapy. For instance, clinicians are encouraged to approach the process of assessment with cultural humility, recognizing their patients' individual histories and experiences. Therapist skills , such as open-ended questioning and reflective statements, help clinicians navigate complex stories that may present, especially in diverse communities with systematic disenfranchisement from access to care, as evidenced in (Price et al., 2025). By identifying these variables and practicing active listening, clinicians not only enhance diagnostic capabilities but also empower patients to be actively invested in their treatment regimens. This collaborative approach develops feelings of agency and autonomy in patients, creating more comprehensive and individualized care plans, as well as improved mental health outcomes in the long term (Figure 2.11).

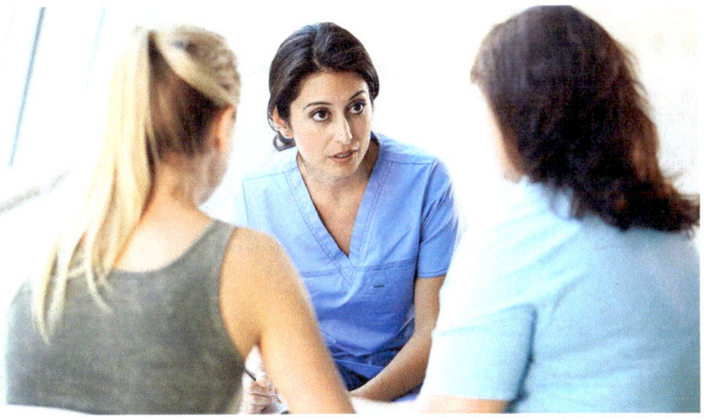

Figure 2.11. Active listening in healthcare.

Source: https://cdn-images.ausmed.com/ausmed-articles/20191113_cover_v2.jpg.

Test Your Knowledge

1. What essential communication skills (e.g., empathy, active listening) are required for effective clinical interviewing?
2. How do history taking, symptom exploration, and risk assessment contribute to a comprehensive clinical interview?

2.4. Introduction to Mental Status Examination (MSE)

Learning Outcome

1. Definition and Importance of MSE.
2. Historical context of MSE.
3. Relationship between MSE and clinical interviewing.

The Mental Status Examination (MSE) is a principal feature of clinical assessment that offers an organized approach to the evaluation of a patient's emotional, intellectual, and behavioral functioning. Conducted as part of a clinical interview, the MSE systematically examines the various areas of appearance, behavior, thought content, mood, and cognitive function. By using this test, clinicians can gather vital information about a patient's mental status to identify psychiatric illness early. Furthermore, the MSE complements the diagnostic interview by producing measurable data that assist clinicians in constructing a fuller picture of the patient's state. The method is particularly useful in cases where verbal communication is challenging, allowing for the overall picture to be constructed on the basis of the patient's physical presentation and actions within the assessment. The relevance of the MSE is also highlighted by its history and efforts towards standardization, as seen in existing literature on psychopathology. Throughout history, practitioners have used descriptive psychopathology to inform their assessment without consensus on standardized methods. In spite of various schools of thought that have composed the MSE instrument, the lack of standardized terms has brought about significant variations in practitioners' practice. This divergence is particularly evident in the Brazilian psychiatric practice, where different psychiatric textbooks assume different meanings of mental functions and atypical presentations. A thorough understanding of the MSE, therefore, necessitates an acknowledgment of these disparate perspectives in trying to maintain stable and reliable means of data collection, hence overall effectiveness in practice (Estellima-Lins et al., 2019). Since the population is growing older and cognitive impairment is becoming a more serious concern, the role of MSE becomes more and more emphasized. Research indicates that older groups, particularly those with cognitive impairment, present with unique challenges across the process of reporting and recall. This group requires specially modified methods, which suit their specific requirements. Recent research has demonstrated that the use of systematic interviewing techniques , such as the Cognitive Interview, can significantly enhance the recall of details by older persons. This is particularly useful in criminal cases and other situations where clear testimony is critical. Together, these results highlight that practitioners need to modify their interviewing approach in order to be able to work with aging populations effectively and make MSE practices develop to respond to the intricacies of contemporary clinical requirements (Wright, 2021) (Figure 2.12).

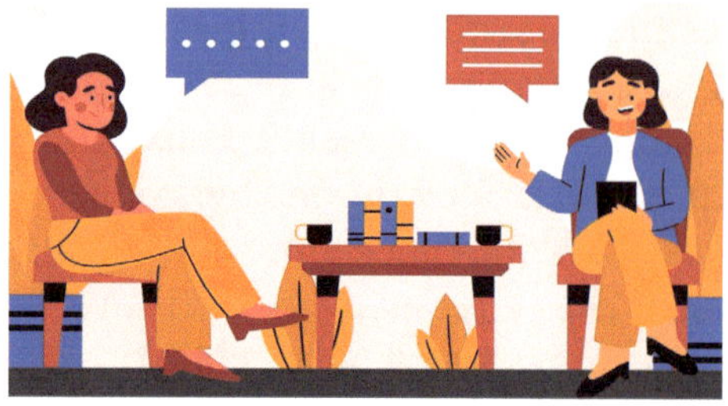

Figure 2.12. The mental status examination (MSE).

Source: https://images.squarespace-cdn.com/content/v1/5c308af3f2e6b1bd0e605a39/1653700871980-6T3URJKTX58QBV8SHD3N/Speech%2C+psychology%2C+Andreas+Astier.

2.4.1. Definition and Importance of MSE

Mental Status Examination (MSE) is an essential tool in clinical psychology, with a formal assessment of a patient's emotional and cognitive functioning. MSE encompasses a variety of fields, including appearance, behavior, thought content, mood, and insight, that altogether provide a full-scale picture of the subject's mental state at a specific point in time. The benefit of conducting an MSE goes beyond simply evaluating symptoms; it also assists practitioners in constructing a differential diagnosis and establishing baselines for continuing evaluations. The MSE allows clinicians to detect alterations in a patient's mental health status, thus enabling them to make proper interventions and adjustments to treatment. This systematic approach results in a deeper understanding of patient needs, which acts as a premise for both acute and more enduring mental health planning. Furthermore, MSE's value lies in its accommodation to practice across a range of clinical settings and patient groups. Research highlights the difficulty of applying MSEs for novice clinicians, with certain reservations regarding the transition from theoretical practices to practice. Candidates may have difficulties managing the interface between structured and unstructured elements of the test, and this may undermine the validity of the results. Cultural aspects, for instance, can significantly influence MSE testing since disparities in age, gender, and ethnicity influence the meanings of certain behavioral signals. Strategies for improving the effectiveness of the MSE, including further training and supervision, can prepare future mental health practitioners to better address these challenges. Closing such training gaps is vital to support competency within the application of MSE, ultimately leading to improved patient outcomes (Seshadri et al., 2019). Importantly, MSE is not merely clinical assessment; it promotes the clinician-client therapeutic relationship to be more appreciated. With rapport-building during the MSE process, clinicians can establish confidence and candor, both which are required to achieve successful treatment. This interpersonal connection emphasizes the MSEs role in not just diagnosis but also in the therapeutic process since patients will reveal crucial information regarding their experience and feelings throughout the interview. Learning a client's cultural background, as noted in literature, can also serve to enhance context for the administration of MSE so that clinicians are able to grasp the complexities of mental health outside of diagnoses. Ultimately, integrating technical and relational components when utilizing the MSE will significantly enhance clinical practice and result in more efficacious therapeutic relationships between practitioners and patients (Niles et al., 2011).

2.4.2. Historical Context of MSE

The Historical Context of the Mental Status Examination (MSE) describes a revolutionary process within the field of clinical psychology and psychiatry. Initially meant to ascertain a patient's cognitive function and emotional state, the MSE has roots dating back to the beginnings of clinical practice when observation was the primary method used to understand mental illness. Over time, the MSE has come to encompass not only direct observation but also systematic evaluation, taking into account a patient's subjective experience. The evolution reflects shifts in how mental health has been conceptualized. Systemic interviewing approaches integrated, as contended by Pollner, identify the importance of respecting people's subjective understanding and experiences, in a manner that suggests their meanings derived from what they have been through are critical in interpreting their state of mind (Gubrium et al., 2011). Alongside history and family functioning, playing an increasing role in the development of MSE throughout history. Psychological theories have increasingly recognized that development is heavily influenced by relationships within the family, which in turn can influence a person's mental health and coping. The stability of memory for things that happened during childhood, and the subtleties of family impact, are crucial aspects of the MSE process. As researchers untangle the complexities of family evaluation, they underscore the implications for understanding mental states in clinical interviews. This shifting perspective highlights the importance of an overall understanding of how family history shapes psychological assessments, revealing the subtlety that clinicians must be mindful of when conducting an MSE (Melchert et al., 1998). Finally, the history of the MSE highlights the importance of the inclusion of various approaches to complement clinical interviewing skills. The MSE is far from a checklist, yet rather a dynamic process that interweaves clinical observation and subtle meaning-making of a client's narrative. Emphasis on "displacement" and not merely "replacement" of meaning enables clinicians to inquire about the contextual origins of their patients and gain a deeper understanding of mental health phenomena. As interviewers refine interviewing and MSE skills, they are also cautioned to keep pace with the dynamic story of psychological understanding that shapes practice. Historical understandings of the MSE guide current methods by building connections between practices of the past and current advances in mental health assessment, ultimately propelling clinicians and their clients forward.

2.4.3. Relationship Between MSE and Clinical Interviewing

The communication between the Mental Status Examination (MSE) and clinical interviewing is at the heart of the accurate assessment of a person's psychological state. Clinical interviewing is the primary tool for gathering comprehensive information about a patient's history, symptoms, and functioning at the time. Through direct contact, clinicians are able to establish rapport and coax patients into disclosure. This symbiotic interchange enhances the quality of information collected, which also supplies the MSE. The delicate pieces of information procured through clinical interviewing, such as the patient's mood, cognition, and behavior, directly supply the MSE's evaluation model, which provides a comprehensive understanding of the mental health terrain under examination. This synergy between clinical interviewing and MSE thereby forms a two-faceted strategy important to a healthy diagnosis process. The inclusion of a number of elements from the clinical interview within the MSE increases its validity and diagnostic usefulness. For instance, some signs in an individual's history, say exposure to trauma or illicit drug use, can have a strong influence on the clinician's observations through the MSE. Research indicates that men who have sex with men, with histories of child sexual abuse, end up experiencing severe mental health challenges like post-traumatic stress disorder and substance addiction (Baker et al., 2015). These should be considered in MSE to understand fully how earlier experiences impact contemporary mental function and behavior. Thus, an effective clinical interview can provide essential contextual information, optimizing the MSE's focus and accuracy, finally resulting in a more well-rounded evaluation and intervention plan. Moreover, the interplay between MSE and clinical interviewing emphasizes the need for familiarity with the psychological constructs that may complicate equitable assessment. For instance, the development of specific assessment tools , such as the Sport Interference Checklists, Sport Specific Screen for Mental Health, points to the merit in addressing specific mental health issues likely to affect performance in various settings (Scott, 2018). This illustrates how clinical interviewing can shape the development of specialized assessment tools based on the recognition of relevant issues that arise through personal narrative. As such, these results can be integrated into the MSE to ensure that an integrative view of a patient's mental health and the effect of context variables is attained. By harmonizing the clinical interview with the MSE, practitioners are able to guarantee that they not only treat the symptoms presented but also the root causes of a patient's condition (Figure 2.13).

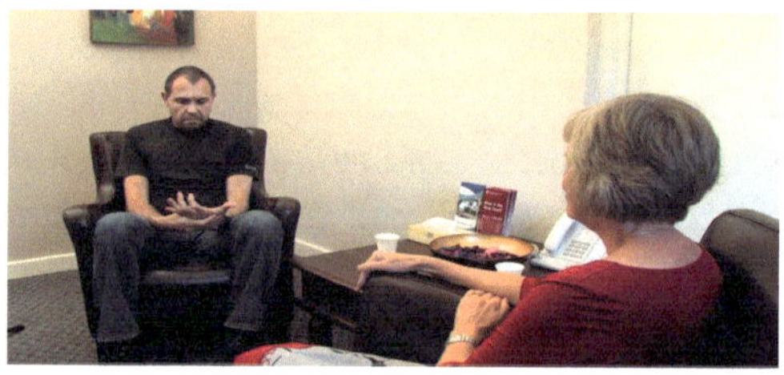

Figure 2.13. Relationship between MSE and clinical interviewing.

Source: https://i.ytimg.com/vi/ktEUiCLu_9s/maxresdefault.jpg.

Test Your Knowledge

1. What is the primary purpose of the Mental Status Examination in psychiatric assessment?
2. How does the MSE complement information gathered during the clinical interview?

2.5. Components of the Mental Status Examination

Learning Outcome

1. Appearance and behavior.
2. Mood and affect.
3. Thought process and content.

Mental Status Examination (MSE) is a structured examination that encompasses a number of items crucial for assessing a patient's cognitive status and affect. MSE is a simple clinical psychiatric instrument that unveils the patient's appearance, behavior, thinking, mood, and intellectual ability. Inspection of these areas assists the clinician in making proper inferences about the patient's mental health status in order to inform diagnosis and treatment. During a systematic scoping review, the emphasis was laid that although MSE is at the center of psychiatric practice, there is still a broad evidence gap in the evidence-based instructional method used in educating healthcare professionals for conducting this assessment (Chivu et al., 2022). Thus, outlining the importance of each factor—along with a systematic process of their transmission—can significantly enhance the outcomes of psychiatric examinations. The other key aspect of the MSE is its emphasis on interpersonal interaction and communication between patient and clinician. How questions are phrased and the clinician's capacity to establish rapport can exert a tremendous influence on the patient's response during the examination. Trainee psychologists, particularly those undergoing psychology courses, are likely to have difficulties with this assessment process, particularly with the application of theoretical knowledge. Evidence indicates that difficulties also come from the MSE's unstructured and structured elements and from client factors, such as age, gender, and cultural diversity (Seshadri et al., 2019). Addressing such difficulties through the use of targeted training modules can potentially enhance trainees' skills in performing thorough MSEs, ultimately leading to more effective appraisals and better patient outcomes. Finally, the interpretation of MSE components should be guided by a sensitive awareness of cultural and contextual factors that may influence both the patient's and clinician's perspectives. A difference in culture influences emotional expression, cognitive functioning, and behavioral presentation so that the clinician must utilize the culturally competent process in performing assessments. Trainees have reported that shared cultural awareness can facilitate rapport development, and cultural or language differences might hinder appropriate evaluation (Seshadri et al., 2019). Thus, instilling an awareness of these dynamics throughout clinical training can create an environment that is conducive to tacit understandings of mental status. By integrating such considerations into the MSE framework, clinicians and educators can enhance both their training methods and clinical interventions, thereby enhancing the quality of psychiatric care delivered overall.

2.5.1. Appearance and Behavior

In Mental Status Examination (MSE) and clinical interviewing, observation of the appearance and behavior of the patient is a helpful diagnostic tool. There are various things that clinicians usually observe, like grooming, choice of clothes, and cleanliness of the body, which indicate the mental status of the individual. For instance, a disheveled appearance would suggest negligence that is normally seen in depressive disorders, while an overly manicured appearance may be indicative of possible mania or obsessive-compulsive behavior. Moreover, observable behavioral anomalies like agitation or somnolence can be signs of hidden psychiatric illnesses. These observations not only assist with identifying existing disorders but also in assessing the patient's daily functioning and coping strategies, hence enabling a comprehensive approach to diagnosis and treatment planning in mental health facilities. Behavioral observations during MSE go beyond appearance and include the patient's mood, facial expressions, and body mannerisms. Clinicians categorize these behaviors in an effort to detect patterns , such as avoidance, aggression, or indifference, that will illustrate the patient's emotional landscape. For example, a patient who exhibits flat affect may be exhibiting profound depression, and labile movement may be a sign of anxiety or thought disorder. The behavior also provides contextual information about the patient's engagement style, for example, the amount of engagement during the interview. Active engagement creates an image of resilience and openness, whereas disengagement constitutes an indicator of distress and resistance to addressing deeper issues. Through decoding behavioral signals, mental health professionals can tailor treatment approaches to the patient's individual needs and issues, leading to more successful intervention. Furthermore, the interplay between patient appearance and behavior can unveil broader psychosocial issues influencing mental status, such as cultural and socioeconomic factors. Having the ability to recognize how these factors motivate one's psychological well-being is central to a knowledgeable assessment. For example, a patient with low income may display reduced concern with appearance based on limited resources, in contrast to indifference to appearance. Similarly, certain cultural practices would influence the behavior of a person within the clinical setting, for instance, not maintaining eye contact or freely showing emotions. Considering all these, the clinical formulation enables practitioners to apply culturally sensitive care methods. Thus, examination of appearance and behavior during the process of the clinical interview is not just vital for diagnosis but for an empathic therapeutic relationship, ultimately culminating in favorable outcomes for the patient's health.

2.5.2. Mood and Affect

Effective clinical interviewing and mental status exams (MSE) depend upon clinicians having an in-depth knowledge of mood and affect, which are of greater importance to assessing a patients emotional health. Mood is the pervasive and enduring emotional state, while affect is the expression of that mood. Clinicians observe both of these when conducting an MSE in order to quantify a patient's psychological well-being.

A person's affect may be flat to either of exuberance, and this connotes some range of underlying illness; for instance, flat affect may imply depression or mood disorders, and excess affect may imply mania. Not only is it useful in diagnosis, but it also helps to establish a rapport between patient and therapist, thereby fortifying the therapeutic alliance so essential to effective treatment. This fundamental ability recognizes the importance of mood and affect differential in clinical decision-making.

The proper understanding of mood and affect requires that clinicians be attentive to potential factors influencing these emotional states. External influences, such as recent history and family considerations, can dramatically influence the mood of a patient, as evidenced in the evolving conception of the influence of family considerations on emotional growth. The complexity of , such assessment is further increased by concerns regarding the accuracy of patients' own descriptions of their emotional state and histories.

Clinicians must use guarded questioning, observation, and proven assessment tools in order to get a better picture of a patient's affect presentation. This careful process ensures clinicians consider dynamic factors impacting mood and affect, thus enabling an informed clinical judgment and intervention plan addressing patients' individual needs, as highlighted in recent literature (Melchert et al.,

1998). Apart from respecting the distinction between mood and affect, professionals should determine how these factors correlate with various psychological disorders. Research has established a robust connection between creativity and mood disorders, particularly among those with bipolar disorder. Therapists who wish to apply therapies to this population face a challenge with this information.

By consolidating findings from different fields, therapists can modify their work to suit creatives with mood disorders, producing safe environments in which they can work and effectively treat their mental illness. As research on these approaches unfolds, ongoing studies will further hone means of adapting existing interventions to the requirements of this subgroup, ultimately informing better treatment outcomes and deepening the therapeutic process (Agopian, 2017) (Figure 2.14).

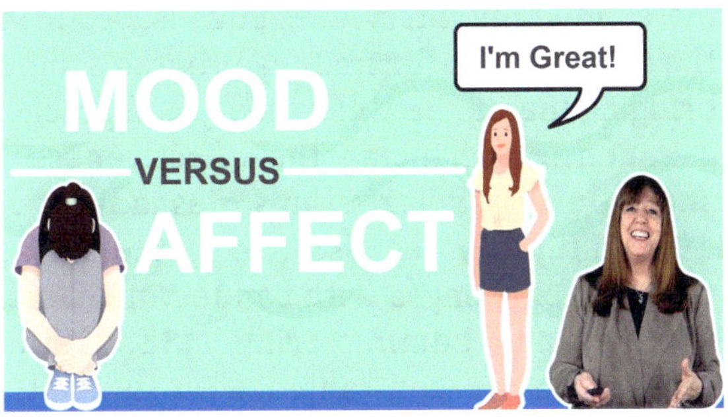

Figure 2.14. Mood and affect.

Source: https://i.ytimg.com/vi/kvvV3Uc2Wkw/maxresdefault.jpg.

2.5.3. Thought Process and Content

The examination of thought content and process is a critical component of clinical interviewing and the MSE. Thought process is used to describe the manner in which a client verbalizes their thoughts, which informs us about the structure, coherence, and continuity of their ideas. Clinicians assess whether the client's thoughts are rational, sequential, and relevant, which provides insight into their cognitive functioning. Furthermore, thought process abnormalities, including tangentiality, flight of ideas, or circumstantiality, can be indicative of hidden mental health issues. These types of evaluations can play a critical role in mood disorders, psychotic disorders, or other cognitive impairments that could occur during the interview, allowing mental health workers to be well-equipped to create effective treatment plans designed to meet the individual's needs. Equally important is the evaluation of thought content, which examines the specific beliefs, themes, or topics that most dominate in a client's narrative. This entails rating for delusions, obsessions, and rumination that can inform the clinician about the client's mental status. Being preoccupied with disturbing or irrational thoughts has a powerful impact on a person's conduct and overall mental status.

It is in the context of content of thought that clinicians can ascertain potential threats, such as suicidal thoughts or self-destructive behavior, to inform treatment at the time of intervention. Moreover, understanding the client's motivation to change is also essential; research has indicated that motivation, broken down into dimensions like importance, confidence, and readiness, is an integral aspect of effective intervention practices. Such integration ensures a wider understanding of the mental state of the client along with more targeted therapeutic treatment (Grodin et al., 2019).

Even greater examination of thought content and process can yield useful insights regarding neurobiological forces that affect mental health. Research from neuroimaging studies reveals the relationship between cognitive appraisal and brain activation, thereby further solidifying the link between cognition and physiology. For instance, studies show that there are some interventions that can enhance motivation to change elements and are linked with activation in areas related to self-reflection and interoceptive awareness. Understanding these neurobiological mechanisms plays a vital role in maximizing therapeutic strategies and planning interventions appropriate to individuals' personalized cognitive profile. Clinicians themselves are encouraged to employ the multidisciplinary approach and integrate qualitative assessments of thought with quantitative neurobiological data to formulate a better framework for effective practice (Bleeker et al., 2006).

Test Your Knowledge

1. What are the major domains assessed in an MSE, such as appearance, mood, cognition, and thought processes?
2. How do abnormalities in speech, perception, or cognition influence the interpretation of MSE findings?

2.6. Challenges in Clinical Interviewing and MSE

Learning Outcome

1. Cultural considerations.
2. Patient anxiety and resistance.
3. Interviewer bias and subjectivity.

The nuances of clinical interviewing and Mental Status Examination (MSE) present numerous challenges that could hinder efficacious practice among trainees. One of them is encountered when mental health practitioners transition from theory to practice, particularly in MSE. Trainee psychologists, for instance, often complain of feeling anxious when attempting to integrate theoretical frameworks with the uncertainty of actual interaction with clients. This is aggravated by internal conflicts, that is, self-doubt or anxiety, which can hamper their capability to perform assessments with confidence. Moreover, the formal and informal aspects of the MSE can be particularly troublesome, leading to unease and potential misinterpretation of responses while conducting interviews. Such issues bring to the fore the need for training programs aimed at bridging the gap between theory and practice, consequently enhancing the effectiveness of trainees during clinical exams (Seshadri et al., 2019). Cultural issues also rise to the surface in terms of challenges with conducting clinical interviews and administering MSE. Trainee psychologists are confronted with difficulties in balancing sensitivity to cultures while trying to establish rapport with diverse clients. To others, shared cultural backgrounds with the clients can be an easy communication, which serves as a ground for mutual understanding. Age, gender, and racial differences, however, can be pitfalls to effective communication, leading to misunderstandings during the assessment process. The two requirements are the reason why cultural competence in clinical training is important; this mandates knowledge of the cultural background of clients to properly assess and come up with effective interventions. It has been highlighted in literature that enhanced cultural sensitivity not only improves the interviewer-client relationship but also improves the quality of care overall (Seshadri et al., 2019). Additionally, external factors , such as pharmacological intervention as well as physical settings may also complicate the process of clinical interviewing further. Literature indicates that pharmacotherapy patients may present varying degrees of perceived sobriety, which influences their engagement and response during the MSE. Such diversity is likely to pose challenges for clinicians in recognizing the impact of medication on clients' mental status. Moreover, distractions from the outside world and even the clinical setting itself may have an impact on interview dynamics and can lead to suboptimal assessments or preconceived notions about the client's mental status. Therefore, clinicians must develop robust skills in managing external influences while conducting thorough assessments. Such abilities will ultimately enhance diagnosis precision and treatment plan efficacy since clients will be accorded full and tailored care (Figure 2.15).

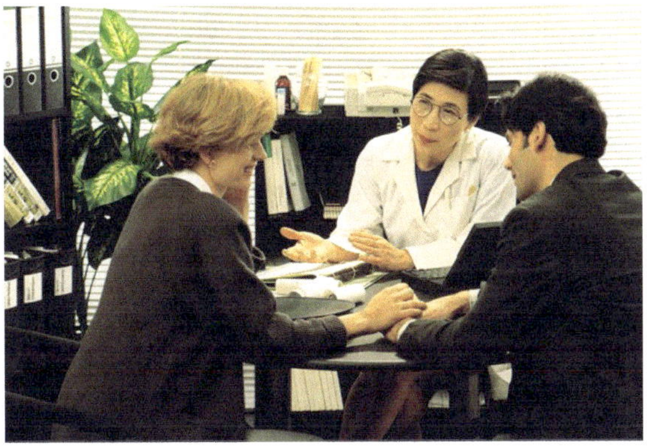

Figure 2.15. The complexities surrounding clinical interviewing and the mental status examination (MSE).

Source: https://external-content.duckduckgo.com/iu/?u=http%3A%2F%2Fimg-aws.ehowcdn.com%2F600x600p%2Fphotos.demandstudios.com%2Fgetty%2Farticle%2F251%2F82%2F78453636.jpg&f=1&nofb=1&ipt=ddbb930f93c5a66fe3b4877221ea1df88f7dedd15ace8d2fa9c28f5ab257b501.

2.6.1. Cultural Considerations

Cultural influences are at the core of the MSE and the clinical interview. With an increasingly diverse population, mental health practitioners must possess the cultural competence to value numerous backgrounds, beliefs, and values, which influence client communication and perception of mental illness. Culture can affect an individual's presentation of distress, his or her reasons for coming in, and his or her responses during clinical assessments. For instance, collectivist culture subjects can emphasize family or community issues in their narratives, while individualistic culture subjects can place more emphasis on personal events. Identification of such perceptions allows clinicians to adjust their style, facilitating more effective and meaningful engagement in the clinical interview. Cultural awareness also encompasses an understanding of specific mental health stigma and its application to client engagement. A few cultural communities might hold beliefs incompatible with dominant mental health paradigms, and this can get in the way of open discussion in assessments. Mental illness in some cultures will be described in terms of the spiritual or the moral, with alternative explanations for psychological misery, which can carry important implications for treatment and client receptiveness. When mental health professionals seek to create a safe and supportive environment, they must work actively to overcome such cultural stigmas and legitimize the experience of the clients to establish trust and rapport. This concordance is not only required for accurate diagnosis and effective treatment but also for enabling general mental well-being in diverse populations as well. Furthermore, the inclusion of cultural elements in the MSE also allows for a holistic appreciation of the client's state of mind. Symptoms of the disorder can differ according to cultural influences because the expression and perception of emotion can vary considerably between cultures. For instance, patients may present with somatic symptoms, such as bodily discomfort, rather than overt emotional distress, depending on cultural rules for feeling expression. , including the knowledge from the cultural frameworks in the MSE not only enriches the clinicians assessment but also aligns with prevailing practices for providing culturally competent care. By changing the evaluation process to include cultural diversity, experts are able to get more detailed information that enhances diagnosis and informs effective treatment methods that consider the individual's personal history and worldview, as can be seen in programs for remediation issues in schools (Escota et al., 2020) (Figure 2.16).

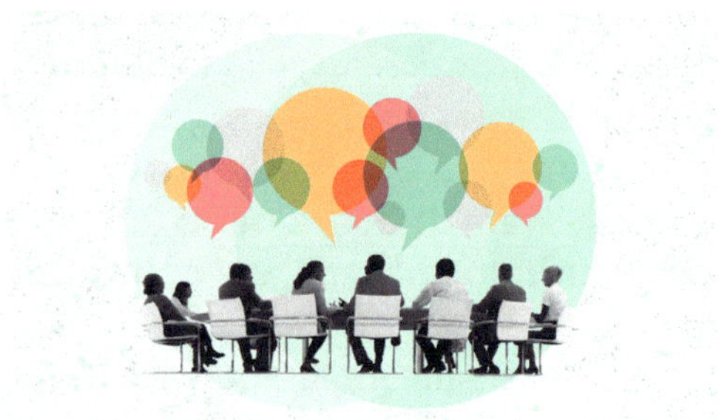

Figure 2.16. Cultural considerations.

Source: https://trainingindustry.com/content/uploads/2018/01/cultural_consideration_thumb.png.

2.6.2. Patient Anxiety and Resistance

Understanding patient anxiety and resistance is crucial in clinical interviewing and mental status examinations (MSE). Patients typically present themselves in clinical settings with diverse anxieties, which can be triggered by fears of being judged, misunderstood, or stigmatized on the basis of a mental disorder. The anxiety could either be verbal or non-verbal, and hence, it is challenging to obtain exact information from the patient. Identification of such anxieties enables a critical context in which to establish a therapeutic alliance, crucial to successful engagement. Therapists must adopt methods of establishing comfort, such as using open-ended questions and empathy, in an attempt to overcome resistance. The therapists ability to identify and resolve such emotional barriers falls significantly on the patients willingness to disclose sensitive information, hence making the entire interview process more effective. Resistance during clinical interactions is usually in the form of patients struggling with the exposure of vulnerabilities. Bad history with healthcare or mental health cultural stigma can intensify this resistance, and as such, clinicians must be culturally sensitive in every case. Building rapport is important; clinicians must strive to create an environment where patients feel free to explore their thoughts and feelings. Existing research underscores the significance of evidence-based interventions when investigating anxiety and resistance in clinical environments, particularly among individuals who experience traumatic life events. For example, those who lost loved ones due to traumatic loss may exhibit considerable resistance through their psychopathological state, and therapeutic interventions ought to be tailored to address their unique experience and needs (Akhonzada et al., 2006). By allowing patients to express their concerns, clinicians can reduce resistance and foster a more collaborative working relationship. Effective management of patient anxiety and resistance has a direct impact on the quality of clinical assessment. Electronic health records (EHRs) may reduce communication and workflow effectiveness, possibly lowering patient anxiety related to treatment procedures. However, the implementation of EHRs has been greeted with ambivalent attitudes among behavioral health providers, as documented in more recent studies (Shank, 2011). Some individual providers acknowledge the potential offered by EHRs in improving patient safety and care, but are concerned with privacy issues and the added workload imposed by EHR systems. These anxieties can inevitably be passed on to patients, who can pick up on clinicians' discomfiture or annoyance at the technology and compound their own anxiety. Clinicians must thus not only negotiate the patient's emotional landscape but also identify the root causes of anxiety within the system so that the clinical setting and use of technology encourage patient participation rather than hinder it during interviews and assessments.

2.6.3. Interviewer Bias and Subjectivity

Interviewer bias and subjectivity are an overarching issue in clinical interviewing and mental status examinations (MSE). Interviewer biases can be due to the interviewer's preconceived notions, attitude, and background, which unconsciously contaminate their interpretation and interaction with the client. This element erodes objectivity and reliability in clinical assessment because the subjective inference of an interviewer can produce misinterpretation of the client's behaviors and statements. Recognizing these biases is essential not only in facilitating fair and unbiased assessment but also in making clients feel understood and accepted throughout the interviewing process. Through active self-reflection and supervision, clinicians can enhance their awareness of personal bias, thus enhancing the validity of their assessments and reducing the potential for biased clinical judgment. Moreover, interviewer-client relationships form an integral part of the incidence of bias in MSE. In the course of the clinical setting, the variables of race, gender, and socioeconomic status can develop and find their way into the relationship. Interviewers may unintentionally project their own experiences upon the client by over-empathizing or maintaining a level of emotional distance, both of which may cause the assessment process to be biased. Besides, through applying creative and embodied research methods, researchers also become exposed to vulnerabilities that shift their role from mere interviewers to co-producers. Such dynamics compound the clinical interviewing complexities because both parties will be required to engage sincerely in their own positionalities. The consequences of such interactions mandate careful consideration of data integrity, therapeutic rapport, and overall process effectiveness of clinical examination (Barnard et al., 2018). In countering interviewer bias, measures to ensure equitable interviewing practice need to be implemented. Standardized interview formats, for instance, may provide a standardized format for clinicians to proceed with, and thereby act as a buffer against personal bias effects on clinical interpretation. Cultural competence training is also necessary, as it equips interviewers with the skills needed to handle a diverse clientele respectfully. Additionally, taking on the reflexive attitude, whereby clinicians evaluate critically their own beliefs and biases, enables them to better understand and acknowledge their potential effect on the outcome of clinical work. As explained by initiatives that aim to incorporate knowledge about disability data collection, it is crucial to adopt best practices in the interviewing process to maintain both data integrity and relational authenticity in clinical settings. Such efforts can help the profession to move towards developing a more inclusive and unbiased setting for all clients (Bleeker et al., 2006).

Test Your Knowledge

1. What factors—such as patient reluctance, cultural differences, or communication barriers—can hinder effective clinical interviewing?
2. How do acute symptoms (e.g., psychosis, severe anxiety) or lack of cooperation affect the accuracy of the Mental Status Examination?

SUMMARY

Clinical interview and mental status examination (MSE) collectively form the backbone of sound mental health assessment and diagnosis. Both facilitate a balanced perception of an individual's psychological state by combining subjective and objective information. Clinical interview allows practitioners to explore a patient's history, symptoms, and problems, whereas MSE provides a systematic evaluation of a patient's cognitive, emotional, and functional status. Both methods are integral to the process of developing a diagnosis and building an appropriate treatment plan, ultimately solidifying the therapeutic relationship between client and clinician. In addition, an awareness of strengths and limitations inherent within the assessment process is needed in order to ensure effective practice. As has been noted by more recent studies, such as those conducted by Mathematica Policy Research, Inc., there is a need to refine data collection to enhance the validity and reliability of data that is collected during clinical evaluation. The results of this study note the necessity of utilizing best practices consistent with clinical interviewing and MSE in order to establish a pathway for greater understanding of patient experience and history. These advances not only train single-case treatment but also inform greater advances in mental health treatment. Finally, with the shifting landscape of psychological testing, future research must contend with ongoing challenges with respect to reliability and validity. The growing concern with the validity of self-report measures, particularly related to family history and early experiences, calls for a reassessment of typical assessment instruments. With the use of the results of recent studies, as outlined in recent psychological literature, clinicians will be better placed to assess the complexity of mental illness disorders. Improved methodologies will not only increase the level of clinical interviewing and MSE but will also have more effective and individualized treatments for patients who are faced with mental health challenges, hence maintaining good health.

In the clinical psychology practice, the Mental Status Examination (MSE) is a key tool for mental health professionals to assess a patient's cognitive functioning, emotional state, and state of mind. MSE contains parameters , such as appearance, behavior, thought process, mood, and insight. It is worth knowing the intricacies of these factors so that a client's mental state can be rightly interpreted. MSE administration requires a balance of structured and unstructured questioning to enable professionals to navigate the intricacies of a client's presentation. Research with trainee psychologists notes some special challenges accompany the shift from theoretical understanding to practice, necessitating extended training in MSE administration (Seshadri et al., 2019). These findings inform teaching approaches so that prospective clinicians can learn the skills that are required for this important aspect of mental health assessment. Additionally, challenges faced by trainee psychologists in conducting the MSE reveal underlying levels of clinical interviewing sophistication. The aforementioned study reveals that not only do trainees have trouble with theoretical models, but they also face interpersonal and intrapersonal barriers to assessment. For instance, age, gender, and cultural differences between the clinician and client can play a big role in affecting the process of interviewing and lead to uneasiness or misinterpretation of responses (Seshadri et al., 2019). These issues need an integrative approach in training programs to equip trainees with skillsets in a position to overcome these issues. As mental health professionals age, it is critical that such barriers be met with reflective practice and personalized training experiences, thus enhancing the quality of clinical assessment and therapeutic relationships. Secondly, the foundation of quality clinical interviewing is the employment of diagnostic criteria as per the DSM-5. An understanding of these categories enables practitioners to conduct knowledgeable diagnostic interviews and write comprehensive assessments, facilitating case management, treatment planning, and intervention strategies. The instructional strategies utilized to educate people, such as lectures, case studies, and interactive activities, assist in reinforcing these skills and linking theory and practice. By doing this experiential work, the learners are better positioned to address real-world scenarios when performing mental health exams, especially in the context of what is described in the experiences of the trainees (Seshadri et al., 2019). Ultimately, equipping future clinicians with a firm understanding of both the MSE and the diagnostic elements underlying opens doors to good practice and improved patient outcomes.

KEY TERMS FROM THIS CHAPTER

- Affect
- Attention
- Clinical interview
- Confabulation
- Hallucinations
- Judgment
- Mental status examination (MSE)
- Appearance
- Behavior
- Cognition
- Delusions
- Insight
- Memory
- Mood

CRITICAL THINKING QUESTIONS

1. **What is the primary purpose of a clinical interview in mental health assessment?**
   a. To perform laboratory tests
   b. To establish rapport and gather information about the patient's psychological state
   c. To prescribe medications immediately
   d. To conduct physical therapy
2. **Which of the following is not a component of the Mental Status Examination (MSE)?**
   a. Appearance and behavior
   b. Thought process and content
   c. Muscle reflexes
   d. Mood and affect
3. **If a patient is oriented to person, place, and time, they are considered:**
   a. Confused
   b. Fully oriented
   c. Depressed
   d. Anxious
4. **In MSE, observing whether a patient's speech is fast, slow, or pressured is part of assessing:**
   a. Perception
   b. Speech and language
   c. Insight and judgment
   d. Cognitive function
5. **Which of the following is an example of assessing insight in a patient?**
   a. Asking about their ability to recall words
   b. Asking if they understand their mental health condition
   c. Checking their heart rate
   d. Observing their clothing style

Short Answer Questions

1. What is the purpose of a clinical interview in mental health assessment?
2. List three key skills a clinician should use during a clinical interview.
3. What are open-ended questions, and why are they important in clinical interviewing?
4. What is the Mental Status Examination (MSE), and what is its primary goal?
5. Name at least five major components of the MSE.

Answer to Critical Thinking Questions

1. (b); 2. (c); 3. (b); 4. (b); 5. (b)

REFERENCES

1. Agopian, Sean, "The development of therapy suggestions for addressing issues of creativity in individuals diagnosed with bipolar disorder" (2017). *Theses and Dissertations*. 764. https://digitalcommons.pepperdine.edu/etd/764(accessed on 28th July 2025).
2. Akhonzada, R., Dillenburger, K., & Fargas, M. (2006). Post-trauma: Is evidence-based practice a fantasy? https://core.ac.uk/download/10041308.pdf (accessed on 28th July 2025).
3. Baker, J. S., Boroughs, M. S., Dale, S. K., et al. (2015). Complexity of childhood sexual abuse: Predictors of current post-traumatic stress disorder, mood disorders, substance use, and sexual risk behavior among adult men who have sex with men. https://open.bu.edu/bitstream/2144/40343/1/nihms-707015.pdf (accessed on 28th July 2025).
4. Barnard, R. A., Cruice, M., & Jones, J. (2018). Researching across two cultures: Shifting positionality. https://core.ac.uk/download/163076789.pdf (accessed on 28th July 2025).
5. Cuchna, J. W. (2017). Measuring outcomes in competence and confidence in clinical skills through the use of standardized patients. https://core.ac.uk/download/217294106.pdf (accessed on 28th July 2025).
6. Deale, A., Heyting, A., Komaroff, A., Strauss, A., Wearden, A., Zigmond, A., Wearden, A. J., et al. (2006). Fatigue Intervention by Nurses Evaluation–The FINE Trial. A randomized controlled trial of nurse led self-help treatment for patients in primary care with chronic fatigue syndrome: Study protocol. [ISRCTN74156610]. https://core.ac.uk/download/52846.pdf (accessed on 28th July 2025).
7. Hayball, F. Z. L., & Pawlowski, C. S. (2018). Using participatory approaches with children to better understand their physical activity behavior. https://core.ac.uk/download/157583047.pdf (accessed on 28th July 2025).
8. Leads, J. (2017). A quantum of solace: An exploratory mixed methods study of online support in the self-management of anxiety in HPV positive women. https://core.ac.uk/download/228199728.pdf (accessed on 28th July 2025).
9. McQueen, T. (2024). Clinical challenges and experiences: Shared knowledge from mental health clinicians. https://core.ac.uk/download/604797092.pdf (accessed on 28th July 2025).
10. Niles, B. A. (2011). Differences between frequency of diagnosis, diagnosis extremity, and Global Assessment of Functioning score in a Euro-American and Alaskan Native client. https://core.ac.uk/download/286999403.pdf (accessed on 28th July 2025).
11. Pogue, J. (2019). Factors associated with return to a Child Advocacy Center for a subsequent sexual abuse allegation: A longitudinal analysis. https://core.ac.uk/download/224735772.pdf (accessed on 28th July 2025).
12. Price, A., McDonald, M., Sanjeevan, S., & Moore, T. G. (2025). Sustained home visiting for vulnerable families and children: A review of effective processes and strategies. https://core.ac.uk/download/pdf/30672646.pdf (accessed on 28th July 2025).
13. Scott, J. (2018). Examination of a screening tool for athletes' mental health and its direct implications to sport training and competition. https://digitalscholarship.unlv.edu/cgi/viewcontent.cgi?article=4386&context=thesesdissertations (accessed on 28th July 2025).

14. Seshadri, S. P., Kishore, M. T., & Udipi, G. A. (2019). Clinical practice guidelines for assessment and management of intellectual disability. *Indian Journal of Psychiatry, 61*, 194. https://doi.org/10.4103/psychiatry.indianjpsychiatry_507_18 (accessed on 28th July 2025).
15. Shank, N. C. (2011). Behavioral health providers and electronic health records: An exploratory beliefs elicitation and segmentation study. https://core.ac.uk/download/17241922.pdf (accessed on 28th July 2025).
16. Smith, C. J. (2016). From patient to student activation: Development of the Student Activation Measure. https://digitalcommons.georgefox.edu/cgi/viewcontent.cgi?article=1218&context=psyd (accessed on 28th July 2025).
17. Wright, A. M. (2021). Use of the enhanced cognitive interview and a modified cognitive interview to improve the eyewitness recall of older adults. https://core.ac.uk/download/384444595.pdf (accessed on 28th July 2025).

DIAGNOSIS AND CASE FORMULATION

3

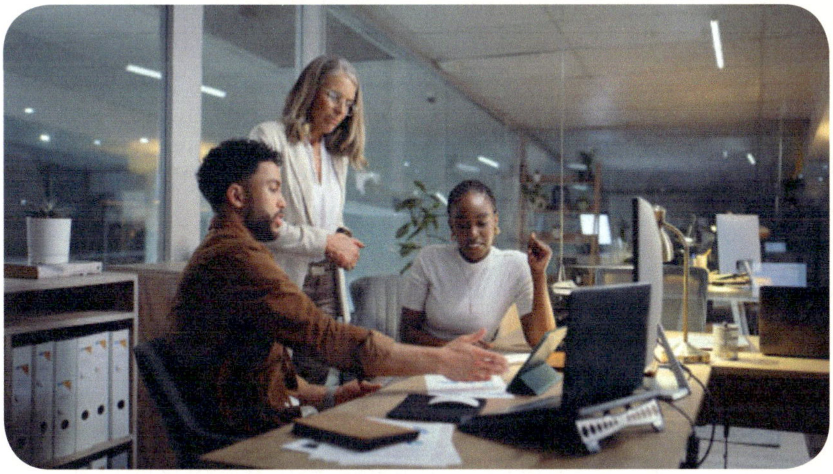

LEARNING OBJECTIVES

After studying this chapter, you will be able to:

1. Give historical context of diagnosis;
2. Describe theoretical frameworks in diagnosis;
3. Explore diagnostic tools and techniques;
4. Define the role of DSM and ICD;
5. List the challenges in diagnosis;
6. Explain case formulation process.

Introduction

The introduction is a critical component in unraveling the complex dynamics of case formulation and diagnosis within the practice of psychology. In mental health, accurate diagnosis provides the foundation for effective treatment, guiding clinicians on the selection of the most appropriate interventions that are best suited to address the specific needs of their clients. The diagnostic process, however, is not problem-free, such as the limits of criterion-based approaches that may overlook the variability of individual experience and narratives. Then, exploring other frameworks, such as narrative comprehension, can enable more understanding of every individual's unique situation to navigate through the intricacy that conventional criteria may not be able to grasp (Thornton 2008). This piece will seek to illuminate the need to integrate holistic approaches in light of the identification of classical model diagnostic schemes. The major aspect of the introduction also encompasses risk assessment principles and the way these impact diagnosis and case formulation. Evaluations are often employed by clinicians in terms of systematic evaluation to establish risk factors to various outcomes, such as harm to others or self. One example of such an instrument is the Short-Term Assessment of Risk and Treatability (START), which shows a model that employs risk and resilience factors to construct individualized assessments for patient groups with different diagnoses.

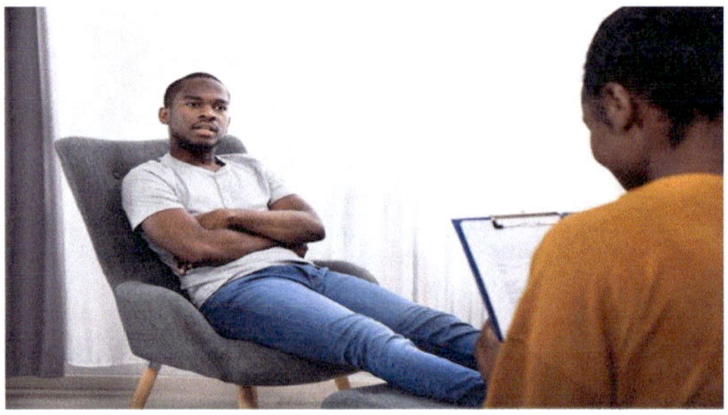

Figure 3.1. Diagnosis and case formulation.

Source: https://sweetinstitute.com/wp-content/uploads/2024/04/Psychodynamic.jpg.

While START has been established to have predictive validity in some groups of patients, its effectiveness in a wider set of diagnoses remains a problem of ongoing investigation (Dickens et al., 2017). This emphasizes the importance of continuous research into making the diagnostic tools more refined and applicable to a culturally diverse patient population, thereby enhancing the process of case formulation and treatment outcomes. Last but not least, an effective introduction leads to an in-depth discussion of the relationship between diagnosis and case formulation. With a critical analysis of existing models and new directions, it becomes simpler to move towards improved mental health diagnosis. The interplay between standardized metrics and individualized assessment techniques will be discussed throughout this chapter, with a focus on how practitioners can resolve the dichotomy to enhance patient care. This exchange not only aims to enhance current practice but also to facilitate the incorporation of diverse assessment methods that honor lived stories, most likely resulting in improved care in mental health settings (Thornton , 2008; Dickens et al., 2017) (Figure 3.1).

Definition of Diagnosis

Understanding the definition of diagnosis is key to effective case formulation in psychiatric and psychological interventions. Diagnosis represents a scientific classificatory system for classifying mental health disorders based on symptoms, cultural background, and personal experiences. It is imperative to understand that diagnosis is greater than merely a label and necessitates a multidimensional process of taking a thorough history of the individual's psychological function and environmental factors. This multi-dimensional personality is placed in the forefront in the field of cultural psychopathology that examines how cultural ideologies and customs dictate the occurrence and significance of psychological disorders. For instance, in some cultures, depression is shown in physical signs rather than in feelings. This aspect calls for a culturally sound diagnostic process that considers the individual's history and allows mental health professionals to offer more accurate and effective care (Heine et al., 2002). Diagnostic implications extend beyond the mere labeling of a disorder; they are part of treatment planning and intervention strategies to meet particular needs. The transdiagnostic framework is increasingly appealing to the profession because it acknowledges that many psychological processes intersect with many mental disorders. According to this perspective, clinicians can develop treatment protocols that address the underlying psychological processes rather than being confined to specific diagnostic conditions. This is preferable, as suggested by studies that argue a common definition of the term "transdiagnostic" can enhance treatment efficacy and accessibility. Furthermore, these treatments can reduce therapeutic regimens to a single form, making them more amenable to various client needs (Barlow et al., 2017). Therefore, clarifying the definition and purpose of diagnosis is crucial in defining good practice in therapy. Lastly, receiving an accurate diagnosis is essential for the patient and clinician and will affect the outcome and success of treatment. Diagnostic processes must encompass consideration of the individual's unique experience, cultural background, and the complex nature of psychological distress. When case formulation is done by mental health practitioners, they are walking the balance between standardized assessment and individualized treatment. By doing so, they are not only assuring the application of evidence-based treatments but also creating a therapeutic relationship that involves engagement and rapport building. The use of many viewpoints, like those highlighted in cultural psychopathology, enables practitioners to solve more complex cases with greater sensitivity and comprehension. Thus, the concept of diagnosis has much to do with how we become involved in mental health care, and it opens up doors to open and effective treatment methods (Heine et al., 2002) (Figure 3.2).

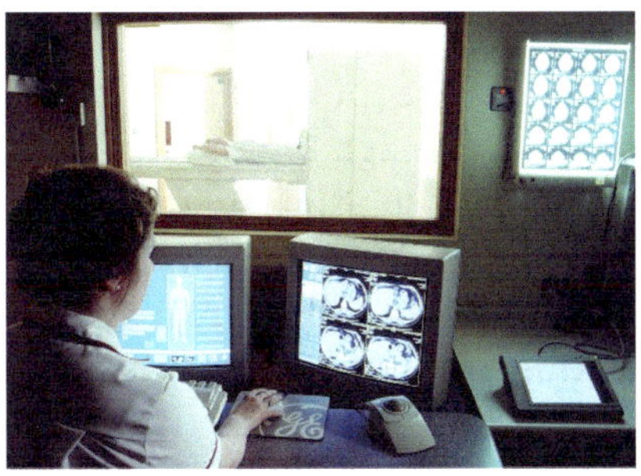

Figure 3.2. The definition of diagnosis.

Source: https://cdn.britannica.com/78/80578-050-BF193014/Magnetic-resonance-imaging-organs-structures-X-rays-radiation.jpg.

Importance of Case Formulation

Case formulation is at the heart of mental health practice since it brings together the data gathered from assessment into a logical description of the client's issues. The structured approach enables clinicians to create individualized treatment plans that address not only the symptoms presented but also the contributing factors underlying the individual's mental health issues. Case formulation aims at the dynamic interplay between a client's background, current functioning, and environmental factors, which allows for an integrated understanding of their psychological picture. As highlighted in ongoing studies, the psychologists highlighted the treatment of the client's complaint while balancing probable classifications and explanations for their state, affirming the usefulness of case formulation as a tool of effective intervention and diagnosis in mental health care, where sound decision-making is critical to a successful outcome (Groenier et al., 2011). In addition, case formulation becomes as significant as the level of therapeutic relationship, shaping the clinicians and clients' conceptualization of the process of therapy. Case formulation, through mutual understanding and collaborative activity, helps to create a therapeutic alliance that is required for effective therapy. When dealing with personality-disordered clients, for example, research finds a high percentage of individuals with multifaceted psychological issues within primary care contexts. The findings indicate that some personality characteristics, like those in emotional distance and aggression, have been found to affect the therapy relationship and make treatment more difficult. Through identifying these traits within an organized and structured case formulation, therapists are capable of predicting probable treatment obstacles and aligning treatment strategies with what each patient needs for heightened participation and outcomes (Burrell-Hodgson et al., 2006). Lastly, case formulation is not just a diagnostic exercise but a comprehensive system that guides and informs treatment selection in different populations within mental health treatment environments. Through the integration of case formulation into practice, clinicians prepare themselves better to anticipate and navigate possible difficulties along the way of the therapeutic process. The iterative nature of case formulation allows constant checking of the client's progress and adjustment of treatment plans to accommodate shifting needs. Case formulation thus not only attains more precise diagnosis and understanding but also makes the therapeutic intervention dynamic and responsive, resulting in better therapeutic relationships and enhancing positive client outcomes in the long term. Through this recursive method, practitioners can maintain diagnoses up to date while simultaneously adjusting treatment modalities to accommodate the complexities of cases.

3.1. Historical Context of Diagnosis

Learning Outcome

1. Evolution of diagnostic criteria.
2. Key figures in diagnostic development.
3. Impact of historical perspectives on current practices.

The historical context of diagnosis has witnessed dramatic transformation over time, influenced by changing social, cultural, and scientific paradigms. Diagnoses in early times tended to be observational in nature and derived from folk wisdom, with physicians relying on a limited interpretation of human pathology and behavior. This led to the development of various medical categorizations, such as the early humoral theory, which sought to explain sickness and wellness through an imbalance of body fluids. As medicine developed, so did the models of diagnosis, driven significantly by advances in technology and a rise in empirical research. The process was one that slowly moved towards increasingly formalized diagnostic criteria, a movement that was essential in establishing mental health conditions in the context of a medical model dominated by biological, psychological, and social determinants. The late 19th and early 20th centuries saw the emergence of significant diagnostic classifications, with the development of the Diagnostic and Statistical Manual of Mental Disorders (DSM) being a pivotal milestone. The DSM provided a systematic approach to diagnosing mental disorders, initially reflecting the prevailing psychoanalytic paradigms. As diagnostic criteria were refined, they began to incorporate a more comprehensive view of mental health, considering environmental and contextual factors. For instance, public attitudes toward mental illness played a major role in the development of diagnostic categories. The resulting historical context emphasizes the worth of learning how cultures, sciences, and political milieus influence the benchmarks for diagnosis, leading up to the advent of incorporating medical practice into intertwinements with broader societal definitions of health and illness. Moreover, one cannot overstate the role of research institutions and universities in this new environment because they serve as key drivers for innovation and the propagation of diagnostic strategies. As explained in literature, local entrepreneurial universities have a potential role to play in strategic activity design that intensifies regional development, particularly in terms of innovation and entrepreneurship (Ferreira et al., 2025). By advancing collaborative research projects, the institutions promote greater learning about diagnosis practices and their implications for health care. Furthermore, exposure to diagnosis history promotes greater insight into how diagnoses reflect not just clinical observations but also societal stories and power dynamics. Therefore, the convergence of the clinical and academic traditions has formed the core of the advancement of innovative diagnostic models, whose applicability and viability in addressing contemporary health issues (Corti et al., 2020) (Figure 3.3).

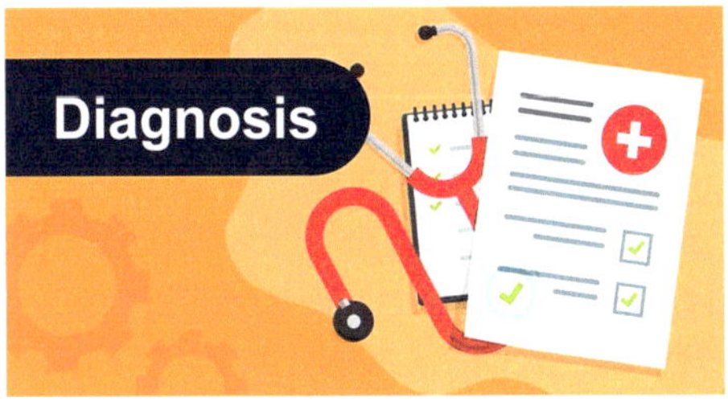

Figure 3.3. The historical context of diagnosis.

Source: https://cdn.myhealthteams.com/graphic/5c3f9af2d9e5c8531c8b9932/woriginal/MyMyelomaTeam_ConditionGuide-2024_Diagnosis_1200x630-bb26f6aa6f251d865a68f04e644f269a.webp?1721339016.

3.1.1. Evolution of Diagnostic Criteria

The evolution of diagnostic criteria in medicine and psychiatry has, over the decades, experienced fundamental transformations, both reflecting improvements in scientific knowledge and shifts in sociocultural orientations. Subjective judgment used to hold a significant predominance in the early systems, resulting in challenges in obtaining consistency and reliability. The innovation of systematic diagnostic manuals, such as the DSM and ICD, was a significant shift since these tried to provide codified criteria for numerous mental health disorders. Standardization through these served to consolidate knowledge about disorders, and practitioners were better able to communicate. As these guides evolved, they increasingly blended empirical findings and clinical experience, an aspect that reinforces the ongoing interdependence of scientific refinement and mundane application in diagnostics. The assimilation of both idiographic and nomothetic approaches into diagnostic criteria has enabled greater insight into individual patients through the integration of individual histories with more universalistic diagnostic paradigms, such as proposed in the evolution post-Psychodynamic Diagnostic Manual (Nancy et al., 2018). Increased complexity in diagnostic criteria has also been an adaptation to the evolving nature of mental health understanding. Previous diagnostic guides were biased toward categorical models, which put disorders into distinct categories according to what could be seen and felt. However, the shift towards dimensional has tried to represent the symptom continuum and the complex nature of mental illness. This is because it acknowledges the diversity among individuals and the fact that mental illness exists along a continuum and not in distinct categories. This evolution is not unique to psychiatry; specialties , such as transplant pathology evidence similar evolution. For instance, the 13th Banff Conference considered the need for more refined diagnostic criteria for antibody-mediated rejection with a focus on the histopathologic markers identifying microvascular injury in a greater level of detail than previous criteria (Angelini et al., 2017). These illustrations emphasize the necessity for continuous revision and refinement of diagnostic models to enhance diagnostic quality and outcomes for patients. Further, the feedback loop provided by research and clinical experience has served to enhance diagnostic criteria. With increasing numbers of studies being released, they not only revise current models but also challenge established concepts to be reconsidered. Criticism by the medical community, whether concerning the simplicity of previous classifications or the need for a change to support new discoveries, is crucial for advancing innovation. The revisions to the Psychodynamic Diagnostic Manual, for instance, are a response to criticism by practitioners regarding its existing usefulness and applicability in practice today, as it brought into focus the need to include emotional, cognitive, and social factors in the formulation of cases (Nancy et al., 2018). This reciprocal interaction between practice, research, and theory depicts that the evolution of diagnostic criteria is not a straight march but a multidimensional dialogue that builds and rebuilds the field of diagnosis in useful language. Such ongoing evolution ensures that diagnostic models are relevant and have the ability to keep up with human health and behavioral complexities (Figure 3.4).

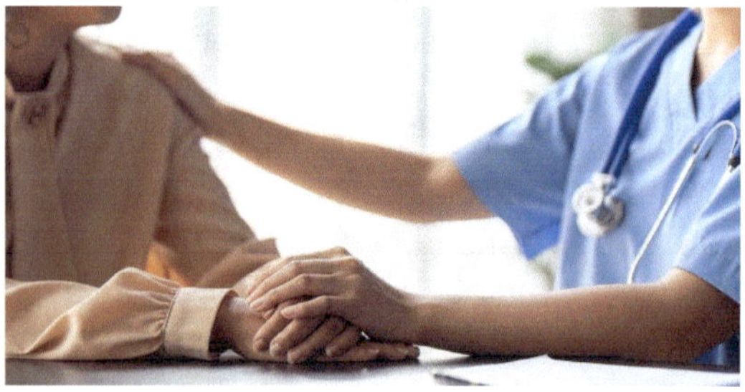

Figure 3.4. Evolution of diagnostic criteria in psychiatry.

Source: https://external-content.duckduckgo.com/iu/?u=https%3A%2F%2Fwww.acpe.org%2Fwp-content%2Fuploads%2F2024%2F04%2Fimage.jpeg&f=1&nofb=1&ipt=8c91b2fbe08b2fefc4061c703132a9bcad8f04cf631c6fac0bc7ded72c7d89ab.

3.1.2. Key Figures in Diagnostic Development

In diagnostic development, key actors emerge as core to the efforts that have transformed practice in contemporary diagnosis and case formulation. Among such actors, clinicians and researchers have employed sophisticated analysis methods to refine diagnostic measures across fields. Such is the case with methodologies involving public participation, which helps enhance diagnostic precision through integration of community intelligence within data collection and formulation. The integration of Public Participation GIS (PPGIS) methods provides a systematic approach to the gathering and analysis of stakeholder input to make the diagnostic development process more enhanced. Highlighted by initiatives from Polish cities Poznań and Łodź, incorporating multiple stakeholders' perspectives optimizes diagnostic challenges' comprehension, as emphasized through the contribution of collaboration for diagnosis and case formulation with innovative approaches (Brudka et al., 2016). Another key player in the diagnostic construction domain is the researcher whose expertise lies in the application of advanced metrics to determine complex environmental phenomena. In constructing a new diagnostic metric in reaction to soil moisture bimodality, this work most clearly depicts ongoing efforts at precision in diagnostic evaluation. The research applies an iterative algorithm on a maximum likelihood estimator, which is a technique that enhances the ability to derive information from probability density functions of soil moisture measurements. The analytical enhancement is significant in that it allows comparative analysis between satellite observations and Earth System Models. Through extensive research of these modalities, it is made evident through understanding land-atmosphere feedback processes how such measurements can be leveraged for informing extended diagnostic frameworks in describing environmental interactions (de Jeu et al., 2017). Notably, the efforts of these instrumental actors disclose the overlap between diagnostic advancement and the employment of interdisciplinary methods, moving towards a more integrated perspective of complex systems. The integration of methodological advances points towards an emphasis on setting and precision in diagnostics, with an eye on the requirement of adaptability in the face of shifting issues. Leaning on new approaches , such as PPGIS and advanced computational techniques, the diagnostic approach becomes more comprehensive, with an eye for a wider array of data and perspectives. This blending of diverse disciplines not only enhances the validity of diagnostic results but also propels the discipline toward more sustainable and effective case formulation practice. Through such a manner, the contributions of these leaders in diagnostic development remain central to influencing accessible, effective, and participatory approaches to diagnosis and case formulation (Figure 3.5).

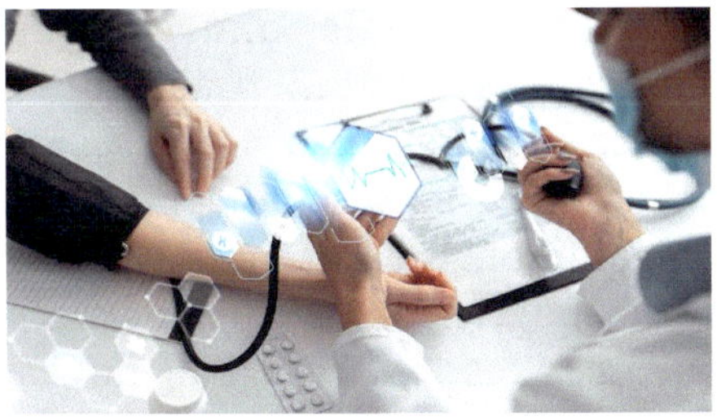

Figure 3.5. Key figures in diagnostic development.

Source: https://draravindan.com/images/blogs/1737434202546126478678f245a3a3ea.jpg.

3.1.3. Impact of Historical Perspectives on Current Practices

The integration of historical perspectives into contemporary practice is important, particularly in fields , such as psychology and social sciences. The knowledge of how the process of diagnosis and case formulation has developed draws attention to the complexity of human behavior and social customs. Historical models provide context through demonstrating how earlier methodologies and paradigms of theory impact contemporary practice. For example, the transition from entirely symptom-focused diagnostic criteria to more sensitive, integrated models is a testament to increased awareness of individual experience complexity. This has been fueled by findings in diverse intellectual traditions, which underline the necessity for an integral understanding in treatment. Overlooking such historical origins has the danger of reinforcing outdated methods and preventing other possible innovative solutions sensitive to diverse client requirements (Merok et al., 2025). Moreover, the interaction between historical frameworks and modern models of education highlights the value of reflective practice in professional training. The construction of narrative methods and common approaches, as revealed in the ICT integration of Teacher Professional Development in Rwanda, offers insight into how prior contexts shape current educational frameworks. Engaging teachers through reflective practice using narratives allows them to engage more deeply with implications from their ideals and methods. Such approaches not only foster a sense of community among the stakeholders but also encourage further equity and inclusivity within pedagogical practices. The historical context aids in gaining a better insight into the challenges and opportunities in current education strategies, hence enriching the outcomes for teachers as well as students (Hooker et al., 2009). Finally, the impact of historical considerations extends economic analysis, particularly in the field of decision-making models. By examining what economic history has to contribute to theory today, practitioners can gain a more complete picture of the richness of economic behavior, determining individual and system choices. Such historical data typically reveal the richness of socio-economic determinants and the history of events that have determined current economic traditions. Overlooking these historical backgrounds can lead to overly reductionist models failing to realize situational limits on decision-making. Therefore, combining historical perspectives not only enriches dominant practices but also equips practitioners with the analytical tools needed to cope with the complexities of modern economic settings and hence enhance the overall efficiency of diagnosis and case formulation (Merok et al., 2025).

Test Your Knowledge

1. How have historical beliefs and cultural perspectives influenced the evolution of psychiatric diagnosis?
2. What major milestones have shaped the transition from early descriptive classifications to modern standardized diagnostic systems?

3.2. Theoretical Frameworks in Diagnosis

Learning Outcome

1. Biological models.
2. Psychological models.
3. Sociocultural models.

The theoretical models of diagnosis play a significant role in the way clinicians understand and interpret symptoms, enable them to make case formulation, and inform their treatment plan. Theoretical models allow clinicians to systematically classify and decode complex patterns of behavior through systematic methods, where cognitive-behavioral models help to understand the interrelation among thoughts, feelings, and behaviors, and help the clinician to identify adaptive cognitive styles that are likely to contribute to some states of mental health. By employing such models, practitioners are more able to identify underlying issues that lie beyond symptomatology. Not only does such a systematic lens avoid more accurate diagnoses, but it also provides a foundation for focused interventions, affirming the value of working with proven theoretical models in clinical practice. Across the diagnostic domain, interdisciplinary approaches embedded within a theoretical model enhance the depth and scope of understanding provided. Advances in fields , such as nanotechnology and bioinformatics have begun to influence diagnostic practice, introducing entirely new approaches that lie outside the conventional. The potential of nanomedicine, as uncovered by present research, demonstrates how interdisciplinarity can facilitate not only diagnosis but also pinpointed treatments. Because nanotechnology deals with interdisciplinary scientific disciplines, such as materials science and biotechnology, its integration offers a wonderful chance to improve diagnostic precision and efficiency in clinical practice. With the convergence of theoretical models and cutting-edge technological innovation, practitioners can maximize case formulation processes in order to offer enhanced patient outcomes in mental health. In addition, the integration of diagnostic models with modern technological advancements raises pivotal questions regarding how success in clinical application can be evaluated. In the same way that the Business and Information Technology Alignment (BITA) model has been pivotal in capturing organizational performance amid digitalization, mental health must embrace such paradigms to quantify the effectiveness of various diagnostic models. By establishing standards that can be measured against these theoretical frameworks, clinicians have a better ability to ascertain the impact of their diagnostic practices on treatment and patient care. By modifying such frameworks, not only is the validity of chosen frameworks enhanced, but constant improvement of diagnostic practice is also ensured. By continuously refining these approaches, practitioners in mental health can guarantee that their models remain effective and applicable in the evolving healthcare and technology landscape.

3.2.1. Biological Models

The information regarding psychological disorders has traditionally been informed by biological models, believing genetic and physiological factors to be key to the diagnosis and treatment of mental illness. The models emphasize the interaction of heredity and neurobiological function in determining individual behavior and mental processes. For example, findings suggest that conditions , such as Attention Deficit Hyperactivity Disorder (ADHD) have a large genetic factor, with those affected being far more likely to have relatives who experience the same symptoms. This biological inclination points to the necessity for incorporating biological perspectives within diagnostic processes to determine the etiology of conditions adequately, as with prevalent disorders like ADHD, which is not yet well understood in child and adult populations (Groenier et al., 2011). Thus, while biological models are pivotal in sharing insight, they also necessitate a more general awareness of psychological and environmental factors. Aside from that, the application of biological models in diagnosis mandates that one has a learned understanding of how environmental factors interact with genetic determinants. For example, psychological assessments most often find that disorders , such as ADHD are not created by heritable traits but are also exacerbated by environmental factors, including prenatal exposures and psychosocial stressors. Diagnosis in this model is not a fixed process; rather, it involves ongoing assessment and adjustment of treatment plans based on the nuances of each case. One recent study examining psychologists' diagnostic processes highlighted that practitioners tended to oscillate between probing categorical classification and questioning causal determinants within the context of interviews. This adaptive approach emphasizes the significance of flexibility in diagnostic strategies in order to accommodate the variability characteristic of clinical disorders like ADHD (Groenier et al., 2011). In addition, biological models have utility beyond their application in early diagnosis to treatment planning and formulation. The neurobiological underpinnings of various disorders assist clinicians in selecting the appropriate type of pharmacological intervention. For instance, methylphenidate has been identified as a first-line treatment for ADHD, with excellent efficacy in about 80% of properly diagnosed instances (Camilleri & Makhoul, 2013). This data not only attests to the applicability of biological models in treatment scenarios but also to the importance of comprehensive diagnostic evaluations encompassing both biological and psychological dimensions. Thus, applying the models to diagnostic and case formulation activity enhances the accuracy of clinicians' judgments and leaves the way open for focused treatment interventions of potentially major benefit to patients (Figure 3.6).

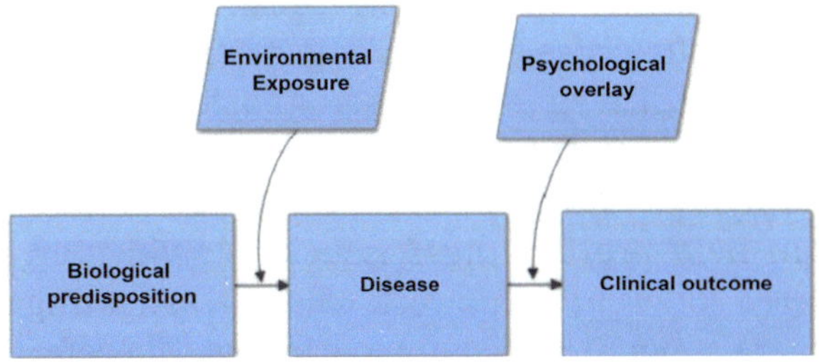

Figure 3.6. Biological models in diagnosis.

Source: https://external-content.duckduckgo.com/iu/?u=https%3A%2F%2Fwww.researchgate.net%2Fpublication%2F323396284%2Ffigure%2Ffig1%2FAS%3A598265657556998%401519649056896%2FBiomedical-model-of-disease.png&f=1&nofb=1&ipt=d8c72cf7e2ed748257be987c2eddb2f762a9889d10f9a5ba8afadfae1f2edf78.

3.2.2. Psychological Models

Psychological model study is at the heart of effective diagnosis and case formulation in mental health care. Models enable the appreciation of human conduct intricacies and psychological disorder complexities. By employing several theoretical perspectives, practitioners can better read patient complaints and underlying causes and thus plan for proper treatment. For instance, cognitive-behavioral, psychodynamic, and humanistic approaches each yield distinct insights into mental health condition processes. Such integrated understanding enhances the psychologists capacity to work through a client's complexity, encouraging a more whole-person practice of care that includes emotional, cognitive, and environmental factors in the process of diagnosis (Groenier et al., 2011). Also, the importance of standardized diagnostic procedures cannot be overstated because they ensure the validity of results and measuring accuracy, as well as testing treatment effectiveness. Lack of uniformity in diagnostic requirements can cause significant variability in classifying psychological disorders, potentially weakening effective intervention programs. By emphasizing consistency in the diagnostic process, psychologists can minimize false positives and misdiagnosis, endemic problems in the field (Larsen et al., 2018). Applying established psychological models can help prevent these issues, allowing for a more coherent framework when investigating a client's symptoms and experiences. Therefore, stability in diagnostic practice and adherence to psychological models become the fulcrum on which practice is enabled to provide quality mental health care that is both contextually sensitive and evidence-based. Fundamentally, the interplay between a psychologist's assessments and continual refinement of understanding concerning the client's status involves a quintessential aspect of effective diagnosis. As they converse with clients, psychologists are continuously forced to update their assessment in the light of new knowledge developed in the course of therapeutic dialogue. It is this cyclical process that facilitates nuanced case formulation that is attuned to the richness of subjective experience and symptomatology. Refocusing attention on the dynamic interplay between observation-based assessment and theoretical application can yield more flexible and adaptive treatment strategies. As conveyed in diagnostic interview research, such fluidity is critical to handling clients' individual presentations and underlying issues and establishing a context in which collaborative exploration of mental health issues will be facilitated (Groenier et al., 2011). This becomes empowering for clients while enabling psychologists to formulate more precise and tailored treatment plans.

3.2.3. Sociocultural Models

Sociocultural models are of vital significance in accounting for mental health disorders, emphasizing the role of social factors and culture in shaping individuals' experiences of distress. Sociocultural models go beyond traditional biomedical treatments by recognizing that mental health has to be examined within the broader sociocultural context. For instance, many researchers have demonstrated that cultural factors not only influence the incidence of certain conditions but also the way people think and respond to their symptoms. Practitioners can form more holistic diagnoses and case formulations, taking into account personal histories as well as societal forces that can potentially influence mental health outcomes, using a sociocultural approach. As a result, sociocultural models encourage an advanced understanding of distress that unites personal experience with the dominant explanations of mental health in given cultural environments. Clinical practice is helped by the establishment of brief "mini-formulations" that distill rich information into therapist- and client-relevant ideas.

By keeping these formulations concise, practitioners are more capable of communicating potential interventions without overwhelming clients. Such models can include linear and cyclical models that illustrate the dynamics of personal distress and cultural setting. Not only does this optimize the therapeutic process, but it also empowers clients by affirming what they experience in a societal context. In a comprehensive case study, the wife caregiver of his husband who was demented showed how minor adjustments to her society's cultural view made living easier for how she managed and for herself, thereby demonstrating the everyday applicability of these sociocultural models (Charlesworth et al., 2004).

Additionally, illustrating the significance of sociocultural contexts, the way diagnostic criteria for disorders, such as Anorexia Nervosa, have evolved through time highlights how societal factors influence pathology within individuals. Early perceptions of the disorder were described largely in terms of a psychological context, but alterations started coming as feminist perspectives provided criticisms of emphasis on individual pathology and instead highlighted attention to social structures and gender relations. This shift has shed light on how external socio-cultural pressures, specifically around femininity, can significantly influence individual mental health trajectories. Through their incorporation of these sociocultural perspectives into diagnosis and case conceptualization, mental health providers can prioritize interventions that target system inequalities and advance larger social change. This deeper understanding helps people make sense of their lives and promotes a critical discussion regarding the societal forces that shape mental health (Till et al., 2011) (Figure 3.7).

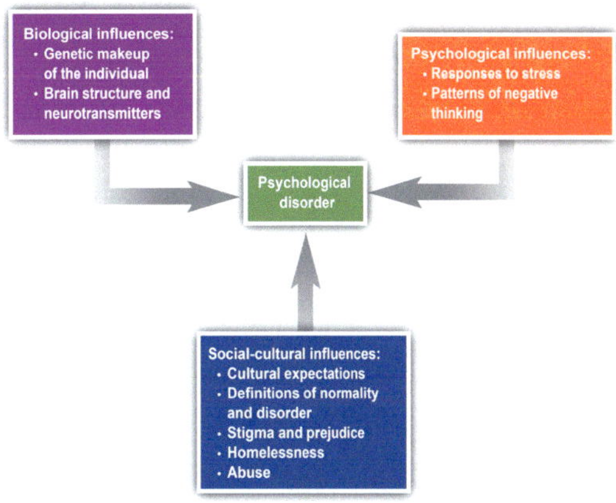

Figure 3.7. Sociocultural models.

Source: https://external-content.duckduckgo.com/iu/?u=https%3A%2F%2Fopen.lib.umn.edu%2Fapp%2Fuploads%2Fsites%2F2%2F2015%2F03%2Ffbc3507df9b56c7daf55386cffaa1595.jpg&f=1&nofb=1&ipt=05b12a5b89c7b941afd6dc52b7c037877a07f1897e21614dcc2dd779784b58de.

Test Your Knowledge

1. How do biological, psychodynamic, cognitive-behavioral, and sociocultural frameworks differ in explaining the origins of mental disorders?
2. Why is it important for clinicians to integrate multiple theoretical perspectives when evaluating complex psychiatric conditions?

3.3. Diagnostic Tools and Techniques

Learning Outcome

1. Clinical interviews.
2. Psychological testing.
3. Observational methods.

Its success in clinical psychology relies significantly on the ability to dissect mental illness into minute details. A few of the most salient tools are standardized tests, such as self-report questionnaires and structured interviews. They help clinicians gather data step by step regarding a patient's feelings, behaviors, and symptoms. By applying these tools, experts are able to make a comprehensive evaluation, leading to a more accurate diagnosis. For example, in diagnosing disorders like Reactive Attachment Disorder (RAD), the deficiencies in currently available diagnostic criteria outlined within the DSM-5 pose a significant challenge. Orthodox methods only capture the complex behaviors that fall under RAD and thus call for a more sensitive method that takes into account the subjective histories and experiences of the children involved, which is critical for effective case formulation and intervention (Owen, 2016). Further, advances in neurobiological research emphasize the benefits of incorporating psychophysiological assessments into models of diagnosis. Procedures , such as skin conductance and heart rate during therapy sessions provide indicators of the physiological responses to distress and traumatic events. In support of new research, these assessments provide an overall picture of the therapeutic process by capturing the underlying reactions lost with more traditional measurements. With this integrative approach, clinicians can better evaluate the efficiency of treatment methods, particularly for trauma-related disorders where dissociation is an important feature. Such evaluation methodology for in-depth assessments highlights the interconnectivity among mental processes and physical reactions, thereby improving the validity and richness of case formulations in making diagnoses for psychological disorders (Palmieri et al., 2015). Finally, the application of modern psychological tests allows for a more dynamic portrayal of patient experience to enrich the case formulation. The integration of projective tests and self-report measures allows multi-dimensional comprehension of a patient's psyche and provides clinicians with the necessary projections of their inner struggles as well as relational patterns. For application in relational trauma contexts, such instruments can highlight the subtle dynamics underlying an individual's clinical presentation. Through examination of the patient's history, symptomatology, and how they interact with their therapist, practitioners are able to develop evidence-based treatment plans with interventions to help treat immediate concerns and underlying issues. This extensive evaluation process not only increases diagnostic accuracy but also results in a therapeutic relationship where patients feel understood and heard, ultimately resulting in better therapeutic outcomes and patient engagement (Palmieri et al., 2015; Owen, 2016).

3.3.1. Clinical Interviews

Clinical interviews are a fundamental aspect of the diagnostic process in mental health care, enabling psychologists to assess clients' grievances in depth. Through clinical interviews, practitioners engage in a systematic discussion that offers them sufficient information regarding the client's experiences and symptoms. The effectiveness of clinical interviews depends on the psychologists' capacity to create a safe and trusting environment, within which clients freely discuss their problems. This interaction process not only involves gathering information with regard to the client's current condition but also probing for possible underlying factors and history. According to recent studies, psychologists are found to respond with a ubiquitous style during such interviews, addressing client complaints as well as potential categorizations, interpretations, and treatments, a sign of the interactive nature of the clinical encounter (Groenier et al., 2011). The multiaxial psychodynamic diagnostic system has been a significant innovation in refining the process of clinical interview structure. Specifically, the operationalized psychodynamic diagnostics (OPD) axes—illness experience, relationships, mental conflicts, and structure—give clinicians a multidimensional view on which to make their diagnoses. Not only are the axes designed to enhance the richness of evaluations, but also the identification of treatment approaches tailored to particular needs. Empirical validation of the OPD in research and clinical contexts demonstrates satisfactory reliability and validity, substantiating its relevance across various settings.

This systematic approach is liberating for clinicians regarding symptom categorization and takes into account the complex interaction between psychological factors in an individual's life, leading to a more accurate examination of the client's mental health (Bellak et al., 2007). In addition, clinical interview practice requires the practitioner to be sensitive to the fluidity of talk and adaptive in style. Psychologists have a tendency to shift between diagnostic activities as new information emerges during the course of an interview, thus triggering modifications to initial impressions about the client's condition. The iterative nature of clinical interviews invites more differentiated diagnostic formulation and emphasizes the requirement for psychologists to be clinically adaptive. By taking into account the interview material and moves made, mental health professionals can improve their diagnostic abilities, ultimately leading to more effective treatment. Such flexibility offers a model of the balance between structured test-taking and the spontaneous development of client-therapist relationships that is essential in the effective handling of mental illnesses (Groenier et al., 2011) (Figure 3.8).

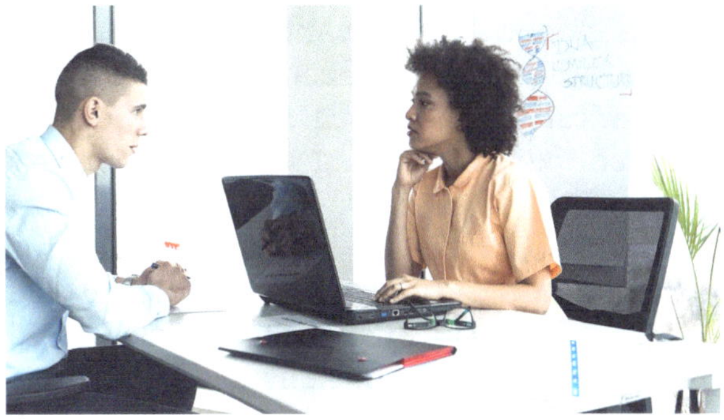

Figure 3.8. Clinical interviews.

Source: https://purosearch.com/wp-content/uploads/How-to-Prepare-for-a-Clinical-Interview-Essential-Tips-for-Success.jpg.

3.3.2. Psychological Testing

Psychological testing is a cornerstone in the case formulation and diagnosis process, producing key data that can illuminate the complexities of an individual's mental health state. Through the use of the structured measurement of psychological concepts , such as intelligence, personality features, and emotional functioning, professionals can make clinical inferences that inform their decisions. For example, the application of standardized testing allows clinicians not only to identify troubling symptoms but also to ascertain their severity and related effect on functioning. This methodical approach to assessment allows psychologists to design individualized treatment plans tailored to the specific requirements of their clients, ultimately improving therapeutic outcomes. Moreover, as the diagnostic operations of different psychologists have commonalities in interviewing and report writing, these tests assist in giving an effective impression of the complaint of the client and treatment concerns, reinforcing the significant position of psychological testing within a connected diagnostic model (Groenier et al., 2011). Psychological testing is critical at the beginning of assessment, that is, for ruling out differential diagnoses and specifying symptomatology. This is especially relevant in areas where false positives can significantly skew research and clinical practice, such as in psychopathy research. As highlighted in contemporary discourses, routine testing tools could report high false-positive rates, which complicate the mental health research and practice world (Larsen et al., 2018). By applying evidence-based testing procedures, clinicians are better able to differentiate among different psychological conditions, reducing misdiagnoses derived from common symptoms. Second, the output of psychological testing provides quantifiable information allowing for monitoring of progress through time and the possibility of making adjustments to treatment strategies along the way. In this manner, psychological testing not only serves the initial function of diagnosis but also facilitates continued evaluation and modification of therapeutic methods. Third, the integration of psychological testing with diagnosis and case conceptualization illustrates the need for a multidimensional strategy. It encourages the integration of information gained from more than one testing modality like clinical interviews, behavioral observation, and standardized questionnaires. It allows psychologists to have interactive engagement with clients through this complete picture, where the two-way exchange of information affects both the diagnostic process and the therapeutic relationship. As observed in diagnostic interviews, psychologists easily switch between assessing symptoms, analyzing causal factors, and arguing treatment plans created based on the individualized profile. This switch highlights the importance of psychological testing to respond to a client's situation changing, hence the entire process of diagnosis and subsequent interventions being more effective (Groenier et al., 2011). Last but not least, the relationship between testing and clinical judgment reiterates the complexity required in diagnosing mental health.

3.3.3. Observational Methods

Observational methods form an essential part of the case formulation and diagnosis process within clinical settings, particularly in observing the behavioral patterns and responses of individuals. As a contrast to explicit questioning or formal tests, observational approaches provide a rich and vivid contextual understanding of patients' behaviors in naturalistic settings. This approach is particularly valuable when evaluating individuals with diverse backgrounds because it allows practitioners to value subtle cues that might represent significant psychosocial difficulties or cultural factors influencing mental health. For instance, augmenting communication in therapy, as discussed in (Bhui et al., 2013), means that observational understanding can support interactions between patients and practitioners and thus lead to increased engagement and understanding during diagnosis. Through close attention to interpersonal dynamics and environmental interactions, practitioners can develop a more holistic diagnosis that considers both individual behavior and contextual variables. The value of observational approaches is also seen in their use across a range of clinical assessments, including those with Black and Minority Ethnic (BME) patients. Research has identified these groups to be often in receipt of inequalities in their care, including over-representation in mental health law detentions and limited access to psychological treatments. Observational methods have the capacity to uncover the underlying reasons for inequalities by pointing out challenges like miscommunication between healthcare staff and patients due to cultural backgrounds. As elaborated in the THERACOM project presented in (Bhui et al., 2013), a major imperative is to create an environment where such observational evidence guides interventions to improve therapeutic communications. Such an environment in practice enhances patient satisfaction and works towards bridging disparities in the delivery of mental health care, thereby making observational methods a key tool in the achievement of equitable treatment outcomes. The application of observational methods requires a rigorous approach, particularly within HTA. Merging observational qualitative and quantitative data has the ability to impact holistic judgments regarding intervention effectiveness, argues. By employing systematic observation frameworks, assessors can standardize findings, and the reliability and comparability of studies improve. This systematic reporting is the foundation of best practice in case formulation and diagnosis, enabling clinicians to construct their understanding of patient conduct on a firm foundation. Thus, through applying strict observation methods, clinicians can reduce more effectively the mysteries attending mental health diagnoses, with subsequent improved patient outcomes as well as improved case formulation within increasingly multicultural surroundings (Figure 3.9).

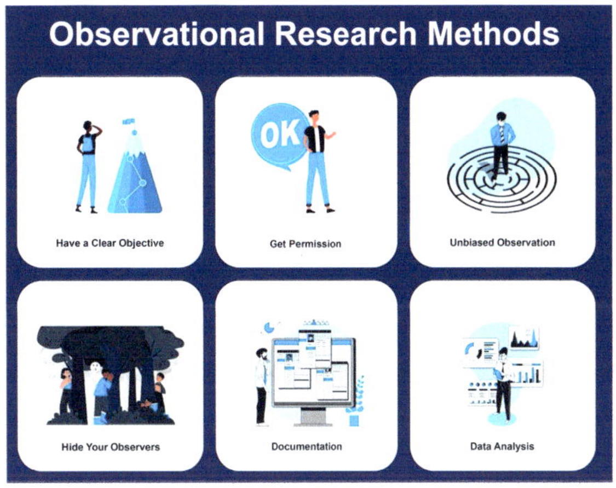
Observational Research Methods
Have a Clear Objective
OK
Get Permission
Unbiased Observation
Hide Your Observers
Documentation
Data Analysis

Figure 3.9. Observational methods.

Source: https://www.questionpro.com/blog/wp-content/uploads/2023/08/observational-research-methods-1.jpg.

Test Your Knowledge

1. What role do clinical interviews, psychological tests, and behavioral observations play in the diagnostic process?
2. How do neuroimaging, lab tests, and standardized rating scales contribute to accurate and comprehensive diagnosis?

3.4. The Role of DSM and ICD

Learning Outcome

1. Overview of DSM (Diagnostic and Statistical Manual of Mental Disorders).
2. Overview of ICD (International Classification of Diseases).
3. Comparison of DSM and ICD.

DSM and ICD are the most prevalent classification systems that are used in mental health diagnosis and formulation. Both classification systems have a systematic approach, which helps clinicians identify and classify psychological conditions. Although the DSM is predominantly utilized in the United States, it has a categorical approach towards the classification, specifying the diagnostic criteria of different mental disorders. By comparison, the ICD, developed by the World Health Organization, is more universally applicable internationally because it encompasses a wider range of health-related conditions, including physical health.

This contrast shows the intricacy of diagnosis, which demonstrates how various cultural paradigms and clinical methods can influence the definition of mental health disorders and thus affect case formulation in therapeutic treatment. Despite the universal acceptance of the DSM and ICD, both classifications have been criticized for oversimplifying the human behavior' complexities. For example, psychodynamic and humanistic clinicians are often beset by the categoric nature of these classifications, which can barely reflect the diverse realities of the individual patient. Their inability to adopt DSM diagnosis labels is due to a resistance to losing the holistic aspects of human individuality that might be sacrificed under categorical diagnoses. Efforts , such as the Psychodynamic Diagnostic Manual (PDM) attempt to integrate these tensions through promoting a more flexible, empirically-grounded model of diagnosis. By integrating clinical nuance with methodological precision, the PDM enables a broader conceptualization of mental health disorders, resisting oversimplification by placing diagnoses within a biopsychosocial framework (Blagov et al., 2015). Furthermore, the limitations of the DSM and ICD precipitate a debate about other concepts of mental health, the most important of which are idiographic and narrative. Idiographic knowledge, rooted in individualized judgment, has been suggested as a panacea for the shortcomings of criteriological diagnoses. However, individuality's nature too frequently becomes hard to explain in terms of pre-established diagnostic grids. Narrative understanding, as presented, could be the better alternative, allowing clinicians to explore patients' individual histories and personal experiences more deeply. This approach facilitates a deeper therapeutic relationship and more nuanced case formulation by enabling clinicians to position the lived experience of their patients as a priority over categorical diagnosis (Thornton, 2008). By integrating narrative methods into the diagnostic process, mental health professionals can expand their perspective into a more diverse one that respects differences while maintaining the underlying structures of the DSM and ICD.

3.4.1. DSM (Diagnostic and Statistical Manual of Mental Disorders) Overview

The Diagnostic and Statistical Manual of Mental Disorders (DSM) is a critical tool for mental health practitioners, defining standardized criteria for the diagnosis of mental disorders. Its development has been a transformative driving force in the history of psychology and psychiatry, offering a global language and structure supporting accurate diagnosis and successful treatment. The development of the DSM follows changing societal attitudes to mental health as well as advances in science. Each edition incorporates new research findings, clinical experience, and an increasing number of disorders, underlining its dynamic nature. By clearly setting out diagnostic criteria, the DSM enables clinicians to distinguish between symptoms and disorders in a systematic way, which is important for good case formulation and effective treatment planning. In the DSM model, diagnostic criteria for disorders are not simply symptom ticklists; they have been researched and clinically developed to a substantial degree. For instance, the current emphasis on Attention Deficit Hyperactivity Disorder (ADHD) reflects its prevalence and impact on both children and adults, as illustrated in recent research (Camilleri & Makhoul, 2013). Comprehending ADHD requires knowledge of its multifactorial etiology, including genetic and environmental factors affecting its expression. The DSM establishes parameters that take into consideration these complexities and require clinicians to consider a broad array of factors in making diagnoses and developing treatment plans. The DSM therefore invites practitioners to think about each case thoroughly and holistically, enabling them to approach mental health diagnosis and care with a subtler understanding.

In actual practice, the processes of diagnosis employed by psychologists must be sequential but also adaptable, as indicated by recent research on psychologists' diagnostic process (Groenier et al., 2011). What emerged from the research is that effective diagnostic interviews involve actively listening to clients' accounts while simultaneously considering potential classifications and treatments. Psychologists must balance the need for detailed appraisals with the dynamism of client interaction. This flexibility ensures that their diagnostic findings are shaped by both the clinical presentation and ongoing controversy in the treatment environment. It is for this reason that the DSM plays a role in aiding these diagnostic processes, as it allows clinicians to chart the probable classifications with room for accommodating also the nuances that may arise under questioning, thus producing more accurate and specific guidelines for treatment (Figure 3.10).

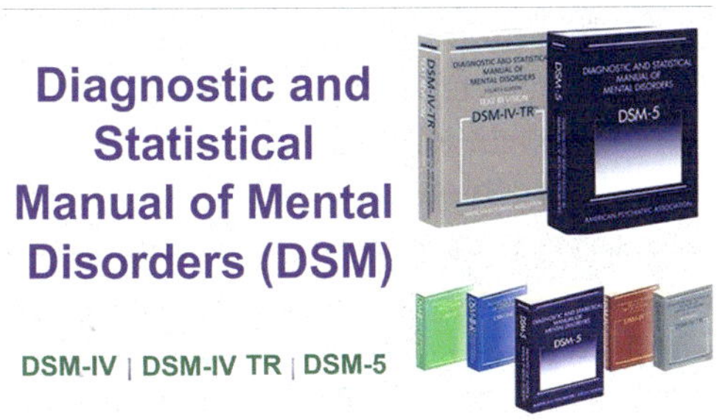

Figure 3.10. The diagnostic and statistical manual of mental disorders (DSM).

Source: https://i.ytimg.com/vi/OMdS5r2QTzc/hq720.jpg?sqp=-oaymwEhCK4FEIIDSFryq4qpAxMIARUAAAAAGAElAADIQj0AgKJD&rs=AOn4CLCL1nn3r6HB-oX92LOulkHsIHduow.

3.4.2. Overview of ICD (International Classification of Diseases)

The World Health Organization (WHO) the International Classification of Diseases (ICD), which is a prominent framework for the classification and diagnosis of health conditions globally. The principal function of the ICD is to facilitate consistent health reporting and international comparability of health information. By its system of universal coding, the ICD allows standardization of diagnoses, essential for epidemiological studies, health services planning, and resource allocation. Transition from ICD-10 to ICD-11 has brought about deep changes due to advancements in medical knowledge, along with shifts in the delivery of health services. Of specific interest is the addition of new hierarchies and classes, which allow greater nuance in the classification of complex health conditions, aligning diagnosis with clinical practice and research objectives. Among the greatest developments in the ICD-11 is the addition of discrete classes for mental disorders, which emphasize the prominence of mental health in healthcare as a whole. These comprise the Obsessive–Compulsive and Related Disorders (OCRD) cluster, demonstrating a trend toward a more clinically relevant classification founded on neurobiological processes underlying the disorders. The rationale for the clustering is based on similarities among disorders like obsessive-compulsive disorder and body dysmorphic disorder that exhibit similarities in clinical presentation and treatment of patients. Emerging evidence from neurochemical and imaging studies underpins this classification, rendering it more credible and useful. The effort of having these disorders clearly defined is intended to improve both diagnostic accuracy and treatment modalities, such that patients are given the most relevant interventions for their conditions (Atmaca et al., 2016). The application of the ICD in practice also has some meaning for documentation and communication among providers. Accurate coding is essential to health information management, particularly with mental illnesses that are likely to be complex and overlapping. Understanding how depression and related disorders are documented in various clinical settings can help identify gaps in data collection and inform best practices for clinicians

(Sheikh et al., 2012). With the continued growth of healthcare systems, making the diagnostic processes consistent with ICD guidelines can ensure continuity of care, facilitate multi-disciplinary working, and ultimately translate into better patient outcomes. The ICD not only serves as a classification tool but also as a bridge between research and clinical practice to ensure a comprehensive understanding of health states and their management (Figure 3.11).

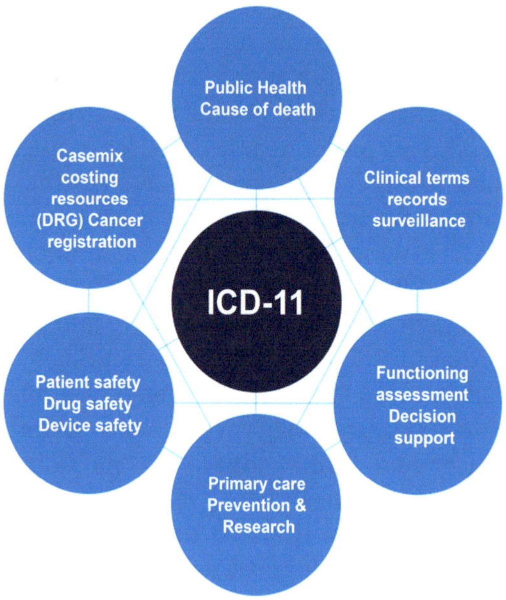

Figure 3.11. The international classification of diseases (ICD).

Source: https://cdn.who.int/media/images/default-source/classifications/icd/icd11/icd-11-uses-cases-.tmb-1920v.png?sfvrsn=2ea3f420_9.

3.4.3. Comparison of DSM and ICD

The Diagnostic and Statistical Manual of Mental Disorders (DSM) and the International Classification of Diseases (ICD) are the most prevalent blueprints for mental health illness diagnosis globally. Even though both manuals share the aim of delivering standardized classification criteria, the two manuals differ significantly in their purpose, format, and use. The DSM is condition-specific for psychiatry, providing detailed descriptions and criteria primarily aimed at mental health practitioners in America. The ICD, on the other hand, is an international, comprehensive system developed by the World Health Organization, classifying a broad range of health conditions, not only mental disorders. This distinction acts to signal the DSM's role in clinical settings and position the ICD in a public health framework, emphasizing the international focus on health it embodies. Consequently, the choice of which system to apply is frequently less a professional decision than driven by geography and sociocultural contexts. Even though they serve distinct purposes, the DSM and ICD share an interest in optimizing the precision of diagnosis and the effectiveness of treatment. Synergies between the two systems are better valued by an appreciation of integrative diagnostic strategies. The DSM criteria, for instance, are used to channel placement of certain disorders into the ICD system, providing for convergence that aids clinicians in comprehending psychiatric diagnosis complexities. In addition, each system's adaptation to fit cultural and contextual differences highlights the ever-evolving nature of the mental health practice. Adaptation in such a manner guarantees that clinicians are attuned to the varying experiences and backgrounds of patients, resulting in increasingly valid and targeted interventions. This connection emphasizes that competition is not the sole correlation between the DSM and the ICD, but one of cooperation towards more enhanced mental health care. Moreover, the cross-cultural applicability of these diagnostic frameworks cannot be overlooked. For example, it has been found that psychiatric classifications dominated from North America tend to unintentionally exclude indigenous systems of conception of mental disorders in different cultures. In exploring these dynamics, it is apparent that while the DSM is most influential, its application is at times selective in recognizing culturally unique expressions of mental disorder. This argument is at the forefront because it captures postcolonial criticism of psychiatric training, opposed to imposing one cultural system on another, as it has been explored in comparative literature on psychiatric training across various global settings. These revelations call for careful examination of the diagnosis's impact on case formulation, with mental health workers having to be on their toes with respect to the local context in using standardized diagnostic manuals. Serious consideration of both the nuances of the DSM and ICD provides a wider and more inclusive framework for diagnosis and case formulation in mental health.

Test Your Knowledge

1. What are the primary functions of the DSM and ICD in standardizing the classification of mental disorders?
2. How do differences between DSM-5-TR and ICD-11 impact cross-cultural diagnosis and clinical practice globally?

3.5. Challenges in Diagnosis

Learning Outcome

1. Misdiagnosis and its consequences.
2. Cultural considerations in diagnosis.
3. The role of stigma in diagnostic processes.

Effective diagnosis is the foundation of mental health therapy; however, there are several complications that make it challenging for practitioners. One primary challenge arises from the inherent complexity of psychological illnesses, which will always be accompanied by intersecting symptoms that lead to misdiagnosis or delayed identification. For instance, depression and anxiety can have both physical and emotional manifestations, making it impossible for practitioners to determine the right diagnosis without a sophisticated appreciation of each client's unique context. This call for personalized assessments underlines the importance of holistic diagnostic approaches that take note of the multifaceted nature of human psychology, as emphasized by the work of Gallagher et al. (2019). The excessive reliance on standardized diagnostic criteria, as important as it is, can have the counterproductive consequence of hiding variations that are essential to effective case formulation. Moreover, the susceptibility to cognitive and communication deficits makes diagnosis highly complicated. Differences in clients' cognition, affect, and communication styles can hinder information exchange on assessments. For example, individuals with brain injury can have poor memory and executive function, which are important in terms of explaining their symptoms and experiences accurately. In such a situation, the revisions to diagnostics and treatment proposed in the review cover how professionals must alter their approach to better accommodate these differences, as referenced in Gallagher et al. (2019). Omitting such barriers can lead to incomplete assessments and ultimately, ineffective outcomes of treatment, underscoring the importance of clinicians being sensitive and adaptable in their assessment processes. Finally, the dynamic nature of mental health diagnoses offers yet another complication. The situational character of client interaction is subject to fluctuation overnight in the course of assessments, as psychologists navigate fluid presentation and client response. This flexibility complicates the diagnostic process because practitioners must continually reconsider their impressions and hypotheses in the moment. Research on psychologists' diagnostic processes revealed that practitioners kept repeatedly going over their considerations when interviewing, demonstrating the challenges of maintaining diagnostic clarity against altering client accounts (as outlined in Groenier et al., 2011). This suggests that there is a requirement for continuous training and support of clinicians so that they can develop flexible styles of diagnosis and case formulation in the context of uncertainty and variability. The issue needs to be addressed to improve mental health diagnostic accuracy and efficacy (Figure 3.12).

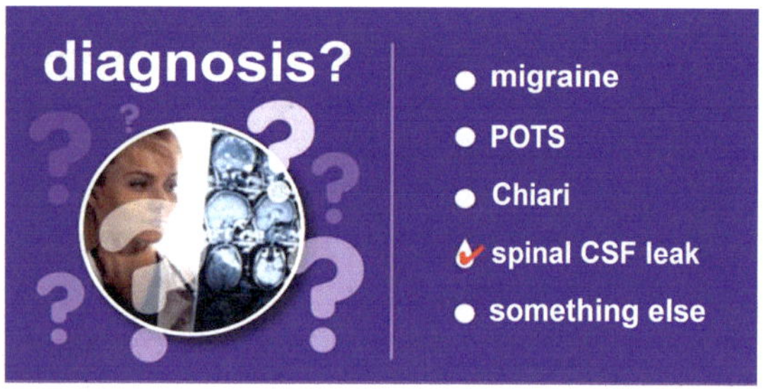

Figure 3.12. Challenges in diagnosis.

Source: https://spinalcsfleak.org/wp-content/uploads/2017/07/Diagnostic-Challenges-e1488119849289.jpg.

3.5.1. Misdiagnosis and Its Consequences

Misdiagnosis is a critical problem in the practice of medicine that has a material impact on patient outcomes. Misdiagnosis is a result of numerous factors, including limited access to diagnostic technology and social determinants of health that influence the diagnostic process. One of concern is that populations in low- and middle-income countries are disproportionately impacted, with access to fundamental diagnostics often lacking. The COVID-19 pandemic revealed the need for accurate and timely diagnosis since rapid transmission and variable presentation of the disease were realized. In this regard, it was understood that reliance on robust diagnostic capability is imperative for best-case formulation and patient management. Inadequate diagnostic access, particularly acutely in primary healthcare, leads to high rates of undiagnosed disease, evidence of a systemic issue in healthcare systems that needs to be addressed in order to reduce the proportion of misdiagnoses and their consequential impact (Fleming et al., 2021). The impact of misdiagnosis resonates far beyond individual patient distress; it resonates throughout healthcare systems, adding to enhanced costs and non-effective treatment strategies. For instance, the patients diagnosed with the incorrect psychiatric disorder will experience delayed treatment and unnecessary stigma, further aggravating their condition. In psychiatric disorders, resistance to treatment is occurring at alarming rates, 20–60% of the patients, hence tremendously increasing the healthcare burden (Howes et al., 2021). This case highlights the importance of an integral grasp of diagnostic issues across various fields, such as mental health, where incorrect diagnosis may mislead therapeutic interventions. Correct diagnoses are essential, as misdiagnosis not only compromises the quality of care delivered but also puts pressure on healthcare resources and impedes proper management of patients. Resolving the excessive rate of misdiagnosis requires a multi-dimensional strategy. Interventions must be designed to improve diagnostics access technologies, training for healthcare providers, and implementing standard guidelines for evaluation. Implementation of diagnostic and case formulation methods, particularly for complex disorders, facilitates patient care-focused thinking directed at achieving correctness in diagnosis. In addition, measures designed to promote teamwork among healthcare providers to collaborate can facilitate the exchange of expertise and reduce overreliance on subjective judgment, which is apt to lead to misdiagnosis. As evoked by today's challenges, including those brought about by the COVID-19 pandemic, increased visibility and prioritization of diagnostic resources are essential to realizing equitable healthcare outcomes (Fleming et al., 2021). In the long run, systemic reforms with the purpose of enhancing diagnostic accuracy will not only reduce individual patient suffering but also improve the overall efficiency of healthcare.

3.5.2. Cultural Issues in Diagnosis

Cultural factors are central to diagnosis, as they have a dramatic impact on how individuals express psychological distress and conceptualize mental health. Ethnicity, socio-economic status, and culture all play a part in the symptomatology of mental illness and the course practitioners take in collecting and interpreting symptoms. For instance, certain cultural groups may exhibit behavior or show affect that deviates from Western normative assumptions and, as such, lead to misdiagnosis or misinterpretation unless cultural circumstances are addressed in a careful manner. Hence, practitioners must be trained in recognizing the nuances of the expressions of distress from the cultural perspective, since otherwise it leads to significant miscommunication and ineffective treatment plans. This cultural competence in diagnosis is part of the growing emphasis on in-depth and compassionate diagnostic practice in psychological assessment. Furthermore, the diagnostic situation is made more complex by varying worldviews about mental illness from culture to culture that may influence the likelihood of treatment-seeking. Other cultures may have different perspectives regarding the causality and meaning of psychological symptoms, defining them as spiritual, social, or physical issues, but not psychiatric illness. As can be seen from studies, psychologists should undertake lengthy and culturally appropriate diagnostic interviews that, in addition to inquiring about prevailing symptoms, explore the cultural narratives about them. This offers mental health professionals ways of modifying their interventions more meaningfully. The importance of applying culturally relevant frameworks in diagnosis cannot be overstated, as this enhances rapport building with clients and enables one to better understand their experiences, resulting in better treatment results (Groenier et al., 2011).

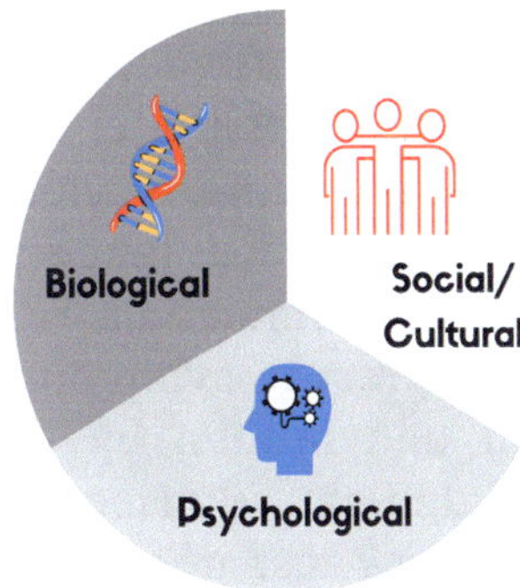

Figure 3.13. Cultural considerations are paramount in the diagnostic process.

Source: https://s3-us-west-2.amazonaws.com/courses-images/wp-content/uploads/sites/5351/2020/08/28140134/Screen-Shot-2020-08-27-at-1.41.29-PM.png.

While recognizing the place that cultural stories occupy in the diagnostic process, there is a requirement to differentiate between idiographic and narrative judgment as frameworks for understanding individual experiences. Narrative judgment encompasses the client's life story and social circumstances, therefore allowing a fuller, more complete understanding of their mental health. Individualistic judgment idiographic approaches, however, compromise the validity of psychiatric diagnoses by simplifying complex cultural influences. According to the World Psychiatric Association, emphasizing narrative constructions helps in situating individual symptoms within broader cultural frames, hence providing more trustworthy diagnoses and effective treatment plans. Focusing on narrative more than on idiographic aspects allows clinicians to construct a broader understanding of clients experience and integrate requisite cultural variables into diagnostic formulations (Thornton, 2008) (Figure 3.13).

3.5.3. The Role of Stigma in Diagnostic Processes

Stigma is also very critical in the diagnosis process in mental health, often influencing the attitudes of the patients and the health professionals. Continuing societal stigma concerning mental disorders hinders definitive diagnosis and case formulation. For instance, individuals will present symptoms that are underreported and hidden by the fear of labeling or judgment. Consequently, such reluctance can skew test outcomes, resulting in over-classification or simplification of complex mental health issues. Application of a diagnostic method poorly adapted to take into account the impact of stigma may lead to a severe deficiency in understanding the intricate nature of mental illnesses. The limitation of traditional categorizations points to the need for changing frameworks that incorporate stigma as well as diagnostic criteria so that mental health assessments can be better made within a clinical context (Dalgleish et al., 2020). Furthermore, as far as contemporary mental health paradigms strive for a more discriminating understanding, the lingering impacts of stigma call for urgent consideration. Stigmatization also overlaps with the cultural domains of mental health, presenting the challenge to practitioners of making a distinction between culturally specific features and true psychopathology. Intersectionality of this overlap provides a challenge to diagnosis because athletes, for example, will present mental health symptoms inextricably intertwined with their performance environments. Inappropriately not making such identifications will lead to interventions that are not holistic or responsive to the person's experience or the biopsychosocial factors. In bypassing rigid diagnostic boundaries, a transdiagnostic model, with greater emphasis on shared underlying processes rather than static categories, might offer a path to reduced stigma and more effective case formulations in clinical practice (Claudia et al., 2019). In consideration of these difficulties, mental health clinicians must navigate stigma sensitively through the diagnosis process. Educating clients and clinicians about the nature of mental disorders can reverse the deleterious effects and build a more embracing treatment environment. Additionally, including stigma-awareness within diagnostic processes allows for a thorough assessment that takes into account an individual's lived experience, rather than merely their symptoms. Stigma in the model of diagnosis is directed not merely to promote a more accurate profile of mental health disease but also to facilitate a therapeutic relationship of positive help. As paradigms for mental health evolve towards less rigid and more open models, responding to the role of stigma is included in improving diagnostic accuracy and consequently the quality of care (Dalgleish et al., 2020).

Test Your Knowledge

1. How do comorbidity, overlapping symptoms, and cultural variations create difficulties for accurate psychiatric diagnosis?
2. What ethical and practical challenges arise from potential diagnostic bias, stigma, and limitations of current classification systems?

3.6. Case Formulation Process

Learning Outcome

1. Gathering relevant information.
2. Identifying key issues and patterns.
3. Developing a treatment plan.

Case formulation is a critical coming together of diagnosis and treatment within mental health practice. It is a reflexive and iterative process, rooted in an integration of knowledge acquired during diagnostic interviews and prolonged client contact. A well-formulated case both detects presenting problems and deals with underlying causation, thereby enabling practitioners to tailor interventions more precisely to the needs of individual clients. When therapists communicate with the patient, they get to know the client's emotional, cognitive, and interpersonal patterns that are part of building a robust and rich assessment of their condition. The Psychodynamic Diagnostic Manual demonstrates this process of integration by placing priority not just on symptom classification, but also on the dynamics underlying (Nancy et al., 2018). This order of analysis informs a treatment plan directed by both nomothetic (typically applicable) and idiographic (individual-specific) knowledge, this dichotomy optimizing the therapeutic effect. Working within the bounds of case formulation, psychologists utilize an orderly but responsive diagnostic procedure to comprehend and manage clients' concerns. An experiment of psychologists engaging in mock diagnostic interviews testifies to the dynamic. The participants underwent comprehensive evaluations that addressed various aspects of clients' presentations, including symptomatic presentations and potential causative factors. Though there was concurrence on classifications, there was variability in the causative factors' explanations and treatment approaches (Groenier et al., 2011). This reflective component to this case formulation emphasizes treatment flexibility; psychologists will be obliged to reassess their knowledge and approach as they react to clients. With such an adaptive diagnostic technique, clinicians create a yet more specific methodology, eventually resulting in a more engaged client and success rate. Furthermore, the process of case formulation is not a linear one but rather a continual dialogue between the clinician and the client. This recurrent looping back and forth creates the space in which to revise the plan for treatment as new insights come to the fore in the course of the therapeutic relationship. Clinicians are required to balance conformity with standardized diagnostic classification with responsiveness to the specificity of each case. Lesson attainment from systematic case formulation can make it possible to identify patterns that are not directly obvious on the surface, thereby illuminating treatment directions that resonate within clients' individual settings. Combining detailed diagnostic assessment with awareness of clients' psychosocial settings also points to the requirement of addressing a range of variables in a client's life as part of effective case formulation (Nancy et al., 2018). Lastly, by creating an open, responsive pattern of diagnosis and case conceptualization, mental health clinicians become more capable of serving their clients, laying the foundation for more authentic and effective therapy.

3.6.1. Gathering Pertinent Information

The process of gathering pertinent information is an essential component in case formulation and diagnosis. It involves a methodical gathering of data that traverses clinical presentations, as well as patient history. Not only does it help make informed diagnoses, but it also guides tailored treatment plans. Among all the sources of data, a patient's account is pivotal in giving information on their experiences, symptoms, and issues. Mental health professionals, for instance, employ systematic interviews and questionnaires to gather comprehensive information. The information efficiently gives a structure for understanding the complexities of a patient's condition, thus enhancing the process of diagnosis. Establishing comprehensive information through such detail-oriented effort also forms a therapeutic relationship, as it informs the patient that their input counts and will finally dictate the direction of their treatment. Complementing subjective patient data, objective data , such as laboratory tests, imaging, and physical examination play a crucial role in the process of gathering relevant information. Such objective measures serve to corroborate or negate clinical assumptions based on patients' own descriptions of their condition. For example, laboratory tests may identify biomarkers for pathologies underlying, and imaging may unveil anatomical malformations not detectable through palpation. This double approach of integrating subjective and objective data not only enhances diagnostic validity but also informs effective intervention. It consolidates practitioners in their case formulation exercise, allowing them to take on a multi-faceted appreciation of the patient's health profile. It is therefore critical that guarded integration of these varied sources of information is at the core of the process of formulating a comprehensive appreciation of the patient's condition. Moreover, during the period of evolving medical technology, advanced methods are revolutionizing the acquisition of relevant information. The formation of nanomedicine is the best model demonstrating the ways in which new technologies can improve diagnostic precision and therapeutic responsiveness. Nanotechnology makes it possible to deliver drugs site-specifically and enhance the therapy efficacy of long-term diseases by facilitating greater targeting of disease targets. This technology is only one of the numerous changes brought by introducing advanced scientific approaches to the clinic. Furthermore, as is being shown in recent studies, the application of nanomedicines to improve the effectiveness of existing drugs and specificity in diagnosing disease is a test of the worth of gathering robust, multidimensional data. As the healthcare sector continues to change, the ability to draw from such new modes of information gathering will be key to guiding effective diagnosis and case conceptualization and ultimately better patient outcomes (Patra et al., 2018 Unger et al., 2020) (Figure 3.14).

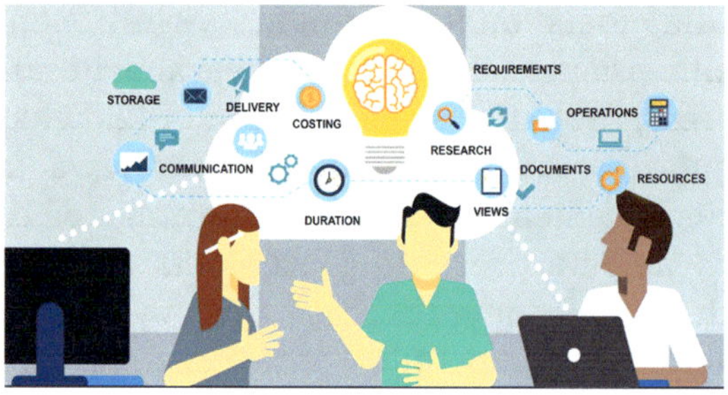

Figure 3.14. The process of gathering relevant information.

Source: https://tigosoftware.com/sites/default/files/2022-09/2004186454_1VIpBEzevOX0YO7Rked6SkA.png.

3.6.2. Identifying Key Issues and Patterns

In case formulation and diagnosis, establishing key themes and issues is a critical pillar of effective clinical understanding. Professionals will be required to perform efficient data collection, such as the history of the patient, presenting complaints, and psychosocial concerns affecting the well-being of the patient. The ability to establish common themes among these factors not only contributes to the development of effective diagnoses but also to the formation of individualized treatment strategies. For instance, trends in a patient's demographic history and lifestyle are generally predictive of emergent underlying risk factors that will influence both the onset and development of mental health issues. Therefore, an empirical method of observing such trends is an essential skill for clinicians to learn, facilitating complete interventions that include symptom and underlying cause. Aside from this, the incorporation of empirical evidence is equally important when it comes to making decisions about the most important concerns regarding patient care. Research has established that several factors , such as genetic predispositions and environmental influences, play significant roles in determining the health trajectory of individuals. Through the integration of findings from recent research, including advances in nanomedicine as characterized by recent reviews, clinicians can optimize their understanding of disease mechanisms as well as treatment efficacy. For example, an understanding of how some nanoparticles may support drug delivery systems is valuable in the pursuit of maximizing therapeutic modalities for long-term conditions (Patra et al., 2018). As such, health professionals must remain abreast with scientific developments and best practices of evidence-based medicine to improve their diagnostic and clinical abilities. Finally, the recursive nature of diagnosis calls for continual reflection and reconsideration of known key issues and patterns. With new data emerging during the process of treatment, clinicians must be adaptable, ready to revise their formulation in response to evolving patient needs. Continual assessment is particularly critical in the case of complicated symptomology, where the interplay of numerous variables will generate non-linear patterns of change in health. Adoption of guideline models, such as those provided by the European Society of Cardiology and the European Society of Hypertension, places particular emphasis on evidence-based care (Williams et al., 2018). By adherence to them, professionals are able to systematically assign priority concerns the highest concerns in patient diagnosis, ultimately contributing to improved evaluation and better health outcomes. Thus, the dynamic nature of the diagnostic and case formulation highlights the necessity to monitor closely the identification of overriding patterns in the process.

3.6.3. Developing a Treatment Plan

Creation of an effective treatment plan is naturally linked with thorough diagnosis and case formulation. The effective treatment plan begins with a clear understanding of the problems of the client, which has to be preceded by a thorough assessment encompassing biological, psychological, and sociocultural elements. Inadequate intake assessment can lead to flaws that render the treatment implemented ineffective. Research indicates that therapists collect key client information but may not always delve into these biopsychosocial variables in depth, making assessments incomplete and weakening case conceptualizations (Jeffrey, 2019).

Clinicians must then refine their intake processes to collect and integrate relevant information in depth, eventually developing a sound foundation for the treatment plan. In addition, treatment plan development should be iterative and adaptive, considering specific client needs and therapeutic objectives. With case formulation as an overarching framework, clinicians can adapt interventions to meet the client's particular context, preference, and culture. Thematic Mapping presents a potential model for structuring treatment plans that not only addresses clinical symptoms but also honors culturally sensitive concerns (Jeffrey, 2019).

The adaptable strategy encourages therapists to engage clients in an active role in the development of treatment plans, which can be used to encourage motivation and increase adherence to recommended interventions. A successful treatment plan is therefore an interactive and collaborative process between client and clinician. Finally, the treatment plan must be regularly monitored and updated according to ongoing reviews and progress of the client. Treatment effectiveness largely relies on the clinician's capacity to monitor outcomes and recognize when changes are necessary. Effective case formulations, as revealed in research, emphasize the requirement for constant integration of new client information into treatment plans (Meyer & Melchert, 2011). This responsive adaptability not only optimizes treatment outcomes but also liberates clients via legitimation of their experience and validation of their agency in recovery. In summary, the development of a treatment plan is an intricate process that requires a reflective balancing of systematic assessment, cultural sensitivity, client involvement, and continuous review (Figure 3.15).

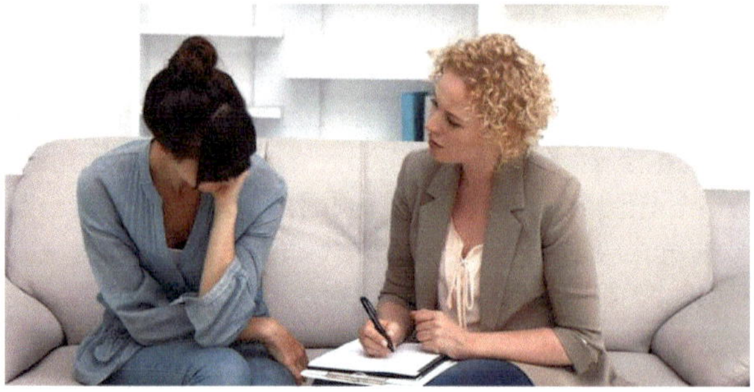

Figure 3.15. Developing a treatment plan.

Source: https://positive.b-cdn.net/wp-content/uploads/mental-health-treatment-plans.jpg.

Test Your Knowledge

1. What essential components make up a comprehensive case formulation, such as predisposing, precipitating, perpetuating, and protective factors?
2. How does case formulation guide individualized treatment planning and improve clinical decision-making?

SUMMARY

A focus on diagnosis and case formulation, it is important to rethink the complexity underpinning clinical practice and methods employed in mental health environments. The utility of diagnostic tools is dependent upon their ability to find true psychopathology and not bogus positives, an issue considered within recent controversy over psychopathy measures. As depicted in Larsen et al. (2018), the research findings' validity is directly related to the specificity of the diagnostic entries. This underscores the importance of using standardized diagnostic criteria capable of precluding discrepancies across studies as well as boosting the trustworthiness of treatment plans. Ultimately, the combined framework for diagnosis helps practitioners develop appropriate interventions tailored to individual cases, which ensures that the therapeutic process remains evidence-based and morally sound. Secondly, integration of idiographic and narrative judgements is crucial to complete comprehension of psychiatric assessment. Promotion by the World Psychiatric Associations of an idiographic strategy intimates the part played by personal narratives in building up clinical understanding. Yet, as cited in Thornton (2008), a combination of idiographic judgement with narrative assessment has the potential to invalidate psychiatric diagnoses. Instead, narrative judgement offers a further way of knowing clinical material by way of a paradigm that acknowledges individual experience alongside broader psychological models. In maintaining this delineation, therapists are better positioned to respond to the complexities of mental health, and thus facilitate more effective diagnostic and formulation strategies that authentically represent the complexity of each patient's experience. Overall, a successful conclusion to diagnosis and case formulation involves a blend of methodological accuracy and individual narrative. The findings of the current investigation make it clear that future innovation in psychiatric treatment must center on the design of accurate assessment tools, with regard to consideration of the significance of individual context in the therapeutic relationship. Emphasizing the necessity of both narrative and criterion-based judgments fits with the evolving nature of mental health treatment and research. Refinement of these methods may decrease the effects of false positives and overall enhance psychiatric diagnosis quality, ultimately resulting in improved patient outcomes and growth in the field of mental health treatment.

The case formulation and diagnostic process of psychological assessment is a thorough investigation of several factors to achieve an understanding of a person's mental health state. Central to the process is the determination of the prevalent disorders of Attention Deficit Hyperactivity Disorder (ADHD), with high heritability and often underdiagnosed in both children and adults. As revealed in recent studies, the rate of prevalence for ADHD is roughly 5.29% among children and 2.5% among adults, which highlights the importance of mental health practitioners being knowledgeable about both the diagnosis and the treatment of the disorder. In addition, comprehension of the multi-factorial etiology of ADHD, including genetics and the environment, is critical to effective case formulation and intervention planning. These results allow more thorough diagnosis so that treatment can be tailored individually to work with patient outcomes and long-term plans for management (Camilleri & Makhoul, 2013). The need for revising diagnostic criteria to accommodate the varied demands of the individual is mentioned in literature on psychological adaptations following brain injury. Cognitive, affective, and interpersonal changes not only complicate assessment but also necessitate adaptation to therapeutic techniques. A critique of suggestions for therapy adjustment demonstrated that CBT therapy is typically in need of alteration when working with post-injury emotional issues. The adjustments involve education in therapy, communication adjustment, and enhancements to assist memory and executive function. By acknowledging these required accommodations, clinicians can apply strategies that more effectively address the distinctive impediments encountered by patients with brain injuries, thus increasing the efficacy of psychological therapies and making treatment more relevant and effective (Gallagher et al., 2019). In conclusion, the connection between diagnosis and case formulation is paramount in the formation of effective treatment plans in mental healthcare. The convergence of successive studies underscores the necessity of clinicians learning the complexities implicated in various disorders, such as ADHD and head injury. This awareness makes it easier to conduct well-rounded assessments that take into account genetic influences as well as environmental factors. Furthermore, the incorporation of evidence-based treatment modifications within therapeutic modalities makes it possible for practitioners to be sufficiently equipped with skills to address the individualistic needs of their patients, resulting in better therapeutic outcomes. This double focus on diagnostic accuracy and personalized treatment plans is a central part of the psychology discipline, driving the best practice and fueling ongoing innovation in mental health interventions (Camilleri & Makhoul, 2013; Gallagher et al., 2019).

KEY TERMS FROM THIS CHAPTER

Antidiuretic hormone (ADH)	Bladder	Bowman's Capsule
Filtration	Glomerulus	Kidneys
Nephrons	Reabsorption	Renal Cortex
Renal Medulla	Secretion	Ureters
Urethra	Urinary system	Urine

CRITICAL THINKING QUESTIONS

1. What is the primary goal of case formulation in clinical practice?

a. To write a prescription

b. To understand and organize information about the client's problems for treatment planning

c. To perform laboratory investigations

d. To provide a legal diagnosis

2. Which of the following is a key component of a diagnostic process in mental health?

a. Identifying physical injuries only

b. Gathering comprehensive history and assessing symptoms

c. Relying solely on psychological tests

d. Administering medication first

3. A differential diagnosis refers to:

a. The process of eliminating alternative diagnoses to reach the correct one

b. A permanent diagnosis made at first meeting

c. Diagnosing only physical illnesses

d. Using only one assessment tool

4. In case formulation, "predisposing factors" refer to:

a. Immediate triggers for the client's problem

b. Long-term vulnerabilities or risks contributing to the problem

c. Protective factors against illness

d. Factors that maintain the problem over time

5. Which model is commonly used for psychological case formulation?

a. Biopsychosocial model

b. Biomedical model only

c. Legal model

d. Mathematical model

Short Answer Questions

1. What is the purpose of diagnosis in clinical practice?
2. Define case formulation and explain how it differs from diagnosis.
3. Why is it important to consider biopsychosocial factors in case formulation?
4. What are the main components of a good case formulation?
5. How can cultural factors influence diagnosis and formulation?

Answer to Critical Thinking Questions

1. (b) 2. (b) 3. (a) 4. (b) 5. (a)

REFERENCES

1. Alexander, J., Baguley, I., Hope, R., et al. (2007). New ways of working in acute inpatient care: A case for change. https://core.ac.uk/download/56059.pdf (accessed on 28th July 2025).
2. Angelini, A., Berry, G. J., Bruneval, P., et al. (2017). The XIIIth Banff Conference on Allograft Pathology: The Banff 2015 Heart Meeting Report: Improving antibody-mediated rejection diagnostics: Strengths, unmet needs, and future directions. https://core.ac.uk/download/323077046.pdf (accessed on 28th July 2025).
3. Anurogo, D., Ikrar, T., & Parikesit, A. A. (2017). Bionanomedicine: A "panacea" in medicine? https://media.neliti.com/media/publications/179998-EN-none.pdf (accessed on 28th July 2025).
4. Atmaca, M., Fineberg, N. A., Fontenelle, L. F., et al. (2016). The classification of obsessive–compulsive and related disorders in the ICD-11. https://core.ac.uk/download/213085588.pdf (accessed on 28th July 2025).
5. Barlow, D. H., Boettcher, H. T., Bullis, J. R., et al. (2017). Current definitions of "transdiagnostic" in treatment development: A search for consensus. https://open.bu.edu/bitstream/2144/40041/1/Current%20Definitions%20of%20Transdiagnostic%20-%206-10%20FINAL.pdf (accessed on 28th July 2025).
6. Beerthuis, R. J., Groenier, M., Pieters, J. M., et al. (2011). Psychologists' diagnostic processes during a diagnostic interview. https://core.ac.uk/download/pdf/11488565.pdf Groenier, M. , Beerthuis, V. , Pieters, J. , M Witteman, C. and Swinkels, J. (2011) Psychologists' Diagnostic Processes during a Diagnostic Interview. Psychology, 2, 917-924. doi: 10.4236/psych.2011.29138. (accessed on 28th July 2025).
7. Bellak, L., Benjamin, L. S., Cierpka, M., Crits-Christoph, P., Fleiss, J. L., Foa, U. G., Rudolf, G., et al. (2007). The operationalized psychodynamic diagnostics system: Clinical relevance, reliability and validity. https://core.ac.uk/download/10115.pdf (accessed on 28th July 2025).
8. Palmieri, Arianna & Kleinbub, Johann & Benelli, Enrico & Sambin, Marco & Broggio, Alice & Bianco, Simone. (2015). THE WORDS OF THE BODY: PSYCHOPHYSIOLOGICAL PATTERNS IN DISSOCIATIVE NARRATIVES. (accessed on 28th July 2025).
9. Bhui, K., Johnson, M., McCabe, R., et al. (2013). THERACOM: A systematic review of the evidence base for interventions to improve therapeutic communications between Black and minority ethnic populations and staff in specialist mental health services. https://core.ac.uk/download/30696864.pdf (accessed on 28th July 2025).
10. Blagov, B., Bornstein, R., Colli, A., Gazzillo, P., Gazzillo, F., et al. (2015). The Psychodynamic Diagnostic Manual–2nd edition (PDM-2). https://core.ac.uk/download/54517792.pdf (accessed on 28th July 2025).
11. Brudka, C., Bąkowska, E., Czepkiewicz, M., et al. (2016). Public participation GIS for sustainable urban mobility planning: Methods, applications and challenges. https://core.ac.uk/download/154444688.pdf (accessed on 28th July 2025).
12. Burrell-Hodgson, G., Fowler, B., Jones, S. H., et al. (2006). Personality disorder in primary care: Factors associated with therapy process and outcome. https://core.ac.uk/download/68622.pdf (accessed on 28th July 2025).

13. Busse, R., Drummond, M., Gurtner, F., et al. (2002). Best practice in undertaking and reporting health technology assessments: Working Group 4 report. https://core.ac.uk/download/58882.pdf (accessed on 28th July 2025).
14. Camilleri, N., & Makhoul, S. (2013). ADHD: From childhood into adulthood. https://core.ac.uk/download/46602345.pdf (accessed on 28th July 2025).
15. Charlesworth, G. M. (2004). Keeping conceptualizations simple: Examples with family carers of people with dementia. https://core.ac.uk/download/1756419.pdf (accessed on 28th July 2025).
16. Corti, L., & Couto, D. (2020). Contextualism in context: Interview with Michael Williams. https://core.ac.uk/download/286357393.pdf (accessed on 28th July 2025).
17. Cox, A. (2021). Clinical case conceptualization skill development and counseling pedagogy: A constructivist grounded theory study. https://core.ac.uk/download/534838714.pdf (accessed on 28th July 2025).
18. Dalgleish, T., Black, M., Johnston, D., & Bevan, A. (2020). Transdiagnostic approaches to mental health problems: Current status and future directions. Journal of Consulting and Clinical Psychology, 88, 179–195. https://doi.org/10.1037/ccp0000482 (accessed on 28th July 2025).
19. Daza-Cardona, J. A. (2022). Las clasificaciones en la formación psiquiátrica: Una aproximación postcolonial. https://core.ac.uk/download/524940337.pdf (accessed on 28th July 2025).
20. de Jeu, R. A. M., Dolman, A. J., Miralles, D., et al. (2017). Global soil moisture bimodality in satellite observations and climate models. https://core.ac.uk/download/84044966.pdf (accessed on 28th July 2025).
21. Dickens, G. L., & O'Shea, L. E. (2016). Use of the HCR-20 for violence risk assessment: Views of clinicians working in a secure inpatient mental health setting. https://core.ac.uk/download/228177613.pdf (accessed on 28th July 2025).
22. Dickens, G. L., Marriott, R., O'Shea, L. E., et al. (2017). Predictive validity of the Short-Term Assessment of Risk and Treatability (START) for multiple adverse outcomes: The effect of diagnosis. https://core.ac.uk/download/228178029.pdf (accessed on 28th July 2025).
23. Etien, A., Nadali, A., van der Raadt, B., Minoli, D., Sledgianowski, D., Őri, D., Umoh, E., et al. (2019). Business and information technology alignment measurement–A recent literature review. http://arxiv.org/abs/1905.02349 (accessed on 28th July 2025).
24. Ferreira, J., Leitão, J., & Raposo, M. (2025). The role of entrepreneurial universities in interfacing competitive advantages: The case of Beira Interior region (Portugal). https://core.ac.uk/download/pdf/6803533.pdf (accessed on 28th July 2025).
25. Fleming, K. A., Horton, S., Wilson, M. L., Atun, R., DeStigter, K., Flanigan, J., Sayed, S., et al. (2021). The Lancet Commission on diagnostics: Transforming access to diagnostics. The Lancet, 398, 1997–2050. https://doi.org/10.1016/s0140-6736(21)00673-5 (accessed on 28th July 2025).
26. Gallagher, M., McLeod, H. J., & McMillan, T. M. (2019). A systematic review of recommended modifications of CBT for people with cognitive impairments following brain injury. https://core.ac.uk/download/74230400.pdf (accessed on 28th July 2025).
27. Heine, S. J., Ryder, A. G., & Yang, J. (2002). Somatization vs. psychologization of emotional distress: A paradigmatic example for cultural psychopathology. https://core.ac.uk/

download/10687096.pdf (accessed on 28th July 2025).

28. Hooker, M. (2009). How can I encourage multi-stakeholder narrative and reflection on the use of ICT in teacher professional development programmed in Rwanda? https://core.ac.uk/download/11310314.pdf (accessed on 28th July 2025).

29. Howes, O., Thase, M. E., & Pillinger, T. (2021). Treatment resistance in psychiatry: State of the art and new directions. Molecular Psychiatry, 27, 58–72. https://doi.org/10.1038/s41380-021-01200-3 (accessed on 28th July 2025).

30. Thornton T. (2008). Does understanding individuals require idiographic judgement?. European archives of psychiatry and clinical neuroscience, 258 Suppl 5, 104–109. https://doi.org/10.1007/s00406-008-5018-y (accessed on 28th July 2025).

31. Jeffrey, C. E. (2019). Thematic mapping in case conceptualization: A test of clinical efficacy. https://core.ac.uk/download/186715173.pdf (accessed on 28th July 2025).

32. McWilliams, N., & Lingiardi, V. (2018). Introduction to the special issue on the Psychodynamic Diagnostic Manual, 2nd edition (PDM-2): The PDM. Yesterday, today, tomorrow. https://core.ac.uk/download/158327594.pdf (accessed on 28th July 2025).

33. Meyer, L., & Melchert, T. P. (2011). Examining the content of mental health intake assessments from a biopsychosocial perspective. *Journal of Psychotherapy Integration, 21*(1), 70–89. https://doi.org/10.1037/a0022907 (accessed on 28th July 2025).

34. Merok, E., & Andresen, N. A. (2025). Back to the future–The marginal utility of history in economics. https://core.ac.uk/download/pdf/6989812.pdf (accessed on 28th July 2025).

35. Owen, C. (2016). PTSD from childhood trauma as a precursor to attachment issues. https://core.ac.uk/download/129592830.pdf (accessed on 28th July 2025).

36. Patra, J. K., Das, G., Fraceto, L. F., Campos, E. V. R., Rodriguez-Torres, M. P., Acosta-Torres, L. S., Díaz-Torres, L. A., et al. (2018). Nano based drug delivery systems: Recent developments and future prospects. Journal of Nanobiotechnology, 16. https://doi.org/10.1186/s12951-018-0392-8 (accessed on 28th July 2025).

37. Reardon, C. L., Hainline, B., Aron, C. M., Baron, D., Baum, A., Bindra, A., Budgett, R., et al. (2019). Mental health in elite athletes: International Olympic Committee consensus statement (2019). British Journal of Sports Medicine, 53, 667–699. https://doi.org/10.1136/bjsports-2019-100715 (accessed on 28th July 2025).

38. Rosenberg Larsen, R. (2018). False-positives in psychopathy assessment: Proposing theory-driven exclusion criteria in research sampling. https://core.ac.uk/download/186331457.pdf (accessed on 28th July 2025).

39. Sheikh, A., Kalra, D., Coyne, J., Cresswell, K., & Morrison, Z. (2012). "There are too many, but never enough": Qualitative case study investigating routine coding of clinical information in depression. https://core.ac.uk/download/16219262.pdf (accessed on 28th July 2025).

40. Thornton, T. (2008). Should comprehensive diagnosis include idiographic understanding? https://core.ac.uk/download/341079.pdf (accessed on 28th July 2025).

41. Till, C. (2011). The quantification of gender: Anorexia nervosa and femininity. https://core.ac.uk/download/29018324.pdf (accessed on 28th July 2025).

42. Unger, T., Borghi, C., Charchar, F. J., Khan, N., Poulter, N. R., Prabhakaran, D., Ramiréz, A. J., et al. (2020). 2020 International Society of Hypertension global hypertension practice guidelines. Journal of Hypertension, 38, 982–1004. https://doi.org/10.1097/hjh.0000000000002453 (accessed on 28th July 2025).

43. Williams, B., Mancia, G., Spiering, W., Agabiti Rosei, E., Azizi, M., Burnier, M., Clement, D. L., et al. (2018). 2018 ESC/ESH guidelines for the management of arterial hypertension. European Heart Journal, 39, 3021–3104. https://doi.org/10.1093/eurheartj/ehy339 (accessed on 28th July 2025).

SCHIZOPHRENIA AND PSYCHOTIC DISORDERS

4

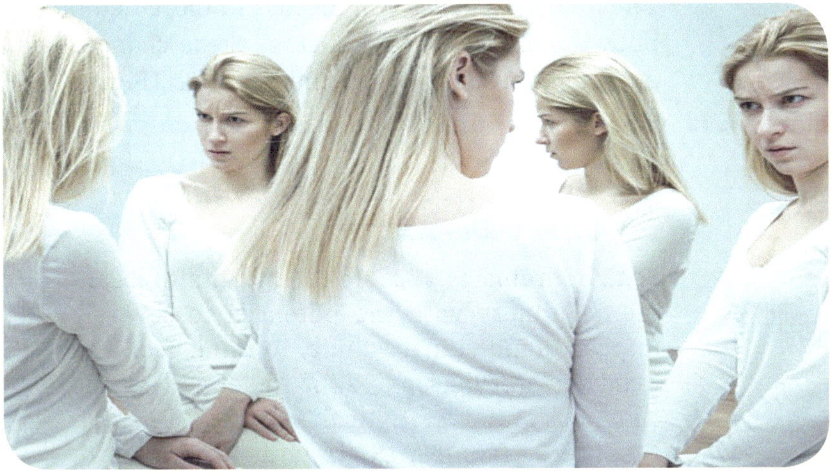

LEARNING OBJECTIVES

After studying this chapter, you will be able to:

1. Give historical context;
2. Identify symptoms of schizophrenia;
3. List the causes and risk factors;
4. Explore diagnosis and assessment;
5. Explain treatment options;
6. List the impact on daily life.

Introduction

Understanding schizophrenia and psychotic disorders entails not only knowledge of their clinical presentations but also the evolving models used in their classification and diagnosis. Schizophrenia, that severe mental illness formerly categorized under the International Classification of Diseases (ICD-10), has had broad revisions since the advent of the newly released ICD-11. These changes encompass a reshuffled structure, new diagnostic criteria, and inclusion of dimensional features like course and symptom qualifiers. With WHO member states beginning to implement these changes, there is a need to consider how the changes will affect clinical practice and patient outcomes. Therefore, the first half of this essay aims to situate these advances in the broader context of psychotic disorders, setting the stage for a critical evaluation of their clinical importance and applicability in modern-day psychiatry (Kerst et al., 2020). The significance of distinguishing between various psychotic disorders lies in the fact that diagnostic criteria formulated in the ICD-10 have been superseded by their updated counterparts in the ICD-11. The literature is consistent regarding how some symptomatological patterns can be utilized to differentiate schizophrenia from other non-affective psychotic disorders. An example of 1,476 in-patients demonstrates that schizophrenia patients are likely to present with severe negative symptoms and lower global functioning compared to patients diagnosed with other disorders , such as persistent delusional disorders and schizoaffective disorders. This distinction not only represents an articulation of the descriptive accuracy of the ICD-10 classification but also reflects the importance of understanding variation in psychotic disorders.

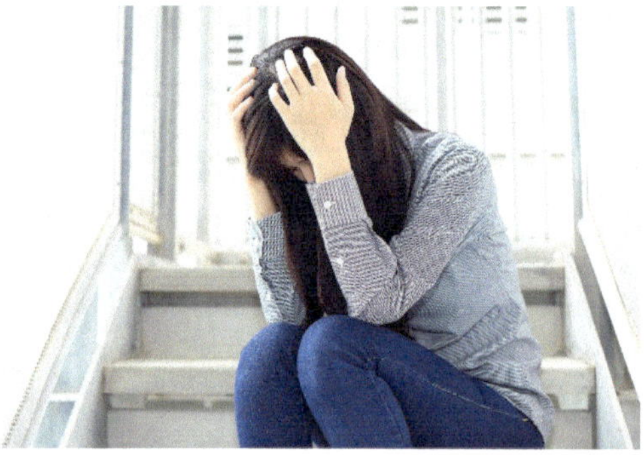

Figure 4.1. Psychotic disorder.

Source: https://medlineplus.gov/images/PsychoticDisorders_share.jpg.

A systematic exposition of schizophrenia and psychotic disorders is thus needed to convey such diagnostic subtleties and their implications for best treatment (Bottlender et al., 2003). In defining the problems of schizophrenia and psychotic disorders, it is also important to take into account the social misconceptions and stigmatization that usually follow such diagnoses. Misconceptions about the condition can lead to fear and stigmatization on the part of society, making it difficult for those who have it to deal with their daily lives and to be treated. Further, the inclusion of ICD-11 offers a chance for more sophisticated public education and campaign efforts. Societal stigma of schizophrenia is the most significant issue to resolve if individuals are to be encouraged to present themselves for intervention. It is not merely about the clinical solution that this introductory section outlines, but also about highlighting the social element of mental illness, which is of greatest significance to the well-balanced perspective of schizophrenia and psychotic disorders in contemporary society. The following pages will discuss in more detail both the clinical significance of these changes and their broader social implications (Figure 4.1).

Definition of Schizophrenia and Psychotic Disorders

Schizophrenia is a complex and multifaceted mental illness with the potential to severely impact an individual's ability to think, feel, and behave. Schizophrenia, as it is defined by the Diagnostic and Statistical Manual of Mental Disorders (DSM-5), exists with symptoms of delusions, hallucinations, disorganized speech, and lack of functionality. These symptoms develop in late adolescence or early adulthood, leading to significant social and occupational impairment. Psychotic disorders, of which schizophrenia is the best-known type, represent a broader group of conditions that encompass distorted thought and perception of reality. Identification of schizophrenia from other psychotic disorders is significant because it allows for the development of customized treatment plans. Overall, knowledge of the clinical presentation of schizophrenia is crucial to proper diagnosis and treatment. The onset of schizophrenia and other psychotic disorders could be extensive, influencing the treatment process and outcome. It has been highlighted in research that recovery from severe mental illnesses (SMI) is multi-dimensional, encompassing both objective and subjective components. In individuals diagnosed with schizophrenia, recovery extends beyond symptom remission, as it is intrinsically linked with meaning-making at the personal level and individual-level experiences of living. From what is known, one of the greatest challenges in recovering knowledge from these disorders arises from the differential operationalization of recovery itself. Some only assess those factors that are quantifiable, while others lay out measures on subjective processes that also need to be targeted within treatment models. Knowledge of the dual nature of schizophrenia allows clinicians to develop more integrated treatment plans that address both the symptoms and underlying emotional and psychological requirements of patients, promoting a more comprehensive recovery process (Hamm et al., 2017). The implications of understanding schizophrenia as both a clinical diagnosis and an intricate subjective experience extend into many of the treatments employed. Clinicians and caregivers must balance objective outcomes against subjective experience to provide the most effective therapeutic effect. This involves not only addressing clinical symptoms of schizophrenia but also establishing environments in which patients can obtain meaning-making processes conducive to recovery. Addressing both sides could prevent harm to a patient's recovery and facilitate resilience. To professionals in mental health and researchers, the study of both objective and subjective accounts in recovery highlights the need for a combined approach to psychotic disorders. It is this integration of objective and subjective recovery mechanisms that will be instrumental to reframing recovery meaning in schizophrenia and psychotic disorders (Giacco et al., 2007).

Importance of Understanding These Mental Illnesses

Understanding schizophrenia and other psychotic disorders is the foundation of successful intervention and support, both for the patients and their families. Not only do these illnesses disrupt the life of the persons that suffer from them, but they also impose a severe emotional and economic burden upon their relatives. A perception of the complexities of these diseases, varying from genetic predispositions, environmental conditions, and psychological fragilities, can enable an integrative treatment and rehabilitation. Mental health professionals must walk the thin line between drug management and personal recovery strategies, as physical health is vital to overall wellness. To guarantee that patients receive enough information and support regarding the treatment options at their disposal, mental health nurses play an important part in facilitating an educated decision-making process. This is indicative of a broader dedication to treating mental health within the framework of whole-person care, thus creating a foundation for healthier populations (Bressington et al., 2015). Furthermore, awareness of psychotic disorders is important in avoiding stigmatization of mental illness. Misunderstanding of diseases like schizophrenia can lead to social exclusion, discrimination, and inappropriate treatment. Education is an effective tool in breaking down such barriers since greater awareness can increase empathy and decrease fear of mental illness. Public health efforts need to focus on mental health literacy, providing communities with information on the symptoms, signs, and treatment available for mental illnesses. This transition towards being more inclusive benefits not only people who have schizophrenia but also encourages a support culture and understanding that is necessary for societal health. Understanding that mental health occurs on a continuum with both illness and wellness can enable patients to access the care they require without suffering from stigma, ultimately enhancing the quality of life for all parties involved (Jenkins et al., 2008). Finally, having these mental illnesses in mind offers methods of research and policy development around effective management strategies. The pathophysiology of schizophrenia and psychotic disorders necessitates ongoing examination of empirical evidence informing optimum treatment and care practice. According to the Foresight Project on Mental Capital and Wellbeing, fixing mental health is a matter of recognizing the interrelatedness of individual and societal factors. Regular exploration of medical, psychological, and socio-economic factors can direct policy to improve mental health service delivery and prevention. Furthermore, as we better realize the risk and protective factors underlying mental health, we are able to create strategic interventions that are proactive and reactive in nature and that enhance the delivery of services for individuals affected by psychotic disorders and reduce their overall burden on society (Jenkins et al., 2008) (Figure 4.2).

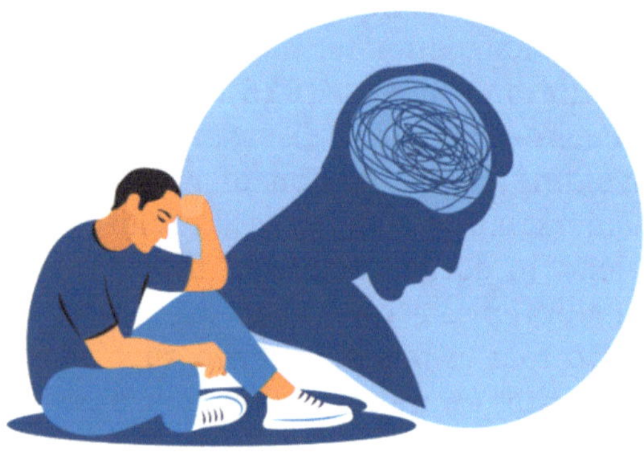

Figure 4.2. Understanding these mental health conditions.

Source: https://www.uab.edu/medicine/news/images/schizophrenia_stock_photo.png.

4.1. Historical Context

Learning Outcome

1. Early perceptions of schizophrenia.
2. Evolution of diagnostic criteria.
3. Key figures in the study of psychotic disorders.

Understanding the history of psychotic disorders and schizophrenia reveals the complex relationship between the societal understanding and clinical practice over time. Originally explained in biomedical terms, the disorder was often attributed to evil spirits or moral failure in ancient times. The stigma of this era has left a continuous story placing individuals with psychotic disorders as other, hence marginalization. Furthermore, revisions in psychiatric diagnostic criteria, particularly with the DSM-III publication, were intended to systematize diagnosis and refine the treatment approach. However, much bias exists both in diagnosis and treatment, particularly among marginalized groups, the necessity of a critical understanding of the historical trajectory in determining mental health illness. This has particularly impacted racialized groups that had in the past faced overdiagnosis and systemic inequalities in mental health care, alluding to the dominant influence of social prejudice on medical choices (Sonya et al., 2023). With the progression of the nineteenth century, the medical field attempted to transcend the moralistic causality of psychosis and instead espoused a scientific direction. But the use of polythetic diagnostic criteria, such as in DSM-IV and DSM-5, has been challenged for their empirical validity. The hoped-for advances in understanding the etiology of schizophrenia and allied disorders have failed to materialize, and this has been followed by criticism of psychiatric nosology. Though the purpose behind all these forms of classification was to improve diagnostic validity, new evidence shows that overreliance on clinical accounts has fallen short in reflecting the intricacies of psychotic illnesses. The lack of anthropological investigations into the practice of diagnosis is a demonstration of the distance between clinical theory and routine practice, and the potential for uncertainties and potentially injurious misdiagnosis. This setting brings forward the pressing need to review diagnostic benchmarks and improve clinician education to offset implicit bias in assessment (Parnas, 2015). With the clinical progress of psychotic illness comes a chronic pattern of racial disparity in diagnosis and treatment. Current research indicates that Black and racialized individuals are excessively diagnosed with schizophrenia compared to their White counterparts. This difference also reflects deeply ingrained social stereotypes and biases that clinicians unconsciously apply to patients. Inadequate race-based care has a long history, further increasing the risk for misdiagnosis, which in turn tends to lead to poor treatment as well as further exposure to the court system. It also complicates the psychiatric treatment process, and such patients may not receive culturally appropriate care. To address these concerns, awareness campaigns and training on the intersection of race and mental health must be accorded top priority. To create an inclusive practice that not only recognizes but also works to dismantle the systemic barriers in mental care, this background needs to be known (Sonya et al., 2023).

4.1.1. Early Views on Schizophrenia

Concepts of schizophrenia in early eras have evolved in great fashion throughout history, usually taking a broad indication of society's beliefs about mental illness. In ancient societies, the symptom-carrying individuals of schizophrenia were usually viewed from the point of view of divine retribution or superstition. This belief assisted in bringing about the stigmatization and isolation of afflicted individuals, who were typically held to be possessed or cursed. The lack of a scientific paradigm to account for these symptoms led to treatments of exorcism or seclusion rather than empathic care. Over time, as medical knowledge changed, attitudes adjusted, permitting a more enlightened perception of schizophrenia as a complex disorder with biopsychosocial etiology. These early perceptions lay the groundwork for current controversies regarding the necessity of dispelling misconceptions and enhancing awareness of psychiatric disorders. Public conceptions of the symptoms of schizophrenia varied broadly, particularly regarding awareness of its associated behaviors and how these influence treatment. The latest studies propose a lack of balance in the public's awareness of some of the symptoms, with minimal positive symptoms , such as hallucinatory behavior and suspiciousness, being readily known by the public to be signs of mental illness. This is restricted knowledge, which may be accompanied by resistance to professional intervention by victims of it, as it is believed that symptoms are not worthy of intervention or treatment by many (Jorm et al., 2013).

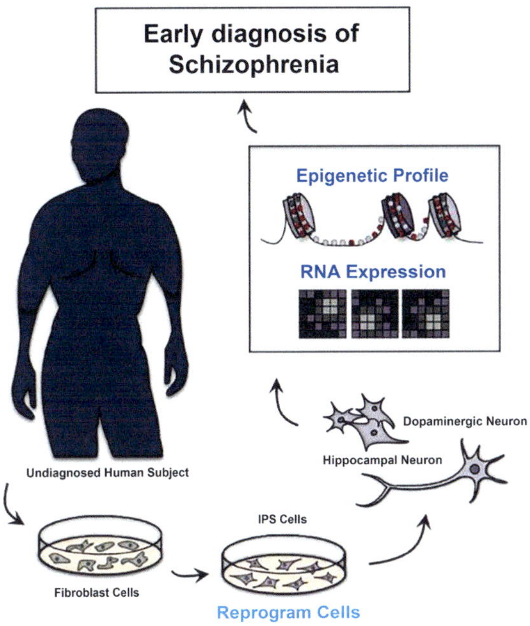

Figure 4.3. The perspectives on early diagnosis of schizophrenia.

Source: https://www.frontiersin.org/files/Articles/756613/fnmol-14-756613-HTML-r1/image_m/fnmol-14-756613-g001.jpg.

Thus, shared understandings can hence hinder early intervention, which is crucial in ensuring the successful management of schizophrenia. Public education and awareness are critical in bridging this gap, for greater understanding of the disorder and in receiving proper help by individuals presenting with symptoms. Moreover, the relationship between illness perceptions and emotional functioning justifies modifying societal attitudes towards schizophrenia. Research has established that negative illness representations predict higher levels of depression and anxiety among individuals presenting with psychosis (Bebbington et al., 2006). This finding underscores the importance of developing healthy recovery and disorder management stories, instead of chronicity and severity. Clinical interventions with insight and healthy treatment attitudes that insist on therapy participation can increase patients' emotional resilience by a significant margin. Reframing initial concepts of schizophrenia, therefore, is not merely a function of familiarity with the disorder, but is essential to facilitate productive coping strategies and support systems that are competent to mediate recovery and improve quality of life (Figure 4.3).

4.1.2. Evolution of Diagnostic Criteria

The evolution of diagnostic criteria for schizophrenia and related psychotic disorders illustrates a complex interplay of medical understanding, cultural context, and scientific advancements. Historically, the classification of psychotic disorders began in the late 19th century, heavily influenced by Emil Kraepelin's systematic approach to psychiatry. His perspectives laid the groundwork for differentiating between distinct forms of mental illness, enabling a more nuanced understanding of psychoses. This historical background has since guided subsequent diagnostic manuals, encouraging the integrationist strategy while addressing the challenge of capturing the disorder's heterogeneity. As researchers have made progress in learning about the neurobiological correlates of schizophrenia, the need for adaptive diagnostic systems has proven critical, attuned to the changing nature of psychiatric theory and science across time. With the emergence of the Diagnostic and Statistical Manual of Mental Disorders (DSM) came an alteration in the diagnostic criteria for schizophrenia and psychotic disorders. Transformations from DSM-III to DSM-5 witnessed significant changes in nomenclature and diagnostic criteria with an aim to enhance specificity and reliability. Interestingly enough, the modern-day definitions have been moving in the direction of emphasis on symptomatology rather than being a historically-based classification, thereby adopting an empirically-oriented approach. However, these changes have not been controversy-free; others indicate that the operationalized criteria lack fidelity to earlier clinical observations. Paranoia and delusional disorders represent paradigmatic cases of this disjunction, in which present criteria do not precisely capture the range of symptoms described in classic psychiatric literature (Kendler, 2017). Moreover, the quest for shared pathogenetic mechanisms of psychotic disorders has given an added perspective to the evolution of diagnostic criteria. On the basis of studies, instead of conceptualizing psychoses as a number of distinct disorders, they can be representations of a single underlying genetic or biological entity, as postulated by new speculations in psychiatric genetics (Crow et al., 1995).

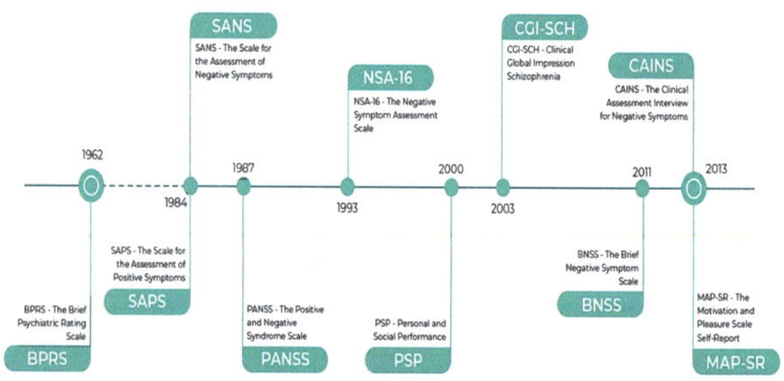

Figure 4.4. The evolution of diagnostic criteria for schizophrenia.

Source: https://schizophrenialife.no/wp-content/uploads/2019/10/Schizophrenia-

Diagnosis_01_Scales_1366px.jpg.

This paradigm shift evokes a more integrated approach in diagnostic practice, perhaps revolutionizing the classification and understanding of these disorders within clinical models. Integrating knowledge from genetics and neuroscience into models of diagnosis may lead to more effective treatment interventions and a deeper understanding of psychotic disorder etiology. Therefore, with the ongoing evolution of the diagnostic criteria, the cross-pollination between past models and today's scientific advancements will remain the most influential factor in shaping the future of schizophrenia and psychotic disorder diagnoses (Figure 4.4).

4.1.3. Key Figures in the Study of Psychotic Disorders

The evolution of psychotic disorders, and more directly schizophrenia, has been determined by the key practitioners in the field whose work has set the benchmark upon which today's knowledge and intervention is based. A primary example is that of Emil Kraepelin, who initially came up with the classification of mental illness and set manic-depressive illness apart from schizophrenia. Kraepelins systematic approach of analysis created a diagnosis classification that has continued to impact. His work emphasized the importance of clinical observation and longitudinal studies, and these vastly enhanced the field. Kraepelin's system of classification, as much as it was amended throughout the years, is still a benchmark in psychiatric diagnosis and informs contemporary methods of studying psychotic disorders. The clarity he introduced to symptomatology and course of illness has allowed subsequent scientists and clinicians to recognize and treat schizophrenia and related disorders more precisely, cementing his position among psychiatry's founders. Sigmund Freud is another essential individual in research on psychotic disorders whose psychoanalytic explanations offered a different perspective on mental illness. Freud's study of the unconscious, repression, and the psychodynamics of internal conflict informed early thinking about schizophrenia. While his methods have been challenged as unsubstantiated, Freud's attention to the subjective experience of people with psychosis has led to additional study of human psychology's complexity. He hypothesized that psychotic behavior could be a reflection of underlying emotional disturbances, thereby laying the groundwork for future psychodynamic therapies. Although some current researchers argue against the relevance of psychoanalytic theory with the advancement of neuroscience, as quoted by Gabbard, the enduring impact of Freud's work on therapeutic practice and understanding patients' experience cannot be dismissed (Lewis, 2008).

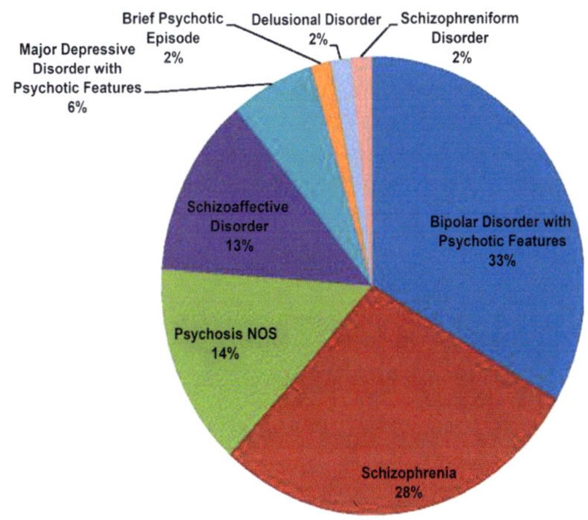

Figure 4.5. Key figures in the study of psychotic disorders.

Source: https://www.researchgate.net/publication/283349096/figure/fig2/AS:293965380243467@1447098216406/Distribution-of-Psychotic-Disorder-Diagnoses-among-EPICENTER-Participants.png.

Furthermore, the regard of pharmacological progress in psychotic disorder conceptualization has been deeply influenced by individuals , such as Albert Hofmann, who originally found lysergic acid diethylamide (LSD). His findings in the 1950s reignited interest in using hallucinogens and the way they could affect mental wellness. The exploration of LSD's impact on perception and cognition has opened the gateways to learning about the neurochemical substrate of schizophrenia, particularly with regard to serotonergic and dopaminergic systems. Since Hofmann's discovery, advances have elucidated how chemicals like LSD interact with brain receptors to yield profound experiences that simulate some psychotic symptoms. Whereas legal restrictions impeded investigation for several decades, more recent research exploits this initial groundwork to examine novel therapeutic use of hallucinogens for the treatment of conditions like anxiety and substance abuse, expanding our knowledge of psychotic illnesses in a larger scientific context (Chan et al., 2013) (Figure 4.5).

Test Your Knowledge

1. How has the understanding of schizophrenia evolved from early medical and supernatural explanations to modern psychiatric models?
2. What major historical developments contributed to changes in how schizophrenia is classified and treated?

4.2. Symptoms of Schizophrenia

Learning Outcome

1. Positive symptoms: hallucinations and delusions.
2. Negative symptoms: emotional flatness and social withdrawal.
3. Cognitive symptoms: impaired memory and attention.

Schizophrenia is characterized by a set of symptoms that can drastically limit one's functioning and quality of life. The primary class of symptoms is positive symptoms, where the prevalence of unusual thoughts and actions are explained. These include hallucinations, where individuals see objects or hear voices that are not present, and delusions, where the existence of beliefs that are false but firmly held in the presence of contrary evidence. For instance, one can be paranoid, having the belief that they are being conspired against or singled out. Such symptoms can lead to upsetting occurrences and also further fuel the people's detachment from reality, complicating their mental illness (Jakovljevi et al., 2009). It is essential to understand such symptoms since they are likely to resonate as guides towards diagnosis and can also direct the treatment strategies aimed at symptom control. Schizophrenia's negative symptoms are also an essential part of the disorder and are more subtle in expression. The symptoms are a loss of emotional response and motivation, leading to social withdrawal and isolation. Anhedonia, or loss of capacity to experience pleasure, and blunting of affects, with a reduced range of emotional expression, are common negative symptoms. Besides cognitive impairment, such as decreased attention and executive function, may complicate the ability of the individuals to effectively respond to their environment. Unlike positive symptoms that are simpler to observe, the negative ones are elusive, making it difficult to identify and treat them. Identification and discrimination among these symptom types are very important in providing complete treatment for individuals with schizophrenia (Boyd et al., 2014). Moreover, the interplay of comorbidities occurring in schizophrenia further complicates the symptomatology of the disorder. Chronic medical illnesses in the majority of schizophrenia patients cause additional somatic symptoms that may simulate or dominate psychiatric ones.

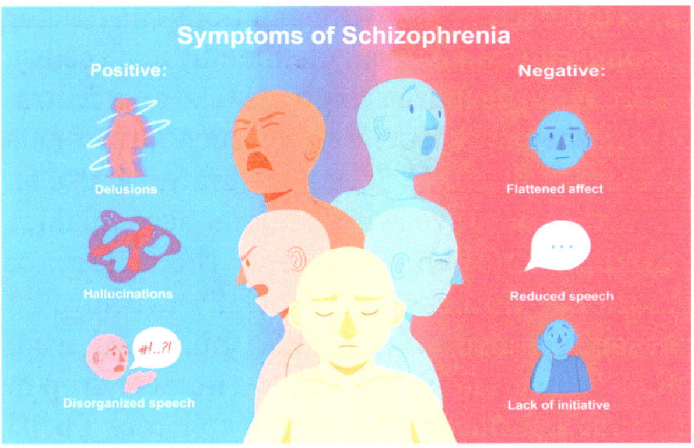

Figure 4.6. Signs and symptoms of schizophrenia.

Source: https://www.verywellmind.com/thmb/UeSbzl7GOSyTejYxQhJBORp58HE=/1500x0/filters:no_upscale():max_bytes(150000):strip_icc()/what-are-the-symptoms-of-schizophrenia-2953120-e15ca22957ec44ff8969cf9b8ac24568.jpg.

This overlap may present diagnostic difficulty since clinicians may find it difficult to determine whether certain symptoms are due to schizophrenia, a comorbid somatic disorder, or even as side effects of antipsychotic drugs (Jakovljevi et al., 2009). Therefore, healthcare providers need to employ a model that incorporates both psychiatric and somatic factors in the planning of treatment. Early detection of this comorbidity may have the ability to reduce exacerbation of symptoms as well as enhance patient overall well-being, allowing for more complete and effective treatment strategies (Boyd et al., 2014) (Figure 4.6).

4.2.1. Positive Symptoms: Hallucinations and Delusions

The hallucinatory state is one of the most striking of the positive symptoms to occur in patients with schizophrenia and other psychotic disorders. Hallucinations can occur across a broad range of sensory modalities, including auditory, visual, and tactile perceptions, but in the most frequent form, as auditory hallucinations, for example, hearing voices, are most often reported. Such states induce great emotional distress and can disrupt an individual's social or occupational functioning. The occurrence of hallucinations not only makes the subjective experience of persons with psychosis more difficult but also makes clinicians' work in devising effective treatment plans more challenging. Knowing how these hallucinations are, in terms of their content and context, is a must to be able to craft therapeutic interventions that match the unique needs of these individuals. Delusions, another characteristic feature of positive symptoms of schizophrenia, consist of fixed false beliefs that resist evidence to the contrary. These are of varying types, for example, paranoid delusions in which individuals are threatened by other people and grandiose delusions in which they will imagine that they possess special talents or rank. Evidence has been reported to indicate that there may be a connection between a history of childhood trauma and the presence of certain delusional ideas. For instance, research found that individuals with a history of physical abuse were at risk of experiencing delusions of grandiosity and feelings (Barker et al., 2009). This suggests that early traumatic exposures have the possibility of shaping delusional content in psychotic disorders and hence integrated assessments taking into account historical trauma are needed in clinical evaluations. The interface between delusions and hallucinations is central to posing basic questions about the cognitive processes underlying psychotic disorders. Individuals diagnosed with schizophrenia generally have compromised Theory of Mind (ToM), or the capacity of an individual to ascribe states of mind to self and others. While there is some evidence that such deficits may play a role in the development and maintenance of psychotic symptoms, it is indicated that ToM impairments do not reliably predict the intensity of positive symptoms , such as delusions and hallucinations (Johnstone et al., 2005). The nuance of this finding only serves to emphasize the necessity of further investigation into the cognitive origins of positive symptoms, as well as the general implications of these findings for treatment approaches. Promoting a comprehensive understanding of the interplay of hallucinations and delusions in cognitive structure is critical to the development of effective therapies that effectively address symptomatic relief as well as underlying cognitive deficits (Figure 4.7).

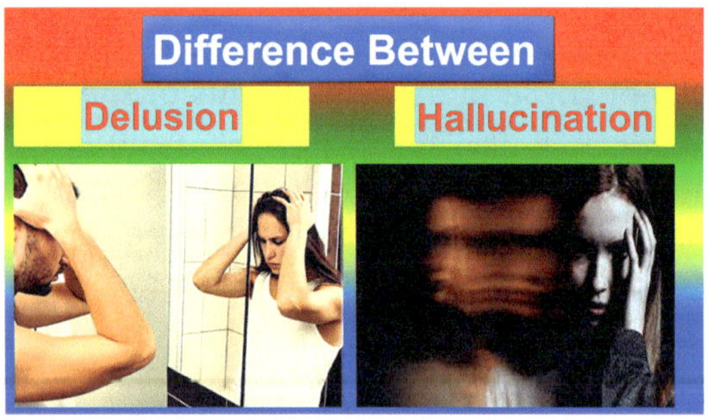

Figure 4.7. Hallucinations and delusions.

Source: https://external-content.duckduckgo.com/iu/?u=https%3A%2F%2Fi.ytimg.com%2Fvi%2F-cmo3MLoXDk%2Fmaxresdefault.jpg&f=1&nofb=1&ipt=5fa81c938635b7d01aab0a229db67ca1aa7e566077bcbea858f5e43aae65f861.

4.2.2. Negative Symptoms: Emotional Flatness and Social Withdrawal

The definition of the negative symptoms of schizophrenia, particularly emotional flatness, identifies a specific area of concern in understanding the complex disorder. Emotional flatness or affective flattening is defined as an apparent reduction in expressiveness and responsiveness to emotions. Patients are observed to exhibit reduced gestures, flat facial responses, and not respond with spontaneous emotional displays, which can severely hinder their ability to communicate with others. This flattening of affects, research indicates, is not merely an idiosyncrasy of the illness but a fundamental shift in the patient's emotional domain, one with significant social ramifications. The decrease in empathy and the loss of the capacity to empathize with emotions can further alienate individuals from their family and society, where these negative symptoms take on a central role in the psychosocial life of such individuals (Maruta et al., 2024). Social withdrawal is also an important negative symptom that accompanies schizophrenia and worsens the effect of emotional flatness. The socially withdrawn person will also avoid contact, pull away from other people, and demonstrate a notable drop in interest in formerly pleasurable activities. Social withdrawal in this instance is not a personal issue but is actually anchored on the overall symptomology of schizophrenia, which has an impaired social cue and emotional processing capacity. The interrelation between impairments of social cognition and negative symptoms is of prime significance, as deviant behavior results from being unable to engage meaningfully with other people. Secondly, prevailing social isolation can reinforce the emotional bluntness of the patients, and therefore, a cycle that enhances misunderstanding and rejection risk does not allow for social contact, making the person's emotional experience worse (Szigeti et al., 2024). The impact of social withdrawal and emotional flatness extends beyond the patient alone to affect the social environment in general. These negative symptoms can lead to diminished quality of life, increased caregiver dependency, and a higher risk for comorbid psychiatric illness. Efforts at seeking therapeutic interventions for these symptoms have also been a long-standing challenge in psychiatry.

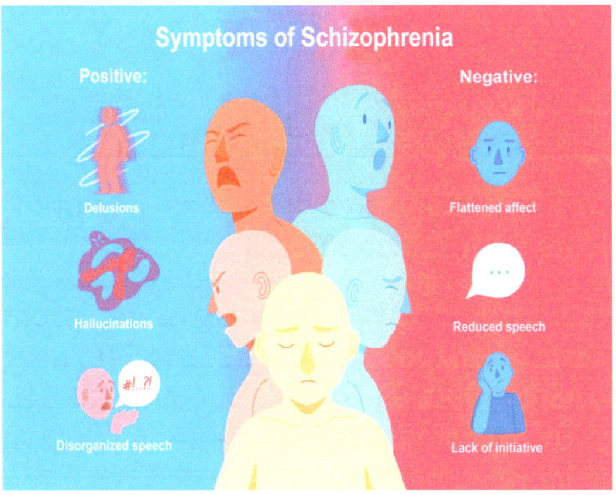

Figure 4.8. Negative symptoms.

Source: https://scontent.fdel11-2.fna.fbcdn.net/v/t1.6435-9/ 123106805_360169617 3208196_19031 9993668980329_n.jpg?_nc_cat=107&ccb=1- 7&_nc_sid=9eae26&_nc_ohc=GCaY1-oNPrQQ7kNvwFCEcsc&_nc_oc=Adl0k9rxLgLyas4AZO IdvQTrKxupS2 6fieX19aaIH GVHf8gmD eUUwYOow rbkULtflRF2VGyAC qf dz08dROLOLpEd&_nc_zt=23&_nc_ht=scontent.fdel11-2.fna&_nc_gi d=Hp-uC53BqxXWqcpq7xfsVQ&oh=0 0_AfRTw 1v6zIPBbcQ6zoyeweGG0rCQ-xawhxHQdHipEpUcWw&oe=689578BE.

The current treatment approaches, including the use of antipsychotics and psychosocial therapy, have been found to have minimal effectiveness in treating the internal motivational and affective deficits in these patients. Research activities, for example, studies on new neurostimulation techniques, aim to enhance outcomes by specifically targeting the neural foundations of negative symptoms (Maruta et al., 2024). As ongoing progress is made in understanding these dimensions, there is a compelling need for more robust clinical methods that can grasp the subtleties in conjunction with emotional flatness and social withdrawal in schizophrenia (Figure 4.8).

4.2.3. Cognitive Symptoms: Impaired Memory and Attention

The neuropsychological deficit of schizophrenia, namely memory and attention deficits, have significant implications for everyday life of individuals so affected. Empirical studies indicate that most schizophrenic patients are impaired on a variety of cognitive operations, including working memory and attentional control, which are fundamental to good problem-solving and decision-making skills. Such profiles of deficits may be part of the overall dysfunction seen in patients, which presents barriers to social functioning and occupational achievements. Specifically, cognitive impairments not only produce the extent of psychotic symptoms but also increase the ease of impairment of everyday functioning. It is essential to comprehend better such cognitive impairments because they are a key element of schizophrenia symptomatology and are susceptible to impacting treatment outcomes. To better explain the specific cognitive impairment that has been observed in schizophrenia, studies have established that patients with the disorder typically exhibit memory patterns of defective memory that are significantly different from those of mentally well individuals. For instance, comparison of cognitive ability reveals that there is severe impairment in auditory and visual learning tasks in individuals with schizophrenia. Deficit in performance is further apparent by comparing people experiencing multisensory hallucinations to those who do not have hallucinations (Bere et al., 2024). In this regard, cognitive testing has proved that people with hallucinations exhibit particular weakness in information processing and hence their cognitive assessment as well as therapy proves to be difficult. This implies that cognitive impairment is not merely an ancillary effect of psychosis but a salient feature in its own right that warrants specific focus in treatment models. Deficient attention in schizophrenia is also a significant contributor to cognitive symptomatology. Findings from eye-tracking techniques have indicated the intricate interplay among attention, prospective memory, and overall cognitive functioning. Schizophrenia patients are likely to demonstrate impairment in cue tracking and distractibility, which results in low accuracy of tasks assessing prospective memory, even when matching symbols appear in regular tests (Li et al., 2024). This means that the traditional tests are perhaps underestimating the extent of cognitive impairment under real-life situations, making it even more complicated in the clinical presentation of schizophrenia. Understanding of these cognitive impairments, particularly attention and memory, is central in developing specially targeted interventions that address the root causes of cognitive dysfunctions and thus enhance the quality of life in individuals with such conditions (Figure 4.9).

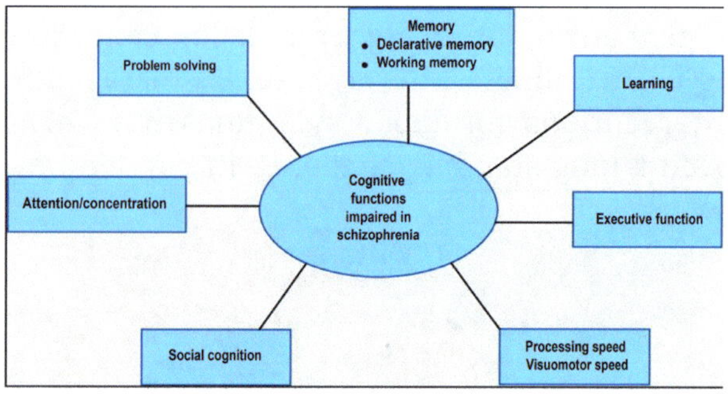

Figure 4.9. Cognitive functions impaired in patients with schizophrenia.

Source: https://www.researchgate.net/profile/Helen-Kitchen/publication/221848546/figure/fig1/AS:386590791749632@1469181835460/Cognitive-functions-impaired-in-patients-with-schizophrenia.png.

Test Your Knowledge

1. What are the key positive, negative, and cognitive symptoms associated with schizophrenia?
2. How do hallucinations and delusions differ, and why are they considered hallmark features of schizophrenia?

4.3. Causes and Risk Factors

Learning Outcome

1. Genetic predisposition and family history.
2. Environmental influences: stress and trauma.
3. Neurobiological factors: brain structure and chemistry.

The identification of risk factors and causes of schizophrenia and psychotic disorders must evolve towards effective intervention and prevention approaches. Predisposition based on genetic factors plays an important role, with research verifying that the risk of schizophrenia is much increased among individuals who have a family history of the condition. Twin studies put the rate of heritability at approximately 80%, highlighting the role of genetic factors. Environmental issues also contribute to this complexity; fetal infection exposure, malnourishment, and psychosocial stress are some factors that can make an individual more susceptible. Childhood adversities, that is, trauma or abuse, have been established as other causative factors that can predispose individuals to psychotic disorders during adulthood and need to be considered to treat and prevent these effects early on in life. Abuse of substances, particularly cannabis, is also a crucial factor involved in the causation of schizophrenia. The research conducted by three Maltese scholars has enlightened the controversial link between the consumption of cannabis and psychosis development, towards the aspect that the consumption of cannabis not only triggers but potentially amplifies the symptoms in vulnerable subjects. The research attempts to determine if cannabis is a causative factor for psychosis or whether its consumption is a risk factor connected with the occurrence of pre-existing mental health issues.

This evaluation is, thus, important because the psychosis history group had exhibited problematic cannabis use patterns, whose tendency to complicate their treatment and recovery processes can easily be exacerbated. On this note, the subtle interplay between substance abuse and psychotic disorder can guide clinical practice in formulating treatment strategies or harm reduction for high-risk groups. Besides environmental and genetic factors, comorbidity of other mental disorders makes the scenario more complex for schizophrenia as well as psychotic disorders. Comorbidity between psychotic disorders and other disorders , such as obsessive-compulsive disorder (OCD), has been put in the limelight in recent years, as such comorbid disorders have the potential to influence the symptomatology as well as the course of the disorders. In accordance with a cross-sectional and longitudinal analysis of associations among such phenotypes, the interaction among such disorders underscores the need for integrated assessment and treatment approaches. Identification and management of the co-morbidities can be a huge difference to the overall efficacy of the therapies, leading to better patient outcomes. Enhanced understanding of these linkages is necessary for clinicians when they formulate holistic treatment plans that incorporate the multidimensional nature of psychotic disorders (Figure 4.10).

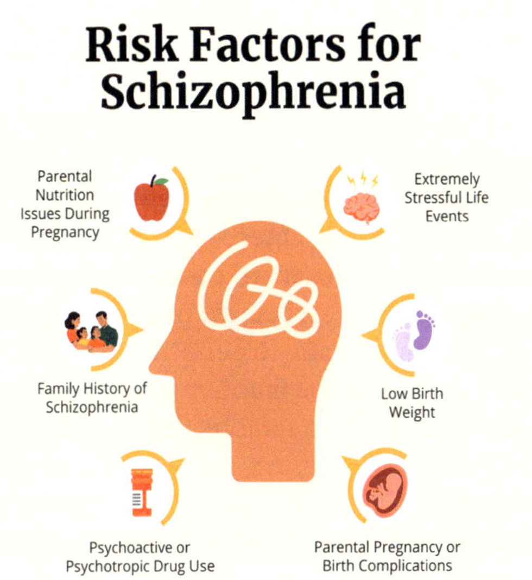

Figure 4.10. Causes and risk factors associated with schizophrenia.

Source: https://images.everydayhealth.com/images/seo-graphic-content-initiative/eh-risk-factors-for-schizophrenia-1080x1080.png?sfvrsn=fab0ef6d_1.

4.3.1. Genetic Predisposition and Family History

Research into the interaction between family history and genetic susceptibility in schizophrenia and other psychotic illnesses is indicative of a multifaceted interaction that influences the outcome and development of the illnesses. Current research has shown that people with a family history of psychotic illnesses are much more likely to develop the same illnesses than people with no such history. This genetic correlation underlines the contribution of genetic elements, which cumulatively constitute the heritability of psychiatric disease. Notably, it is also essential to realize that while there is a very strong genetic influence, there are also very influential environmental determinants over the progression of mental illness health. This interaction between genetics and environment makes it crucial to realize both the hereditary and setting considerations in risk factor evaluation and prevention strategies for psychosis. The simplicity of genetic etiology is also shown in evidence for a homogeneity of the pathogenesis of psychotic disorders. Because it has been argued that a single genetic entity may be in charge of the heterogeneity of psychotic symptomatology observed between families and individuals. This perspective not only highlights the operation of a single genetic predisposition but also speaks to the manner in which selective pressures function in establishing the expression of such disorders across different populations. Clarification of this single genetic basis may provide avenues for more focused research on the specific genes involved and their functional roles within the neurobiological pathways to schizophrenia. Consequently, detection of shared genetic susceptibility among diverse disorders can enhance personalized therapeutic interventions for patients with psychosis family histories patients and eventually enhance the prognosis of patients. Cognitive alterations in patients with non-affective psychotic disorders have also been detected, not only in affected family members but also in their unaffected parents and siblings, indicating inherited cognitive vulnerability among families. By assessing cognitive impairments in these relatives, researchers can achieve an image of the earlier signs that may likely ante-date psychosis. This kind of family cognitive style may be an effective potential biomarker for the identification of at-risk individuals and thus enable early intervention. The resulting understanding of family patterns justifies the importance of a nuanced attitude in the clinical diagnosis of schizophrenia, with genetic susceptibility and family history being essential components of patient evaluations. Eventually, this consideration of familial factors demands a broader discussion of the way genetic susceptibility runs its course through potential environmental interactions, possibly exacerbating or countering risks associated with psychotic illness, as an essential element of mental health research.

4.3.2. Environmental Influences: Stress and Trauma

The environment of schizophrenia and psychotic disorder is strongly determined by environmental elements, particularly by trauma and stress. Participation in negative experiences , such as child abuse or neglect, could lead to compromised brain development and risk of psychiatric disease at a later age. Scientific research shows that 70% of patients with schizophrenia have undergone some form of trauma, illustrating the main argument of confluence between environmental influences and genetic susceptibilities. As these associations become understood, it is clear that although genetic influences play a role in the risk of contracting schizophrenia, environmental stressors can synergistically interact with such genetic susceptibilities to affect the onset and course of the disorder. For example, including gene × environment interactions in psychiatric studies shows the way in which external stressors can synergistically amplify genetic predisposition, highlighting the multifaceted etiology of psychotic disorders (Frydecka et al., 2018). In addition, bullying has emerged as a major environmental predictor of psychotic symptoms. There is research to prove that individuals exposed to bullying in their formative years exhibit higher risks of psychosis. As victims of bullying tend to experience long-term stress and social rejection, these situations cause psychological distress, which leads to a range of mental illnesses like schizophrenia. The psychodynamics of bullying and psychosis operate through various processes , including developmental, biological, and cognitive ones. For instance, chronic victimization stress may disrupt neurobiological processes to impair emotional regulation and cognitive processing and hence lead to psychotic expression. Furthermore, the shared risk factors of psychosis and bullying emphasize the multidimensionality of these disorders, implying that not only is bullying causally implicated in psychosis but also has a wider impact on mental health (Broome et al., 2017).

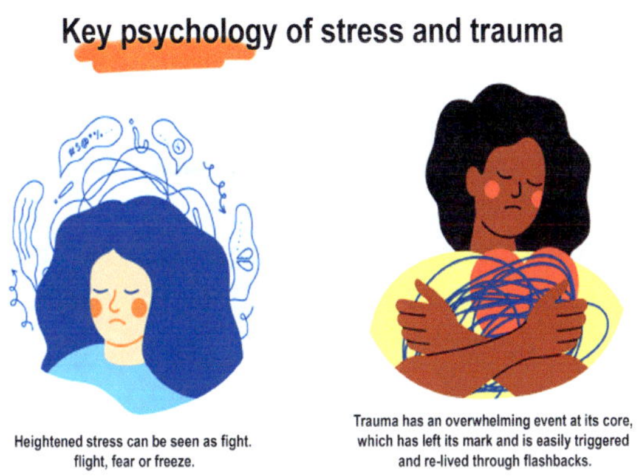
Key psychology of stress and trauma
Heightened stress can be seen as fight. flight, fear or freeze.
Trauma has an overwhelming event at its core, which has left its mark and is easily triggered and re-lived through flashbacks.

Figure 4.11. Stress and trauma.

Source: https://www.educationsupport.org.uk/media/hrxbjv3o/education-support_diagrams_1080x1920_1b.png.

Enclarity regarding the contribution of environmental factors , such as trauma and stress, is imperative in the development of preventive and therapeutic strategies for schizophrenia and psychotic disorders. By realizing that individuals are often shaped by their experiences, mental health professionals can adopt holistic treatment approaches that take into account biological and environmental factors. The interfacing of trauma-informed treatment and resilience-based interventions may prevent early life stress and trauma from developing, potentially altering the trajectory of psychotic disorders. In addition, research on the interaction between genetic vulnerabilities and environmental pressures can guide the creation of individualized interventions, with potential for more effective strategies in the treatment and prevention of schizophrenia. A combined approach that identifies both environmental and genetic components is required to fully address the complexities of psychotic disorders and improve patient care (Figure 4.11).

4.3.3. Neurobiological Factors: Brain Structure and Chemistry

The neurobiological basis of schizophrenia and psychotic disorders is complex and multifactorial, and it is largely made up of chemical and structural brain abnormalities. It has been found that schizophrenic patients are likely to exhibit striking changes in brain morphology, especially in brain areas , such as the prefrontal cortex and the hippocampus. These structures have a crucial role in cognition, memory, and emotional regulation, the functions of which are typically impaired in patients with psychotic disorders.

Specifically, a reduction in hippocampal volume has been correlated with the severity of cognitive impairment and negative symptoms, suggesting a pivotal involvement of neuroanatomical organization in the manifestation of these diseases. Moreover, disorganization of neural interconnectivity across different brain regions could be the basis of the pervasive disorganization of thinking and perceptual disturbances typically experienced by schizophrenia patients, and thus, it is possible to gain a detailed understanding of the neurobiological substrate of these ruinous diseases. Concomitant to the structural alterations, neurochemical imbalances also account for schizophrenia heterogeneity. The dopamine hypothesis, suggesting overactivation of dopaminergic circuits, the mesolimbic system in particular, as being accountable for positive symptoms of hallucination and delusion, is strongly supported by empirical evidence. As opposed to this, hypofunction of glutamate circuits, the prefrontal cortex in particular, is thought to be accountable for negative symptoms and cognitive impairment.

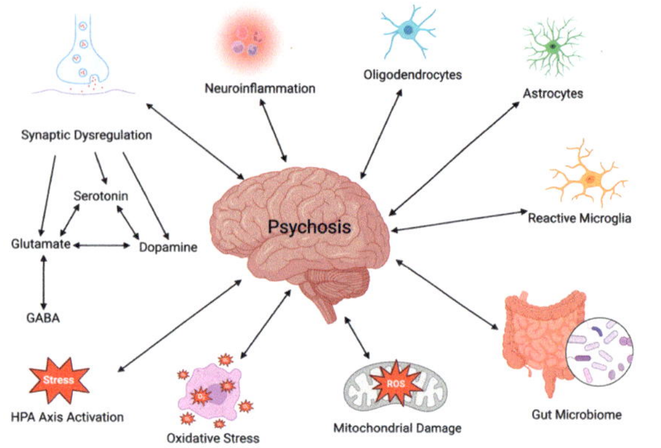

Figure 4.12. Neurobiological factors in schizophrenia.

Source: https://www.mdpi.com/antioxidants/antioxidants-13-00709/article_deploy/html/images/antioxidants-13-00709-g001.png.

This imbalance involving two neurotransmitters implies that schizophrenia is not merely an overabundance of dopamine but rather a complex interrelationship between multiple neurochemical systems. Notably, neuroimaging studies, specifically positron emission tomography (PET) scanning, have also demonstrated support for aberrant dopamine synthesis and release and have established a biological substrate for symptom-related behavior in psychotic patients. Infection of the mother during pregnancy has also emerged as a key aspect of the explanation of the neurodevelopmental origins of schizophrenia.

Epidemiological work has demonstrated that there is a correlation between exposure to infection and an increased risk of neurodevelopmental disorders, such as schizophrenia, in offspring. As an example, nonhuman primate models of maternal immune activation (MIA) have shown that offspring possess higher striatal dopamine levels, a biomarker widely associated with schizophrenia—during late adolescence, illustrating long-term effects of prenatal immune disturbance. These results indicate that neurobiological mechanisms defining schizophrenia go beyond the deficits in the function of single neurons to include prenatal environmental impacts on brain development. These observations underscore the necessity for insight into the interplay between neurochemistry, genetics, and the environment in the etiology of psychotic disorders and thereby shed directions for future research and possible therapy on a multifaceted and elusive field (Figure 4.12).

Test Your Knowledge

1. What genetic, neurobiological, and environmental factors are believed to contribute to the development of schizophrenia?
2. How do prenatal complications, substance use, and family history increase the risk of schizophrenia?

4.4. Diagnosis and Assessment

Learning Outcome

1. Diagnostic criteria from the DSM-5.
2. Role of clinical interviews and psychological testing.
3. Challenges in diagnosing schizophrenia.

Diagnosis for schizophrenia and other psychoses is complex and multi-step, employing broad assessment techniques to accurately assess the existence of symptoms and their severity. Practitioners employ a combination of structured interviews, self-reports, and collateral information from family members or friends. The DSM-5 criteria for schizophrenia emphasize the presence of predominant symptoms of delusions, hallucinations, and disorganized thinking for at least six months. It should also rule out other psychiatric disorders because symptoms may overlap in this respect with mood disorders and anxiety disorders. According to the most recent studies, there has also been advocacy for the fact that temporal dynamics of psychotic experiences can guide the diagnosis and improve the treatment recommendations for systematically optimizing patient outcomes. Assessment strategies also consider not only the occurrence of symptoms but also how they impact functioning in a number of areas of life. Assessment of cognitive deficits is particularly relevant, as cognitive impairment has been found to significantly impact the course and recovery trajectory of the schizophrenic subject. Cognitive impairment can be measured by neuro-psychological tests, and it measures the extent of impairment, which is largely associated with poorer outcomes and higher disability. Additionally, the interrelation of psychotic disorders and comorbid states, such as obsessive-compulsive disorder (OCD), necessitates a complicated diagnosis and treatment. Research shows that individuals presenting with common symptoms must be evaluated using proper measures considering the capacity of symptom covariance across time, which further aids the clinicians in creating proper, personal treatment plans (Van Daelet al., 2011). An additional complication arises with the consideration of developmental factors and their role in the diagnosis and assessment of psychotic disorders. For instance, adolescents born preterm are at greater risk for mental illnesses like schizophrenia. It has been revealed through research that such patients not only acquire psychotic symptoms but also a variety of emotional disorders, ADHD, and other neurodevelopmental problems, all of which are essential to monitor carefully and have intervention tactics. Such heightened susceptibility necessitates clinicians incorporating developmental history and risk factors into their assessment frameworks for better prediction of long-term outcome in these high-risk groups. Early identification and active treatment are critical, since a large percentage of preterm teens are afflicted with psychiatric disorders, setting the stage for repeated assessment at critical developmental phases (Johnson et al., 2013).

4.4.1. Diagnostic Criteria from the DSM-5

Diagnostic and Statistical Manual of Mental Disorders, Fifth Edition (DSM-5) is a landmark in the diagnosis and classification of schizophrenia and other psychotic disorders. DSM-5 requires specific diagnostic criteria that insist on the existence of characteristic symptoms , such as delusions, hallucinations, disorganized thinking, and significant impairment in functioning. To be considered schizophrenia, the patients should have a minimum of two of the aforementioned symptoms for a significant portion of a month, with some degree of disturbance persisting for six months. The extremely specific time frame and the emphasis on functional decline indicate the chronic nature of the disorder, distinguishing it from transient psychological disturbances. As the study shows, proper and integrated diagnostic models, such as those found in the DSM-5, aid in understanding the onset and potential outcome of schizophrenia, with accuracy for treatment and management plans. In addition to the main symptoms, the DSM-5 emphasizes the ruling out of other mental illnesses that could manifest with similar psychotic phenomena. That is significant, since the diagnostic challenge is distinguishing between schizophrenia and affective disorders, such as major depression or bipolar disorder, in which there can be psychotic symptoms as well. The conservative method utilized by the DSM-5 is designed not to misdiagnose, particularly with overlap from transient and episodic psychotic disorders. The diagnostic criteria really split symptoms into categories based on duration and severity of the symptoms, which not only enhances clinical specificity but also directs treatment plans that can be quite different depending on the causative disorder.

This specificity fits with evidence that observes that to enable targeted interventions, it is important to distinguish between chronic conditions like schizophrenia and other episodic disorders (Bottlender et al., 2004). Also, DSM-5 recognizes the pivotal position of negative symptoms, like diminished emotional expression, avolition, and anhedonia, in the diagnostic picture of schizophrenia. The negative symptoms are generally persistent and may lead to an overall worsening of the patient's quality of life, wherefore integrative treatment interventions beyond mere control of positive symptoms are needed. Current studies have documented that negative symptoms can have a significant effect on everyday functioning and social interaction, thus supporting the DSM-5's position to include a full range of the disorder. The amalgamation of these intricate criteria is in accordance with the intention of providing clinicians with an evidence-based model for treatment and diagnosis. These models not only help to distinguish schizophrenia from other non-affective psychoses but also enhance the descriptive validity of schizophrenia as a distinct clinical disorder (Bottlender et al., 2003) (Figure 4.13).

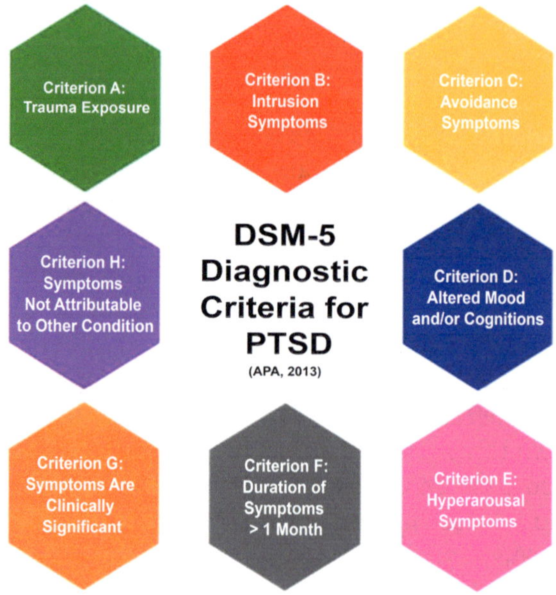

Figure 4.13. Diagnostic criteria from the DSM-5.

Source: https://external-content.duckduckgo.com/iu/?u=https%3A%2F%2Fwww.researchgate.net%2Fpublication%2F361280781%2Ffigure%2Ffig2%2FAS%3A1166872733065240%401655215547915%2FSummary-of-DSM-5-diagnostic-criteria-for-PTSD-There-are-eight-diagnostic-criteria.png&f=1&nofb=1&ipt=1e7979a68fde78e62535706a144373f5057213f64bb18af8194ecfa5677a02f7.

4.4.2. Role of Clinical Interviews and Psychological Testing

The role of clinical interview and psychological testing in the diagnostic process of schizophrenia and other psychotic illnesses is paramount, and it is the foundation for effective assessment and management. Clinical interviews provide mental health professionals with the opportunity to understand patients' experience, history, and symptomatology in a context of some detail. They allow clinicians to probe the nuances of psychotic symptoms , such as hallucinations, delusions, and thought disorder, which manifest differently in different patients. The interviews can also identify critical psychosocial variables affecting the patient's status, including family history and environmental stressors. The interview ability of clinical interviews also facilitates a therapeutic relationship, with patients more likely to disclose their symptoms freely, thereby enhancing diagnostic yield and shaping treatment planning. Psychological testing complements clinical interviewing by offering standardized measures to assess various domains of cognition and emotion, critical in unearthing the complexities of psychotic disorders. Cognitive function, personality, and symptom severity can be assessed through tests that provide objective information to guide diagnosis and treatment. Tests can establish cognitive deficits that are common among schizophrenia patients, such as deficient attention and memory. Also, standardized testing is capable of distinguishing between schizophrenia and other conditions with psychotic disorder-like symptoms and contributing towards the correct differential diagnosis. The psychological testing combined with clinical interviews not only strengthens the assessment but is also consistent with new conceptualizations in psychopathology, such as the Hierarchical Taxonomy of Psychopathology (HiTOP) model, which emphasizes dimensional rather than the traditional categorical diagnoses (Kotov et al., 2017). With the multifaceted nature of schizophrenia and the difficulty of its diagnosis, the compatibility of clinical interviews and psychological testing must be the priority in clinical practice. Using thorough evaluations, practitioners are able to create a very personalized treatment plan that is specially crafted for each patient according to their special needs. This dual approach facilitates a better grasp of the patients mental outlook, guiding any appropriate therapeutic intervention. In this regard, the evolving context of mental health treatment, particularly in response to the COVID-19 pandemic, highlights the increasing need for formal evaluations to achieve optimal treatment and address mental health inequities (Zhou et al., 2020). Amid the emerging challenges surrounding the delivery of mental health care, the process of optimizing clinical interviews and psychological testing remains integral in furthering effective care for psychotic disorders (Figure 4.14).

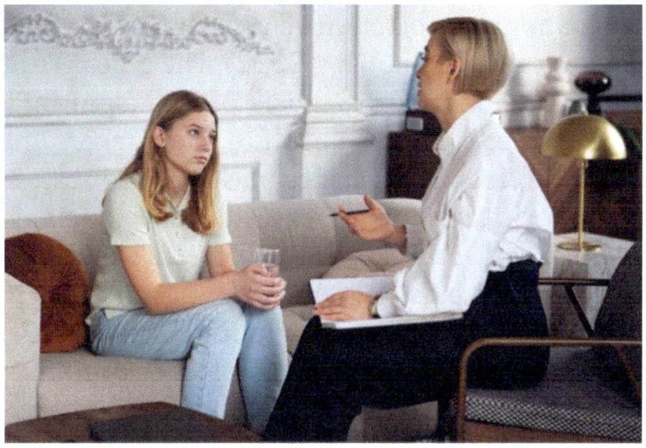

Figure 4.14. Role of clinical interviews and psychological testing.

Source: https://external-content.duckduckgo.com/iu/?u=https%3A%2F%2Fsouthjerseycopingclinic.com%2Fwp-content%2Fuploads%2F2024%2F02%2FTherapy-and-Counseling-1.jpg&f=1&nofb=1&ipt=005ddbca54e8c2a41c83d16fc93bb4e53dcdff2f30fcdab9452f9210da4a6146.

4.4.3. Challenges in Diagnosing Schizophrenia

Schizophrenia diagnosis is a challenging endeavor, partly due to its symptom similarity with other psychiatric disorders. Delusions, hallucinations, and cognitive impairments are not pathognomonic for schizophrenia but can occur in bipolar disorder and major depressive disorder as well. The overlap between the symptoms poses a problem in making an accurate diagnosis, leading to misdiagnosis or delayed diagnosis. The experts have to practice in an intricate environment where they evaluate the nuances of every patient's presentation, because inconsistency within the manifestation of symptoms can hide the true disease. An integration of evaluation from more than one angle, clinical evaluation and history from the patient, can lead to a more accurate diagnosis. Also, the historical and measurable criteria for the diagnosis of psychotic disorders might not accurately manifest the ongoing change in psychiatric characteristics across different populations and hence need continuous revision of the criteria (Cummings, 2012). The other great impediment to the diagnosis of schizophrenia is that there are no absolute biomarkers or objective tests. The reliance on subjective scales, based primarily on observation by clinicians and interviews with patients, inevitably involves some risk of bias and lack of uniformity. Each clinician has a unique view, and this may color the interpretation and ranking of symptoms. Cultural factors, for example, influence reporting of symptoms and the clinician's impression of them, sometimes leading to a misunderstanding of culturally normative behaviors as pathology. It is necessary to have a comprehensive diagnostic process, employing more than one source of information and considering the patient's history and environment. As schizophrenia typically presents with irregular severity and symptomatology across time, the need for a dynamic process of assessment becomes all the more urgent to achieve an accurate diagnosis and adjust interventions accordingly (Adadzi et al., 2024). Apart from the intrinsic complexity of the disease, sociocultural determinants also significantly add to the diagnostic challenge faced by healthcare workers. Stigmatization against mental illness, particularly schizophrenia, can discourage individuals from seeking assistance or lead to underreporting. This issue is further exacerbated in certain societies where mental health discussions are stigmatized. In addition, the age of onset of schizophrenia can be variable, and late-onset schizophrenia can show differential symptom sets that make it difficult for general diagnostic criteria Incorporation of cutting-edge research into practical disorders could further knowledge and description of schizophrenia's symptomatology, with possible insight into diagnostics (Cummings, 2012). Clarifying these sociocultural nuances is essential for improving diagnostic precision and giving affected patients the right therapy, precisely for their respective needs and circumstances (Adadzi et al., 2024).

Test Your Knowledge

1. What clinical criteria are used to diagnose schizophrenia in systems such as DSM-5-TR and ICD-11?
2. How do clinical interviews, psychological testing, and functional assessments assist in confirming a diagnosis of schizophrenia?

4.5. Treatment Options

Learning Outcome

1. Pharmacological treatments: antipsychotic medications.
2. Psychotherapy approaches: cognitive-behavioral therapy.
3. Supportive services: rehabilitation and community support.

Treatment of schizophrenia and other psychotic illnesses is multifaceted, consisting of pharmacological, psychological, and community treatments. Antipsychotic medication is often the cornerstone of treatment, aimed at relief from delusional and hallucinatory symptoms. The medications can be categorized into first-generation (typical) and second-generation (atypical) antipsychotics, each with varying efficacy and side effects. Moreover, adjunctive treatment like psychotherapy is relevant in management, including cognitive behavioral therapy (CBT), which can assist in coping and shatter distorted perceptions. The integration of medication management and psychosocial assistance is vital because studies have shown that combined approaches lead to better treatment outcomes and quality of life for patients with schizophrenia and psychotic disorders. Community-based treatment has become increasingly recognized as an essential element in the treatment of schizophrenia. Treatment of choice for such patients often includes assertive community treatment (ACT) programs, which provide intensive individual treatment with interdisciplinary teams. Hospital and emergency care rates have been found to decrease with these programs, reflecting the need for ongoing support outside hospitals. Symptom management is not just the goal, but also social skill augmentation and return to society. Research has revealed that these encompass elements , such as social awareness and can affect the success of community-based interventions, particularly in establishing trust and cooperation among treatment participants. Therefore, linking clinical treatment with community services could enhance the sustainability of treatment among patients facing the challenges of psychotic disorders (Fett et al., 2019). Cost considerations in inpatient and outpatient treatment are also extensively explored in terms of schizophrenia management. Existing research has highlighted the enormous economic impact of inpatient treatment, underlining the importance of such variables as the duration of stay and complexity of treatment plan in defining total costs. In particular, psychosis and the application of specialized interventions, like electroconvulsive therapy or clozapine, have been proven to increase costs significantly and imply that targeted intervention can enhance clinical efficacy as well as cost-effectiveness (Baldessarini et al., 2016). As a result, research needs to continue identifying effective, affordable treatment modalities that can be incorporated into comprehensive treatment planning. This will make the people with schizophrenia empowered and improve their overall mental well-being as they deal with the economic impact of their therapy.

4.5.1. Pharmacological Treatment: Antipsychotic Medication

Antipsychotic medications are the pillar of pharmacological therapy for schizophrenia and other psychotic conditions. Antipsychotics primarily exert their effects by modulating the dopamine systems that are involved in the pathogenesis of psychotic symptoms. Though highly effective in managing positive symptoms , such as hallucinations and delusions, antipsychotic treatment has long been associated with a range of side effects , including weight gain, metabolic syndrome, and extrapyramidal symptoms. Psychiatric professionals must contend with such issues in clinical work to promote medication regimen compliance with a reduction in side effects. Additionally, treatment with antipsychotics must consider the patient's individual health history carefully, where shared decision-making between patients and clinicians must be promoted to facilitate well-informed pharmacological treatment decisions (Bressington et al., 2015). The discovery of the atypical antipsychotics has opened up the pharmacologic frontier, bringing with it alternatives that may relieve the side effect burden of traditional antipsychotic therapy. The medications not only alleviate the positive symptoms of psychoses but also the negative symptoms of anhedonia and social withdrawal, which are often overlooked in treatment. Of special mention among these are medications like clozapine, which although typically reserved for use in treatment-resistant situations, has proven effective at improving overall function and preventing suicidal ideation in schizophrenia patients. Although these medications have their utility, they are not without danger, having the potential to continue triggering metabolic abnormalities and other medical problems, which is why ongoing monitoring and support throughout therapy are indicated (Chwaliszewski et al., 2025). Mental health clinicians are uniquely placed to effect the reconciliation between pharmacological management of psychotic conditions and more general measures stressing the health of the individual patient. Physical morbidity concerns assume amplified importance as a result of the nature of the untreated symptoms. An integrative approach that includes psychoeducation, lifestyle modification, and adjunct therapies , such as exercise, can enhance outcomes by addressing both somatic and mental symptoms. Such a wide focus is an indication of a redefinition of mental health nursing practice, in which managing physical health and informed patient choices are paramount. Finally, making patients aware of their treatments promotes compliance, breeds trust, and promotes improved clinical outcomes in the treatment of schizophrenia and other psychotic disorders (Bressington et al., 2015) (Figure 4.15).

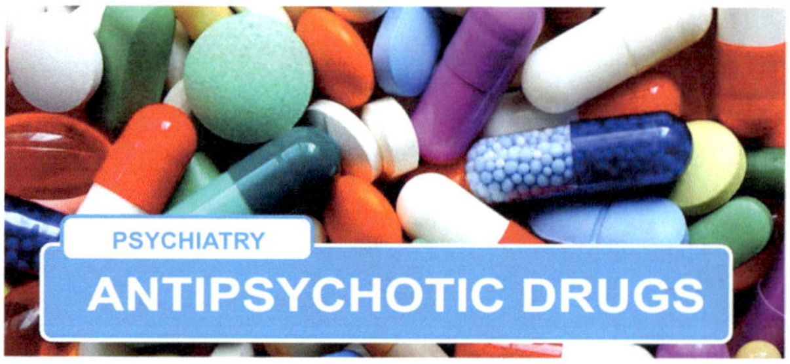

Figure 4.15. Antipsychotic drugs.

Source: https://external-content.duckduckgo.com/iu/?u=https%3A%2F%2Fimage.prepladder.com%2Fprepladder%2F2024%2F04%2F16114439%2FAntipsychotic-Drugs.webp&f=1&nofb=1&ipt=cf7e9cee5b5ca804458189bcb4d9c2c6eb6b7b6a3fbada8d3fa4576f1c6d8de1.

4.5.2. Psychotherapy Approaches: Cognitive-Behavioral Therapy

Cognitive-behavioral therapy (CBT) has been a corner stone treatment of patients with schizophrenia and other psychotic disorders. In aiming to advance patients' functioning in general, CBT addresses distorted thought processes and increased emotional regulation. This is particularly significant considering the risk of partial remission of symptoms or side effects discouraging compliance with the use of traditional pharmacological interventions. Through directed sessions, therapists help clients to become sensitized and challenge irrational beliefs, building healthier adaptive mechanisms necessary to deal with day-to-day issues. The technique of CBT allows it to be adapted to suit the unique experiences of psychosis sufferers, creating a therapeutic environment where patients are able to delve into challenging cognitions and feelings safely. Recent advancements have demonstrated the potential of merging CBT with other new approaches to enhance treatment efficacy. For example, Hybrid treatment models combine standard CBT with new technologies , such as virtual reality and neurofeedback in opposition to symptoms like auditory verbal hallucinations, one of the most disabling characteristics of psychotic disorders. This kind of combination represents a transition toward multimodal treatments that value the complexity of psychotic symptoms as simultaneous psychological and physiological phenomena. Initial findings from these ongoing studies suggest that this hybrid approach not only increases acceptability and treatment feasibility but also engages patients more comprehensively in their own recovery process. Such custom-made, hybrid designs are essential to respond to the multifaceted needs of patients with schizophrenia, potentially paving the way for more integrated care.

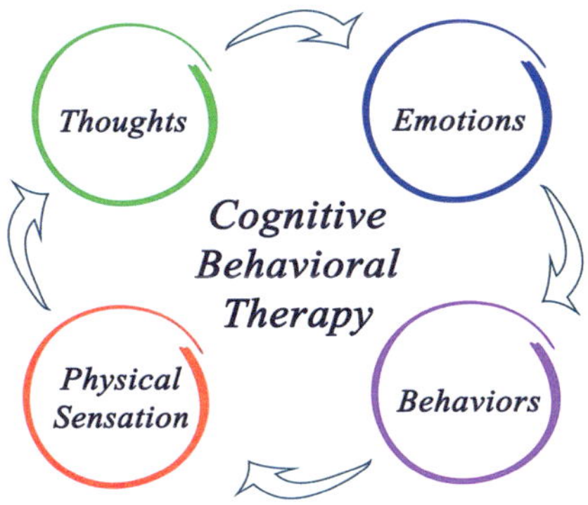

Figure 4.16. Cognitive-behavioral therapy.

Source: https://external-content.duckduckgo.com/iu/?u=https%3A%2F%2Ftheinternationalpsychologyclinic.com%2Fwp-content%2Fuploads%2F2018%2F12%2FAdobeStock_106546247-1-1024x880.jpeg&f=1&nofb=1&ipt=e63b06f844347983d93951aba1a1489a53a143bfa05a161f061fbaafe8233a41.

Moreover, the exploration of CBT for insomnia (CBT-I) among patients with psychotic disorders also points to a key therapeutic treatment area. Disturbances in sleep are pervasive among individuals with psychosis and tend to enhance the disorder's symptoms and slow down recovery. Recent meta-analyses illustrate that CBT-I significantly influences better sleep quality as well as reduced insomnia, simultaneously improving overall psychotic symptoms and mental health. By providing the patient with practical skills to manage sleep patterns, CBT-I complements the primary CBT treatment and emphasizes the significance of treating comorbid illnesses in psychotic treatment. Although new findings persist in supporting the integration of CBT-I into treatment strategies, it underscores the flexibility and modernity of CBT methods toward improving patient outcomes for schizophrenia and psychotic disorders as a progressive trend in psychotherapy practice in mental health interventions (Mustafa et al., 2024; Spark et al., 2025) (Figure 4.16).

4.5.3. Supportive Services: Rehabilitation and Community Support

Community rehabilitation and support are extremely crucial parts of schizophrenia and psychotic disorder management, with the overall aim of improving the quality of life of the patients with these disorders. Support services entail a variety of methodologies, ranging from therapy to social support systems and vocational rehabilitation, which synergistically interact towards recovery and recovery augmentation. The Mental Health Recovery Star (MHRS) is precisely that kind of tool that emphasizes collaborative care planning and building communication between users and providers to assess and measure recovery outcomes. Though the MHRS is satisfactory in terms of test-retest reliability, concerns have been raised regarding its interrater reliability, a sign that more work is needed to ensure that social functioning and recovery assessment in clinical practice are accurate (Killaspy et al., 2012). Hence, the use of methodologies that confirm the robustness of outcome measures is essential to the effective design of rehabilitation programs. One of the evidence-based interventions in community care among schizophrenia patients is occupational therapy, which focuses on functional skills and the promotion of independence. A pilot randomized controlled trial proved the effectiveness of occupational therapy in the promotion of social functioning as well as the relief of negative symptoms for individuals with psychotic disorders. During a 12-month interval, participants who were given individualized occupational therapy made clinically significant improvement on a number of the subscales of the Social Functioning Scale, such as relationships and independence (NC et al., 2008). Such findings highlight the adoption of individualized, community-based interventions that aim for the relief of psychiatric symptoms as well as for the learning of life skills. These high-intensity interventions can facilitate individuals to become more engaged in their communities and improve their overall quality of life. In addition, integrating rehabilitation interventions with community care systems affords a more integrated model for responding to the needs of individuals with schizophrenia. Mental health services cannot simply respond to symptom relief but also design settings that facilitate social inclusion and stability. By the combination of therapeutic modalities with a strategic purpose, such as cognitive-behavioral therapy with vocational interventions, service providers can ideally optimize the process of recovery. This is attributed to the MHRS findings that confirm that even though this instrument is beneficial in assessing social function, it must not replace the necessity for diverse, multidimensional support systems that address the various needs of individuals (Killaspy et al., 2012). Thus, an interactive strategy that incorporates numerous types of supportive services has the potential to improve living conditions among individuals with psychotic disorders dramatically.

Test Your Knowledge

1. How do antipsychotic medications differ in their role and effectiveness in managing schizophrenia symptoms?
2. What non-pharmacological treatments—such as psychotherapy, psychoeducation, and social skills training—are used to support recovery?

4.6. Impact on Daily Life

Learning Outcome

1. Effects on personal relationships and social interactions.
2. Challenges in employment and education.
3. Stigma and misconceptions surrounding psychotic disorders.

Having schizophrenia or other psychotic disorders significantly impacts a person's daily life, typically far beyond the psychiatric symptom itself. Interference with their thought process is often difficult for people, and it can interfere with their ability to do ordinary tasks , such as taking care of their money or being employed. Cognitive issues, which may vary from difficulties in concentrating, memory, and organizational skills, can be a significant barrier to daily functioning. This is particularly significant as many individuals who suffer from psychotic illness are reliant on routine predictability to manage their condition effectively. Reducing productivity and making social interaction harder, this cognitive impairment not only impacts life satisfaction but also enhances feelings of isolation that typically accompany the condition. The daily realities of patients can thus precipitate drastic lifestyle and social interaction changes. Furthermore, the intricate symptomatology of schizophrenia, including delusions and hallucinations, consistently alters individuals' interpersonal relationships and social capacity. Day-to-day interactions may be punctuated by miscommunication or heightened tension, leading to social withdrawal or avoidance of previously pursued activities. At a point when psychotic symptoms emerge, the ability to establish and maintain friendships can decline precipitously, forcing individuals into emotional isolation. Such withdrawal is occasionally more than a side effect of the illness; it fuels stigmatization cycles, reinforcing social myths and resulting in greater alienation. Over time, the cumulative impact of such social challenges can result in a low quality of life, as impacted individuals may find themselves ever more burdened or believing the world to be hazardous. These shifting social dynamics highlight the necessity for specially designed interventions that deal with both clinical symptoms and social reintegration. In addition to cognitive and social impairment, individuals with schizophrenia often have profound deficits in daily living skills. The characteristic symptoms of psychotic disorders can influence fundamental self-care activities like cleanliness, eating, and maintenance of health. Daily routines, which are taken for granted by most people, are too much to bear for those with disabling symptoms. This is compounded by the stigma of mental illness, which may discourage others from seeking treatment or adhering to treatment protocols. Incorporating support systems—that is, family, peer support, and community resources—is thus the key to optimizing their capacity to effectively function in daily routines. Establishing structured environments that facilitate self-efficacy and autonomy can be an important component of increasing resilience and general quality of life for individuals with schizophrenia. Knowledge of the intersection of mental illness and daily life can lead to more compassionate and efficacious interventions in treatment, essentially bridging the gap between clinical and daily life (Sharma et al., 2018; Borsboom, 2017).

4.6.1. Effect on Personal Relationships and Social Interactions

The impact of schizophrenia and other psychotic disorders on interpersonal relationships and social functioning can be highly disruptive, often leading to isolation and decreased social networks. Such conditions have the potential to yield symptoms of delusions, hallucinations, and impaired emotional control, which can undermine the abilities of individuals for successful interpersonal connections. Such challenges may result in misunderstanding, strained relationships, and social support withdrawal, hence making loneliness worse and contributing to the condition of the individual. Indeed, a systematic review demonstrated that loneliness and inadequate perceived social support are significant predictors of adverse outcomes among individuals experiencing mental health disorders, depicting the critical role interpersonal relationships take in recovery and well-being (Wang et al., 2018). Good communication and good network are particularly required since not achieving this results in a vicious cycle of isolation that further complicates social recovery and functioning. Lastly, the quality of relationships is also impacted by psychotic disorder and schizophrenia stigma. Individuals are given society's incorrect presumptions about them that define them as unstable or dangerous, and their friends and family members start avoiding being in contact with them. Stigma can potentially serve as a barrier to help provision and social activity participation, which in turn exacerbates isolation. Perceived social support is revealed to be related to enhanced symptom and social functioning outcomes, and therefore, it is possible that strengthening social relationships is an integral part of the treatment process (Wang et al., 2018). Also, the stigmatizing emotional cost has the potential to create feelings of shame, which contribute to already complicated relationship dynamics one has to deal with. Public education and awareness of schizophrenia are thus key in a bid to foster a more tolerant environment where social interactions can take place without the fear of rejection or misunderstanding. Interventions towards social skill and relationship enhancement can be a significant factor in helping individuals afflicted with schizophrenia and other related disorders.

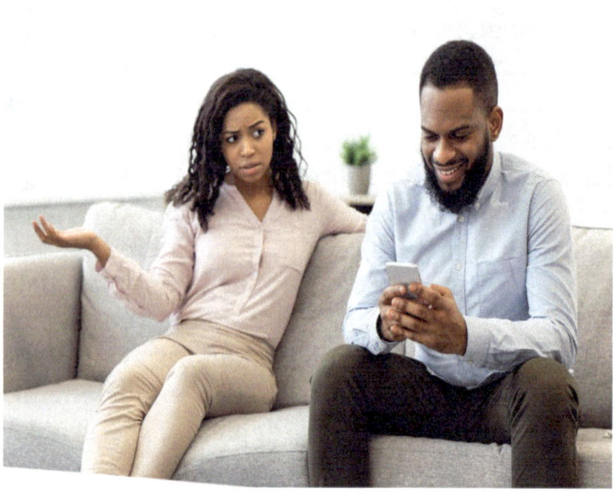

Figure 4.17. Effects on personal relationships and social interactions.

Source: https://external-content.duckduckgo.com/iu/?u=https%3A%2F%2Fmindbodycounselingreno.com%2Fwp-content%2Fuploads%2F2023%2F08%2Fhow-social-media-affects-relationships.jpg&f=1&nofb=1&ipt=a1e82d85170bb41db683c51892e8d0210b455004ba05508fbfab01dbfbe62234.

Social interaction-based therapies and support groups can help enhance self-esteem and general relationship skills, providing individuals with a platform to express their experiences and feelings. Such interactions are crucial since they not only dispel the stigma surrounding mental health conditions but also enable the establishment of a conducive social environment. Research shows that the increase in perceived social support leads to better recovery outcomes; thus, the development of opportunities for socialization becomes a priority in treatment (Wang et al., 2018). Also, combating loneliness through communal engagement and forming relationships can avert relational effects of psychotic disorders and eventually enhance the quality of life of the individual as well as integrate them into society more effectively. Social support and mental health interaction again emphasizes the role of relational processes in schizophrenia and psychotic disorders, showing that recovery highly relies on holistic approaches (Figure 4.17).

4.6.2. Challenges in Employment and Education

The interrelation of schizophrenia, psychotic disorders, and work and learning capability is crucial in achieving the broader picture of mental health. Individuals with such disorders usually have very severe barriers to employment as unemployed individuals or to maintaining employment. Employer attitudes remain influenced by stereotypes regarding mental illness, leading to discrimination and a lack of awareness of the capabilities of individuals afflicted with such disorders. Moreover, the random nature of symptoms accompanying schizophrenia is likely to introduce additional challenges to normal job function, and employers will likely view it as a lack of ability or dedication. Such system-based discrimination, apart from striking the individual's economic situation, further reinforces feelings of stigmatization and isolation, ultimately affecting mental health. Education is also equally problematic for patients with schizophrenia and other psychotic disorders. The affective and cognitive manifestations can impair learning procedures, making the victims incapable of learning in schools. Academic institutions, in most cases, are not equipped to provide the necessary support, such as accommodation for individuals with mental disorders, which results in high school dropout. Additionally, teachers' lack of knowledge and awareness of schizophrenia may be the cause of providing a derogatory academic environment. Because educational success is often tied to employment opportunities, the barriers that an individual faces in school environments can lead to chains of disadvantage, making it impossible for an individual to be capable of doing well academically and professionally. Furthermore, expense also presents another difficulty to the problems of people with schizophrenia in terms of work and learning. Others are able to have disability benefits act as a backstop, which by definition limits their career options because they risk losing their health care benefits and income. Work opportunities that are compatible with individuals who are fighting mental illness do not usually have good health benefits, so it is a dilemma in that looking for employment jeopardizes necessary medical care. The interaction between limited employment opportunities, stigma and economic issues tends to result in low employment rates of labor force individuals with psychiatric disabilities (Wittenburg et al., 2005). It requires radical system shifts in corporate culture, educational support systems, and greater awareness to provide the atmosphere of inclusiveness and compassion within all sectors.

4.6.3. Stigma and Misconception Regarding Psychotic Disorders

The stigma of psychotic disorders, particularly schizophrenia, is general and detrimental, vastly impacting the lives of those afflicted with the conditions. Beliefs related to stigma can be manifest in various ways, both socially and as internalized stigma among individuals with schizophrenia. Internalized stigma's effects can also be extremely cruel because individuals begin to internalize negative attitudes, which bring hopelessness and low self-esteem. Research indicates that individuals with greater social power have lower internalized stigma and negative symptoms. This suggests that empowering schizoaffective disorder patients through psychosocial interventions would encourage resilience to stigma, consequently enhancing their psychosocial functioning and quality of life (Campellone et al., 2014). Strategies for enhancing the social power of these patients can therefore be a successful method for combating stigma and the resulting negative effects. Media representations help add significantly to the myths surrounding psychotic disorders and have a tendency to portray them in negative terms.

Review of South African press reports illustrates that an astonishing 79% of articles surveyed generally reported on matters on schizophrenia and other psychotic disorders rather than suggesting solutions or explaining the intricacies involved with such conditions. This portrayal belongs to a public perception that reflects exaggerated focus on the risks and unpredictability of individuals who suffer from schizophrenia, which could contribute to stigma and fear among communities. Secondly, media reportage's tendency to label causes rather than report well-informed feedback consolidates misinformation about these disorders (Masinga, 2017). This review emphasizes the necessity of responsible reporting that gives a balanced portrayal of mental health to bring about increased understanding and hopefully relieve stigma. Stigma and stigma-related myths regarding psychotic illness must be countered by a multi-pronged approach that includes both policy and community education strategies. Increased portrayal of psychotic disorder sufferers in secondary roles within media reports can contribute to the breaking down of negative stereotypes, as well as to empowering those with the conditions. Further, public, medical practitioner, and media employee education campaigns can potentially have a significant impact on opinion by providing evidence-based information about the nature of psychotic disorders. Through empowering society with enhanced knowledge, one can create an environment in which acceptance and support become more common than fear and misconstruction. These methods not only aim to reduce stigma but also generally seek to secure the welfare of individuals suffering from schizophrenia and co-occurring disorders and identify the worth of social engagement in advocacy for mental illness (Figure 4.18).

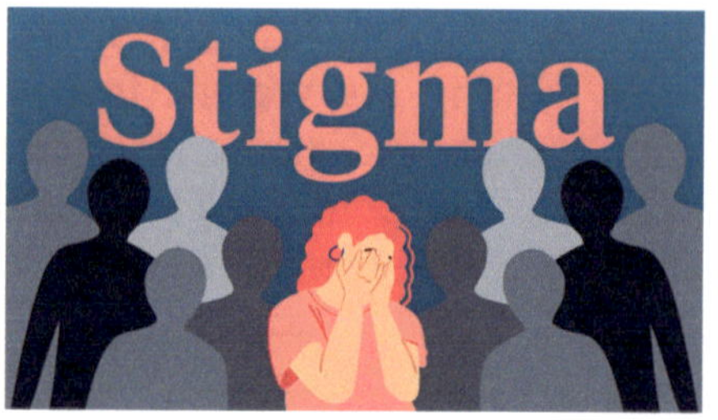

Figure 4.18. Stigma and misconceptions surrounding psychotic disorders.

Source: https://external-content.duckduckgo.com/iu/?u=https%3A%2F%2Fausmed-images.s3.ap-southeast-2.amazonaws.com%2Fausmed.com%2Fausmed-lecture%2FAUSLEC1852v1.0.jpg&f=1&nofb=1&ipt=dae62c68fddc3ff63dffb456f27de621331bb51fb47ca42e10706a97edbdd01c.

Test Your Knowledge

1. How do symptoms of schizophrenia affect an individual's ability to perform daily activities, maintain relationships, or hold employment?
2. What challenges do individuals with schizophrenia face regarding social stigma, independence, and long-term functioning?

SUMMARY

Any definitive analysis of schizophrenia and psychotic disorders must emphasize the multidimensionality and complexity of these disorders. Realization that schizophrenia is not one disease but a cluster of manifestations that have something in common enables one to comprehend its etiology and treatment more effectively. This view is consistent with the premise that the manifestation variability of psychoses derives from a common pathogenesis. This stance encourages the scientific community to venture beyond the solitary symptom, encouraging an integrated position in addressing diagnosis and intervention. In this context, awareness of the interaction of the genetic, environmental, and sociocultural factors that contribute to the emergence of psychotic disorders is essential, which eventually results in more effective therapeutic strategies. The interaction between schizophrenia and comorbid somatic disorders must be addressed cautiously as well. One of the most important findings is the link between schizophrenia and chronic medical illnesses, which complicates the clinical presentation and may also hinder effective treatment. Adverse effects of antipsychotic medication can mimic or exacerbate underlying somatic illnesses, generating diagnostic challenges that must be navigated by healthcare providers. Thus, mental health practitioners must place a high value on comorbidity identification at early stages, as heightened awareness can lead to improved patient outcomes. This emphasis on the intersection of mental and physical care is a progressive move toward mutual treatment models that address the whole individual, rather than severing mental from bodily issues, so providing a more comprehensive model of care for affected individuals. Generally, the future trajectory of treating schizophrenia and psychotic disorders requires the acceptance of joint biological and psychosocial facets of these disorders. As more and more evidence accumulates towards a unitary genetic origin of heterogeneity of psychotic presentations, future research must investigate in more detail the genes and pathways involved. Furthermore, the discovery of factors resulting in comorbidity with somatic conditions aids the justification of the requirement for an integrated treatment approach encompassing pharmacological as well as psychosocial measures. The combination of mentalities has the potential to serve the needs of schizophrenia and other associated diseases, bringing about improved quality of life for sufferers of these challenging disorders. Collectively, mental health workers can progress toward a broader concept of psychosis, instilling hope and improved outcomes for those it affects.

In exploring schizophrenia and psychotic disorders, several significant points present themselves that are well-suited to comprehensive knowledge of these conditions. First and foremost is a greater awareness of the scope of psychotic experiences that individuals can be exposed to, particularly in reference to their adolescence and childhood. The research has established that psychotic disorders, such as schizophrenia spectrum disorders, manifest differently in the young than in adults and, therefore, necessitate a consideration of the particular developmental context of youth. Of particular interest, the research indicates the prevalence of psychotic experiences within community as well as clinical samples, thus necessitating early intervention as well as risk assessment in youths. As noted by current studies, their capture and treatment can yield much improved results as well as reduce the long-term impact of such disabling disorders (Kelleher, 2025). Second, proper diagnosis and treatment are the greatest concerns while treating schizophrenia and related psychotic disorders. The development in psychometric tests and symptomology has made more accurate and timely diagnoses possible, which is most important in formulating proper treatment plans. The identification of key risk factors and the implementation of psychiatric interventions emphasize a multifaceted approach to treatment through pharmacological and psychotherapeutic management. Present evidence favors a combination of medication, cognitive behavioral therapy, and psychoeducation as a strategy for enhancing coping skills among the afflicted population. The successful integration of these variables into treatment plans illustrates a commitment to personalized care that addresses the specific needs of each patient (Manfredini et al., 2024). Also, the treatment of schizophrenia and psychotic disorders is constantly evolving because of ongoing research and theoretical advances. Emerging studies explore the biological, psychological, and social determinants of these conditions, noting their interaction in psychosis development and progression. With an increasing number of professionals recognizing the value of a biopsychosocial approach, there is a trend towards preventative methods and aiming to prevent risks early before they develop into full-scale disorders. This proactive approach is underscored by conclusive evidence necessitating early detection methods and community intervention. The lessons learned from clinical and community research support a shared responsibility from families, educators, and healthcare providers to create mental health-supporting environments and to initiate timely intervention for at-risk individuals (Kelleher, 2025).

KEY TERMS FROM THIS CHAPTER

- Anhedonia
- Avolition
- Catatonia
- Delusional disorder
- Disorganized speech
- First-episode psychosis
- Hallucinations
- Antipsychotic medication
- Psychotic disorder
- Cognitive impairment
- Delusions
- Extrapyramidal symptoms
- Flat affect
- Negative symptoms

CRITICAL THINKING QUESTIONS

1. **Which of the following is a positive symptom of schizophrenia?**
   a. Flat affect
   b. Social withdrawal
   c. Hallucinations
   d. Lack of motivation
2. **Delusions are best described as:**
   a. Visual perceptions of things not present
   b. Strongly held false beliefs not based in reality
   c. Repetitive behaviors like hand-washing
   d. Temporary confusion
3. **Which neurotransmitter is most commonly associated with schizophrenia?**
   a. Serotonin
   b. Acetylcholine
   c. Dopamine
   d. GABA
4. **The onset of schizophrenia most commonly occurs during:**
   a. Childhood (under 12)
   b. Adolescence to early adulthood
   c. Middle age (40–60 years)
   d. Old age (over 65)
5. **A common feature of schizoaffective disorder is the presence of:**
   a. Only mood symptoms
   b. Only psychotic symptoms
   c. Both mood disorder and psychotic symptoms
   d. Only anxiety symptoms

Short Answer Questions

1. What is the primary characteristic that defines psychotic disorders?
2. Name three common positive symptoms of schizophrenia.
3. What are negative symptoms in schizophrenia? Provide two examples.
4. What is the difference between hallucinations and delusions? Give an example of each.
5. Which neurotransmitter is most implicated in the development of schizophrenia?

Answer to Critical Thinking Questions

1. (c) 2. (b) 3. (c) 4. (b) 5. (c)

REFERENCES

1. Adadzi, J., Anderson II, J., Azi, C. I., et al. (2024). Mental health in later life: Clinical insights and management strategies for late-onset psychiatric conditions. https://core.ac.uk/download/621451783.pdf (accessed on 28th July 2025).
2. Addington, J., Andreasen, N. C., Anselmetti, F., Appels, M., Bediou, B., Benton, T., Bilder, R., et al. (2012). Cognitive alterations in patients with non-affective psychotic disorder and their unaffected siblings and parents. https://core.ac.uk/download/pdf/12979984.pdf (accessed on 28th July 2025).
3. Agius, M., Grech, A., & Zammit, S. (2010). Cannabis and psychosis: The Maltese contribution. https://core.ac.uk/download/46602245.pdf (accessed on 28th July 2025).
4. Andreasen, N. C., Brintnell, E. S., Cook, S., Corporate Policy Unit SCC., Creek, J., Department of Health., Chambers, E., et al. (2008). Occupational therapy for people with psychotic conditions in community settings: A pilot randomized controlled trial. https://core.ac.uk/download/1594196.pdf (accessed on 28th July 2025).
5. Van Dael, F., van Os, J., de Graaf, R., ten Have, M., Krabbendam, L., & Myin-Germeys, I. (2011). Can obsessions drive you mad? Longitudinal evidence that obsessive-compulsive symptoms worsen the outcome of early psychotic experiences. Acta psychiatrica Scandinavica, 123(2), 136–146. https://doi.org/10.1111/j.1600-0447.2010.01609.x (accessed on 28th July 2025).
6. Baldessarini, R. J., Centorrino, F., Curto, M., et al. (2016). Factors associated with costs of hospitalization of severely mentally ill patients. https://core.ac.uk/download/154948434.pdf (accessed on 28th July 2025).
7. Barker, G., Bebbington, P., Beck, A., Bernstein, E., Brett, E., Fink, G., Goff, D., et al. (2009). Childhood abuse and the content of delusions. https://core.ac.uk/download/1639599.pdf (accessed on 28th July 2025).
8. Baskin-Sommers, A. R., & Fonteneau, K. (2016). Correctional change through neuroscience. https://core.ac.uk/download/144231726.pdf (accessed on 28th July 2025).
9. Bauman, M. D., Carter, C. S., Cherry, S. R., et al. (2019). Preliminary evidence of increased striatal dopamine in a nonhuman primate model of maternal immune activation. https://core.ac.uk/download/323070440.pdf (accessed on 28th July 2025).
10. Bebbington, P. E., Dunn, G., Fowler, D., et al. (2006). Emotional dysfunction in schizophrenia spectrum psychosis: The role of illness perceptions. https://core.ac.uk/download/1670764.pdf (accessed on 28th July 2025).
11. Jenkins, R; Meltzer, H; Jones, PB; Brugha, T; Bebbington, P; Farrell, M; Crepaz-(accessed on 28th July 2025).
12. Bere, M., Rossell, S. L., Tan, E., Carruthers, S., Gurvich, C., Neill, E., Sumner, P., et al. (2024). Exploring the cognitive profiles related to unimodal auditory versus multisensory hallucinations in schizophrenia-spectrum disorders. *Cognitive Neuropsychiatry, 29*, 55–71. https://www.semanticscholar.org/paper/9c39c67668d142abe61a7f096699aaf7a437a77f (accessed on 28th July 2025).
13. Borsboom, D. (2017). A network theory of mental disorders. *World Psychiatry, 16*, 5–13. https://doi.org/10.1002/wps.20375 (accessed on 28th July 2025).

14. Bottlender, R., Jäger, M., Möller, H. J., et al. (2003). On the descriptive validity of ICD-10 schizophrenia: Empirical analyses in the spectrum of non-affective functional psychoses. https://core.ac.uk/download/16432279.pdf (accessed on 28th July 2025).

15. Bottlender, R., Jäger, M., Möller, H. J., et al. (2004). Classification of functional psychoses and its implication for prognosis: Comparison between ICD-10 and DSM-IV. https://core.ac.uk/download/16432278.pdf (accessed on 28th July 2025).

16. Boyd, A., Fossati, A., Johnson, A. D., Cardno, A. G., Fanous, A. H., Fanous, A. H., Fanous, A. H., et al. (2014). Are genetic risk factors for psychosis also associated with dimension-specific psychotic experiences in adolescence? https://core.ac.uk/download/20117926.pdf (accessed on 28th July 2025).

17. Bressington, D., White, J., et al. (2015). Recovery from psychosis: Physical health, antipsychotic medication and the daily dilemmas for mental health nurses. https://core.ac.uk/download/151156871.pdf (accessed on 28th July 2025).

18. Broome, M. R., Catone, G., Lennox, B., et al. (2017). Bullying victimization and psychosis: The inter-dependence and independence of risk trajectories. https://core.ac.uk/download/132201613.pdf (accessed on 28th July 2025).

19. Campellone, T. R., Caponigro, J. M., & Kring, A. M. (2014). The power to resist: The relationship between power, stigma, and negative symptoms in schizophrenia. https://core.ac.uk/download/323311082.pdf (accessed on 28th July 2025).

20. Chan, R. H. A. (2013). Hallucinogens: Mechanisms and medical complications. https://open.bu.edu/bitstream/2144/12070/6/Chan_Ryan_2013_nosig_nocv.pdf (accessed on 28th July 2025).

21. Chwaliszewski, K., Fikas, K., Goliszek, Z., et al. (2025). Exploring the therapeutic role of physical activity in psychotic disorders: Cognitive, somatic, and mental health impacts. https://core.ac.uk/download/636385728.pdf (accessed on 28th July 2025).

22. Crow, T. J. (1995). A continuum of psychosis, one human gene, and not much else–The case for homogeneity. https://core.ac.uk/download/pdf/86082.pdf (accessed on 28th July 2025).

23. Cummings, L. (2012). Establishing diagnostic criteria: The role of clinical pragmatics. https://core.ac.uk/download/30643850.pdf (accessed on 28th July 2025).

24. Faber, S. C., Khanna Roy, A., Michaels, T. I., & Williams, M. T. (2023). The weaponization of medicine: Early psychosis in the Black community and the need for racially informed mental healthcare. *Frontiers in Psychiatry, 14*. https://doi.org/10.3389/fpsyt.2023.1098292 (accessed on 28th July 2025).

25. Fett, A. K. J., Krabbendam, L., Lemmers-Jansen, I. L. J., et al. (2019). Social mindfulness and psychosis: Neural response to socially mindful behavior in first-episode psychosis and patients at clinical high-risk. https://core.ac.uk/download/185244505.pdf (accessed on 28th July 2025).

26. Frydecka, D., Gawęda, Ł., Misiak, B., et al. (2018). Interactions between variation in candidate genes and environmental factors in the etiology of schizophrenia and bipolar disorder: A systematic review. https://core.ac.uk/download/161229507.pdf (accessed on 28th July 2025).

27. Giacco, D., McCabe, R., Kallert, T., et al. (2007). Friends and symptom dimensions in patients with psychosis: A pooled analysis. https://core.ac.uk/download/30696662.pdf (accessed on 28th July 2025).

28. Hamm, J. A., Hasson-Ohayon, I., Huling, K., et al. (2017). Recovery and serious mental illness: A review of current clinical and research paradigms and future directions. https://core.ac.uk/download/96883617.pdf (accessed on 28th July 2025).

29. Jakovljević, M., Kozumplik, O., & Uzun, S. (2009). Psychotic disorders and comorbidity: Somatic illness vs. side effect. https://core.ac.uk/download/14420499.pdf (accessed on 28th July 2025).

30. Johnson, S. J., & Wolke, D. (2013). Behavioral outcomes and psychopathology during adolescence. https://core.ac.uk/download/9847191.pdf (accessed on 28th July 2025).

31. Johnstone, E. C., Lawrie, S., MacIntyre, D., et al. (2005). A Theory of Mind investigation into the appreciation of visual jokes in schizophrenia. https://core.ac.uk/download/pdf/3566533.pdf (accessed on 28th July 2025).

32. Jorm, A. F., Jorm, A. F., Yung, A. R., Dell'Osso, B., Lauber, C., Lincoln, C., Morgan, C., et al. (2013). Are lay people good at recognizing the symptoms of schizophrenia? https://core.ac.uk/download/18488559.pdf (accessed on 28th July 2025).

33. Kelleher, I. (2025). Annual research review: Psychosis in children and adolescents: Key updates from the past 2 decades on psychotic disorders, psychotic experiences, and psychosis risk. *Journal of Child Psychology and Psychiatry, and Allied Disciplines, 66*, 460–476. https://www.semanticscholar.org/paper/b9057ae57ca75460e7b948123422062e496553c2 (accessed on 28th July 2025).

34. Kendler K. S. (2017). The Clinical Features of Paranoia in the 20th Century and Their Representation in Diagnostic Criteria From DSM-III Through DSM-5. *Schizophrenia bulletin, 43*(2), 332–343. https://doi.org/10.1093/schbul/sbw161(accessed on 28th July 2025).

35. Kerst, A., Stricker, J., & Gaebel, W. (2020). Classification and diagnosis of schizophrenia or other primary psychotic disorders: Changes from ICD-10 to ICD-11 and implementation in clinical practice. https://core.ac.uk/download/388187411.pdf (accessed on 28th July 2025).

36. Killaspy, H., King, M., Taylor, T. L., et al. (2012). Psychometric properties of the Mental Health Recovery Star. [No link provided for access date].

37. Kotov, R., Krueger, R. F., Watson, D., Achenbach, T. M., Althoff, R. R., Bagby, R. M., Brown, T. A., et al. (2017). The Hierarchical Taxonomy of Psychopathology (HiTOP): A dimensional alternative to traditional nosologies. *Journal of Abnormal Psychology, 126*, 454–477. https://doi.org/10.1037/abn0000258 (accessed on 28th July 2025).

38. Lewis, A. J. (2008). Neuropsychological deficit and psychodynamic defense models of schizophrenia: Towards an integrated psychotherapeutic model. http://hdl.handle.net/10536/DRO/DU:30016990 (accessed on 28th July 2025).

39. Li, H., Wang, Q., Hou, W., Chen, D., Ding, Y., Zhang, Z., Hou, W. W., et al. (2024). Further clarification of cognitive processes of prospective memory in schizophrenia by comparing eye-tracking and ecologically-valid measurements. *Schizophrenia, 10*. https://www.semanticscholar.org/paper/622b7f09bcd9efed5982e5404210faf3b9e7a3f6 (accessed on 28th July 2025).

40. Manfredini, D., Häggman-Henrikson, B., Al Jagshi, A., Baad-Hansen, L., Beecroft, E., Bijelic, T., Bracci, A., et al. (2024). Temporomandibular disorders: INfORM/IADR key points for good clinical practice based on standard of care. *CRANIO®, 43*, 1–5. https://www.semanticscholar.org/paper/6872d48a634f04904ee405af21357149df90a15f (accessed on 28th July 2025).

41. Maruta, N., & Kushnir, Y. (2024). Characteristics of the affective sphere in patients with negative symptoms in schizophrenia. *Lviv Clinical Bulletin*. https://www.semanticscholar.org/paper/b9a00afe1ddd106bd362f157cf8826476e085a5d (accessed on 28th July 2025).

42. Masinga, N. (2017). Representations of the schizophrenia spectrum and other psychotic disorders in South African newspapers. https://core.ac.uk/download/304374268.pdf (accessed on 28th July 2025).

43. Orban Szigeti, B., Farkas, K., Hermán, L., Zsigmond, R., Réthelyi, J., & Csukly, G. (2024). Theta-burst rTMS in schizophrenia to ameliorate negative and cognitive symptoms: A double-blind, sham-controlled, randomized clinical trial. *European Psychiatry, 67*, S212. https://www.semanticscholar.org/paper/ab5a8cbd81f77075f6ee49e771a52aa04e14b5dc (accessed on 28th July 2025).

44. Parnas, J. (2015). Differential diagnosis and current polythetic classification. *World Psychiatry, 14*, 284–287. https://doi.org/10.1002/wps.20239 (accessed on 28th July 2025).

45. Sharma, M., Sivakumar, P. T., Rao, G. P., & Paul, N. (2018). Clinical practice guidelines for management of dementia. *Indian Journal of Psychiatry, 60*, 312. https://doi.org/10.4103/0019-5545.224472 (accessed on 28th July 2025).

46. Sideli, L., Trotta, G., Spinazzola, E., La Cascia, C., & Di Forti, M. (2020). Adverse effects of heavy cannabis use: Even plants can harm the brain. *Pain, 162*, S97–S104. https://doi.org/10.1097/j.pain.0000000000001963 (accessed on 28th July 2025).

47. Spark, J., Rowe, E., Alvarez-Jimenez, M., Bell, I., Byrne, L. K., Dzafic, I., Ellinghaus, C., et al. (2025). Integrating virtual reality, neurofeedback, and cognitive behavioral therapy for auditory verbal hallucinations (Hybrid): Protocol of a pilot, unblinded, single-arm interventional study. *JMIR Research Protocols, 14*. https://www.semanticscholar.org/paper/d8bdbf82dc994a8d9b19738e7320405eaef60ea6 (accessed on 28th July 2025).

48. Uğurlu, M., Uğurlu, G., Kabadayi Sahin, E., Kamış, G. Z., & Caykoylu, A. (2024). Short and long-term effects of cognitive behavioral therapy on sleep problems and psychotic symptoms in patients with psychotic disorders: A meta-analysis study. *Revita Brasileira de Psiquiatria*. https://www.semanticscholar.org/paper/3bcfff49cd64bced3c3aadfa5f735d742ee11ee9 (accessed on 28th July 2025).

49. Wang, J., Mann, F., Lloyd-Evans, B., Ma, R., & Johnson, S. (2018). Associations between loneliness and perceived social support and outcomes of mental health problems: A systematic review. *BMC Psychiatry, 18*. https://doi.org/10.1186/s12888-018-1736-5 (accessed on 28th July 2025).

50. Wittenburg, D., Aron, L. Y., & Burt, M. R. (2005). Recommendations to the Social Security Administration on the design of the Mental Health Treatment Study. https://core.ac.uk/download/71340972.pdf (accessed on 28th July 2025).

51. Zhou, J., Liu, L., Xue, P., Yang, X., & Tang, X. (2020). Mental health response to the COVID-19 outbreak in China. *American Journal of Psychiatry, 177*, 574–575. https://doi.org/10.1176/appi.ajp.2020.20030304 (accessed on 28th July 2025).

MOOD DISORDERS

5

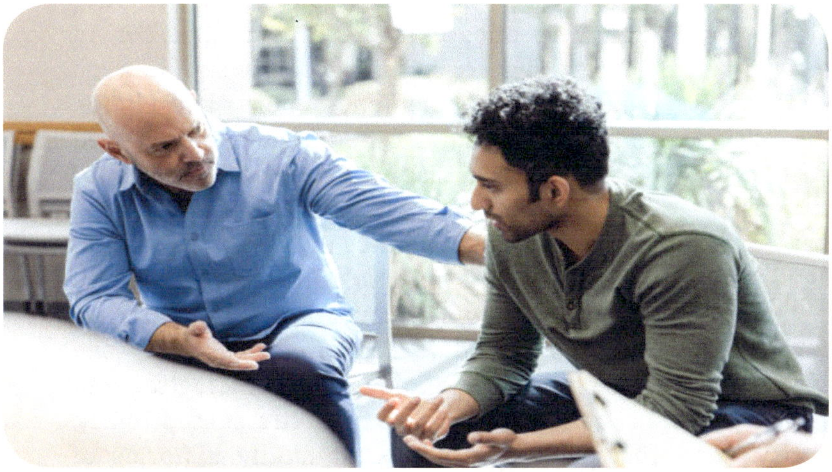

LEARNING OBJECTIVES

After studying this chapter, you will be able to:

1. Give historical context;
2. List the symptoms and diagnosis;
3. Describe the causes and risk factors;
4. Explain the types of mood disorders;
5. Focus on the impact on daily life;
6. Explore the current research trends;
7. Define stigma and public perception.

Introduction

Mood disorders are a leading category of mental illness that entail the suffering of alterations in an individual's emotional state. They represent a set of disorders impacting how a person feels, thinks, and behaves, leading to alterations in functioning in daily life. Major depressive disorder, bipolar disorder, and dysthymia are the most commonly recognized mood disorders, among others. These are not discrete episodes of sullenness or irritability but rather a constellation of emotional disturbances capable of causing severe impairment in social, occupational, and personal functioning. An understanding of these disorders begins with the acknowledgment that mood changes may result from an array of biological, psychological, and environmental factors, which highlight the complexity of every individual's experience. Diagnostic symptoms for mood disorders encompass a wide range of symptoms beyond transient happiness or sadness. For instance, major depressive disorder is characterized by an extended period of depressed mood lasting two weeks or more with various accompanying symptoms , such as appetite, sleep, and loss of interest in once pleasurable activities. Bipolar disorder, however, includes depressive and manic episodes, which lead to extreme mood changes that can significantly disrupt an individual's life. The mental health care providers have a model for diagnosis that takes note of how these illnesses can be very dissimilar in presentation and how symptom persistence and intensity are also deciding factors in distinguishing between several mood disorders. Apart from their clinical definition, mood disorders have far-reaching implications for global health. Individuals afflicted by such disorders typically experience problems in relationship maintenance, work performance, and daily activities. On top of that, stigmatization of mental illness can additionally perpetuate perceptions of loneliness and hopelessness, making recovery challenging. As such, comprehensive treatment approaches, incorporating psychotherapy, medications, and behavior modifications, are needed to effectively manage mood disorders. Through having a clearer understanding of these illnesses, society can assist in reducing stigma and promoting supportive environments that enable individuals with mood disorders to come forward and receive the help that they need to attain recovery and an improved quality of life (Figure 5.1).

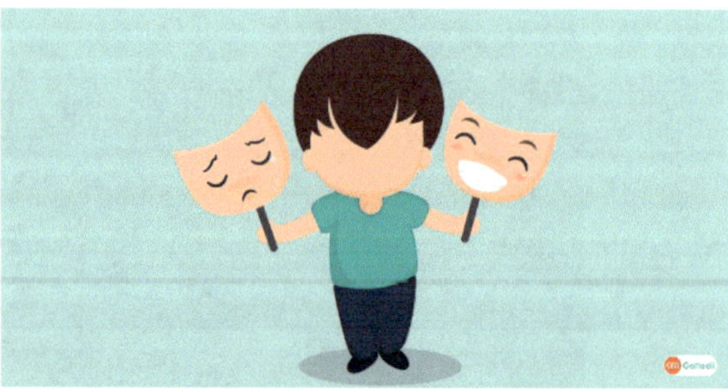

Figure 5.1. Mood disorders.

Source: https://english-blog.s3.amazonaws.com/uploads/2018/06/Bipolar-Disorder-in-Children-Symptoms-Signs-and-How-to-Manage.jpg.

Overview of Mood Disorders

Mood disorders are a broad category of psychological conditions that are characterized by extreme disturbances in the mood state of an individual, leading to impairment in daily functioning. The three main types of mood disorders include major depressive disorder, bipolar disorder, and persistent depressive disorder (dysthymia). Major depressive disorder is characterized by extreme sadness, hopelessness, and loss of interest in activities that were once enjoyed. Bipolar disorder, in contrast, involves extreme mood swings between manic highs of heightened energy and elation and depressive lows. Differentiating the nuanced features of each disorder is essential to proper diagnosis and effective treatment, highlighting the complex dynamic between emotional regulation and psychological well-being in these disorders. The causation and persistence of mood disorders are often shaped by the interplay among biological, psychological, and environmental factors. Genetic susceptibility, too, plays a role in that family histories of mood disorders are risk factors. Beyond that, imbalances in neurotransmitters , such as serotonin and norepinephrine are also frequently mentioned in depressive disorders. Additionally, environmental stressors , such as traumatic events or chronic stress are frequent causes of the exacerbation of pre-existing mood conditions or of their development. Hence, comprehensive assessments considering an individual's current and previous life circumstances are crucial in constructing intervention plans and modifying treatments according to the specific needs of individuals, testifying to the fact that a multidimensional approach is most critical in treating mood disorders. Emerging treatment trends have introduced new methods to maximize the effectiveness of interventions among individuals suffering from mood disorders. One such field is horticultural therapy, which entails the use of plant-based activities to provide therapy. This process has been discovered to have promising results, particularly in specific populations, such as military veterans with post-traumatic stress disorder (PTSD) stemming from their exposure activities (Nadeau, 2019). Horticultural therapy is a possible adjunct treatment for mood disorders, engaging patients in goal-oriented activities resulting in emotional recovery and resilience. The network model of thinking about mood disorders therefore, is important for illustrating the interconnectedness of symptoms, whereby changing a single factor of emotional wellness can affect the broad disorder structure and support recovery and relapse prevention (Curtiss et al., 2016). It emphasizes the worth of multidimensional treatment models integrating mainstream and alternative treatments to achieve the highest level of psychological well-being (Figure 5.2).

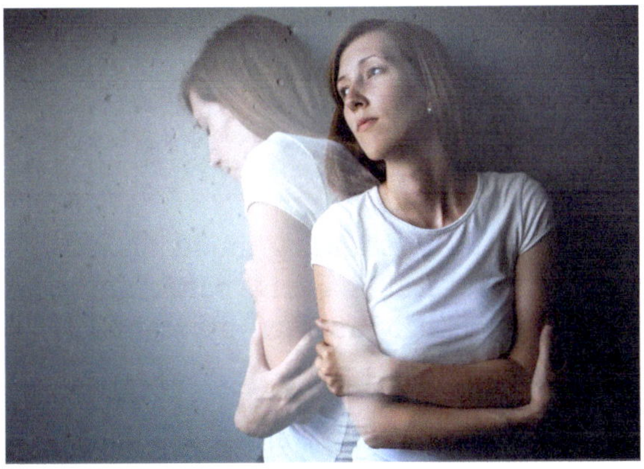

Figure 5.2. Mood disorders encompass a broad spectrum of psychological conditions characterized by significant disturbances in an individual's emotional state, leading to dysfunction in daily life.

Source: https://atlanticbehavioralhealth.com/wp-content/uploads/2024/09/local-woman-suffering-from-mood-disorder.webp.

Types of Mood Disorders

The mood disorder category includes three types of conditions characterized by major depressive disturbance in an individual's mood. In these, major depressive disorder (MDD) is probably the most common type, characterized by chronic sadness, hopelessness, and loss of interest in activities previously found pleasing. Patients with MDD typically experience incapacitating symptoms that may interfere with their daily functioning, thus making it a priority concern for mental health services. Research indicates that mood disorders like MDD are prevalent among various groups, and research has indicated that they form a considerable proportion of referrals to mental health services (Bedford 53.8%, Perugia 48%, Magione 45%, Bastia 38%) (Agius et al., 2013). This statistic brings forth the necessity of proper interventions and support systems to address such widespread mental illness. Bipolar disorder, including fluctuations between depression and mania or hypomania, ranks as yet another top category in mood disorders. Patients of bipolar disorder may experience extreme mood swings that disrupt their professional and personal lives. The manic phases can generate impulsivity, high mood, and enhanced energy, while the depressive phases can be similar to the major depression symptoms. This swing between the mood states demands personalized treatment modalities that will target both the ends. Along with that, the stabilization of mood and enhancement in the ability of patients to function normally in day-to-day life is usually demanded with the combination of medication and psychotherapy for the treatment of bipolar disorder. Complexities of bipolar disorder need to be realized in order to develop effective mental health care interventions that are able to adequately address those who are afflicted. Dysthymia, or chronic depressive disorder, is a mood disorder in which a patient feels a chronic condition of depression for two years or longer. Major depressive disorder is different from dysthymia in the sense that dysthymia is capable of presenting as a lighter but more enduring symptom of depression. The people afflicted by dysthymia feel inadequate and lack self-worth, also experiencing chronic tiredness and the inability to appreciate life. Dysthymia does not get noticed, as its effects might pass for aspects of an individual's personality or outlook in life. Dysthymia does need to be recognized and treated, however, since people might go on for years without help, even making things worse. The impact of mood disorders like dysthymia on personal well-being as well as on the overall systemic systems warrants more awareness and preventive treatment strategies (Biesok et al., 2024).

Significance of Knowing Mood Disorders

It is essential to understand mood disorders for many reasons, especially within an increasingly mentally health-affected society. Mood disorders, such as depression and bipolar disorder, have profound effects on individuals' day-to-day functioning and interpersonal relationships. The better that practitioners are able to understand the lived experience of this population, the more effectively they can craft interventions and support structures that address this population's unique needs. For instance, a study has been able to recognize vital themes , such as the process of acceptation of the diagnosis and the negative effect it has on relationships, which are capable of enhancing practitioners' empathy and competence (Cooke et al., 2016). This delicate framework not only benefits directly diagnosed individuals but also enables effective communication and interpretation between peers and family members, thereby creating an overall more supportive-oriented environment for individuals facing mood disorders. The social implication of the acknowledgment of mood disorders goes beyond treatment at the patient level. As the conditions would disrupt family life, it is important to comprehend how they affect child development and parenting. For example, parents with depressive disorder would be unable to offer adequate caregiving, with detrimental impacts on the emotional and psychological development of their children (McCauliff et al., 2007). Increased awareness of these challenges can lead to the development of targeted outreach and education programs that address the particular needs of mood disorder-affected families. Some examples of such programs are workshops for parents, community support groups, and accessible mental health clinics, in effect bridging the gap between need and availability of resources. As communities make the knowledge of mood disorders a priority, they help not only those affected but also promote greater general stability and welfare in society.

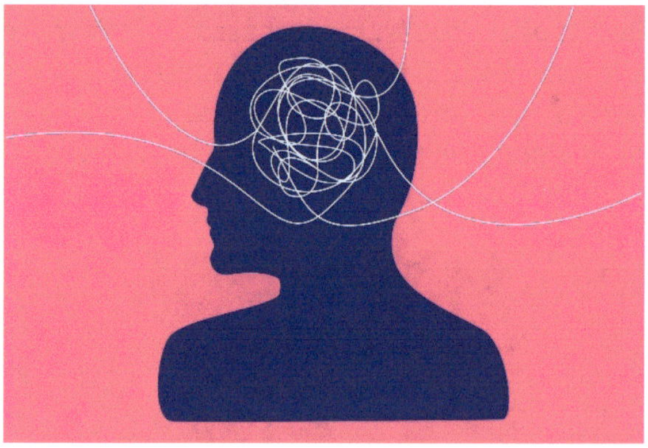

Figure 5.3. Understanding mood disorders is critical for several reasons, particularly in a society increasingly affected by mental health issues.

Source: https://neurowellnessspa.com/wp-content/uploads/2024/04/what-causes-mental-illness.jpg.

Additionally, increased knowledge of mood disorders can also bring changes in how people perceive them, breaking down stigma and creating a culture that supports frank discussion of mental illness. This is important in persuading people to come forward and seek help and assistance without fear of rejection. As studies reveal, stigma related to mood disorders tends to dissuade individuals from proper treatment and support, exacerbating their symptoms (Cooke et al., 2016). By encouraging mental health awareness and education, society can make individuals feel comfortable enough to openly discuss their struggles. This sharing of experiences empowers individuals with mood disorders as well as friends and family members, using shared experience to create a feeling of belonging and resilience. Ultimately, embracing a more expansive view of mood disorders is key to building a more empathetic and compassionate society, ushering in improved mental health for all (Figure 5.3).

5.1. Historical Context

Learning Outcome

1. Understand hotel maintenance management and its impact
2. Perform preventive maintenance
3. Discuss about breakdown maintenance

The history of mood disorders illustrates the complex evolution of mental health knowledge that has evolved radically over the centuries. Mood disorders have been attributed to supernatural forces or the balance of body humors in ancient cultures, for instance. Hippocrates formulated theories that associated the emotional with the physical, setting the stage for a rudimentary medical classification system. This conceptualization set the stage for later psychiatric models, though it lacked a current empirical basis. In the course of time, centuries later, the development of psychiatric hospitals in the 19th century marked a turning point where mood disorders were systematized under categories. The advent of diagnostic criteria and the definition of mental health as a field for medical inquiry represented the start of a transition to an increasingly medicalized understanding of such illness, indeed shaping the way psychiatric practice and research developed. In the course of the 20th century, advances in psychology and psychiatry were tremendous, with a more nuanced understanding of mood disorders. The development of the Diagnostic and Statistical Manual of Mental Disorders (DSM) during the mid-20th century made standardized diagnosis criteria possible, and it was possible to apply uniformity to the classification of mood disorders , such as major depression and bipolar disorder. The DSM became core in clinical practice as it enabled doctors to diagnose and treat patients more effectively. Nonetheless, there has been mounting criticism of the categorical differences in the DSM. Critics argue that such strict definitions generally fail to take into consideration the subtleties of personal experience. This nascent skepticism paved the way to more integral approaches, aimed at understanding the integration of biological, psychological, and social factors acting on mood disorders, thereby violating traditional nosological models and enhancing treatment approaches. Now, the restriction of categorial models has fostered transdiagnostic models' popularity, where syndromes are explained more in terms of how they are connected than in opposition to one another. The aim here is to address the dimensionality and the comorbidity that define mood disorders, rooted in growing awareness that patients tend to present with syndromes that are prevalent across disorders. Emerging research emphasizes the need for early detection and intervention employing novel methods , such as social media analysis to track behavioral markers linked with mood changes. Evidence suggests that public health initiatives must transform accordingly to develop more responsive diagnostic tools and treatment mechanisms. With the development of the field of psychiatry, an emphasis on a transdiagnostic approach can have limitless scope for enhancing clinical effectiveness as well as leading to increased knowledge about mood disorder development and maintenance, as highlighted in (Dalgleish et al., 2020; Choudhury et al., 2021).

5.1.1. Evolution of Mood Disorder Concepts

The mood disorder concept has evolved significantly over the past few decades from simple to complex models encompassing biological, psychological, and social factors. Mood disorders were traditionally dealt with in a clinically oriented manner where the focus was laid on observable symptoms and their categorization in diagnostic manuals. This reductionist approach has been challenged, however, since researchers and clinicians recognize the limitation that it imposes on understanding the full complexity of these disorders. In particular, the establishment of biopsychosocial models highlights the importance of recognizing emotional and cognitive factors in addition to traditional pharmacological views. Such an expanded vision creates opportunities for more robust interventions that acknowledge the interplay between intrinsic vulnerabilities and extrinsic stressors, further advancing the literature on mood disorders and their etiology. With science demanding to know more about the intricacies of mood disorders, early life experience and adverse environment have taken center stage. Evidence implies that childhood adversities have a strong impact on emotional regulation and mood-related predispositions to mental disorders in adulthood. And family turmoil's contribution to the development of mood disorders is increasingly supported by empirical work showing how these experiences affect both cognitive and noncognitive abilities. Delving deeper, macroeconomic factors further complicate this landscape; for instance, transitions into economic recessions correlate with heightened instances of disconnection among youth, thereby potentially exacerbating mood disorders in this vulnerable demographic. As our understanding of these various influences grows, it becomes increasingly evident that a multifaceted approach is essential for comprehensive treatment and prevention strategies. In addition, the conceptual development of mood disorders transfers over to the field of treatment modalities, identifying personalized interventions integrating pharmacological and psychotherapeutic elements. Theoretical definition of mood disorders not merely within the domain of their symptoms but also under the umbrella of neurobiological processes presents a more effective treatment modality to the therapeutic field. Current studies highlight the necessity of exploring both environmental stressors and genetic vulnerabilities to obtain an integrated view of mood disorder management. Moreover, with the developments in neuroscience that unveil the intricacies of neural circuits and their implication in mood control, novel treatment modalities are being formulated that extend beyond traditional pharmacotherapy. This sustained progression obviously shows heightened sensitivity that the management of mood disorders needs a comprehensive understanding of the dynamic interaction among biological, psychological, and social factors, ultimately translated into better treatment outcomes among affected populations (Figure 5.4).

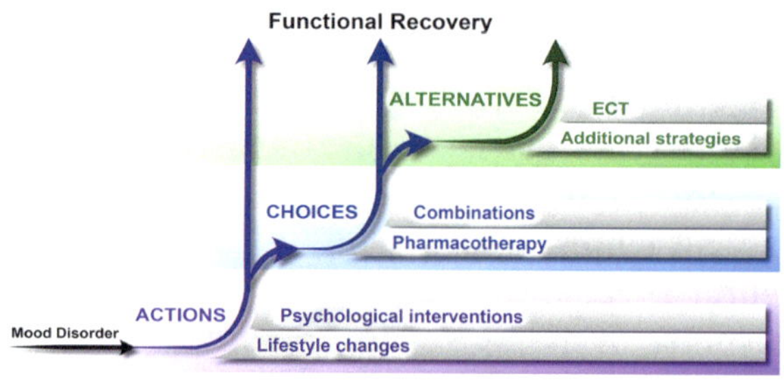

Figure 5.4. Historically, mood disorders were often viewed through a purely clinical lens, with emphasis placed on observable symptoms and their categorization in diagnostic manuals.

Source: https://journals.sagepub.com/cms/10.1177/0004867420979353/asset/images/large/10.1177_0004867420979353-fig18.jpeg.

5.1.2. Key Figures in Mood Disorder Research

The research history of mood disorders has been significantly dictated by some of the major players whose contributions have helped both the treatment and the comprehension of these diseases. Among those is Aaron T. Beck, who became a major player after discovering cognitive therapy, which revolutionized the strategy that clinicians employ to address mood disorders, with depression being a central component. His classic book proposed the concept that cognitive distortions are central to causing and maintaining emotional issues. By separating these errors in worldview and self-concept, Beck's theories laid the foundation for a model for therapy that emphasized the necessity of altering skewed patterns of thinking. Beck's lasting clinical practice legacy is observed in the broad acceptance of cognitive behavioral therapy, which remains one of the most empirically supported treatments for mood disorder today. Such an emphasis on cognitive function has led the door to further study in this field. Another prominent researcher of mood disorder study is Emil Kraepelin, whose initial system of classification of psychiatric disorder has influenced the field for centuries. By creating precise diagnostic criteria for mood disorders like major depressive disorder and bipolar disorder, Kraepelin's work allowed for more systematic treatment and investigation. His classification of manic-depressive illness as a distinct category allowed for greater understanding of the cyclical pattern of mood disorders and their varied presentations. Further, Kraepelin's emphasis on the biological underpinnings of psychiatric disorders encouraged subsequent investigators to explore neurobiological factors in mood disorders. This has led to a myriad of studies examining the role of neurotransmitters, genetic markers, and other physiological factors in mood dysregulation. Kraepelin's system is still widely used in contemporary psychiatry as a framework on which contemporary diagnostics are built. Field research has also gone on to explore the microbiota-gut-brain axis, a new finding that connects gut health with mood disorders. Researchers have come to understand how the composition of gut microbiota can influence neurobiological processes, showing new avenues of treatment for diseases like depression and anxiety. Notably, various microbial metabolites influence brain function through a number of pathways, including the immune system and neural signaling. These aspects show the necessity for an integrated treatment of mood disorders in light of food, environmental, and psychological factors. As the field evolves further, the prospect for the identification of microbiome-derived interventions for mood disorders is a prime area for future studies. By merging these biological components with typical psychological approaches, current and future researchers make every effort to develop further insight and extend deeper therapeutic interventions for individuals afflicted by mood disorders (Livingston et al., 2020).

5.1.3. Changes in Diagnostic Criteria Over Time

The evolution of mood disorder criteria demonstrates the increasing nature of mental health knowledge. Previously, mood disorders used to be divided on the basis of strict labels based on manifest symptoms without the provision of richness in diagnosis. Time has witnessed more open criteria focusing on subjective experience and cultural context for determining the description of mood disorders. This shift is significant because it acknowledges that disturbances of mood manifest differently across various populations and settings. Thus, the classification systems, including the Diagnostic and Statistical Manual of Mental Disorders (DSM) and the International Classification of Diseases (ICD), have been modified to be more descriptive of the nuances of mood disorders. The updates in the diagnostic criteria will continue to inform successful treatments and enhance clinicians' capacity to address varying presentations of mood disorders successfully. In recent years, there has been a clear expansion of the definition of a mood disorder, reflecting a broader approach to diagnostics. This shift is one of the recognition of non-substance behavioral addictions, such as compulsive gambling and shopping, as part of the mood disorder spectrum. These behaviors have been found by research to have underlying symptoms , such as impulsivity and dyscontrol that are akin to traditional substance use disorders and destabilize the earlier separation of behavior and substance-based disorders. The studies of these overlaps, as indicated within comparison addiction studies, highlight the need for the broadening of diagnostic definitions to more accurately represent the whole range of mood-related disorders. Treatment implications of this are immense, in that an identification of these connections can serve to establish more integrative and effective therapeutic interventions, which are crucial to individual recovery and overall mental health improvement (McLachlan & Starkey, 2012). The latest developments in the practice of diagnosis, particularly the rollout of ICD-11 by the World Health Organization, are indicative of the ongoing evolution of the mental health community. The new policy is centered on world application and usefulness to clinicians, a radical shift toward greater reflection of real-world clinical environments within diagnosis. The revisions aim at enhancing the accuracy of diagnoses while concurrently acknowledging the multitudes of cultural contexts in which these disorders occur. The reconception is to facilitate the application of these guidelines among mental health practitioners in various settings, such that they are not only applied in specialist care but also in primary care and community health programs. These improvements in diagnostic criteria have the potential to solidify evidence-based treatments, ultimately leading to improved outcomes for individuals suffering from mood disorders (Berk et al., 2020).

Test Your Knowledge

1. How have cultural and historical views on sadness, melancholy, and mania shaped modern understanding of mood disorders?
2. What key developments in psychiatry led to the differentiation between depressive and bipolar disorders?

5.2. Symptoms and Diagnosis

Learning Outcome

1. Understand hotel maintenance management and its impact
2. Perform preventive maintenance
3. Discuss about breakdown maintenance

The symptoms of mood disorder can also vary significantly in terms of the type of disorder, such as Major Depressive Disorder (MDD) or Bipolar Disorder (BD). Common symptoms include persistent sadness, hopelessness, lethargy, and changes in sleep and appetite. For MDD, lack of interest in previously enjoyable activities is accompanied by cognitive impairment in the form of reduced concentration ability. Bipolar Disorder, in contrast, is a broader spectrum of symptoms with manic or hypomanic experiences of elated mood, increased energy, and impulsive behavior. These contrasting symptomatologies reflect the nuances of mood disorders necessitating thoughtful examinations for accurate diagnosis. Besides, an understanding of the symptom presentation of every disorder is crucial in preventing misdiagnosis, which could lead to incorrect treatment interventions and further complicate the disorder, as observed in many clinical situations (Bahn et al., 2021). Mood disorder diagnostic evaluation typically depends on extensive clinical interviews and rating scales. Instruments , such as the Patient Health Questionnaire-9 (PHQ-9) provide a systematic way of measuring symptoms and their severity to make effective diagnoses. The World Health Organization Composite International Diagnostic Interview (CIDI) can be utilized in studies to classify mood disorders appropriately. Within a study of individuals who experience low mood, incidence rates of BD and MDD within the sample population were extremely high, at 24% and 36%, respectively, detected in a baseline low mood sample (Bahn et al., 2021). This indicates the problem practitioners are faced with in making the correct diagnosis and demonstrates excessive under- and misdiagnosis of mood disorders, which has a detrimental effect on treatment outcomes and patient wellbeing.

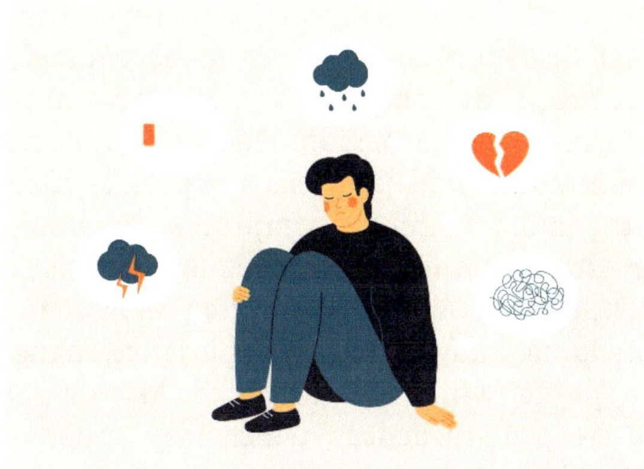

Figure 5.5. The symptoms of mood disorders can vary significantly depending on the specific type of disorder, such as Major Depressive Disorder (MDD) or Bipolar Disorder (BD).

Source: https://clearbehavioralhealth.com/wp-content/uploads/2024/09/depression-symptoms.jpg.

The identification of comorbid conditions is crucial in an attempt to make a correct diagnosis and effectively intervene. For instance, adult patients complaining of symptoms associated with Attention-Deficit/Hyperactivity Disorder (ADHD) would manifest an increased risk of mood disorders when the condition occurs alongside conditions like MDD. Research in an inpatient adult population revealed that while there was no such direct correlation between ADHD symptoms and suicidality, when mood disorders were present, the relationship was significant. This suggests the importance of evaluating mood disorder symptoms in full, as overlapping disorders make it harder to diagnose and increase the risk of negative outcomes, such as suicidality. These complications are a concern of close attention within clinical work, emphasizing the necessity for better diagnostic accuracy and individually tailored treatment approaches to address the multiaxial nature of mood disorders (Figure 5.5).

5.2.1. Common Symptoms of Mood Disorders

Mood disorders are a group of psychological illnesses encompassing major mood disturbances in a person, leading to an array of emotional and physical symptoms. A few of the most common symptoms encompass persistent sadness or a lack of interest in activities previously enjoyed, often referred to as anhedonia. Individuals may experience changes in appetite, which lead to weight loss or gain, and sleep disturbances, which may appear as insomnia or hypersomnia. These are not only side effects but also contribute to the overall impact of the disorder on everyday functioning. Recognition of these symptoms is most crucial for early identification and treatment, as individuals with such symptoms may find it challenging to maintain social relationships and fulfill occupational demands, which can worsen their emotional issues. Instability in mood (MI) is another prevalent symptom encountered with mood disorders that notably aggravates the clinical presentation. There are reports that indicate that MI is highly associated with disorders like depression and post-traumatic stress disorder (PTSD). Patients with mood instability may experience unpredictable and sudden shifts in their emotional state, and such shifts will exacerbate the feeling of anxiety and contribute to suicide ideation. Contrary to expectations, suffering from MI actually increases the risk of suicide, and research has indicated that it increases suicidal ideation by nearly five times in some patients (Chanen et al., 2013). This points to the importance of the incorporation of mood fluctuation assessment in clinical diagnosis since treatment for MI can be decisive in formulating appropriate treatment strategies and avoiding harmful outcomes in vulnerable groups. Lastly, common symptoms of some mood disorders, such as bipolar disorder, illustrate the severity and complexity of these disorders.

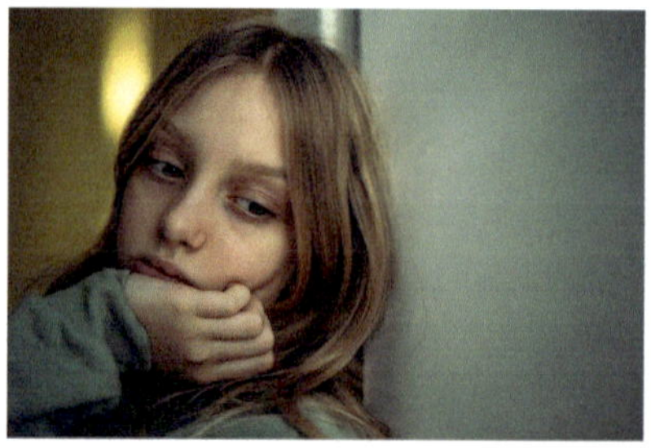

Figure 5.6. Among the most common symptoms are persistent feelings of sadness or a lack of interest in previously enjoyed activities, often referred to as anhedonia.

Source: https://www.helpguide.org/wp-content/uploads/2024/09/Anhedonia-Causes-Symptoms-and-Treatment-.jpg.

Bipolar disorder is characterized by unstable periods of mania and depression, with highs and lows that range from extreme elation to debilitating lows. Rapid cycling is the term applied when patients report moving rapidly from one mood state to another, which can be debilitating and distressing. A significant percentage of patients with bipolar disorder will also be faced with comorbid conditions, such as anxiety or substance abuse, further complicating treatment (Biedermann et al., 2002). An understanding of the varied manifestations of these symptoms not only enhances the comprehension of mood disorders but also stresses the importance of individualized therapy addressing both the core mood disturbances and any resultant psychological complications (Figure 5.6).

5.2.2. Diagnostic Tools and Criteria

Mood disorder etiology is multifactorial and thus needs a multidimensional diagnostic process with the use of various tools and criteria. The foundation of the diagnostic process is the Diagnostic and Statistical Manual of Mental

Disorders (DSM), which provides the specific criteria for the diagnosis of mood disorders, including Major Depressive Disorder and Bipolar Disorder. The DSM not only assists in providing a framework for the diagnosis of such disorders but also ensures that clinicians consider the full spectrum of symptoms and how they impact the day-to-day functioning of an individual. A full evaluation typically involves the use of standardized screening instruments, for example, the Mood Disorder Questionnaire (MDQ), which serves as a first step in the identification of the presence of mood disturbance symptomatology. The MDQ is particularly valuable in distinguishing mood disorders from other psychiatric illnesses and focusing the diagnostic process and guiding treatment interventions. The MDQ's effectiveness is noted through research in its application to the identification of those presenting with dysregulation symptoms of the mood, even if without a clinically diagnosed mood disorder. A study determined that individuals with a positive MDQ, without a comorbid mood disorder, had lower health-related quality of life (HRQoL) ratings compared to a matched control group. Such findings raise the critical question of how to interpret positive MDQ scores, since they may reflect an underlying "Dysregulation of Mood, Energy, and Social Rhythms Syndrome" (DYMERS). This syndrome suggests that even subclinical presentations of mood symptomatology have considerable distress and impairment, outlining an area of concern worthy of additional consideration by mental health specialists and primary care providers alike. Thus, the MDQ's use is more than screening, characterizing our understanding of mood disorders as a spectrum rather than categorical. While screening tools like the MDQ are valuable in yielding critical information, the complexity of mood disorder diagnoses necessitates a fuller assessment approach. Secondary assessments typically include clinical history and standardized interviews to confirm the diagnosis and rule out other concurrent illnesses. Existing research determines that primary care physicians most frequently address mood disorders, which points to the utility of effective diagnostic approaches in these settings, where early treatment is crucial. Due to the intricate pattern of mood disorders, reliance on screening alone is not sufficient. An assessment must be multi-dimensional in consideration of both biological and psychological factors influencing mood management. Here, effective collaboration between primary care and mental health professionals becomes essential in a bid to facilitate adequate assessment with the ability to inform appropriate treatment modalities, including pharmacotherapy and psychotherapy, thus improving outcomes for patients across different environments (Smith et al., 2023).

5.2.3. Diagnosis Challenges

The challenge of diagnosing mood disorders is considerable, as many of the symptoms overlap, making them challenging to diagnose or treat. Of particular concern, depression and bipolar disorder have overlapping sets of affective symptoms, which further complicates diagnosis. Clinicians are frequently compelled to navigate the subtle presentation of the disorders, frequently requiring careful evaluation to exclude one from the other.

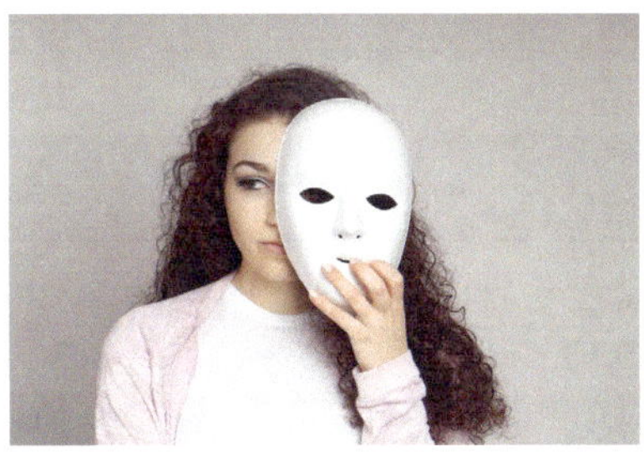

Figure 5.7. The complexity of diagnosing mood disorders is noteworthy, as numerous overlapping symptoms can lead to misdiagnosis or delayed treatment.

Source: https://atlanticbehavioralhealth.com/wp-content/uploads/2024/07/woman-with-a-mood-disorder.webp.

This process may be difficult due to patient history, emotional state, and even cultural nuances, for possible diagnostic errors. Overcoming these obstacles requires a detailed diagnosis and by interaction with the patient, so that both conditions can be acknowledged and later managed with ease. Lack of resources is also a major obstacle in the diagnosis of mood disorders, particularly if that area is rural and underprivileged. As per the National Institute of Mental Health, almost 1 out of 5 adults suffers from a diagnosed mental disorder, that is, around 43 million Americans. However, access is limited by some barriers , such as insufficiency of trained psychiatrists, especially in Vermont, limiting timely and adequate mental health care access. It leads to long waiting lists for evaluation and treatment that, in turn, continue to perpetuate the severity of mood disorders. In this context, primary care practitioners are likely to be at the forefront in the diagnosis of mood disorders, and therefore high-quality screening instruments have to be employed to maximize their restricted consultation time (Cooper et al., 2017). Moreover, access and usage of standardized screening measures can have a strong influence on diagnostic precision and treatment effectiveness. Other tools like the Mood Disorder Questionnaire (MDQ) have also been found to be helpful for the detection of bipolar spectrum disorders among outpatient populations. The usefulness of the MDQ is seen in its cited sensitivity and specificity, although it does reveal limitations in specific scenarios. Practitioners must, thus, navigate the nuances of such devices while being conscious of their limitations and the specific requirements of a given set of patients. In regions where resources for mental health are scarce, such as Vermont, the MDQ can be a valuable starting point for diagnosis, allowing for the identification of risk individuals despite the desperate resource constraints of mental health care (Cooper et al., 2017) (Figure 5.7).

Test Your Knowledge

1. What are the common symptoms used to diagnose major depressive disorder and bipolar disorder?
2. How do diagnostic criteria in DSM-5-TR help clinicians distinguish between normal emotional changes and clinical mood disorders?

5.3. Causes and Risk Factors

Learning Outcome

1. Understand hotel maintenance management and its impact
2. Perform preventive maintenance
3. Discuss about breakdown maintenance

The causes and risk factors for mood disorders need to be known if prevention as well as effective intervention is to be achieved. Genetic predisposition is also a significant factor, with individuals who have had a family history of mood disorders being more susceptible to developing mood disorders. Biological factors, including neurochemical imbalance, are also believed to play a role in these disorders. These imbalances will affect mood regulation and general psychological well-being, making people susceptible to conditions like depression and bipolar illness. External causes, such as traumatic life experiences, trauma, or chronic stress, can trigger this susceptibility, further contributing to the complexity of the way mood disorders manifest in individuals. Psychosocial factors create a richly textured history of risk regarding mood disorders. Such chronic stressors as bullying, family adjustment, or loss may also significantly contribute to mental health. Of greatest note, emotional disturbance in periods of development critical for adjustment, such as childhood, can have long-standing effects on mood regulation. Research indicates that children with adverse exposure are at risk for mood disorders in adulthood. In particular, connectivity between factors , such as urbanization, noise, and environmental pollution also contributes to social and emotional stressors, thereby increasing risks among younger individuals and making them vulnerable to experiencing mood disorders (Pitti et al., 2024). Unhealthy lifestyle also emerges as a prominent predictor of risks for mood disorders. Inactive lifestyles, unhealthy diets, and irregular sleeping patterns may lead to a decline in physical and mental well-being. These lifestyle factors not only impact mood but may also interact with biological vulnerabilities to produce an elevated risk for mood disorders. Additionally, substance abuse and other such behaviors are unhealthy for mental health and perpetuate a vicious cycle that continues to reinforce mood instability. The interaction between psychosocial and environmental factors with these life decisions forms a sophisticated web influencing the development and the course of mood disorders (Alvarez-Pitti et al., 2023). Explanation of such sophisticated interactions is significant in designing appropriate interventions and treatment.

5.3.1. Biological Factors

Biological factors play a significant role in the etiology of mood disorders, or rather how genetic influence affects the risk of developing mood disorders. It has been discovered that those with a family history of mood disorders are at significant risk of their own diagnosis, which means that there is significant contribution by genetics to vulnerability of these disorders. For instance, the transmission patterns of uni- and bipolar disorders show a family pattern that cannot be solely attributed to environmental influences. Genetic studies have begun to unravel the complexities of these predispositions, showing variations of neurobiological processes that can lead a subject to mood dysregulation. It is important to establish these genetic vulnerabilities as it leads the way to the potential for more specific interventions and early detection plans, in the end designing a road map for future research into the hereditary nature of mood disorders. Further investigation into the biological underpinnings of mood disorders reveals the significant role that neurochemicals play in mood regulation. Neurotransmitters , such as serotonin, norepinephrine, and dopamine have been implicated in the pathophysiology of these conditions as playing a role in mood regulation but also in maintaining a myriad of physiological functions. Dysregulation of these systems may express as symptomatic presentations of mood disorders , including depression and mania. The Mood and Resilience in Offspring (MARIO) cohort study underscores the importance of examining these biological measures alongside clinical and environmental measures in order to better understand the multicenter aspect of mood disorders. By searching for how levels of neurotransmitters interface with gene expression and environmental stresses, scientists aim to know why some individuals get mood disorders and why others, being equally biologically equipped, remain unaffected (Beerthuizen et al., 2024; Beerthuizen et al., 2024). Also important is the investigation of the interplay between biology and environment in the etiology of mood disorders. Whereas genetic susceptibility creates the underlying risk, extrinsic stressors , such as chronic stress, trauma, and psychosocial stressors may act as provoking agents, pushing the balance towards inherent biological vulnerabilities. The MARIO study highlights the necessity of considering these factors together since it is conceivable that what is known about how environmental stressors converge with biological vulnerability might tell us something about the multiplicative mechanisms of mood disorders. Through the accrual of rich data over long intervals, researchers can observe patterns that better explain how these biological variables are involved in the intergenerational transmission of mood disorders. Identifying this interaction can ultimately be used to inform prevention and treatment strategies and allow for improved outcomes in people at risk based on their family history (Beerthuizen et al., 2024) (Figure 5.8).

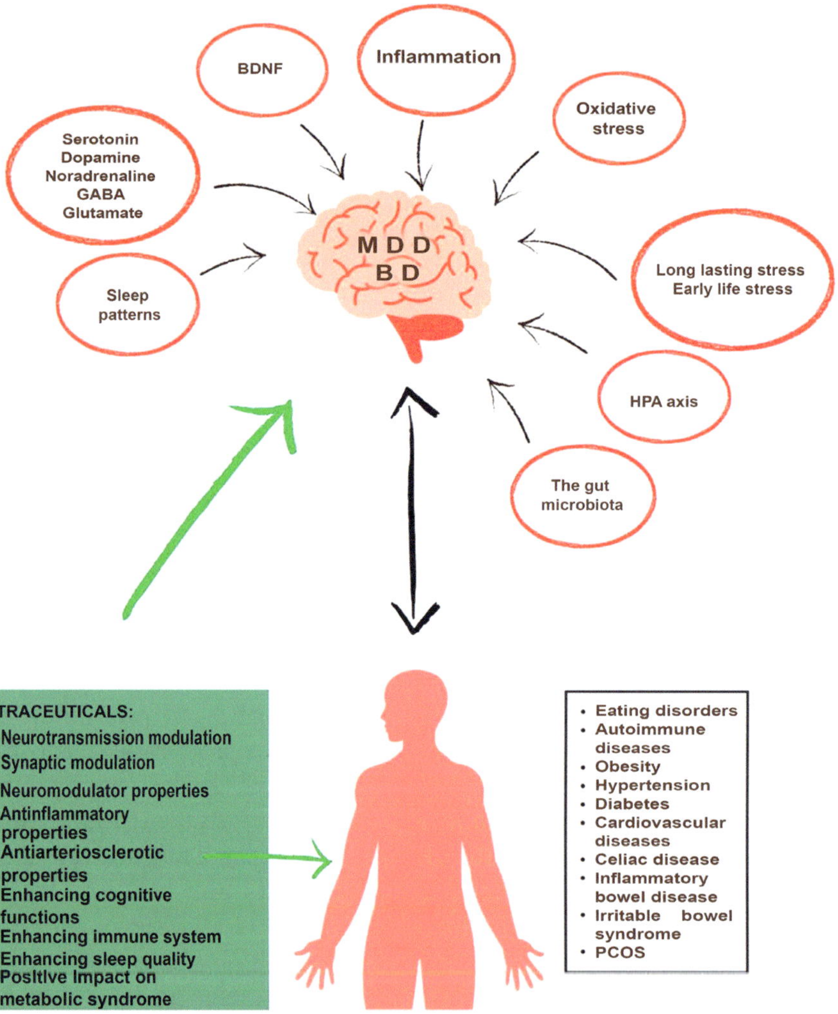

Figure 5.8. Biological factors play a crucial role in understanding the etiology of mood disorders, particularly in recognizing how genetic predispositions influence the likelihood of developing such conditions.

Source: https://pub.mdpi-res.com/brainsci/brainsci-13-01262/article_deploy/html/images/brainsci-13-01262-g002.png?1693392822.

5.3.2. Psychological Factors

Understanding the psychological contributors to mood disorders is highly relevant, as they greatly impact individuals' emotional well-being. Cognitive distortions in the form of maladaptive beliefs and negative thoughts are the building blocks in the etiology and maintenance of mood disorders like depression and anxiety. These distortions can lead individuals to interpret their experience in extremely pessimistic terms and hence enhance feelings of despair and hopelessness. Furthermore, studies indicate that emotional processing and regulation are required in mood moderation; those who cannot sense and control their emotions are inclined to develop disorders. In this case, cognitive restructuring-based interventions provide potential paths towards symptom decrease, with an emphasis on the intersection of cognition and mood moderation. Lastly, psychological states regarding the stress response are also paramount in mood disorders. Environmental stressors, particularly chronic stress, have been shown to exacerbate dysregulation of mood and to cause the onset of depressive symptoms. Research suggests a significant correlation between stress levels and a number of psychological outcomes, including anxiety and depressive disorder. Individuals with high levels of stress become trapped in a feedback loop of heightened emotional response that further heightens their stress, and they develop a profound sense of mental fatigue and helplessness. By looking at the interaction between mood disorders and stress, it's clear that treatments targeting stress reduction can improve general mood and emotional coping. The connection between physical and mood disorders cannot be underestimated since psychological issues tend to be expressed through somatic symptoms. New studies have established correlations between physical conditions , such as erectile dysfunction and psychological distress, which have identified the effects of mood disorders on numerous aspects of physical health. For instance, the association of poor semen analysis parameters and mood disorders, as in current literature, indicates that stress, anxiety, and depression have tangible effects on physical health. This underscores the need for a holistic therapeutic approach, integrating medical treatment and counseling. Therapy for mood disorders based on a holistic principle can not only improve emotional health but may even foster better physical health, reiterating the sheer importance of psychological factors in physical well-being and quality of life.

5.3.3. Environmental Influences

The environment plays a very significant role in the evolution of mood disorders: it will influence the onset and course of illness. Of the environmental influences on circadian rhythms, which is a key determinant of stability or otherwise of mood, irregular exposure to light could be associated with dysregulation of mood. Research has consistently found that disruptions , such as shift work, jet lag, or seasonal fluctuations in daylight can trigger or exacerbate symptoms of disorders , such as major depressive disorder and seasonal affective disorder. By seeing how environmental signals correlate with internal circadian clocks, we get a better sense of the systemic desynchronizations responsible for mood instability. This is an indication of the necessity for integrated treatment approaches, addressing not just the psychological dimensions but also the environmental dimensions that can disrupt mood regulation at the biological level, as reported in research on the intricate interplay between exposure to light and mood disorders (Rahim et al., 2025). Also, the environmental dimensions are more than circadian disturbances, interlocking with other developmental and psychosocial dimensions that foster mood disorders. Children exposed to negative environmental situations , such as neglect, trauma, or instability, are more prone to mood-related issues. The onset of conduct disorders in teenagers is also usually simultaneous with the onset of mood disorders, suggesting a shared neurobiological substrate underlaid by environmental factors. As indicated in literature, the comorbidity of mood disorders and conduct disorder underscores the interactive complexity with which environmental stressors can function to amplify behavioral and emotional problems, creating a cascade effect of mental health problems that requires multiplicity in intervention methods. The interactivity of these dynamics underscores the significance of considering environmental elements in the development of effective prevention and treatment protocols for mood disorders (Altable, 2023). Also, the dynamic interaction of the external environment with genetics plays a powerful role in mood disorders and their occurrence. Genetic vulnerabilities can establish a foundation of risk, but most commonly, it is the external environment that triggers or calms these latent risks. Adversive environments, such as those characterized by socio-economic disadvantage or pathological family environments, often trigger underlying genetic vulnerabilities to the onset of a number of mood disorders. The reciprocal interaction between organismal dispositions and environmental stressors highlights the necessity of a multifactorial approach in explaining mood disorders. Thus, interventions that counteract deteriorating environmental stressors alongside intensive treatment for biological aspects can maximize benefits for individuals with mood disorders, accepting a more holistic approach to mental health treatment that recognizes the profound role environmental aspects play as described in the past research (Rahim et al., 2025) (Figure 5.9).

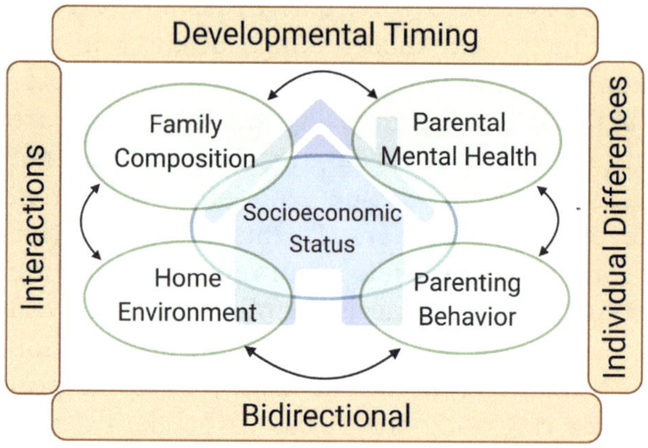

Figure 5.9. The environment plays a critical role in shaping mood disorders, influencing both the onset and progression of these conditions.

Source: https://www.frontiersin.org/files/Articles/504260/fpsyt-11-00547-HTML/image_m/fpsyt-11-00547-g001.jpg.

Test Your Knowledge

1. How do biological factors such as genetics and neurotransmitter imbalances contribute to mood disorders?
2. What environmental and psychosocial factors—such as trauma, stress, and lifestyle—serve as risk factors for developing mood disorders?

5.4. Types of Mood Disorders

Learning Outcome

1. Understand hotel maintenance management and its impact
2. Perform preventive maintenance
3. Discuss about breakdown maintenance

The research on mood disorders comprises a spectrum of states with their own individual emotional dysregulation. Of these, major depressive disorder (MDD) is one of the most prevalent, with tens of millions of victims worldwide. MDD manifests as constant feelings of sadness, hopelessness, and insufficient interest in previously enjoyed activities. Patients present with fluctuations in appetite and sleep, along with severe impairment of cognitive function. It is critical to recognize the nuances of MDD since it commonly co-exists with other psychiatric conditions, thereby complicating diagnosis as well as treatment. In realizing the intricacies in MDD, researchers focus on the necessity of its identification of biological, psychological, and social factors that contribute to its emergence, therefore enhancing the efficacy of therapeutic measures. Bipolar disorder, the second severe mood disorder category, is characterized by cyclical occurrences of mania or hypomania and depression. Bipolar disorder has a characteristic cyclical pattern that extensively affects an individual's daily functioning and interpersonal relationships. Manic episodes in this condition are characterized by elevated mood, energy, and impulsivity, leading to risky behavior. Conversely, depressive attacks in bipolar disorder can replicate the major depressive symptom, exhibiting a rich contrast between contradictory emotional states. Awareness of bipolar disorder's implications transcends individual experiences as communities and families struggle with unpredictability around mood swings. Acceptance of bipolar disorder's bipolarity is pertinent in creating awareness and reducing stigmatization, enabling afflicted populations to receive assistance and care. Beneath the mood disorders falls a category of conditions, including dysthymia and cyclothymia, involving chronic but mild emotional disturbance. Dysthymia, or persistent depressive disorder, involves two or more years of chronic depression symptoms that significantly affect quality of life despite their blunted intensity.

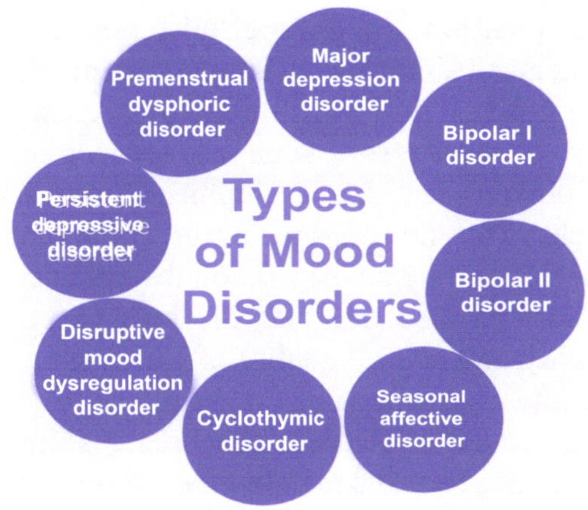

Figure 5.10. Types of mood disorders.

Source: https://www.simplypsychology.org/wp-content/uploads/Types-of-mood-disorders-1.jpg.

On the other hand, cyclothymia is characterized by frequent episodes of hypomanic symptoms interrupted by depressive symptoms, which, although less intense than those that occur in bipolar disorder, can lead to functional impairment in the long run. Most recent research has begun examining the relationship between mood disorders and attachment styles, for instance, as suggested in studies of borderline personality disorder patients (Hobson et al., 2007) and their multiple narrative structures in attachment interviews. Similarly, adult studies with autism spectrum disorders suggest the nuanced interaction between emotional regulation and attachment security (Charman et al., 2008). These results contribute further richness to the discussion of the heterogeneous environment of mood disorders (Figure 5.10).

5.4.1. Major Depressive Disorder

Major Depressive Disorder (MDD) refers to a severe psychiatric illness characterized by frequent low mood, anhedonia, and a range of cognitive and somatic symptoms. The etiology of MDD is multifactorial, involving a broad category of factors , including genetic predisposition, environmental stressors, and biochemical abnormality. Biogenic amine theory hypothesizes the involvement of a change in neurotransmitters , such as serotonin and norepinephrine in the development of depressive attacks. This multifaceted interaction renders MDD not merely an easy mood disturbance but a disabling disorder that disables functional capacity and overall quality of life. This insight into these mechanisms is required to treat the disorder effectively and create sufficient treatment protocols to help affected individuals in their recovery process. Recurrent Major Depressive Disorder is an essential element of its clinical presentation. Depressed patients have heightened chances of experiencing subsequent bouts of depression. Research has established that recurrence is proportional to the number of previous episodes, particularly where residual symptoms are present during the interepisode intervals. Depressed patients typically grapple with helplessness, and a vicious cycle of relapse can become habitual without intervention. For instance, a 40-year-old female patient with a background of severe chronic depression revealed the cyclical behavior typical of MDD, dismissing traditional therapies due to their side effects (Mahalle, 2024). This indicates the merit of individually adapted therapy approaches that consider not only the medical history of the patient but also their individual preferences in managing this multifactorial disorder. Despite the severe consequences of Major Depressive Disorder, misdiagnosis and delayed treatment are major barriers to effective treatment. The reasons for such problems range from overlapping symptoms with other mental diseases to societal stigma that prevents people from seeking help in a timely manner. A study of depressed mood participants revealed predictors of misdiagnosis , such as the level of depressed mood and the nature of previous psychiatric evaluations (Benáček et al., 2024). These results underscore the necessity of greater awareness and detection of mood disorders by clinicians since early and precise diagnosis has the potential to unveil treatment possibilities to the fullest and a better prognosis in those suffering from MDD. By addressing these system-level issues, it is possible to alleviate the disabling effects of Major Depressive Disorder and provide a more humane setting for those in need (Figure 5.11).

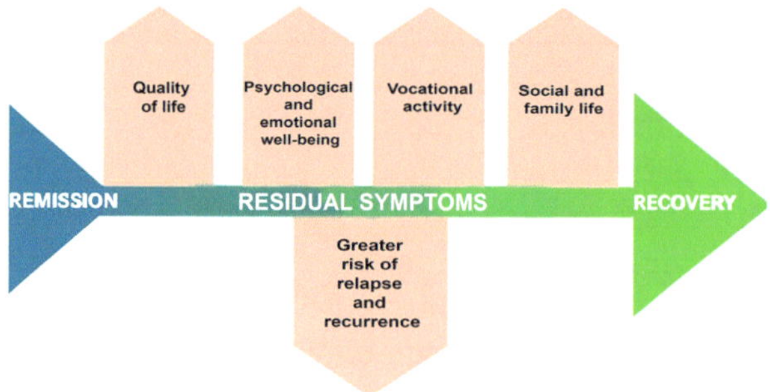

Figure 5.11. Major Depressive Disorder (MDD) represents a significant psychiatric condition characterized by pervasive low mood, anhedonia, and a variety of cognitive and physical symptoms.

Source: https://www.mdpi.com/jpm/jpm-14-00828/article_deploy/html/images/jpm-14-00828-g002.png.

5.4.2. Bipolar Disorder

Bipolar disorder is an affective disorder characterized by fluctuations in moods to extremes, coupled with variations in energy and activity levels. Episodic mania or hypomania is most often preceded or followed by periods of depression. Bipolar disorder has the potential to lead to extreme interference with daily functioning and interpersonal relationships. The coordination of neurobiological, environmental, and genetic factors in the development and evolution of bipolar disorder is thus the subject of a lot of research and interest. The capacity of individuals with bipolar disorder to process emotion is of crucial significance to understand. It has been revealed in studies that mood disorders, including bipolar disorder, have changed emotional reactions patients, which can influence their social behavior and general well-being, particularly emphasized in studies of facial recognition of expressions during different episodes of mood. Furthermore, recent studies have introduced the conceptual model of Dysregulation of Mood, Energy, and Social Rhythms Syndrome (DYMERS), which is centered on the disruption of normal emotional control in bipolar disorder. The idea is salient because it addresses the way that disturbance of mood could become intertwined with sleep and behavior patterns to create more potential for other illnesses. In comparing bipolar disorder to systemic illnesses , such as systemic lupus erythematosus (SLE), more positivity on the Mood Disorder Questionnaire (MDQ) was observed in SLE patients. This correlation not only provides information about co-occurring symptomatology but also suggests a shared pathway in dysregulation of mood that would be interesting to study further. The implications of these results are profound, requiring more careful screening practice to better identify those at risk for bipolar disorder, especially in multicultural medical populations (Gonzales et al., 2024). Lastly, the treatment situation for bipolar disorder highlights the importance of a conjoint strategy that includes pharmacological treatment and psychotherapy. Drugs , such as mood stabilizers and antipsychotics aim at stabilizing mood swings, while psychotherapeutic interventions aim at cognitive-behavioral approaches to alter inappropriate thought processes. Even psychoeducational interventions of a supportive nature by education can empower the patient to manage their symptoms successfully. Because bipolar disorder is multifactorial in nature, ongoing studies are required to better know its mechanisms, to obtain a more accurate diagnosis, and to improve treatment outcomes. By considering both the psychosocial and biological aspects of the disorder, more integrated treatment tailored to the specific challenges faced by those with this condition can be provided by clinicians (Gonzales et al., 2024) (Figure 5.12).

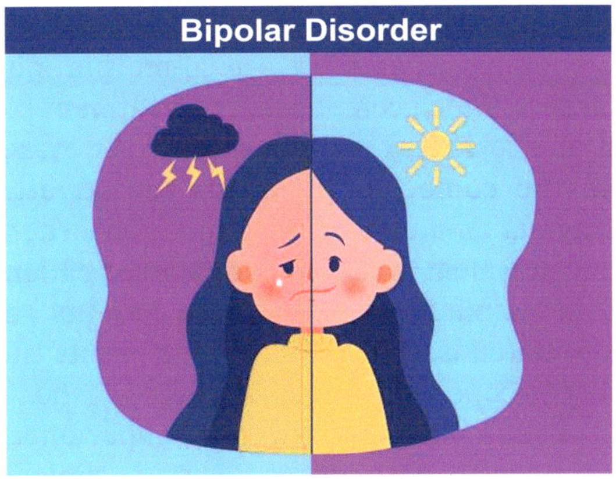

Figure 5.12. Bipolar disorder.

Source: https://drdeepakaiims.com/wp-content/uploads/2024/01/Bipolar-Disorder-Symptoms-Causes-Types-and-Diagnosis.jpg.

5.4.3. Dysthymia and Other Mood Disorders

Dysthymia, or chronic depressive disorder, is a serious but often underappreciated mood disorder consisting of chronic, low-grade depressive symptoms occurring for at least two years in adults. While less severe than those accompanying major depressive disorder, the symptoms can severely impair an individual's functioning in the majority of areas of life. The attacks which involve dysthymia are typically less intense but are characterized by their duration and chronicity, which can lead to a relentless deterioration of individual and workplace functioning. The chronic state of dysthymia necessitates an extensive treatment course, often combining pharmacotherapy with a series of psychotherapeutic approaches to optimize overall outcomes and mitigate the influence of the disorder on daily functioning, as delineated in research on treatment outcomes and patient satisfaction (Portilla et al., 2023). The coaction of dysthymia with comorbid mood disorders , such as major depressive disorder and anxiety disorders, adds additional complexities to diagnosis and treatment. Research further indicates that dysthymia patients also develop an exacerbation of symptoms when there are co-morbid mood disorders, which complicate the treatment plan and add to functional impairment. As evident from the comorbidity pattern investigation, dysthymia as a co-occurring mood disorder is highly prevalent in alcohol use disorder patients, and the implication is that these patients have drug-related issues that might complicate their ability to cope with mood disorders (Roshchina et al., 2021). This emphasizes the importance of a correct evaluation process, wherein clinicians must take into account the full spectrum of mood disorders to develop effective and patient-specific intervention strategies. In addition, the longitudinal course of dysthymia has significant implications for research and clinical practice. The chronic condition of dysthymia raises deep challenges since, if left untreated, it can evolve into more severe forms of depression , such as double depression, which contributes to the extent of functional impairment and complicates treatment even further. There is a critical need for effective interventions, especially when standard serotonin reuptake inhibitors are not satisfactory for all patients. New models of treatment, including the potential benefits of atypical antipsychotic medications like aripiprazole, are being studied in an effort to offer alternative means of symptom management. Through continued research and development of treatment models, mental health professionals can better equip themselves to treat those who are experiencing dysthymia and its comorbidity with other mood disorders (Portilla et al., 2023) (Figure 5.13).

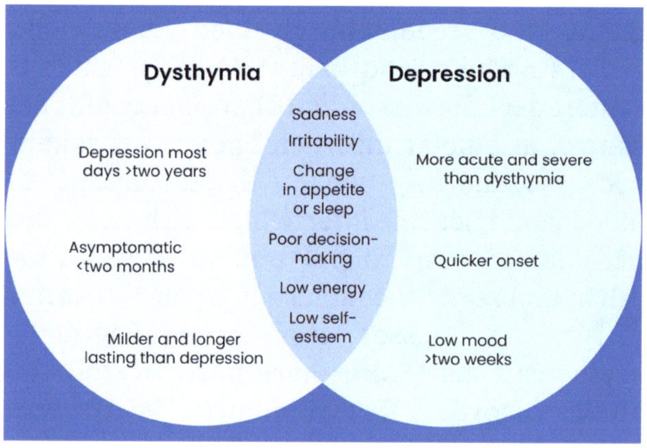

Figure 5.13. Dysthymia versus depression.

Source: https://images.ctfassets.net/yixw23k2v6vo/4L3AqTodoMN0MdM3YcCaBO/1178249a02cb658c20536bfa00726b38/large-dysthymia-depression-venn-diagram.jpg.

Test Your Knowledge

1. What distinguishes major depressive disorder, persistent depressive disorder, and bipolar disorders from one another?
2. How do cyclothymic disorder and bipolar II differ in severity and symptom patterns?

5.5. Impact on Daily Life

Learning Outcome

1. Understand hotel maintenance management and its impact
2. Perform preventive maintenance
3. Discuss about breakdown maintenance

The influence of mood disorders on daily life is immense, covering a wide range of different areas , including social interaction, work ability, and overall health. Individuals with disorders , such as depression or bipolar disorder have an immense loss of ability for routine tasks. This may manifest as low levels of motivation, concentration problems, and a general feeling of hopelessness. These symptoms not only hinder interpersonal relationships but also lead to isolation, where the people with such disorders withdraw from social activities due to feelings of inferiority or fear of being judged. Over time, these problems create a cycle in which the social withdrawal generates more mood disorders, making the people's challenges even worse. Mood disorders may also play a huge role in hindering one's work performance. Individuals may struggle to meet job-related responsibilities due to cognitive impairment, lack of energy, and increased absenteeism. This may lead to a chain effect of undesirable outcomes, including workplace problems, reduced productivity, and even termination from employment. Inability to perform job duties often results in economic challenges, further exacerbating the mood disorder symptoms. Thus, the relationship between work and mental health affects not only the individual but the organization's effectiveness and the workplace dynamics as well. In response to this, employers must create supportive environments that hold the importance of their workers' mental health in the consideration it is accorded. The effects of mood disorders extend beyond the individual to family patterns and interpersonal relationships in the community. Family members may be under extreme emotional pressure as they attempt to assist their loved one, resulting in caregiver burnout and feelings of helplessness for many. The resulting stress of living with or interacting with an individual suffering from a mood disorder can produce anxiety and depression among family members. Moreover, such dynamics may also affect children in the family unit, who may struggle to understand their parents' emotional state, leading to confusion or acting out issues. For these reasons, successful intervention methods are critical for the individual who is suffering from mood disorders as well as for the larger familial group in an effort to create a healthier interaction and reduce stigma surrounding mental health.

5.5.1. Impact on Personal Relationships

Mood disorders also have a strong influence on interpersonal relationships, and they usually lead to tension and distance within family and friends. Individuals with disorders , such as depression or anxiety can experience repeated fluctuations in mood that are misunderstood by other people. Most of the time, loved ones react in anger and frustration, and this exacerbates the feelings of isolation experienced by the person with the disorder. A study that targeted depressive and anxiety disorders highlighted that family functioning is essential; namely, girls who lacked good maternal support experienced a greater number of these disturbances in mood. This shows how relational factors , such as maternal support, not only influence the emotional well-being of the person but also the health of interpersonal relationships within the family (Monck, 1996). If left unaddressed, these shifting dynamics are likely to produce long-term relational cleavages and position mood disorders as causes of familial conflict. The effects of mood disorders extend beyond dyadic familial relationships, influencing friendships and social networks. Friends may not feel competent to provide assistance, leading to frustration and helplessness. Moreover, individuals afflicted with mood disorders tend to withdraw from social interactions due to the overwhelming feeling of sadness or anxiety, thus perpetuating the feeling of abandonment among peers. Withdrawal continues to repeat a cycle of segregation because the lack of social interaction reinforces negative thoughts and distorts interpersonal perception further. As recorded in the literature on mental health, depression of a parent can compromise effective parenting, hence affecting the emotional and developmental impacts on children (McCauliff et al., 2007).

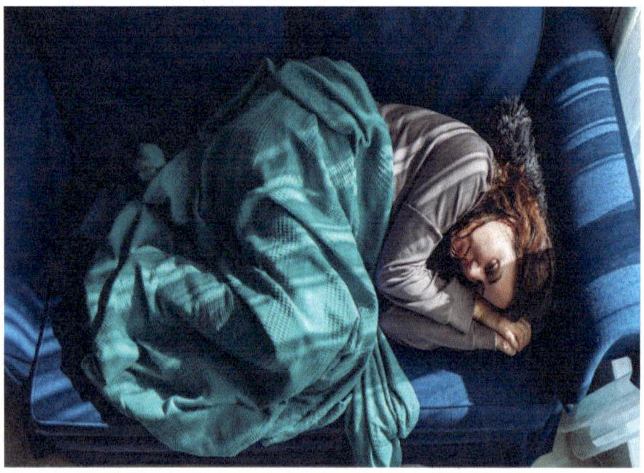

Figure 5.14. Individuals suffering from disorders , such as depression or anxiety can experience emotional fluctuations that may be misinterpreted by those around them.

Source: https://media.post.rvohealth.io/wp-content/uploads/2024/07/sad-depressed-woman-lying-on-couch-blanket-sofa-1296x728-header.jpg.

Such processes help to highlight the need for an understanding of mood disorders' multi-level impacts on relationships, along with the need for responsive interventions for repairing and strengthening social bonds. The discussion of the influence of mood disorders on interpersonal relationships must be an integrated one that addresses mental health care and education. An increased awareness among family and friends about the nature of mood disorders will help them offer a better understanding and supportive help. Apart from that, family and counseling therapy are crucial in helping individuals and their families understand issues of mood swings and emotional distress. Research shows that if appropriately treated and provided with proper support services, people with the condition have greatly improved interpersonal relationships that bring about healthier relationship dynamics and a generally better quality of life. They must place higher emphasis on outreach services and programs to reach the victims of mood disorders with the treatment they need, which will prove to be as helpful for the individual as for their entire social network (Monck, 1996; McCauliff et al., 2007) (Figure 5.14).

5.5.2. Influence on Work and Productivity

The interface of work productivity and mood disorders underscores a powerful social and economic problem. Those whose illnesses involve depression or anxiety often experience compromised mental performance, decreased motivation, and exacerbated fatigue, all of which directly contribute to on-the-job impairment. For instance, the signs that are common to these mood disorders have the potential to lead to an inability to concentrate on tasks, meet deadlines, and communicate effective with colleagues. This decrease in work functioning not only harms individuals but also has a cost for organizations in terms of greater turnover and medical expenses. Also, the involved may end up being disproportionately targeted by organizational stigma regarding mental illness, further exacerbating their work functioning problems. Thus, it is important to accept mood disorders as actual health problems to design supportive work environments that enable individuals to thrive despite their illnesses.

The effect of mood disorders does not only extend to the individual but also to family life and relationships. Family members, including children with atopic dermatitis, caring for individuals with mood disorders, experience high levels of tension and disruption of their home environment. Symptom surveillance and management of treatment routines are caregiving activities that can take much physical and emotional energy. When added to family work demands, this heavy load has the effect of lowering job performance and improving absenteeism. Family members are also plagued by issues of keeping personal relationships intact because mood disorders tend to induce misconceptions and tensions in the household.

The impact is two-fold; caregivers may be asked to deal with lengthy care with job duties alongside dealing with their own emotional responses, leading to a dynamic impact on work and overall productivity (Yang et al., 2018). Disturbed sleep that comes with mood disorders is a significant predictor of reduced work productivity as well. Sleep disorders, particularly insomnia, have emerged as a commonly recognized symptom as well as a consequence of mood disorders, significantly impairing cognitive functions essential for effective job performance. Sleep loss not only leads to decreased alertness and bad judgment, as per research, but also becomes a risk factor for many chronic diseases. For mood disorders, the sleep problems are compounded by the problems like the reduction of hormone levels in menopause, which have the tendency to contribute to the mood disturbances and impact the capacity to work (Schaedel et al., 2021). This formed a vicious cycle of reciprocation in which sleep quality and mood disorders blended together to become a perfect mix, leading to formed added stress and more sleep problems, eventually affecting professional satisfaction and overall quality of life.

5.5.3. Physical Health Consequences

The connection between body health and mood disorders is intricate and profound because the psychological disorders seem to have real physical impacts. In people with mood disorders, symptoms , such as fatigue, sleep changes, and appetite disturbances are sufficiently distressing that they can interfere with daily life seriously. It is more than a question of being miserable; it can exacerbate existing conditions and precipitate new disease, setting up a cycle of deterioration. Notably, research has shown that people with depressive symptoms tend to report heightened physical pain and discomfort, which could lead them not to engage in routine physical activities, thus worsening the effect on their overall health and creating a decline in their quality of life related to health (Agrell et al., 2010). Therefore, identifying this overlap between mental and physical health is significant in order to develop holistic treatment plans that address both. The impact of mood disorders on physical health can also be seen in some groups, such as pregnant women, who are potentially vulnerable to a heightened susceptibility during this significant period of their lives. In particular, pregnancy evokes varied physiological alterations, thus enhancing the psychological suffering of women with pre-existing mood disorders. Sleep disturbances, a common condition in this group of women, have been associated with various mental disorders , including anxiety and depression. Through research, it was confirmed that a large percentage of pregnant women suffer from insomnia, which has a significant relationship with the presence of mental disorders (Babaie et al., 2015). The interaction of mood disorders and insomnia also affects not just mental health but physical health, such as increased fatigue, compromising maternal and fetal health outcomes. Thus, detection of such interactions is essential for effective prenatal care and intervention. Further, the deleterious effects of mood disorders on physical health tend to be extended to the quality of life in general.

Such individuals tend to become less likely to engage in physical work, adopt dietary habits that maintain good health, or maintain proper management of chronic disease. Such neglect can prove hazardous to one's health, varying from obesity to heart disease and weakening of the immune system. The overall effect of these lifestyle changes ultimately decides the overall health trajectory for an individual, underlining the importance of healthcare professionals adopting a holistic approach towards addressing mood disorders. By focusing on both mind and body, professionals are able to promote greater overall wellness and improve quality of life for those with mood disorders. The practice offers a system not only for symptom reduction of the type associated with mood disorders but also for mitigating their ill effects on physical outcomes (Figure5.15).

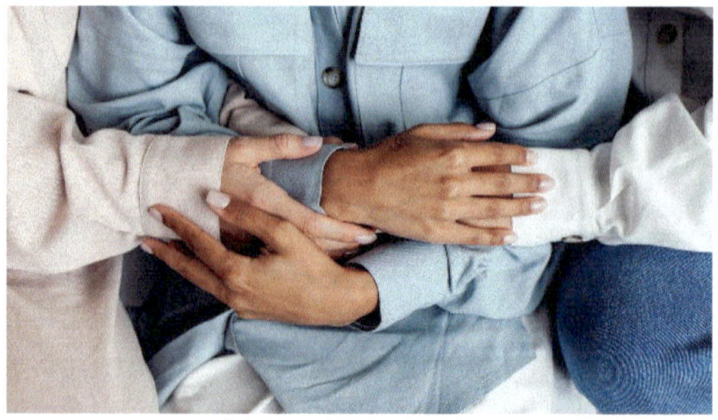

Figure 5.15. For individuals grappling with mood disorders, symptoms , such as fatigue, altered sleep patterns, and changes in appetite can disrupt daily functioning significantly.

Source: https://images.everydayhealth.com/images/emotional-health/anxiety-disorders/helping-a-loved-one-with-anxiety-disorder-1440x810.jpg.

Test Your Knowledge

1. How do mood disorders affect an individual's functioning in areas such as work, education, and interpersonal relationships?
2. What challenges do individuals with mood disorders face in maintaining routines, decision-making, and emotional regulation?

5.6. Current Research Trends

Learning Outcome

1. Understand hotel maintenance management and its impact
2. Perform preventive maintenance
3. Discuss about breakdown maintenance

New advances in non-invasive neuromodulation methods have appeared in the treatment of mood disorders, notably through such methods as transcranial focused ultrasound (tFUS). The novel method is promising for mood and emotional regulation modulation, an essential aspect of mood disorder treatments. Research indicates that tFUS is superior to traditional methods , such as transcranial magnetic stimulation (TMS), in having larger spatial resolution and capacity to activate deeper brain structures. In clinical trials examining its effects on healthy volunteers, right inferior frontal gyrus (rIFG) tFUS resulted in improved self-reported mood states and alterations in functional connectivity within networks of mood regulation. Collectively, these findings attest to the potential of tFUS as an innovative method in mood disorder treatments, pushing the boundaries of existing therapeutic paradigms (Allen et al., 2020). Research into another interesting field includes examining spontaneous thinking modes, encompassing mind-wandering and spontaneous memory recall. Understanding the dual nature of spontaneous thoughts has the potential to reveal their adaptive and maladaptive effects in individuals susceptible to mood disorders. Notably, spontaneous thinking is geared to unattained goals, and this results in negative affective states as individuals reflect on mismatches between desired outcomes and current situations. This persistence can actually increase cognitive vulnerabilities , such as rumination and low self-esteem, hence raising the possibility of obtaining or aggravating mood disorders. Investigation of these higher-order processes provides insightful information about the mechanisms of depression and bipolar disorder, raising important questions concerning the application of therapeutic interventions based on cognitive restructuring approaches (Marchetti et al., 2016). As more research continues to unpack the nuances of mood disorders, increasingly it is clear that interdisciplinary treatment is successful. For instance, the integration of data from neuroscience, psychology, and cognitive science can facilitate a multidisciplinary understanding of the etiology and treatment of mood disorders. The interface between innovative neuromodulation techniques, for example, tFUS, and cognitive therapies for spontaneous thinking is a future direction worth exploring. Such interdisciplinary merging not only improves our insight into mood disorders but also paves the way for personalized treatments. The objective remains one of developing more unified treatment approaches that fully address the biological and cognitive aspects of mood disorders, ultimately increasing patient outcomes in this multidisciplinary field of mental health research.

5.6.1. Advances in Genetic Studies

New advances in the genetic studies have significantly increased our understanding of mood disorders. Studies have shown that psychiatric disorders like these are highly heritable, and genetic polymorphisms are largely responsible for predisposing to development. There has been a paradigm shift in research that is fundamental, moving away from a monogenic model emphasizing solitary genes to a polygenic risk model that gained prominence from about 2015. This shift has been mounted alongside the increasing preponderance of genome-wide association studies, which have facilitated a more precise examination of the intricate genetic structure of mood disorders. Data obtained from such studies reveal that various genetic factors interact, hence a complex interplay of influences that highlights the importance of examining multiple genes simultaneously in mood disorder studies (Bonacina et al., 2023). The areas of overlap between mood disorders and other psychiatric conditions have also become an area of the highest interest. These overlaps have been shown to be crucial to the study of comorbidities, for example, those that are common in conditions , such as cardiovascular diseases (CVDs). Research shows that patients with mood disorders, major depressive disorder in particular, have enhanced mortality and morbidity in relation to CVDs. Such a connection highlights a remarkable genetic correlation whereby genetic mechanisms underlying mood disorders also predispose individuals towards cardiovascular disease. Besides, exploration of the genetic interaction of mood disorders with other conditions provides an avenue to comprehending long-range implications of genetic research in the realm of psychiatry (Chen et al., 2023). Incorporation of new findings provides an anticipatory perspective of the research environment regarding mood disorders. Key trends emerging through the thematic clustering of genetic studies reflect the need to investigate both the genetic etiology and the contribution of the environment in such conditions. The interaction between genetic predispositions and environmental precipitants has come to the forefront, with evidence suggesting that extrinsic determinants may be capable of significantly altering genetic risk. Such a holistic understanding is essential to the creation of customized interventions aimed at the pathological biological mechanisms of mood disorders in the background of individual patients. Thus, while genetic research remains ongoing, it can potentially unfold additional knowledge and contribute to the creation of more effective treatment methods, ultimately reformulating the treatment of mood disorders (Bonacina et al., 2023).

5.6.2. Neurobiological Research Findings

Neurobiological foundation of mood disorders gives tremendous understanding into the pathophysiology that causes their initiation and relapse. Findings attest to the fact that depression is characterized by a profound neurobiological alteration, particularly in the prefrontal cortex and subcortical regions like the amygdala. Specifically, decreased prefrontal activity, perhaps influenced by serotonin metabolism under the regulation of the HPA axis, is responsible for impairments in emotional regulation and attentional control. These neurologic changes are associated with the hyperactivation of the amygdala over prolonged durations in response to environmental stress, thus rendering an individual more susceptible to adverse emotional states. Understanding these neurological mechanisms is extremely crucial to the development of effective interventions that target the cognitive and biological mechanisms of mood disorders, especially following multiple occurrences of depression, in which vulnerability can substantially increase, as evidenced by the mounting empirical data of attention deficits and rumination in depressed patients (Raedt et al., 2010). Furthermore, the effect of spontaneous thinking has been recognized as an important area in the research on cognitive vulnerabilities for mood disorders. This cognitive process, such as mind-wandering and daydreaming, has adaptive and maladaptive influences, particularly when a person experiences failed goals. Spontaneous thought, for instance, is particularly prone to highlight the gap between one's actual emotional state and the target one's goal, causing hopelessness and self-deprecation. These cognitive vulnerabilities, such as rumination, can enhance negative affect and elevate risk for the emergence of depressive symptoms. This connection between spontaneous cognition and mood disorders underscores the need for an integrative model that incorporates cognitive processes into the neurobiological model, acknowledging how cognitive styles can be involved in creating and maintaining mood disturbance (Marchetti et al., 2016). In conclusion, the use of neurobiological discoveries to explain cognitive and emotional processes gives a complete picture of mood disorders. The point at which the focus is both on the disrupted neurobiological function in regions which are correlated with mood regulation and the contribution of cognitive vulnerabilities highlights the complexity of the conditions. Since researchers have been searching into the interplay between these factors more and more, it is increasingly evident that treating both cognitive and neurobiological factors is essential in the development of effective therapies. By being aware of the interplay between brain function and cognitive processes in both directions, interventions can work to reverse the effects of both neurobiological deficits and unconstructive thinking styles, ultimately leading to healthier outcomes for mood disorder sufferers (Raedt et al., 2010; Marchetti et al., 2016).

5.6.3. Innovations in Treatment Methods

As the prevalence of mood disorders is on the rise, new treatments have evolved to address the expanding demand for effective interventions. Digital therapeutics have been one of the most notable advancements in addressing this emerging need. Digital therapeutics are technology-delivered interventions on evidence-based mental health care. They utilize AI and machine learning to provide individualized, adaptive treatment regimens, optimizing patient engagement and monitoring. This integration not only complements the rising trend towards personalized medicine but also circumvents traditional hurdles , such as accessibility and stigma regarding accessing help. Additionally, the potential for real-time data analysis within online systems facilitates clinicians to make informed decisions for altering treatment, thus optimizing therapeutic returns. Overall, the shift towards technology-facilitated treatment is a significant improvement in being able to properly treat mood disorders (Isa, 2024). One of the most important innovations among mood disorders is Internet-based use of cognitive behavior therapy (CBT), as with guided self-help programs. These treatments have proved to be effective for a variety of mood-related issues, including binge-eating disorder (BED), by providing guided therapeutic content in an active, accessible form. Research indicates that these online classes work, particularly for people who may otherwise avoid traditional therapy due to its stigma or logistical issues. A key discovery is the role of emotion regulation issues as a better predictor of therapy effectiveness when utilizing online CBT. This suggests that the augmentation of clients' emotion regulation ability has direct implications for treatment effectiveness and compliance, and thus underscores the importance of certain therapy modalities in the age of the internet (Forrer et al., 2024). Moreover, the integration of wearable technology into mood disorder therapy is a new development. Such devices, aimed at quantifying somatic and emotional indicators, can give instant feedback to patients as well as clinicians. This data can include changes in heart rate, sleep activity, and activity levels, all of which are important variables in mood disorder understanding and regulation. With these wearables taking data continuously, they allow a more active mental health management course, with interventions being made in a timely fashion to prevent worsening of mood symptoms. The capability of such technology to offer information in addition to therapeutic intervention enables the possibility of better understanding a patient's overall health. By embracing these technologies, the treatment of mental illness can expand to not only be reactive but also proactive, ultimately improving the quality of care administered to individuals with mood disorders.

5.7. Stigma and Public Perception

Learning Outcome

1. Understand hotel maintenance management and its impact
2. Perform preventive maintenance
3. Discuss about breakdown maintenance

The intersection of stigma and public opinion directly influences the understanding of mood disorders. Stigmatization often results from poorly informed feelings and myths regarding mental illness, leading to negative feelings towards individuals with such states. Mood disorder patients, such as depression or bipolar disorder, may experience prejudices that decrease their confidence in obtaining treatment. This fear can be added to by fear of discrimination or judgment, and then creates a cycle of pain and silence. Moreover, the opinions of the public can perpetuate these issues; public discussion of mental health in constraining or negative terms will contribute to fostering a society where people feel they do not have a safe space for articulation of their afflictions. Recent research shows the change in public attitudes towards the treatment of mental illness over time. An important study illustrated that perceived treatment obstacles increased from the early 1990s to the early 2000s, particularly negative attitudes toward treatment need itself (Chartier et al., 2016). This shift in perception reflects a broader cultural misperception of mood disorders and the efficacy of treatments presently available. With evolving social attitudes, sufferers of mood disorders have a conflict of interest between their health needs and the prevalent public opinion, which will dissuade them from seeking the necessary help. This is the push for mass education for mental health with the intention of demolishing stigma and encouraging increased acceptance. In the long run, people's perception of mood disorders has an impact on their mental health outcomes. Most individuals with conditions like tuberous sclerosis complex (TSC) have neuropsychiatric manifestations but are excluded from seeking mental health treatment due to various obstacles. Even though the necessity for treatment is recognized, costs are a strong obstacle that mirrors general societal attitudes toward mental health treatment (Mowrey et al., 2018). Stigma surrounding mental health can influence public attitudes toward the validity and necessity of seeking care, which disproportionately affects low-income individuals who indicate self-stigma. Through greater public awareness and targeted interventions, these barriers can be overcome to enable individuals to seek the care they need without fear of stigma.

5.7.1. Societal Attitudes Towards Mood Disorders

Societal attitudes towards mood disorders significantly influence the experiences of individuals navigating these conditions. Historically, stigma has overshadowed mental health issues, often framing individuals with mood disorders as weak or flawed. This negative perception can lead to social isolation and a reluctance to seek help, as individuals fear judgment or discrimination. Current evidence indicates that societal understanding of mood disorders is gradually evolving; however, challenges remain. Efforts to initiate open discussions around mental health have helped demystify these conditions and foster empathy. Additionally, public awareness campaigns aim to educate communities about the biological and psychological aspects of mood disorders, reducing misconceptions that contribute to harmful stigmas. As awareness increases, so does the potential for social acceptance and support, which are critical for recovery and mental well-being. The role of education in shaping societal attitudes towards mood disorders cannot be overstated. Educational initiatives often target both general audiences and specific sectors, such as healthcare professionals, to promote a deeper understanding of these disorders. Research has shown that better-informed individuals are more likely to exhibit compassion and support towards those affected by mood disorders. For instance, the European Network Adult ADHD highlights that educational efforts can significantly combat stigma, leading to improved treatment and diagnosis outcomes. Such initiatives emphasize the need for accurate knowledge and the importance of addressing common misconceptions surrounding mood disorders. By equipping society with factual information, it becomes possible to dispel myths and foster an environment conducive to support and understanding, ultimately enhancing the quality of life for those affected. Despite progress in improving societal attitudes towards mood disorders, several hurdles persist, particularly concerning marginalized groups. Cultural factors often exacerbate stigma, leading to underdiagnosis and undertreatment. In communities where mental health is stigmatized, individuals may experience heightened shame and fear, hindering their willingness to seek help. Furthermore, there remains a lack of available resources and mental health professionals trained to address the unique needs of diverse populations. The complexities of these societal attitudes emphasize the necessity for comprehensive strategies that not only promote awareness but also ensure equitable access to mental health care. As highlighted in the ongoing discussions about ADHD and its societal implications, understanding how societal attitudes impact various mood disorders is essential for crafting effective interventions. Increased efforts are needed to create an inclusive narrative that respects and accommodates the varied experiences of individuals facing mood disorders.

5.7.2. The Role of Media in Shaping Perceptions

The media have a pivotal role in shaping perceptions in society, even more so for complex disorders like mood disorders. Individuals gain conceptual frameworks from media platforms , such as television, social media, and advertising, which inform their perceptions of mental health. The representation of mood disorders within these media typically deviates from clinical experience, resulting in skewed perceptions that generate stigma and misunderstanding. For example, when individuals identify with individuals who exhibit symptoms of mood disorders, they have a tendency to internalize these descriptions, shaping their impressions regarding such individuals. Studies have shown that extensive exposure to media images could have negative emotional effects, thus uncovering an essential relationship between media consumption and personal experiences of mood disorders, particularly among young people and young adults, as they are more vulnerable to media control and peer relationships (Maria et al., 2017). In addition, the prevalence of direct-to-consumer (DTC) advertising of antidepressants serves to reinforce a distorted understanding of mental illness and treatment. These advertisements tend to make mental health issues so common that viewers will infer an exaggerated prevalence of mood disorders. This can result in a misdirected sense of need for treatment, since it affects people's perceptions of their own mental health risk. The research indicates that exposure to DTC advertisements is associated with increased perceived prevalence and life-time risk of depression, which means that media not only teaches but also constructs public social realities regarding mood disorders. Therefore, the saturation of these advertisements across the various forms of media can have significant implications on public awareness and response toward mood disorders (Grow et al., 2008). Apart from influencing knowledge of mood disorders among individuals, the media also plays a pivotal role in shaping public perceptions of mental illness. The information conveyed through the media can either foster stigma or enhance understanding. Positive portrayal of mood disorders contributes significantly to depopularizing the disorders and reducing social stigma, encouraging people to reach out for assistance. Sensationalized or false impressions, however, foster myths and fear about mental illness. The cultivation of empathy and sensitivity in media narratives is thus of paramount importance in influencing public attitudes. Lastly, the dynamic reciprocal relationship between media depictions and public attitudes emphasizes the responsibility of content creators to address mental health concerns responsibly and sensitively, recognizing that their narratives have the potential to inform people's information regarding mood disorders and vulnerability to talk about mental illness.

5.7.3. Efforts to Reduce Stigma

Techniques for reducing the stigma of mood disorders play a pivotal role in the encouragement of tolerance and understanding of mental illness. Throughout history, mental illness has been mystified and feared, placing it off-limits for those who suffer from it. Social stigma raises formidable barriers to seeking treatment, which increases the severity of the mood disorders. Numerous campaigns and organizations have emerged, aiming at reshaping people's attitudes toward mental illnesses through relaying human stories and encouraging open debate on the conditions. Raising awareness and education messages, such campaigns progress to combat stereotypes and myths and later establish an acceptance culture crucial for healing and recovery. Policy frameworks have also been instrumental in combating stigma by promoting the rights of individuals with mental illness. The International Labour Organization (ILO) raises the issue of comprehensive policies that allow people with physical, psychiatric, and intellectual disabilities to achieve their career dreams. These policy reform efforts are informed by the terms of the ILO Convention 159, relating to equal treatment and employment opportunities of disabled persons. It is by way of such sensitization of policymakers, employers, and trade unions to the problems caused by individuals suffering from a mood disorder that the removal of barriers to engagement in society is made possible. Since mental health is recognized as a genuine issue that deserves attention and support, the stigma typically accompanying it is removed. In addition, integrating the treatment of mental health into overall health programs, such as HIV treatment and prevention platforms, is an enlightened movement toward stigma elimination. By associating mental health care with physical health care, specialists are capable of treating the complexity of mood disorders as a part of comprehensive health strategies. This multifaceted strategy not only increases the level of mental health care but also normalizes discussing mental illness in the health system. Through the promotion of Sylvia Kaaya and others, having platforms that offer integrated care creates mental health awareness as a vital component of one's overall well-being. Initiatives , such as these serve to decrease stigma by reaffirming the validity of mental illness and emphasizing the intersectionality of mental health and other illnesses, ultimately toward a more integrated understanding of health.

Test Your Knowledge

1. What recent advances in neuroscience and genetics are influencing the understanding and treatment of mood disorders?
2. How are digital mental health tools and personalized medicine shaping emerging research in mood disorder management?

SUMMARY

The research on mood disorders sheds light on the importance of such disorders in influencing individuals and society at large. As indicated, the mental health landscape has been influenced increasingly by issues beyond mental health, particularly in times of crisis , such as the COVID-19 pandemic. The fact that students have experienced various levels of depression, ranging from slight to severe, validates the necessity of addressing mental health in the classroom. The findings reveal a disconcerting prevalence of depressive symptomatology and confirm that interventions must be put into practice to encourage students' emotional well-being. Multidisciplinary mental health practice should be utilized to counteract these effects and prevent the long-term morbidity associated with mood disorders in vulnerable groups (Aisah et al., 2020). Moreover, the relationship between mood disorders and broader lifestyle factors , such as diet and exercise, cannot be overlooked. Current studies, particularly those focusing on the gut-brain axis, suggest that exercise and probiotics both have a beneficial impact on mental health outcomes. Exercise not only enhances the symptoms of mood disorders like depression and anxiety, but could even be used as an adjunct to psychological interventions. This highlights the necessity for multidimensional treatment plans, considering the complex interactions between psychological, biological, and lifestyle determinants of mood disorders (Grant & Baker, 2016). Understanding such interactions will enable healthcare workers to prescribe full and integrative approaches responding to individual needs. In conclusion, the treatment of mood disorders involves a wide, integrative approach considering both physical and psychological health. It is vital to build awareness and promote effective interventions that address the unique challenges of mood disorders, particularly in contexts aggravated by societal stressors like the pandemic. Interagency collaboration between mental health professionals, educators, and policymakers can go a long way towards concrete improvements in mental health practices. By putting mental health awareness at the forefront and promoting new treatments, society can better equip individuals to deal with the issues of mood disorders and enhance overall quality of life, leading towards a time when mental health is looked upon as highly important as physical health (Grant & Baker, 2016).

It is only with thorough examination of symptomatology that the understanding of mood disorders can be developed, having a significant impact on the daily life and well-being of individuals. Mood disorders encompass several conditions, with major depressive disorder and bipolar disorder being the most recognized. Underlying all the disorders are widespread depressive symptoms manifesting as persistent sadness, hopelessness, and loss of pleasure in activities once found enjoyable. Additionally, mood disorders are often followed by anxiety, complicating diagnosis and treatment. A critical review of the existing literature sheds light on the distinctive presentation of the disorders, pointing toward the need for certain therapeutic approaches. In such conditions, it is necessary to review authoritative actions to enable the evaluation of mood disorder complexity and provide appropriate treatment outcomes. The validity of certain depression screening instruments has been extensively explored, particularly in specialty populations , such as cancer patients. A meta-review of over 50 depression tools revealed key information in the context of their applicability and usefulness in various medical environments (Andersen et al., 2015). Of the tools analyzed, the Hospital Anxiety Depression Scale (HADS) was found to be popular but hampered by inconsistencies in cutpoints, making it less useful in late-stage cancer situations. In contrast, the Beck Depression Inventory proved to be more adaptable across cancer types and stages, highlighting its utility in practice settings. Interestingly, the Center for Epidemiologic Studies Depression Scale was identified as the most sensitive, requiring health practitioners to utilize the best measure to find and treat people with mood disorders in a holistic manner. Novel forms of therapy like community-based cognitive behavioral therapy (CBT) interventions also provide promising avenues to mood disorder treatment, particularly in preventing discontinuities in access to care. A more recent randomized controlled trial reviewed the "Living Life to the Full" (LLTTF) classes as a supported CBT self-help intervention, aimed at those with low mood symptoms (McClay et al., 2013). By means of support in the community, the intervention covers both the hurdle of waiting lists for mental health care and the treatment gap among those who steer clear of access in the usual sense. The trial assesses a number of outcomes, including depression, anxiety, and social functioning, ultimately assessing the effectiveness and cost-effectiveness of the interventions. Such community outreach programs have the potential to become crucial in enhancing access to psychological therapies, which would be a significant step towards the treatment of mood disorders.

KEY TERMS FROM THIS CHAPTER

- Anhedonia
- Bipolar disorder
- Bipolar II disorder
- Depression
- Hypomania
- Mania
- Mixed features
- Atypical depression
- Bipolar I disorder
- Cyclothymic disorder
- Euthymia
- Major depressive disorder (MDD)
- Melancholic features
- Mood disorder

CRITICAL THINKING QUESTIONS

1. **Which of the following is a key symptom of Major Depressive Disorder (MDD)?**
   a. Elevated self-esteem and grandiosity
   b. Delusions and hallucinations
   c. Persistent sadness or loss of interest in activities
   d. Rapid shifts between anxiety and euphoria
2. **Which mood disorder is characterized by alternating periods of depression and mania?**
   a. Generalized Anxiety Disorder
   b. Bipolar Disorder
   c. Schizophrenia
   d. Persistent Depressive Disorder
3. **In Bipolar I Disorder, the individual must have experienced at least one:**
   a. Hypomanic episode
   b. Panic attack
   c. Manic episode
   d. Depressive episode
4. **What is a common symptom of a manic episode?**
   a. Low energy and fatigue
   b. Slow speech
   c. Increased goal-directed activity and decreased need for sleep
   d. Social withdrawal
5. **Persistent Depressive Disorder (Dysthymia) differs from Major Depressive Disorder in that it:**
   a. Is more severe but lasts for a shorter time
   b. Includes episodes of psychosis
   c. Is a chronic form of depression lasting at least 2 years
   d. Involves alternating manic and depressive episodes

Short Answer Questions

1. What are mood disorders, and how are they broadly categorized?
2. What is the difference between unipolar and bipolar mood disorders?
3. Describe the main symptoms of Major Depressive Disorder (MDD).
4. What is the difference between dysthymia (Persistent Depressive Disorder) and major depression?
5. What are the key features of Bipolar I Disorder and Bipolar II Disorder?

Answer to Critical Thinking Questions

1. (c) 2. (b) 3. (c) 4. (c) 5. (c)

REFERENCES

1. Agrell, A., American Psychiatric Association, Appelros, A., Bays, A., Bell, A., Chia, A., Craig, A., et al. (2010). Health-related quality of life in people with aphasia: Implications for fluency disorders quality of life research. https://core.ac.uk/download/5230590.pdf (accessed on 28th July 2025).
2. Aisah, N. A., Ardi, W. R., Dwidiyanti, M., Handayani, et al. (2020). Tingkat depresi mahasiswa keperawatan di tengah wabah COVID-19. https://core.ac.uk/download/352146090.pdf (accessed on 28th July 2025).
3. Allen, J. J. B., Daft, C. M. W., Hameroff, S., et al. (2020). Transcranial focused ultrasound to the right prefrontal cortex improves mood and alters functional connectivity in humans. https://core.ac.uk/download/288435742.pdf (accessed on 28th July 2025).
4. Marchetti, I., Koster, E. H. W., Klinger, E., & Alloy, L. B. (2016). Spontaneous Thought and Vulnerability to Mood Disorders: The Dark Side of the Wandering Mind. *Clinical psychological science : a journal of the Association for Psychological Science*, *4*(5), 835–857. https://doi.org/10.1177/2167702615622383(accessed on 28th July 2025).
5. Altable, M. (2023). Psychiatric comorbidities in conduct disorders and neurobiological bases. *World Journal of Advanced Research and Reviews*. https://www.semanticscholar.org/paper/351b3943f52917088422a55dfa5ca2c1df9ebf60 (accessed on 28th July 2025).
6. Alvarez Pitti, J., Borghi, C., Brzeziński, M., et al. (2024). Psychosocial and environmental risk factors of obesity and hypertension in children and adolescents—A literature overview. https://diposit.ub.edu/dspace/bitstream/2445/208707/1/fcvm-10-1268364.pdf (accessed on 28th July 2025).
7. Alvarez-Pitti, J., Borghi, C., Brzeziński, M., Drożdż, D., Fernández-Aranda, F., Gabbianelli, R., González Lopez-Valcarcel, B., et al. (2023). Psychosocial and environmental risk factors of obesity and hypertension in children and adolescents—A literature overview. https://core.ac.uk/download/597999376.pdf (accessed on 28th July 2025).
8. Amiri, A., Andrade-Machado, A., Barba, A., Blanchet, A., Bleuler, A., Blumer, A., Blumer, A., et al. (2016). The interictal dysphoric disorder of epilepsy: Legend or reality? https://core.ac.uk/download/46166233.pdf (accessed on 28th July 2025).
9. Andersen, A., Becker, A., Carey, A., Carlson, A., Carlson, A., Cella, A., Cella, A., et al. (2015). Patient-reported depression measures in cancer: A meta-review. https://core.ac.uk/download/42138163.pdf (accessed on 28th July 2025).
10. Angelo Maria, A., Saliani, A., Baiocco, R., Barcaccia, B., et al. (2017). Dysfunctional eating behaviors, anxiety and depression in Italian boys and girls: The role of mass media. https://core.ac.uk/download/127586647.pdf (accessed on 28th July 2025).
11. Annagur, A., Annagur, A., Beck, A., Benson, A., Cronin, A., Dennett, A., Dowdy, A., et al. (2018). Polycystic ovary syndrome across the life span of women: A wellness-based integrative intervention. https://core.ac.uk/download/213088882.pdf (accessed on 28th July 2025).
12. Asarnow, J. R., Hughes, J. L., Langer, D. A., et al. (2017). Family-focused treatment for childhood depression: Model and case illustrations. https://open.bu.edu/bitstream/2144/24312/1/2015%20Accepted%20Tompson%20Langer%20Hughes%20Asarnow.pdf (accessed on 28th July 2025).

13. Attanasio, F., Barbini, B., Bosia, M., Cavallaro, R., Colombo, C., Fregna, L., Manfredi, E., et al. (2022). Non-pharmacological treatments. https://core.ac.uk/download/559263292.pdf (accessed on 28th July 2025).

14. Aviles Gonzales, C. I., Carrà, G., Carta, M. G., et al. (2024). Mood Disorder Questionnaire positivity in systemic lupus erythematosus and other chronic diseases , including screen bipolar disorders or rhythm and energy dysregulation syndromes (DYMERS). https://core.ac.uk/download/621423022.pdf (accessed on 28th July 2025).

15. Babaie, N. A., & Purhashemi, S. (2015). Investigating the relationship between mental health and insomnia in pregnant women referred to health centers in Estahban. https://media.neliti.com/media/publications/151697-EN-investigating-the-relationship-between-m.pdf (accessed on 28th July 2025).

16. Baconi, Daniela Luiza; Ciobanu, Anne-Marie; Vlăsceanu, Ana Maria; Cobani, Oana Denisa; Negrei, Carolina; and Bălălău, Cristian (2015) "Current Concepts on Drug Abuse and Dependence," *Journal of Mind and Medical Sciences*: Vol. 2: Iss. 1, Article 4. DOI: https://doi.org/10.22543/2392-7674.1008 (accessed on 28th July 2025).

17. Bahn, S., Barton-Owen, G., Bell, E., et al. (2021). The Delta Study–Prevalence and characteristics of mood disorders in 924 individuals with low mood: Results of the World Health Organization Composite International Diagnostic Interview (CIDI). https://core.ac.uk/download/475646921.pdf (accessed on 28th July 2025).

18. Grant, M. C., & Baker, J. S. (2017). An overview of the effect of probiotics and exercise on mood and associated health conditions. Critical reviews in food science and nutrition, 57(18), 3887–3893. https://doi.org/10.1080/10408398.2016.1189872 (accessed on 28th July 2025).

19. Balogh, L., Taguchi, S., Tanaka, M., Török, N., & Vécsei, L. (2021). Crosstalk between existential phenomenological psychotherapy and neurological sciences in mood and anxiety disorders. https://core.ac.uk/download/592568728.pdf (accessed on 28th July 2025).

20. Beerthuizen, A., Bergink, V., Boks, M. P. M., et al. (2024). The Mood and Resilience in Offspring (MARIO) project: A longitudinal cohort study among offspring of parents with and without a mood disorder. https://core.ac.uk/download/610616199.pdf (accessed on 28th July 2025).

21. Benáček, J., Lawal, N., Ong, T., Tomasik, J., Martin-Key, N., Funnell, E., Barton-Owen, G., et al. (2024). Identification of predictors of mood disorder misdiagnosis and subsequent help-seeking behavior in individuals with depressive symptoms: Gradient-boosted tree machine learning approach. *JMIR Mental Health, 11*. https://www.semanticscholar.org/paper/a864dae63fa4b95a9fb8f3142f427f2cded5c5c5 (accessed on 28th July 2025).

22. Berk, M., Brewin, C., Briken, P., et al. (2020). Mental, behavioral and neurodevelopmental disorders in the ICD-11: An international perspective on key changes and controversies. https://core.ac.uk/download/287582535.pdf (accessed on 28th July 2025).

23. Biedermann, N. C., Dittmann, S., Forsthoff, A., et al. (2002). The Stanley Foundation Bipolar Network: Results of the naturalistic follow-up study after 2.5 years of follow-up in the German centres. https://core.ac.uk/download/16432437.pdf (accessed on 28th July 2025).

24. Biesok, M., Lewoniuk, N., Macherski, M., et al. (2024). Analysis of the effects of regular yoga on the adaptive capacity of the nervous system. https://core.ac.uk/download/620863318.pdf (accessed on 28th July 2025).

25. Bonacina, G., Carollo, A., & Esposito, G. (2023). The genetic side of the mood: A scient metric review of the genetic basis of mood disorders. *Genes, 14*. https://www.semanticscholar.org/paper/3103b55f3438f685b3d99f9e28e87414415f9502 (accessed on 28th July 2025).

26. Brooks, S. K., Webster, R., Smith, L., Woodland, L., Wessely, S., Greenberg, N., & Rubin, G. J. (2020). The psychological impact of quarantine and how to reduce it: Rapid review of the evidence. *The Lancet, 395*, 912–920. https://doi.org/10.1016/s0140-6736(20)30460-8 (accessed on 28th July 2025).

27. Brown, E. L. (2017). Postpartum depression screening of women veterans in Alaska quality improvement project. https://core.ac.uk/download/286607496.pdf (accessed on 28th July 2025).

28. Chartier, K. G., Miller, K., Harris, T. R., & Caetano, R. (2016). A 10-year study of factors associated with alcohol treatment use and non-use in a U.S. population sample. *Drug and alcohol dependence, 160*, 205–211. https://doi.org/10.1016/j.drugalcdep.2016.01.005 (accessed on 28th July 2025).

29. Cardona, F., Chiarotti, F., Pellico, A., et al. (2018). A randomized controlled trial comparing behavioral, educational, and pharmacological treatments in youths with chronic tic disorder or Tourette syndrome. https://core.ac.uk/download/188827600.pdf (accessed on 28th July 2025).

30. Carta, M., Kalcev, G., Fornaro, M., Pinna, S., Avilés González, C. I., Nardi, A., & Primavera, D. (2023). Does screening for bipolar disorders identify a "Dysregulation of Mood, Energy, and Social Rhythms Syndrome" (DYMERS)? A heuristic working hypothesis. *Journal of Clinical Medicine, 12*. https://www.semanticscholar.org/paper/56862b2f11358531ae03b4a4fe4a9eceb303eab0 (accessed on 28th July 2025).

31. Carter, J. D., Crowe, M., Douglas, K. M., Frampton, C. M. A., Gallagher, P., Gray, V., Inder, M., et al. (2024). The effect of age on emotion processing in individuals with mood disorders and in healthy individuals. https://core.ac.uk/download/603541120.pdf (accessed on 28th July 2025).

32. Cavaye, J. (2009). Service users' views of therapeutic care. https://core.ac.uk/download/3433.pdf (accessed on 28th July 2025).

33. Chanen, A. M., Bagge, C., Henry, C., McConville, C., McConville, C., Brewin, C. R., Brewin, C. R., et al. (2013). Mood instability, mental illness and suicidal ideas: Results from a household survey. https://core.ac.uk/download/16663950.pdf (accessed on 28th July 2025).

34. Charman, T., Target, M., & Taylor, E. (2008). Attachment in adults with high-functioning autism. https://core.ac.uk/download/pdf/83316.pdf (accessed on 28th July 2025).

35. Chen, C. J., Liao, W. Y., Chattopadhyay, A., & Lu, T. P. (2023). Exploring the genetic correlation of cardiovascular diseases and mood disorders in the UK Biobank. *Epidemiology and Psychiatric Sciences, 32*. https://www.semanticscholar.org/paper/b4b12d558981aaf09d4bb38073629903f5a3765d (accessed on 28th July 2025).

36. Cooke, N., Corcoran, J., Crooks, P., et al. (2016). The lived experience of bipolar disorder: A systematic review and meta-synthesis. https://core.ac.uk/download/79821865.pdf (accessed on 28th July 2025).

37. Cooper, S. (2017). Implementing a community bipolar screening questionnaire in VT. https://core.ac.uk/download/84397750.pdf (accessed on 28th July 2025).

38. Creese, A., Jaquet, A., Van Rie, A., Thota, A. B., Owe-Larsson, B., Sherbourne, C. D., Gilks, C. F., et al. (2013). Grand challenges: Improving HIV treatment outcomes by integrating interventions for co-morbid mental illness. https://core.ac.uk/download/pdf/16666900.pdf (accessed on 28th July 2025).

39. Cryan, J. F., O'Riordan, K. J., Cowan, C. S. M., Sandhu, K. V., Bastiaanssen, T. F. S., Boehme, M., Codagnone, M. G., et al. (2019). The microbiota-gut-brain axis. *Physiological Reviews, 99*, 1877–2013. https://doi.org/10.1152/physrev.00018.2018 (accessed on 28th July 2025).

40. Curtiss, J., Hofmann, S. G., & McNally, R. J. (2016). A complex network perspective on clinical science. https://open.bu.edu/bitstream/2144/21704/3/PERSPECTIVES_Complex_Network.pdf (accessed on 28th July 2025).

41. Dalgleish, T., Black, M., Johnston, D., & Bevan, A. (2020). Transdiagnostic approaches to mental health problems: Current status and future directions. *Journal of Consulting and Clinical Psychology, 88*, 179–195. https://doi.org/10.1037/ccp0000482 (accessed on 28th July 2025).

42. De Choudhury, M., Gamon, M., Counts, S., & Horvitz, E. (2021). Predicting depression via social media. *Proceedings of the International AAAI Conference on Web and Social Media, 7*, 128–137. https://doi.org/10.1609/icwsm.v7i1.14432 (accessed on 28th July 2025).

43. De Raedt, R., & Koster, E. (2010). Understanding vulnerability for depression from a cognitive neuroscience perspective: A reappraisal of attentional factors and a new conceptual framework. https://core.ac.uk/download/55843012.pdf (accessed on 28th July 2025).

44. Forrer, F., Rubo, M., Wyssen, A., Meyer, A. H., & Munsch, S. (2024). The predictive value of emotion regulation difficulties and negative mood on short and long-term treatment outcomes in an online guided self-help programmed for adults with binge-eating disorder. *European Eating Disorders Review, 33*, 163–173. https://www.semanticscholar.org/paper/b9da9a553f20260b13ca12788cfd8f1f299296a6 (accessed on 28th July 2025).

45. Forte, A., Erbuto, D., Orri, M., Orri, M., Pompili, M., & Sarubbi, S. (2021). ADHD symptoms and suicide attempts in adults with mood disorders: An observational naturalistic study. https://core.ac.uk/download/589948373.pdf (accessed on 28th July 2025).

46. Gabriel, P., & International Labor Office. (2000). *Mental Health in the Workplace: Situation Analyses, United States*. https://core.ac.uk/download/5129345.pdf (accessed on 28th July 2025).

47. Getz, M., Sebrow, L., Lacritz, M., Maeda, K. I., Palmeri, M. J., & Seng, E. (2024). B-95 Cogniphobia and psychological factors in episodic migraine: A correlational analysis. *Archives of Clinical Neuropsychology*. https://www.semanticscholar.org/paper/44b75be0ce48f997068b93653cab198a78c848c4 (accessed on 28th July 2025).

48. Grow, J. M., & Park, J. S. (2008). The social reality of depression: DTC advertising of antidepressants and perceptions of the prevalence and lifetime risk of depression. https://core.ac.uk/download/213086329.pdf (accessed on 28th July 2025).

49. Hobson, R. P., Lyons-Ruth, K., Melnick, S., et al. (2007). A controlled study of hostile-helpless states of mind among borderline and dysthymic women. https://core.ac.uk/download/103202.pdf (accessed on 28th July 2025).

50. Isa, A. K. (2024). Exploring digital therapeutics for mental health: AI-driven innovations in personalized treatment approaches. *World Journal of Advanced Research and Reviews*. https://www.semanticscholar.org/paper/53bfe9b7411354ba8686b608bf132c47324a7a5f (accessed on 28th July 2025).

51. Kooij, J. J. S., Bijlenga, D., Salerno, L., Jaeschke, R., Bitter, I., Balázs, J., Thome, J., et al. (2018). Updated European consensus statement on diagnosis and treatment of adult ADHD. *European Psychiatry, 56*, 14–34. https://doi.org/10.1016/j.eurpsy.2018.11.001 (accessed on 28th July 2025).

52. Livingston, G., Huntley, J., Sommerlad, A., Ames, D., Ballard, C., Banerjee, S., Brayne, C., et al. (2020). Dementia prevention, intervention, and care: 2020 report of the Lancet Commission. *The Lancet, 396*, 413–446. https://doi.org/10.1016/s0140-6736(20)30367-6 (accessed on 28th July 2025).

53. Mahalle, M. (2024). Treatment of patient with recurrent major depressive disorder: A case report. *Scientia Psychiatric*. https://www.semanticscholar.org/paper/753020a0bfd7e6dda488af6c861c500b44c1d8ea (accessed on 28th July 2025).

54. McCauliff, K. (2007). The effects of mood disorders on families and their well-being. https://core.ac.uk/download/56323768.pdf (accessed on 28th July 2025).

55. McClay, C. A., McConnachie, A., Morrison, J., Williams, et al. (2013). A community-based group-guided self-help intervention for low mood and stress: Study protocol for a randomized controlled trial. https://core.ac.uk/download/16461280.pdf (accessed on 28th July 2025).

56. McLachlan, A. D., & Starkey, N. J. (2012). The classification of substance and behavioural addictions: A preliminary investigation. *New Zealand Journal of Psychology, 41*(1), 7–18. (accessed on 28th July 2025).

57. Moghadam, M. N., Ghaemi, M., Delfan, S. E., Afshari, M., Kaveh, M., Eshraghi, N., & Shahraki, Z. (2024). Mood disorders and sexual function in infertile men: Exploring the relationship with semen analysis results. *Andrologies*. https://www.semanticscholar.org/paper/0641f89a900d5ab7411f1eebb121be2e9797b34d (accessed on 28th July 2025).

58. Monck, E. M. (1996). Family and social factors associated with depression and anxiety disorders in late adolescent girls. https://core.ac.uk/download/323206759.pdf (accessed on 28th July 2025).

59. Mowrey, K. (2018). Psychiatric impact of tuberous sclerosis complex and utilization of mental health treatment. https://core.ac.uk/download/212897094.pdf (accessed on 28th July 2025).

60. Nadeau, M. (2019). The role of horticultural therapy in the treatment of refugees with post-traumatic stress disorder. https://core.ac.uk/download/213463622.pdf (accessed on 28th July 2025).

61. Ogando Portilla, N., Bañón González, S. M., Agudo Urbanos, M., Martínez Cortés, M., & Sobrino Cabra, O. (2023). Use of aripiprazole in dysthymic disorders. Purposely a case. *European Psychiatry, 66*, S839–S840. https://www.semanticscholar.org/paper/46c2fea33e8e2ef022aaca2dd0ee8fffd032c946 (accessed on 28th July 2025).

62. Payne, T. D. W. (2016). Social, emotional, and behavioral functioning for transitional-aged youth with autism. https://digitalcommons.georgefox.edu/cgi/viewcontent.cgi?article=1222&context=psyd (accessed on 28th July 2025).

63. Pfeiffer, F., & Seiberlich, R. R. (2025). A socio-economic analysis of youth disconnectedness. https://core.ac.uk/download/pdf/6935641.pdf (accessed on 28th July 2025).

64. Price, C. A. (2017). Tai Chi/Qi Gong in mental health treatment and prevention: A review of meta-analytic evidence and an analysis of evidence congruence with training practices. https://core.ac.uk/download/84397718.pdf (accessed on 28th July 2025).

65. Rahim, A. R., Will, V., & Myung, J. (2025). Mood variation under dual regulation of circadian clock and light. *Chronobiology International*. https://www.semanticscholar.org/paper/5e22201f171b2a46b03ffe34e69fe786ac42aca2 (accessed on 28th July 2025).

66. Roshchina, O., Simutkin, G., & Bokhan, N. (2021). Clinical-dynamical features of alcohol use disorder and mood disorders considering the chronology of their comorbidity formation. *Psikhiatriya*. https://www.semanticscholar.org/paper/5b4e3947d01ef4794b2da5865238e1898a5231b5 (accessed on 28th July 2025).

67. Schaedel, Z., Holloway, D., Bruce, D., & Rymer, J. (2021). Management of sleep disorders in the menopausal transition. *Post Reproductive Health, 27*, 209–214. https://doi.org/10.1177/20533691211039151 (accessed on 28th July 2025).

68. Visseren, F. L. J., Mach, F., Smulders, Y. M., Carballo, D., Koskinas, K. C., Bäck, M., Bénétos, A., et al. (2021). 2021 ESC guidelines on cardiovascular disease prevention in clinical practice. *European Heart Journal, 42*, 3227–3337. https://doi.org/10.1093/eurheartj/ehab484 (accessed on 28th July 2025).

69. Yang, E., Beck, K. M., Sekhon, S., Bhutani, T., & Koo, J. (2018). The impact of pediatric atopic dermatitis on families: A review. *Pediatric Dermatology, 36*, 66–71. https://doi.org/10.1111/pde.13727 (accessed on 28th July 2025).

70. Zarate, C. A., Wheeler-Castillo, C., Latov, D., Salvadore, G., Henter, I. D., Baumann, J., Ibrahim, L., et al. (2010). New therapeutic targets for mood disorders. https://core.ac.uk/download/pdf/26905733.pdf (accessed on 28th July 2025).

ANXIETY DISORDERS

6

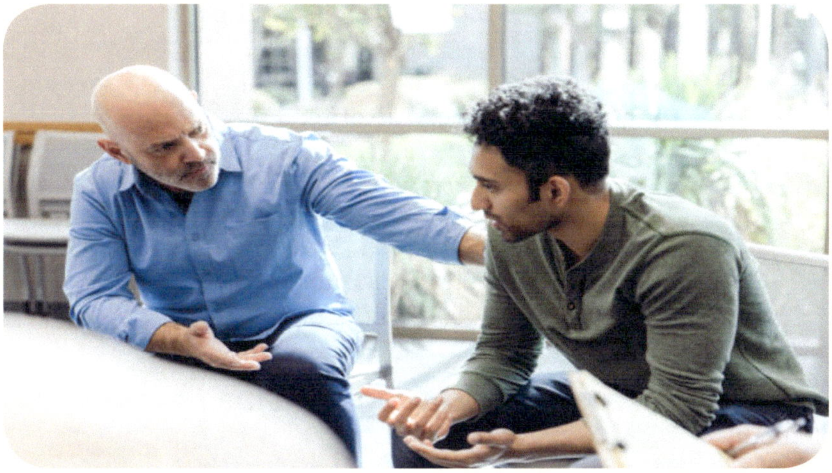

Introduction

Anxiety disorders are a prevalent and intricate category of mental disorders that take an enormous toll on the lives of tens of millions of individuals across the world.

The disorders, characterized by excessive fear or worry, present in a variety of forms, including generalized anxiety disorder, panic disorder, and social anxiety disorder, each with varying symptoms and etiology. With rising mental health awareness in society, the overall knowledge that undermines the stigma surrounding anxiety disorders improves, and people find it less challenging to seek assistance and freely speak about their condition. There is a need to be familiar with the nature and complexities of anxiety disorders, not only for those suffering but also for trained mental health professionals and society at large. The heightened incidence of anxiety disorders emphasizes the need for effective treatments and management interventions, with a high value placed on both psychological

LEARNING OBJECTIVES

After studying this chapter, you will be able to:

1. List the types of anxiety disorders;
2. Describe the causes and risk factors;
3. Explore the symptoms and diagnosis;
4. Focus on the treatment and management.

and holistic approaches in enhancing resilience and quality of life. Diagnostic features, etiology, and treatment modalities of anxiety disorders will be discussed in this chapter (Figure 6.1).

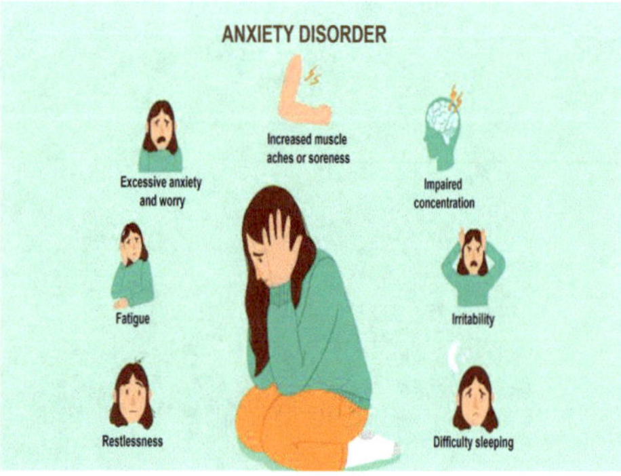
ANXIETY DISORDER
Increased muscle aches or soreness
Excessive anxiety and worry
Impaired concentration
Fatigue
Irritability
Restlessness
Difficulty sleeping

Figure 6.1. Anxiety disorders.

Source: https://www.bestpsychiatristindelhi.com/blog/wp-content/uploads/2020/12/Anxiety-Disorder1.png.

Definition of Anxiety Disorders

Anxiety disorders refer to a collection of mental conditions characterized by excessive fear or worry that gets in the way of an individual's daily functioning. Anxiety disorders may appear in a variety of forms , including generalized anxiety disorder, panic disorder, social anxiety disorder, and specific phobias, among others. According to recent epidemiological data, anxiety disorders manifest early in life and have high rates of sufferers experiencing symptoms at ages below 14 and 18, supporting the need for early intervention therapies (Solmi et al., 2021). The encounters that accompany anxiety disorders tend to generate incapacitating symptoms that hamper interpersonal relations, academic achievement, and overall quality of life. Also, they co-occur with other comorbid conditions , such as depression and drug disorders, which make them more challenging to treat and diagnose (Liu et al., 2021). Thus, an in-depth comprehension of anxiety disorders is paramount for the development of effective therapy and prevention programs that tackle their impact on an individual and society (Figure 6.2).

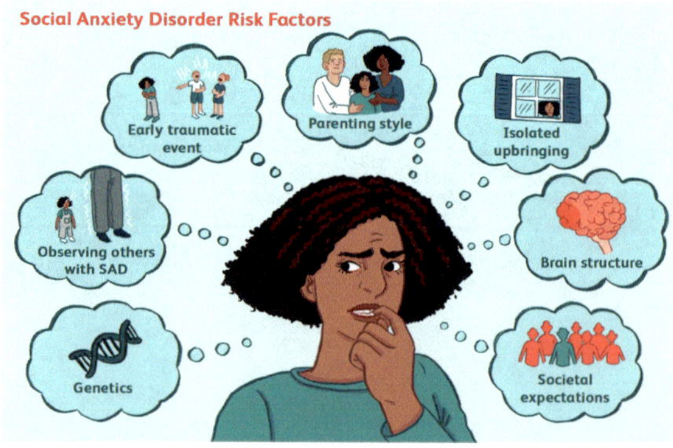
Social Anxiety Disorder Risk Factors
Early traumatic event
Parenting style
Isolated upbringing
Observing others with SAD
Brain structure
Genetics
Societal expectations

Figure 6.2. Anxiety disorders.

Source: https://www.verywellmind.com/thmb/S9_JXKoBxUTY_S7Eo3S4odeBtwA=/1500x0/filters:no_upscale():max_bytes(150000):strip_icc()/social-anxiety-disorder-causes-3024749-5c3b8f7bc9e77c0001bffa28.png.

Prevalence and Significance in Society

Anxiety disorders are a significant public health concern, with prevalence rates that attest to the insidious extent of their impact upon the community. Current estimates indicate that almost 19.1% of adults in the United States experience an anxiety disorder within any single year, a figure that clearly illustrates its prevalence. Such a somewhat alarming number serves not only to highlight the individual distress of anxiety disorders but also to point towards broader implications for social productivity and healthcare costs. The interaction between comorbid disorders, such as depression and cardiovascular disease, and anxiety contributes to the complexity, highlighting the need for integrated mental health care. Therefore, the social burden of anxiety disorders is not only illustrated by research findings on prevalence but also by its potential to affect daily life functioning and quality of life. Treatment of these disorders through preventive interventions and appropriate therapy is essential to making healthier communities and helping to decrease the financial burden they have on healthcare.

Overview of Types of Anxiety Disorders

Anxiety disorders comprise a variety of specific disorders, with each having distinct symptoms and triggers. Generalized Anxiety Disorder (GAD) is marked by excessive and persistent concern with many aspects of life, whereas Panic Disorder is defined by recurrent panic attacks that bring on extreme fear and physical symptoms. Social Anxiety Disorder is marked by fearful dread in social contexts, wherein people fear criticism or humiliation. In contrast, specific phobias trigger intense fear responses to particular objects or circumstances, for example, heights or spiders. Besides this, Separation Anxiety Disorder is primarily observed in children and is characterized by pathological distress when separated from caregivers. Present statistics indicate that anxiety disorders have grown globally, particularly fueled by circumstances like the COVID-19 pandemic that introduced increased stressors giving rise to these disorders, according to evidence on a 25.6% increase in anxiety disorders during this period (Andrade et al., 2019). Understanding these diverse manifestations is key to successful intervention and support.

Why Understanding Anxiety Disorders Is Important

It is important to understand anxiety disorders for several reasons, especially considering their high prevalence and dramatic impact on quality of life. Conditions in this broad category include generalized anxiety disorder, panic disorder, and specific phobias and other notable conditions, each of which can severely impair most aspects of daily functioning and emotional quality of life. Appreciation of the mechanisms involved—, such as hormonal shifts accentuated by ongoing research linking stress response to the BNST PACAP system—is valuable in guiding treatment design to individual needs. Furthermore, knowledge of the unique presentation of anxiety disorders among diverse populations, such as increased risk of symptoms in females exposed to stressors, highlights the need for directed investigation. By analyzing the subtlety of anxiety disorders, clinicians and researchers are able to create nuanced interventions, ultimately fostering resilience and enhancing psychosocial adjustment in those affected.

Historical Overview of Anxiety Disorders in Psychology

The notion of anxiety disorders in psychology has altered significantly in the past century, tracing a path from early moral and social model-based thinking to an increasingly mature bio-psychosocial conceptualization. Early on, anxiety was explained in moral terms, being blamed for spiritual or character defects; but with the advent of psychoanalytic theory by the likes of Sigmund Freud, all that began to shift towards intrapsychic conflict and unconscious processes. The publication of diagnostic manuals , such as the DSM, has subsequently influenced these classifications and definitions further, although it too has been accused of failing to incorporate new neurology research (Thomas et al., 2010). This divide highlights the long-standing challenges in the area, highlighting the need for such systems as the Research Domain Criteria (RDoC) project to provide a framework based on pathophysiology rather than symptomatology, thus ensuring improved understanding and more effective treatment for anxiety disorders (Benjamin et al., 2015).

Key Terms and Concepts

It is necessary to familiarize oneself with the key terms and concepts related to anxiety disorders to properly cover their complexity. Anxiety itself most often means a heightened state of worry about potential threats, which can manifest itself in various psychological and physiological responses. Discrimination between worry and anxiety is therefore important in this context; the literature appears to indicate that worry is most commonly associated with positive self-concept and interpersonal relationships, but anxiety is more likely in association with feelings of inferiority and overconcern with impending threat (Muijs & Stoeber, 2001). The difference clearly guides practice but also serves to highlight the necessity for proper nomenclature in clinical use. Moreover, the implementation of Buddhist-derived interventions (BDIs) is a significant step in the field of psychotherapy, promoting mindfulness and compassion as essential pillars to alleviate symptoms of anxiety. Nevertheless, clinical implementation of such concepts should be done with care not to cause misunderstandings that hamper their effectiveness (Griffiths et al., 2014).

6.1. Types of Anxiety Disorders

Learning Outcome

1. Generalized Anxiety Disorder (GAD)
2. Panic Disorder
3. Social Anxiety Disorder
4. Specific Phobias
5. Obsessive-Compulsive Disorder (OCD)
6. Post-Traumatic Stress Disorder (PTSD)
7. Separation Anxiety Disorder
8. Agoraphobia
9. Other Specified Anxiety Disorders

Anxiety disorders are a range of conditions characterized by excessive fear or worry that significantly impairing everyday life. Among the most common are generalized anxiety disorder (GAD), panic disorder, and phobias. GAD consists of ongoing worry across multiple aspects of life, while panic disorder features recurrent panic attacks, sudden moments of intense fear that result in extreme physical responses. Specific phobias, in contrast, refer to irrational fear of specific things or circumstances that lead individuals to avoid them at all costs. Social anxiety disorder, another significant disorder, creates excessive fear of social situations, which could initiate avoidance behavior that restricts one's social life. The National Mental Health Survey recommends that anxiety disorders are prevalent mental disorders that impact numerous people from different sections of society, making it imperative to understand and treat the conditions holistically (Murthy, 2017). Understanding the heterogeneity of anxiety disorders, we can apply interventions and support systems to the patients more suitably (Figure 6.3).

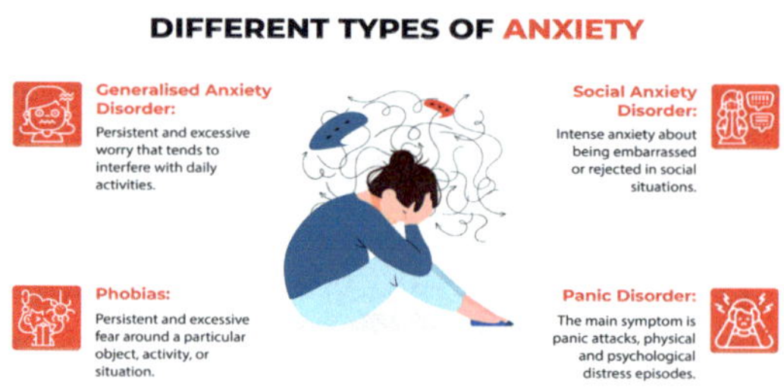

Figure 6.3. Types of anxiety disorders.

Source: https://www.australiawidefirstaid.com.au/media-library/infographic-on-different-types-of-anxiety-disorders.png.

6.1.1. Generalized Anxiety Disorder (GAD)

Generalized Anxiety Disorder (GAD) is a severe disorder in the anxiety disorders category that is accompanied by persistent and intrusive worry, interfering with daily life. GAD patients usually present with negative somatic symptoms like tension and fatigue, which tend to result in severe limitations in personal and occupational activities. Recent research emphasizes the role of monitoring underlying psychological variables, such as mindfulness and self-compassion, that may prove to be instrumental in the reduction of disability associated with GAD. Studies have indicated that GAD patients score lower on both mindfulness and self-compassion compared to control subjects, while these variables are inversely related to anxiety and worry scales (Britta et al., 2013). Most notably, mindfulness has also been found to be a better predictor of disability than traditional anxiety symptom ratings (Britta et al., 2020). Therefore, the inclusion of mindfulness-based treatment may significantly enhance treatment outcomes for curing the prevalent disorder.

6.1.2. Panic Disorder

Panic disorder, an anxiety disorder with recurrent, unprovoked panic attacks, significantly impacts people's functioning and overall quality of life. The attacks are primarily felt as abrupt, acute fear periods with a concomitant physical symptom complex of palpitations, shortness of breath, and dizziness.

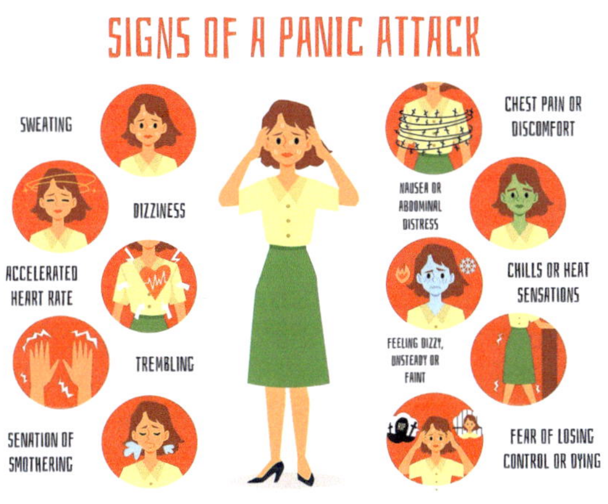
SIGNS OF A PANIC ATTACK
SWEATING
DIZZINESS
ACCELERATED HEART RATE
TREMBLING
SENATION OF SMOTHERING
CHEST PAIN OR DISCOMFORT
NAUSEA OR ABDOMINAL DISTRESS
CHILLS OR HEAT SENSATIONS
FEELING DIZZY, UNSTEADY OR FAINT
FEAR OF LOSING CONTROL OR DYING

Figure 6.4. Panic disorder.

Source: https://www.simplypsychology.org/wp-content/uploads/panic-attack-symptoms.jpg.

Significantly, research has indicated that panic disorder has the propensity to coexist with other psychiatric diseases, multiplying mental health morbidity. For instance, a study of young men revealed extensive prevalence of anxiety disorders in that 35.9% of them met the criteria for such disorders, demonstrating extensive existence of panic-related symptoms (Chang et al., 2008). Secondly, one needs to understand the development course of anxiety disorders, for instance, panic disorder, because symptoms not only emerge but also become more evident during childhood and adolescence, which is an intervention window period (Kara, 2022). Recognizing these patterns allows for more effective diagnostic and therapeutic strategies, ultimately leading to improved results for the individuals involved (Figure 6.4).

6.1.3. Social Anxiety Disorder

Social Anxiety Disorder (SAD), another prevalent anxiety disorder, handicaps daily functioning due to excessive fear of social situations and potential embarrassment. SAD individuals may feel highly anxious in everyday encounters, such as public speaking or meeting new people, and this prompts them to engage in avoidance behaviors that further worsen their condition. The disorder usually develops in childhood or during adolescence, coinciding with significant developmental milestones during which social relationships are more complicated and stressful (Kara, 2022). Comorbidities are common; SAD is likely to co-exist with other disorders like generalized anxiety disorder and depression, complicating treatment and recovery (Reid et al., 2017). The importance of early diagnosis and intervention cannot be overestimated, as early intervention can minimize the disorder's long-term effect on an individual's occupational and social functioning. Understanding the nuances of SAD is thus important to formulate better prevention, diagnosis, and treatment approaches in the overall context of anxiety disorders.

6.1.4. Specific Phobias

Specific phobias are a type of anxiety disorder that involves the development of an intense, irrational fear of a particular object or situation, causing marked distress and impairment in functioning. Cognitive behavioral therapy (CBT) has been reported by research to be the gold standard treatment for anxiety disorders, including specific phobias. A scoping review revealed that exposure to feared stimuli, a fundamental component of CBT, is effective in the treatment of such anxieties, although substantial gaps in literature exist regarding its application in the younger age groups between 14 and 24 years (Teunisse et al., 2022). Moreover, benzodiazepines, though commonly employed in cases of anxiety-related conditions, carry dependency and abuse risks, particularly with patients suffering from specific phobias (Zaami et al., 2021). Hence, there is a need to comprehend both therapeutic methods as well as potential pharmacological treatment constraints to create comprehensive treatment plans tailored to individuals with specific phobias.

6.1.5. Obsessive-Compulsive Disorder (OCD)

Obsessive-Compulsive Disorder (OCD) is a significant subtype of anxiety disorders characterized by the occurrence of recurring, intrusive ideas (obsessions) and ritualistic actions or mental rituals (compulsions) that one undertakes in a bid to reduce the ensuing anxiety caused by these obsessions. Etiology of OCD is multifaceted, with genetic and environmental factors contributing roles that predispose the individual to OCD. Recent studies have examined various treatment modalities, with a focus on cognitive-behavioral therapy (CBT), which has been effective but often inadequately so for many patients, making the search for augmentation techniques continue in order to maximize the treatment outcome (Torbecke et al., 2024). Nutritional interventions have also been suggested with innovations, for example, explored with trout fish that is rich in tryptophan to possibly impact serotonergic systems and offer a new treatment pathway (Salloum et al., 2024). Such studies bring into focus the requirement for diversified treatment regimes tailored according to the individual needs of individuals with OCD (Figure 6.5).

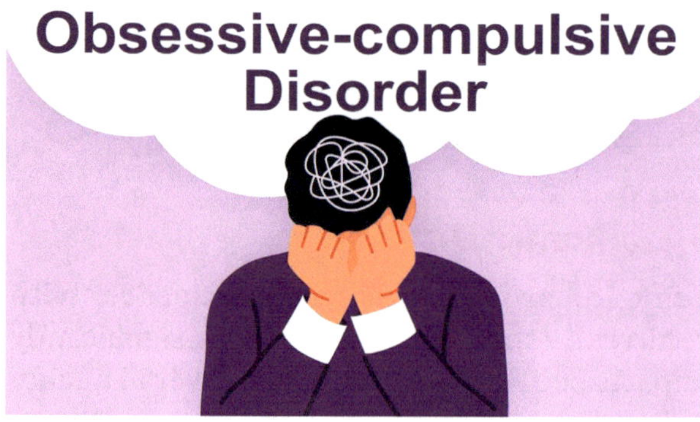

Figure 6.5. Obsessive-compulsive disorder (OCD).

Source: https://cdn-images.ausmed.com/ausmed-articles/20191127_cover_v2.1.jpg.

6.1.6. Post-Traumatic Stress Disorder (PTSD)

Post-Traumatic Stress Disorder (PTSD) is a significant manifestation of anxiety disorders that arises among individuals following the occurrence of traumatic experiences. Characterized by persistent symptoms of hyperarousal, intrusive thoughts, and numbing of emotion, PTSD is rather difficult to diagnose and treat (Ayers et al., 2010). The disorder not only affects psychological well-being but also poses physical health risks as it has been found to lead to a higher risk for heart disease and other comorbidities (Ayers et al., 2010). This exchange emphasizes the need for healthcare providers to implement a multimodal approach in the treatment of PTSD, involving cognitive-behavioral therapies, psychotropic medication, and alternative treatments , such as cannabinoids that target endocannabinoid systems to lower symptoms of anxiety (Chiappini et al., 2019). In addition, initial treatment and comprehensive care systems are also critical in forestalling the long-term effects of PTSD, ultimately promoting quality of life for the afflicted individuals in the big picture of anxiety disorders.

6.1.7. Separation Anxiety Disorder

Separation Anxiety Disorder (SAD) is a prevalent disorder, particularly in children, wherein there is pathological fear or anxiety concerning separation from an attachment figure. It exists in various forms, for example, distress when separation is impending, excessive preoccupation with harm to loved ones, or physical complaints , such as stomachaches and headaches upon separation being achieved. Research indicates that certain developmental characteristics influence the expression of anxiety disorders, as children have a much higher rate of SAD diagnosis compared to adolescents. For instance, research with 200 subjects indicated that children aged between 6 and 12 years were much more vulnerable to this disorder than the same individuals in the advanced stages of their age, who were prone to developing other kinds of anxiety syndromes and comorbidities, such as social anxiety disorder (Albano et al., 2014). It is necessary to know the details of SAD within the big picture of anxiety disorders to adapt effective treatments, and this suggests the necessity for age and symptomatology-differentiated therapeutic approaches (Białas et al., 2022).

6.1.8. Agoraphobia

Agoraphobia, a complex anxiety disorder, is characterized by intense or avoidance of circumstances in which it would be difficult to escape or assistance unavailable, particularly in public places or open areas. The illness typically emerges alongside panic disorders, where patients develop an enhanced sensitivity to fear of having panic attacks in public places and thus impose restrictive lifestyle constraints. Interestingly, studies show that agoraphobic individuals have very distinct interactions with their children in contrast to non-anxious mothers, with behaviors like higher verbal control and criticism, which can impact child development and relationships negatively (Goldstein et al., 2009). Moreover, the effectiveness of treatment is promising with the application of the Unified Protocol for Transdiagnostic Treatment of Emotional Disorders since it has proved equivalent symptom reduction compared to conventional single-disorder treatments (Ametaj et al., 2017). Overall, these studies bring out the significant interaction among agoraphobia, interpersonal relationship problems, and treatment in the overall context of anxiety disorders (Figure 6.6).

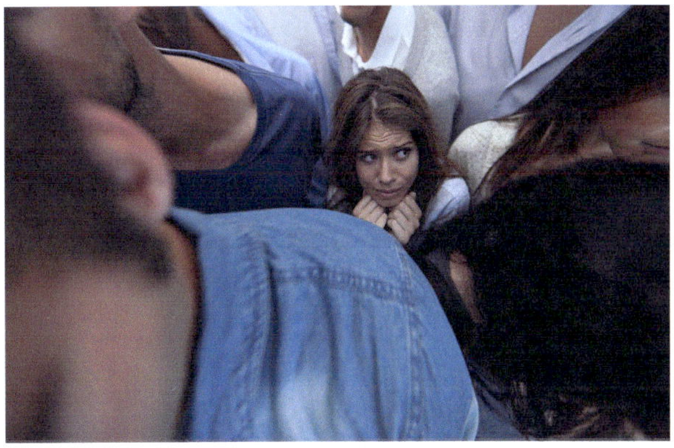

Figure 6.6. Agoraphobia.

Source: https://goodhealthpsych.com/wp-content/uploads/2023/04/how-to-overcome-agoraphobia-quickly.jpg.

6.1.9. Other Specified Anxiety Disorders

Other specified anxiety disorders (OSAD) represent a range of anxiety presentations that do not meet the full criteria of recognized disorders but still significantly impair a person's functioning. These presentations usually share symptoms consistent with generalized anxiety disorder, social anxiety disorder, or specific phobias, but manifest in unique and diverse ways that reflect the individual's specific provocations and experiences. Such conditions include presentation , such as:

- Adjustment disorder.
- Other presentation.

For instance, individuals may develop extreme anxiety regarding a specific situation, like public speaking or success on an exam that does not fall under the strict diagnostic guidelines for an accepted disorder, but interferes with functioning significantly and triggers avoidance. Current research emphasizes the place of particular intervention , such as cognitive-behavioral therapy, on the mentioned particular symptoms, as in research on therapeutic interventions in children battling related issues (Galán-Luque et al., 2023). Understanding of OSAD emphasizes the necessity of a multifaceted approach to evaluation and intervention options, giving comprehensive mental health care to all parties involved.

Test Your Knowledge

1. What distinguishes generalized anxiety disorder (GAD), panic disorder, and social anxiety disorder from one another?
2. How do phobias, OCD, and PTSD differ in terms of their core symptoms and underlying anxiety patterns?

6.2. Reasons and Risk Factors

Learning Outcome

1. Genetic Predisposition
2. Neurobiological Factors
3. Environmental Influences
4. Psychological Factors
5. Life Experiences and Trauma
6. Stressful Life Events
7. Co-Occurring Mental Health Conditions
8. Cultural Influences

Differences by Age and Gender

The risk factors and etiology for anxiety disorders are complex, with a complex interplay of genetic, environmental, and psychological elements. Etiology has proposed that family patterns matter, with patients who have a family history of anxiety disorders being at increased risk of developing related disorders themselves (Vineetha et al., 2019). In addition, prenatal and perinatal states, for example, maternal pregnancy emotional state, have been established as correlates of child anxiety, with early life experience being particularly emphasized. Environmental stressors , including trauma, life-threatening events, and chronic stress, also play a role in the etiology of anxiety disorders, particularly in vulnerable individuals (Hastuti et al., 2008). Psychological factors , such as personality traits, that is, neuroticism, also maintain vulnerability to anxiety. Such complicated associations help clinicians identify at-risk patients better and implement preventive interventions to mitigate the impact of such contributing elements to mental illness (Figure 6.7).

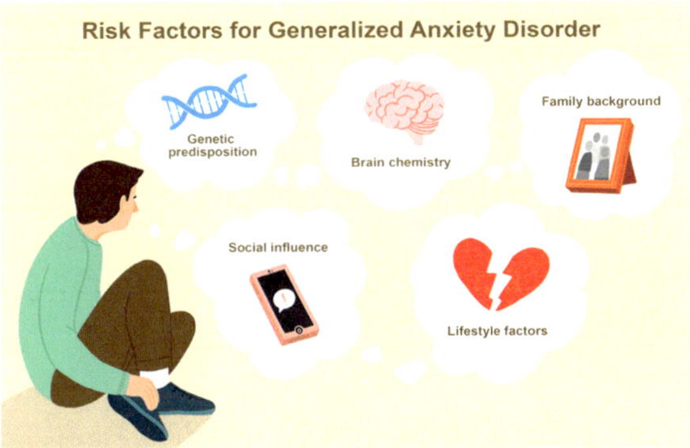

Figure 6.7. Causes and risk factors of generalized anxiety disorder.

Source: https://www.verywellmind.com/thmb/FjDm8DIOnNO84UhMv0RMPVvtBYk=/1500x0/filters:no_upscale():max_bytes(150000):strip_icc()/gad-causes-risk-factors-1392982-488cca43a0484ff7804288f6129035f9.png.

6.2.1. Genetic Predisposition

In studying anxiety disorders, the contribution of genetic predisposition is an important line of investigation that explains the intricate interplay between genes and environment. Research has repeatedly demonstrated that genetic contribution plays a large part in determining how likely a person is to develop these disorders, and there are multiple genomic loci implicated in multiple anxiety phenotypes. For example, studies on the serotonin transporter gene (5-HTT) have identified associations between gene variation and increased anxiety symptoms, highlighting its significance in anxiety pathology (Morris-Rosendahl, 2022). Mendelian randomization analyses have further indicated that socioeconomic determinants and genetic markers can act as protective factors against anxiety disorders, pointing toward a complex genetic profile (Gu et al., 2024). This supports the fact that although genetics provides the foundation for susceptibility, environmental interaction further influences the expression of anxiety disorders, pointing toward an involved genetic and phenotypic correlation.

6.2.2. Neurobiological Factors

Neurobiological processes are also of major importance for the emergence and expression of anxiety disorders, emphasizing the interplay among genetic, epigenetic, and environmental determinants of mental well-being. Studies have also shown that genetic variations in genes like the adenylate cyclase-activating polypeptide receptor (ADCYAP1R1) are associated with increased amygdala reactivity, especially in females, indicating that a genetic disposition can enhance susceptibility to anxiety symptoms and posttraumatic stress disorder (PTSD). Also, maternal anxiety disorders have been recognized as risk factors across generations, wherein stress during pregnancy affects neurodevelopment and attachment patterns, potentially predisposing offspring to anxiety disorders (Newman et al., 2016). This fact highlights the importance of considering early neurodevelopmental processes since they play a crucial role in the onset of mental health disorders. Through the synthesis of these neurobiological findings, scientists can create specialized interventions to minimize the occurrence of anxiety disorders through generations (Figure 6.8).

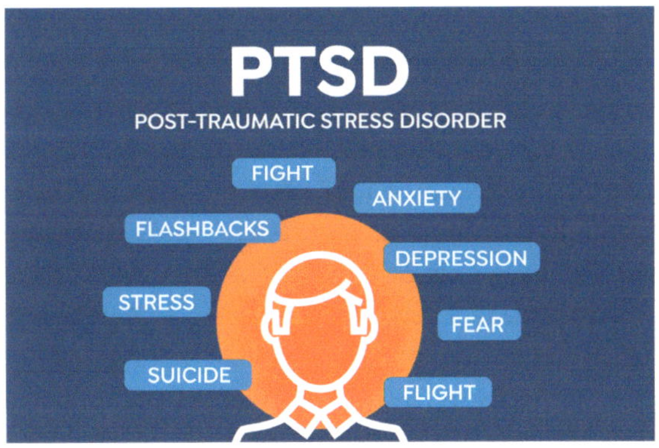

Figure 6.8. Posttraumatic stress disorder (PTSD).

Source: https://images.squarespace-cdn.com/content/v1/5c7961434d8711e9cca81d33/1572639071052-JR12NJ2DVXG799KMZFJL/9.20_PTSD_Blog.png.

6.2.3. Environmental Influences

Environmental influences play a critical role in the causation and exacerbation of anxiety disorders, particularly through stress and decision-making mechanisms. From research, it is expected that stressful environments will result in anxious symptoms, with variations in susceptibility among people influencing these findings (Bond et al., 2015). For instance, individuals with low-trait anxiety may employ harm-avoidant tactics in their reaction to stress, thus exposing themselves to fewer further stressors. Conversely, highly anxious individuals can be involved in risk-taking activities, which will accumulate more issues in their mental health (Bond et al., 2015). Moreover, the environment in which children are exposed to anxiety influences their emotional and psychological strength, and various risk and protective factors have been identified based on the environments around them. This acknowledgment highlights the necessity of a clear exploration of how environmental stressors influence individual traits and shape the trajectory of anxiety disorders throughout development.

6.2.4. Psychological Factors

Involvement of psychological factors significantly influences causality and persistence of anxiety disorders. Research has shown that childhood experiences, such as insecurity and low self-esteem, can exacerbate symptoms of anxiety as individuals develop into adolescents and adults (Nuruddaroini et al., 2021). For instance, adolescent individuals with negative attitudes towards parental attitudes can develop a negative self-concept, further aggravating anxiety and depression. In addition, studies have shown that having a healthy classroom community is linked to reduced anxiety, and this shows the importance of social contexts in building resilience to psychological distress (Amrai et al., 2011). The intricate nature of these psychological aspects points to the necessity of targeted interventions that address these elements. By offering coping mechanisms and enhancing self-esteem in youths through encouragement, teachers and parents can mitigate the risk of developing anxiety disorders. Understanding the psychological basis is thus crucial in creating effective prevention strategies within mental health discourse.

6.2.5. Life Experiences and Trauma

Life experiences, particularly those that expose an individual to trauma, are instrumental in the occurrence and manifestation of anxiety disorders. Trauma-related experiences like community violence have profound psychological impacts that extend beyond immediate reactions, impacting individuals' long-term mental health. In some, the cumulative effect of existing in risk environments is to instill a pervasive sense of anxiety and terror, ultimately translating to heightened vulnerability to anxiety disorders. Such a link is most evident within the older cohorts who might have endured historical traumas that resonate through their lifespan, shaping their emotional adjustment and coping mechanisms. Identification of the impact of life events on mental health is important, not only at the time of treatment but in planning preventive interventions to minimize the effects of trauma. Recognition of these connections enhances our knowledge about anxiety disorders and highlights the importance of integrative therapies to the treatment of mental illness.

6.2.6. Stressful Life Events

Stressful life events (SLEs) are reputed to play key roles in the development and severity of anxiety disorders, particularly within high-risk groups , such as adolescents. It is revealed that SLEs vary in nature and impact and encompass important dependent interpersonal events that have strong links with externalizing problems as well as attention-deficit/hyperactivity disorders (Francisco et al., 2024). These events are capable of provoking a sense of helplessness and anxiety, lowering subjective well-being, further complicating mental health implications. In addition to this, resilience has also emerged as a major mediating variable because research states that SLEs negatively affect resilience and hence psychological well-being (Fayez Mahamid et al., 2021). This indicates that an increase in resilience can counter the negative effects of SLEs, thus providing a protective shield against anxiety disorders. Thus, an understanding of SLEs' interaction with resilience and mental health can inform the interventions to reduce symptoms of anxiety and psychological well-being in those exposed to extreme SLEs.

6.2.7. Co-Occurring Mental Health Conditions

The phenomenon of co-morbidity, and particularly that of anxiety disorders, is quite problematic with regard to diagnosis and treatment paradigms. The evidence indicates that anxiety patients are likely to experience cumulative stressors when they present with other mental illnesses, such as depression or substance abuse disorders.

For instance, anxiety and college students' patterns of binge drinking demonstrate how participants might utilize maladaptive coping styles to alleviate their feelings of anxiety, but these coping styles might eventually contribute to their psychological distress (Kays, 2018). Integrated care models, such as those built in New Hampshire, underscore the importance of both behavioral and physical health being addressed simultaneously, thereby optimizing treatment success and overall patient outcome (Bartels et al., 2016). With the application of a holistic model, the clinician is better positioned to help people cope with the dual impairment of anxiety and its co-occurring disorders, thereby establishing a more successful pathway to mental wellness (Figure 6.9).

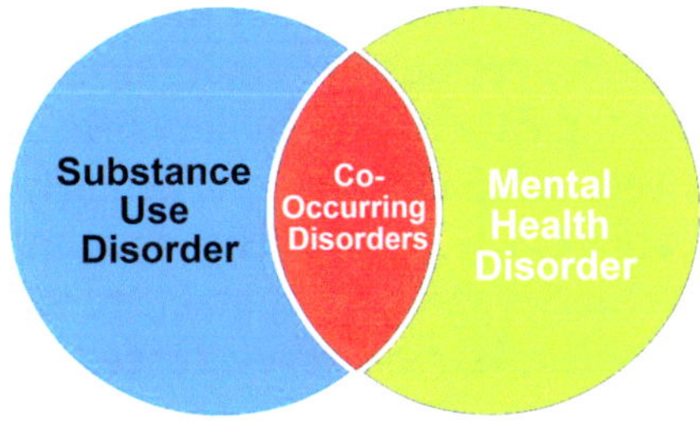

Figure 6.9. Co-occurring mental health conditions.

Source: https://acmionline.com/wp-content/uploads/2021/09/coccurring-v7-2021-09-09_16-47-20.jpg.

6.2.8. Cultural Influences

Cultural forces play a significant role in shaping the expression and interpretation of anxiety disorders in various populations. Cultural norms define acceptable behavior and how feelings are expressed, which in turn influence people's experiences of anxiety. As such, in collectivist cultures, attention to social harmony can lead to heightened social interaction anxiety and family role-related concerns, whereas in individualist cultures, achievement and independence can produce performance anxieties. Moreover, mental illness stigma may vary culturally and impact whether or not a patient is treated, as well as their understanding of the symptoms. This is illustrated in an instance of cyberchondria, whereby hypochondria can be exacerbated by internet research on health, particularly in such cultures where health is a taboo subject (Starčević et al., 2015). Therefore, awareness of such cultural foundations is of paramount importance in developing culturally sensitive interventions for treating anxiety disorders across populations (Sivertsen et al., 2015).

6.2.9. Differences by Age and Gender

The interaction of age and gender has a profound effect on the occurrence and manifestation of anxiety disorders, most notably across developmental periods like emerging adulthood. Evidences indicate higher anxiety levels among females compared to males, particularly across the age range of 18–28 years. Higher vulnerability among women is partly attributable to variations in developmental strengths; evidences show that lower positive values and higher negative values tend to exacerbate anxiety in young women (Gómez Baya et al., 2022). Besides, age factors, such as experience and maturity, can also impact anxiety symptomatology. For instance, gender differences have been observed in attention-deficit/hyperactivity disorder (ADHD), where female adolescents exhibit more symptoms of depression and anxiety, showing that there is a complex interaction between comorbid mental health issues, gender, and age (Boecker et al., 2023). These findings point to the need for developing prevention and intervention methods specifically geared towards these differences.

Test Your Knowledge

1. How do genetic predisposition, neurotransmitter imbalances, and brain structure contribute to the development of anxiety disorders?
2. What environmental and psychosocial factors—such as trauma, stress, and early childhood experiences—increase the risk of anxiety disorders?

6.3. Symptoms and Diagnosis

Learning Outcome

1. Common Emotional Symptoms
2. Physical Symptoms of Anxiety
3. Behavioral Symptoms
4. Diagnostic Criteria (DSM-5)
5. Importance of Accurate Diagnosis
6. Role of Mental Health Professionals
7. Self-Assessment Tools
8. Diagnosis Challenges
9. Misdiagnosis and Its Implications

Anxiety disorders are typically difficult to identify because symptoms differ among individuals and among diagnostic classes. Importantly, common symptoms , such as worry, restlessness, and physical symptoms of increased heart rate must be carefully analyzed in order to make appropriate connections between anxiety and diagnoses. Research indicates that low resting-state heart rate variability (HRV) is strongly correlated with symptoms of worry and anxiety rather than the clinical diagnosis per se, so HRV can be a transdiagnostic biomarker for symptoms of anxiety (Camm et al., 2016). In addition, high comorbidity is noted in hair-pulling disorder and anxiety disorders, thus pointing out the complex inter-relationship between the two conditions and their similarity in symptoms, including depression and other behavioral disorders (Compton et al., 2016). The complexity of symptoms and diagnosis helps in creating effective interventions to counter the unique experiences of individuals with anxiety disorders.

6.3.1. Common Emotional Symptoms

General emotional symptoms of anxiety disorders usually appear as long-standing feelings of distress, apprehension, and unease. Individuals with anxiety can be excessively worried and experience an overpowering fear that can disrupt normal functioning. Research uncovers that sensitivity to anxiety, or the fear of being anxious, is one of the central factors in the development and emergence of these emotional symptoms (Uluyol & Meterelliyoz, 2023). In addition, repetitive negative ruminations, as worry and rumination, also complicate patients' emotional states because they are strongly linked with both symptoms of anxiety and depression (Harvey et al., 2013). This interplay between cognitive activity and emotional states demonstrates how maladaptive schemas contribute to the maintenance of anxiety symptoms, producing a cycle that is sometimes hard to break. Therefore, realizing and treating such emotional expressions is essential for efficient intervention and treatment plans for people with anxiety disorders.

6.3.2. Physical Symptoms of Anxiety

Anxiety disorders also manifest themselves outside of emotional issues in numerous physical complaints that strongly impact people's daily lives. The somatic presentation can vary from a rapid heart rate, muscle tension, gastrointestinal symptoms, and fatigue, all of which can add up to a compromised quality of life. Research has also shown that there is a high correlation between physical symptoms of anxiety and patients' physical and psychological well-being, emphasizing the convergence of psychological and physical health (Lomper et al., 2023). For instance, coronary artery disease (CAD) patients are known to express physical symptoms that may be either a byproduct of co-existing anxiety or depression, emphasizing their entangled nature (Peng et al., 2022). Understanding these bodily responses is crucial, as they make diagnosis and treatment challenging, necessitating an integral approach that both heals the mind and body to maximize outcomes in anxiety disorder patients (Figure 6.10).

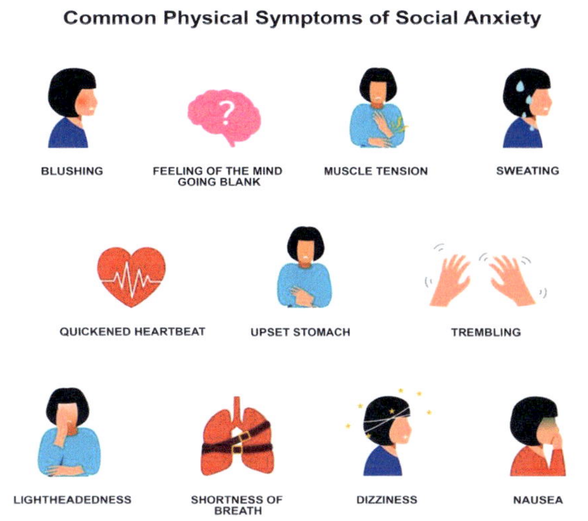

Figure 6.10. Physical symptoms of anxiety.

Source: https://www.drugwatch.com/wp-content/uploads/Common-Physical-Symptoms-of-Social-Anxiety-1.jpg.

6.3.3. Behavioral Symptoms

Behavioral manifestations are a critical part of the identification of anxiety disorders, in that they present themselves in ways that significantly affect everyday functioning. Anxiety patients can exhibit avoidance behaviors, like the avoidance of social interactions or places that trigger their fear, as demonstrated in social anxiety disorder (SAD) (Matsumoto et al., 2023). Moreover, overconcern can result in compulsive behavior to neutralize perceived danger, common in generalized anxiety disorder (Paul Farrand et al., 2023). These behaviors not only characterize the psychological distress suffered by such people but also act as coping strategies to deal with paralyzing anxiety. By identifying and confronting these behavioral manifestations, therapeutic approaches can be adjusted to promote improved responses. For instance, therapies like cognitive behavioral therapy have been shown to minimize such symptoms and improve overall well-being, and consequently, the quality of life for people with anxiety disorders.

6.3.4. Diagnostic Criteria (DSM-5)

The Diagnostic and Statistical Manual of Mental Disorders, Fifth Edition (DSM-5) presents extensive criteria for the identification of various forms of anxiety disorders of prime significance in clinical assessment and intervention. All the disorders, such as Generalized Anxiety Disorder (GAD), Social Anxiety Disorder (SAD), and Specific Phobias, require the presence of some symptoms to result in serious impairment or bring about important distress (Greiner et al., 2022). For instance, GAD is defined as excessive worry on more than half the days of a period of at least six months, along with three or more somatic symptoms like restlessness or difficulty concentrating. Similarly, SAD's criteria are repeated fear in social situations, intruding on people's ability to carry out common tasks. The wide range of these criteria not only guides clinicians in the diagnosis of anxiety disorders but also facilitates the transferability of effective therapeutic interventions, emphasizing the importance of proper diagnostic systems in mental health care.

6.3.5. Importance of Accurate Diagnosis

Proper identification is critical in the management of anxiety disorders since improper identification may result in inappropriate treatment and continued distress. Quick and proper identification is paramount, particularly for common conditions like Generalized Anxiety Disorder (GAD) that are common among the majority of the population, as outlined by the World Health Organization (Prajesha & Veni, 2023). Accurate assessment enables clinicians to tailor interventions of maximal efficacy to particular patients, reducing the prevalence of comorbidities and achieving better long-term results. Development of integrated diagnostic tools, such as the Anxiety Assessment Scale (AAS), illustrates the need for multicomponent assessment methods that capture the pervasive subtlety of symptoms of anxiety (Malakcioglu, 2022). Finally, proper diagnosis will not only result in an improved therapeutic intervention but also give power to the patient with a better insight into his/her mental state, thereby opening the gates to his/her recovery.

6.3.6. Role of Mental Health Professionals

Mental health professionals play a vital role in the treatment and diagnosis of anxiety disorders, exercising immense impact on patient outcomes through evidence-based interventions and therapeutic strategies. Not only do they facilitate the diagnosis of various anxiety disorders, but they also build personalized treatment plans that include psychotherapy, medication management, and lifestyle counseling.

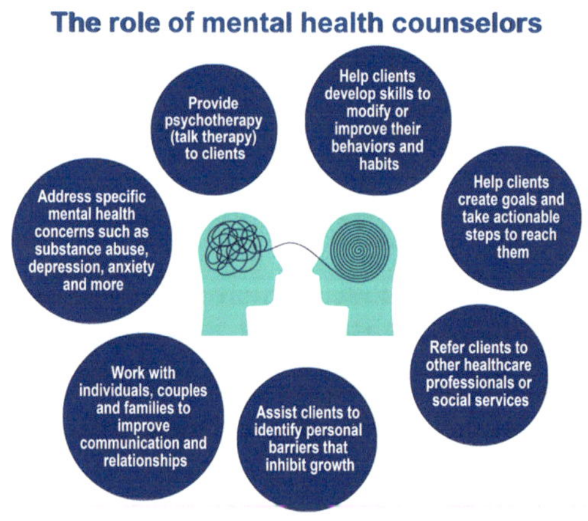
The role of mental health counselors
Provide psychotherapy (talk therapy) to clients
Help clients develop skills to modify or improve their behaviors and habits
Help clients create goals and take actionable steps to reach them
Address specific mental health concerns such as substance abuse, depression, anxiety and more
Refer clients to other healthcare professionals or social services
Work with individuals, couples and families to improve communication and relationships
Assist clients to identify personal barriers that inhibit growth

Figure 6.11. Role of mental health professionals.

Source: https://www.allpsychologyschools.com/wp-content/uploads/2024/10/Mental-health-counselor-job-duties.webp.

The integration of mental health professionals, especially general practitioners

(GPs), is vital in early symptom detection and successful management. For example, GPs tend to disentangle the subtleties of perinatal mental health, concentrating on psychosocial aspects of anxiety rather than merely classifying disorders. Their application of clinical acumen, as noted in research, facilitates more personalized care, which enhances patient-informed decision-making (Ayers et al., 2017). Moreover, bringing GPs and specialist mental health clinicians together can bridge gaps in provision for excellent psychological treatments, ultimately enhancing the overall quality of care for anxiety disorder sufferers (Woodie, 2009) (Figure 6.11).

6.3.7. Self-Assessment Tools

Self-assessment tools are useful tools in the management of anxiety disorders since they allow individuals to quantify their psychological condition and identify symptoms effectively. These tools, such as questionnaires and rating scales, provide template structures where the users can reflect on their emotional and cognitive responses and, therefore, easily identify trends characteristic of anxiety. For instance, the Generalized Anxiety Disorder 7-item scale (GAD-7) has been widely applied in research and clinical practice in screening and measuring the severity of generalized anxiety disorder. Also, self-reports can be wonderful resources under crisis situations, such as the latest COVID-19 pandemic, which has increased levels of anxiety among many individuals (Monaghesh & Hajizadeh, 2020).

By facilitating self-awareness, these tools not only facilitate early interventions but also prompt individuals to seek professionals when their self-reported symptoms highlight the necessity for timely intervention (Ellemarije Altena et al., 2020). Through this medium, self-assessment tools play a significant role in the general knowledge and treatment of anxiety disorders.

6.3.8. Diagnosis Challenges

The diagnostic difficulties of the anxiety disorders are multifaceted and based on profound historical and methodological foundations. One of the significant ones is excessive dependence on the Diagnostic and Statistical Manual of Mental Disorders (DSM), which, as a diagnostic key to defining criteria, has prioritized interrater reliability at the expense of the validity of its diagnoses. Described here are the DSM-IV's limitations as hindrances in the attainment of precise diagnoses, as these specifications can generate "epistemic blinders" that constrain clinical understanding and therapeutic advancement (Am. Psychiatr. Assoc. et al., 2010). The application of internet-based cognitive behavior therapy (ICBT) with younger clients has also demonstrated issues about program adherence and intervention effectiveness. Evidence has shown that without explicit guidance and support structures, most children find it difficult to interact effectively with self-directed therapies, further making the diagnostic process complex (Baldwin et al., 2019). The challenges thus serve to highlight the need for constant improvement in both diagnostic tools and therapeutic approaches.

6.3.9. Misdiagnosis and Its Implications

Misdiagnosis of anxiety disorders carries significant implications for patients, typically in the form of inappropriate treatment and prolonged suffering. For instance, illnesses , such as generalized anxiety disorder (GAD) are mixed up with other psychiatric ailments, leading to drug treatment that exacerbates the condition instead of alleviating it. Misdiagnosis can potentially overlook underlying biological causes, such as monoamine oxidase (MAO) neurotransmitter dysregulation, which have been linked to anxiety susceptibility and symptomatology (Ravikant Sharma et al., 2023). Moreover, if patients are misdiagnosed, they will likely experience extreme emotional distress and frustration, thus undermining their trust in healthcare professionals. Inadequate treatment and the cycle of misdiagnosis can perpetuate worsening of mental health, highlighting the necessity of healthcare professionals using reliable assessment processes. Accurate handling of such nuances not only enhances the effectiveness of treatment but is indispensable in improving the overall level of care administered to individuals grappling with anxiety disorders (Luise Pruessner et al., 2024) (Figure 6.12).

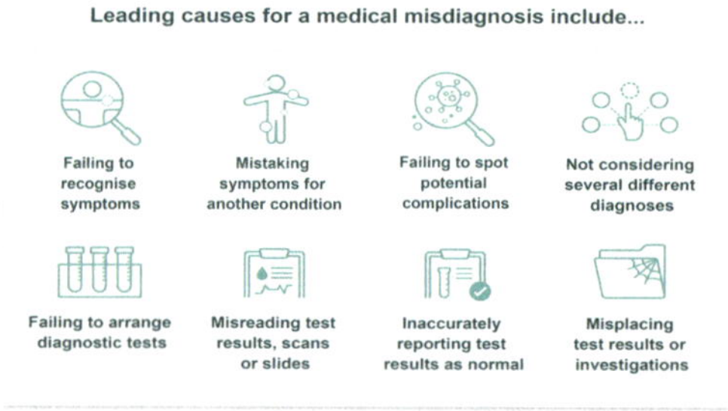

Figure 6.12. Misdiagnosis and its implications.

Source: https://www.gadsbywicks.co.uk/media/gadsby-wicks-leading-causes-for-a-medical-misdiagnosis-include.jpg.

Test Your Knowledge

1. What physical, cognitive, and behavioral symptoms are commonly associated with anxiety disorders?
2. How do clinicians use clinical interviews, DSM-5-TR criteria, and standardized assessment tools to diagnose different anxiety disorders?

6.4. Treatment and Management

Learning Outcome

1. Psychotherapy Options
2. Medication Types and Their Effect
3. Coping Behavior and Lifestyle Changes
4. Role of Support Groups
5. Alternative Treatments (e.g., Yoga, Mindfulness)
6. Importance of a Personalized Treatment Plan
7. Barriers to Treatment Access
8. Long-Term Management Actions
9. New Therapies and Research

Treatment and management of anxiety disorders need to be multi-modal, including both pharmacological and non-pharmacological modalities. It is found that cognitive behavioral therapy (CBT) can be particularly effective; in conjunction with customized management methods, including those that are customized to college students, it delivers amazing outcomes. To cite an example, a study comparing the usual treatment approaches to an association of CBT with university-based support indicated a whopping 96.15% rate of effective treatment among the latter group, as compared to a meager 76.92% among the former (Sun, 2023). These findings highlight the importance of psychoeducation and shared decision-making (SDM) during treatment, considering patients' preference for psychological treatment over medication (Chen et al., 2024).

Overall, these integrative strategies aim not just to reduce symptoms but also to encourage greater patient engagement in their mental health work, ultimately constructing a more adaptive and resilient strategy for anxiety disorders (Figure 6.13).

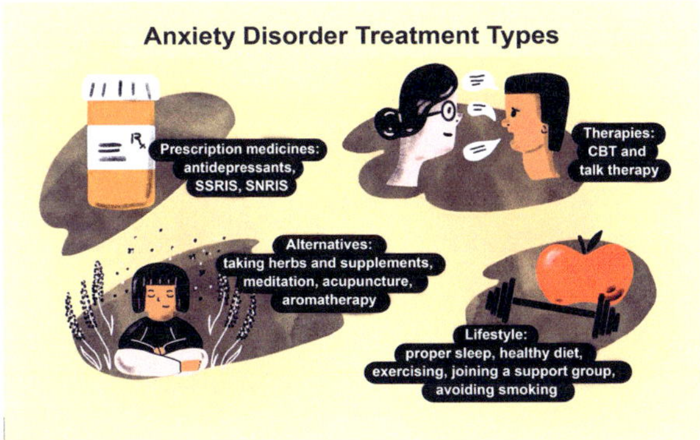

Figure 6.13. Anxiety disorder treatment.

Source: https://www.verywellhealth.com/thmb/GezodDeFZYYCbFc_TO_P6SX1PbY=/1500x1000/filters:no_upscale():max_bytes(150000):strip_icc()/anxiety-disorder-treatment-5114725_final-0eefc1d56cec4bdf91acb6df706931e7.jpg.

6.4.1. Psychotherapy Options

Psychotherapy treatment for anxiety disorders is diverse, with many modalities being tailored to individual needs and treatment goals. Cognitive Behavioural Therapy (CBT) is a mainstay treatment and targets the modification of maladaptive thought patterns that perpetuate anxiety. Through structured sessions, patients learn skills to manage anxiety-evoking fears and alter unhelpful thinking. Psychoanalytic psychotherapy offers another option with the investigation of unconscious processes underlying behaviour. While classically blamed for a lack of empirical support, it has raised debate concerning research integration into clinical practice, insisting on the demonstration of research-based efficiency in psychotherapeutic treatment (Wood, 2010). Moreover, behavioral treatment for particular anxiety-related diseases , such as headaches in children, has been efficacious, pointing to the benefit of integrating consideration of psychosocial elements and an increase in quality of life (Arruda et al., 2016). Taken together, these psychotherapy options provide valuable avenues for relief-seeking patients in need of anxiety alleviation, emphasizing individually tailored and evidence-based treatment.

6.4.2. Medication Types and Their Effect

Treatments of anxiety disorders usually involve a combination of drugs that work through diverse mechanisms and effects. SSRIs , such as fluoxetine and fluvoxamine are frequently utilized because they significantly enhance serotonin levels and thus alleviate anxiety symptoms. Benzodiazepines become effective immediately by augmenting the function of GABA receptors, but their liability for addiction means it is hard to sustain their use over time. A meta-comparison of pharmacotherapy and psychotherapy on outcomes implies that both are beneficial but perhaps vary in the degree of their benefit on certain disorders; for example, pharmacotherapy is more beneficial in dysthymia, but psychotherapy might be superior for obsessive-compulsive disorder. Newer treatments, including neurostimulation techniques, also provide alternatives, though with less solidly established usage rates. Such treatment modality diversity emphasizes the need for individualized interventions to efficiently deal with anxiety disorders.

6.4.3. Coping Behavior and Lifestyle Changes

The emergence of anxiety disorders during the COVID-19 pandemic has ushered in a huge trend in lifestyle changes and adaptation mechanisms among those affected. Some students, for instance, reported increased stress and anxiety linked with medical issues and interference with day-to-day life, as evidenced by research indicating 71% of surveyed college students felt more anxious during this period (Son et al., 2020). As a coping mechanism to these issues, the individuals employed both healthy and unhealthy coping strategies, where most of them employed healthier lifestyle adaptations like exercise, healthy eating, and mindfulness training as a defense mechanism against stress. Others employed unhealthy adaptations , such as drug use or isolation (Brenda, 2020). Such adaptations highlight the need for specialized interventions that promote effective coping mechanisms and emphasize the need to maintain a balanced life in an attempt to strengthen mental health resilience when dealing with anxiety disorders (Figure 6.14).

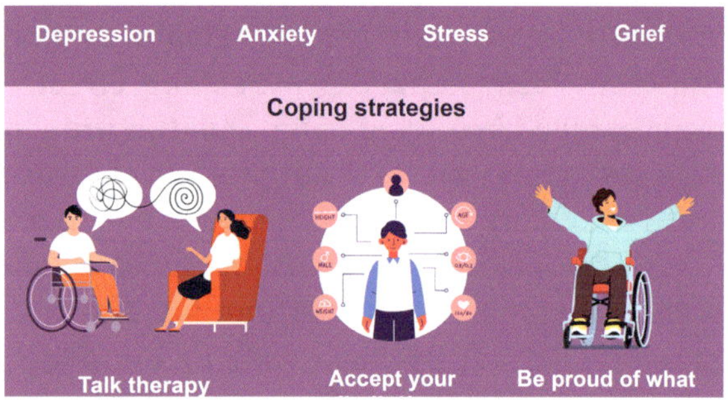

Figure 6.14. Lifestyle changes and coping strategies.

Source: https://smanewstoday.com/wp-content/uploads/2023/09/Coping-strategies-to-improve-SMA-mental-health-1200x630-cropped.png?p=85612.

6.4.4. Role of Support Groups

Support groups play a key role in the management of anxiety disorders, as they provide sufferers with an important venue to exchange experiences and coping mechanisms. Support groups provide members with a feeling of belonging and community, which diminishes feelings of isolation that accompany anxiety issues. Through their interaction with other individuals who understand their challenges, the participants are able to gain valuable insights and emotional guidance, something that can significantly enhance their capacity to manage symptoms. Research indicates that peer support significantly lowers levels of anxiety and promotes recovery, lending credence to the theory that sympathy and association are central to mental wellness.

Additionally, within these social support systems, individuals can establish effective coping abilities and gain practical coping strategies to deal with situational stressors, a requirement that is increasingly present in today's ever-changing world. Lastly, support groups are an essential component of broad-based treatment for anxiety disorders, promoting resilience and recovery.

6.4.5. Alternative Treatments (e.g., Yoga, Mindfulness)

Other forms of treatment, such as yoga and mindfulness, have been in the spotlight as complementary therapy for managing anxiety disorders. Both therapies emphasize the body-mind connection in reducing tension and emotional instability through certain practices like conscious breathing and posture exercises. Research has also demonstrated the power of yoga in reducing symptoms of anxiety in a randomized controlled trial where participants who participated in a six-week yoga intervention showed statistically significant decreases in anxiety scores compared to a waitlist control condition (de Manincor et al., 2017).

Furthermore, the holistic approach of mindfulness enhances self-awareness and resistance to stress so that individuals can manage situations that provoke anxiety better. Although problems with the methodological limitations and heterogeneity of intervention exist, the promising outcomes of these treatments show that they can be valuable components of a total treatment plan for anxiety, enhancing overall quality of life and happiness for individuals with such disorders (Contreras et al., 2019).

6.4.6. Importance of a Personalized Treatment Plan

In the management of anxiety disorders, the significance of a tailored treatment approach cannot be overemphasized. Anxiety disorders are heterogeneous and need to be managed by a tailor-made strategy that is responsive to the patient's specific needs, choices, and responses to previous interventions. Since research has established, prescribing regular treatments , such as selective serotonin reuptake inhibitors or cognitive-behavioral therapy is not sufficient since such treatments may be effective to varying extents in patients (Dan et al., 2021). Personalized treatment programs enable practitioners to alter treatment strategies, using varied modalities and handling co-morbidities effectively. Moreover, the evolution of decision-support tools accentuates individualized care as an aspect, which allows for a careful analysis of the suitable domains which are fundamental in the management. The personalization not just enhances the therapy outcome but also enhances patient engagement and satisfaction, leading ultimately to resilience in anxiety disorder management and its intricacies (Frank et al., 2021). Personalization thus marks a turning point in clinical practice (Figure 6.15).

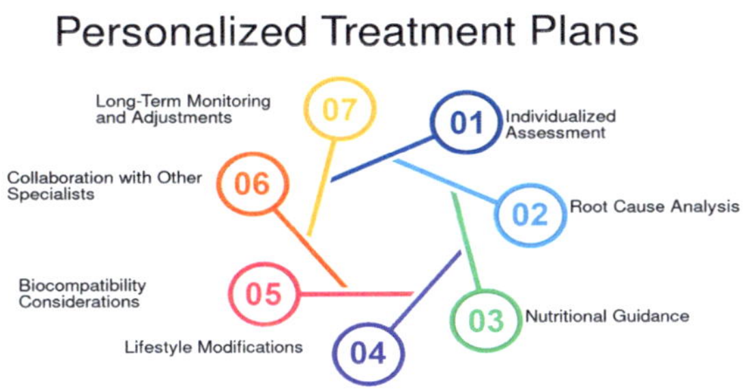
Personalized Treatment Plans
Long-Term Monitoring and Adjustments
07
01
Individualized Assessment
Collaboration with Other Specialists
06
02
Root Cause Analysis
Biocompatibility Considerations
05
03
Nutritional Guidance
Lifestyle Modifications
04

Figure 6.15. Understanding the importance of personalized treatment plans.

Source: https://fastercapital.co/i/Dental-functional-medicine-Revolutionizing-Dental-Health--How-Functional-Medicine-is-Changing-the-Game--Personalized-Treatment-Plans.webp.

6.4.7. Barriers to Treatment Access

Anxiety disorder barriers to treatment access present a complex phenomenon preventing an intervention with a level of success, especially in children and adolescents. A study indicates that professional intervention is acquired by only a fraction of the anxious children, casting a serious hindrance created by parents in the process of searching for assistance (Creswell et al., 2018).

The barriers occur at four phases: identification with the anxiety, acceptance of the need for professional assistance, reaching out to providers, and finally getting adequate care. These are parental beliefs about the child's problem as being severe, unfamiliarity with existing services, and lack of knowledge about navigating the treatment system. Furthermore, structural aspects , such as stigma in the treatment of mental health and economic constraints exacerbate the situation (Burns et al., 2004). With efficient barrier elimination to improve care access, the care for those in vulnerable populations will be required for effective management.

6.4.8. Long-Term Management Actions

Effective long-term treatment of anxiety disorders is crucial to enhancing the quality of life of patients. The secret to such treatment lies in the integration of therapy and self-management techniques, which most often involves cognitive-behavioral therapy (CBT) as a cornerstone therapy.

There is evidence that technologies like smartphone apps have the potential to provide ongoing support, though ongoing engagement often requires interpersonal connectivity features and incentive mechanisms, such as messaging and reward-based features for the attainment of personal objectives (Fleddermann et al., 2023).

Additionally, the need for tailoring treatment plans arises, as individuals may not engage with resources that are not attuned to their own circumstances or experiences. As has been outlined in post-viral wellness studies, there is a need to address mental health issues with personalized interventions to ensure continued treatment for symptom management after recovery (Visco et al., 2022). For the most part, a multifaceted, patient-centered approach will be required to thrive in treating the complexity of anxiety disorders in the long term.

6.4.9. New Therapies and Research

New insights into the management of anxiety disorders have helped fuel research into new treatments beyond standard pharmacology. These new therapies include the use of neurofeedback, relying on real-time feedback of brain activity to allow patients to learn enhanced emotional regulation skills. Also, the incorporation of technology, such as use of mobile apps for mindfulness and cognitive-behavioral therapy, has the potential to make treatment interventions more accessible and individualized. As pointed out in recent reviews, there is burgeoning interest in the therapeutic role of psychobiotics—probiotics that influence mental health through gut-brain interactions—emphasizing the complex interaction between gastrointestinal health and anxiety (Kaye et al., 2024). Research also increasingly explores the possible efficacy of plant compounds, such as cannabidiol, in the alleviation of symptoms of anxiety. All together, these new treatments are a cutting-edge approach to the treatment of anxiety disorders, and further research is warranted to validate and enhance their effectiveness (Han Grezenko et al., 2024) (Figure 6.16).

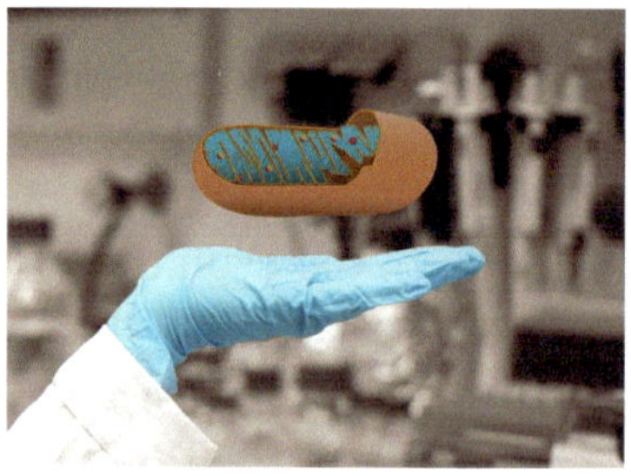

Figure 6.16. Emerging treatments and research on anxiety disorders.

Source: https://maxplanckneuroscience.org/wp-content/uploads/2015/12/img_2995_bgsepiagloveblueyellowmitoextract1-810x588.jpeg.

Test Your Knowledge

1. How do pharmacological treatments—such as SSRIs, SNRIs, and benzodiazepines—help manage anxiety disorders?
2. What role do psychotherapies like CBT, exposure therapy, and mindfulness-based approaches play in long-term anxiety management?

SUMMARY

The research on anxiety disorders illustrates a complex interplay among biological, psychological, and social factors that underlie their expression and prevalence among diverse populations. Evidence is that while some theories would anticipate an autonomic dysregulation of reactions in anxious subjects, current research refutes this by pointing to the fact that anxious children can show identical patterns of physiology to that of their non-anxious peers during stress, which implies a role of subjective anxiety levels (Alkozei et al., 2015). Additionally, the high prevalence rates of anxiety disorders in regions , such as north-eastern Uganda offer proof that contextual socio-demographic factors, along with exposure to trauma, are important in the development of these disorders (Abbo et al., 2013). Therefore, it is necessary to treat anxiety in a multi-faceted context, encompassing the environmental factors as well as the psychological experiences of the individual, since methods of prevention and treatment are in demand among various cultures.

Anxiety disorders comprise a heterogeneous collection of conditions characterized by heightened fear, worry, and related behavioral dysfunction severely interfering with daily functioning. A vital aspect of understanding these disorders is the recognition that they have a multifactorial genesis with biological, psychological, and environmental factors being involved. For example, individuals with previous or traumatic mental health histories are more likely to develop conditions , such as post-traumatic stress disorder (PTSD) (Kennedy-Moffat, 1997). Furthermore, evidence-based practices (EBPs) have been found to be effective against the treatment of anxiety disorders, yet their implementation remains difficult in practice environments due to several systemic barriers (Barlow et al., 2018). Knowledge of anxiety disorders and health care use is essential, as the patients present with severe symptoms that necessitate increased medical care, also pointing towards the necessity of proper interventions in curbing the impact of these disorders promptly.

KEY TERMS FROM THIS CHAPTER

- Acute stress disorder
- Anxiety disorder
- Cognitive distortions
- Generalized anxiety disorder (GAD)
- Intrusive thoughts
- Obsessive-compulsive disorder (OCD)
- Panic disorder
- Agoraphobia
- Avoidance behavior
- Compulsions
- Hypervigilance
- Obsessions
- Panic attack
- Post-traumatic stress disorder (PTSD)

CRITICAL THINKING QUESTIONS

1. **Which of the following is a hallmark feature of Generalized Anxiety Disorder (GAD)?**
   a. Recurrent panic attacks
   b. Excessive worry about various aspects of life for at least 6 months
   c. Fear of specific objects or situations
   d. Alternating periods of mania and depression
2. **A person who experiences sudden episodes of intense fear, palpitations, sweating, and a sense of impending doom is likely suffering from:**
   a. Obsessive-Compulsive Disorder (OCD)
   b. Social Anxiety Disorder
   c. Panic Disorder
   d. Specific Phobia
3. **Which of the following best describes a phobia?**
   a. Persistent, excessive fear of a specific object or situation
   b. Generalized worry about multiple issues
   c. Recurrent intrusive thoughts and repetitive behaviors
   d. Periods of low mood and energy
4. **In Social Anxiety Disorder, the individual fears:**
   a. Heights and closed spaces
   b. Being in situations where they may be judged or embarrassed
   c. Losing control in public places
   d. Contamination from germs
5. **Which of these symptoms is NOT typical of anxiety disorders?**
   a. Muscle tension
   b. Excessive worry
   c. Hallucinations
   d. Restlessness

Short Answer Questions

1. What are anxiety disorders, and how are they different from normal feelings of anxiety?
2. List at least four types of anxiety disorders and briefly describe each.
3. What are the main symptoms of Generalized Anxiety Disorder (GAD)?
4. How does Panic Disorder differ from other anxiety disorders?
5. What is a phobia, and how is it different from general fear? Give an example.

Answer to Critical Thinking Questions

1. (b) 2. (c) 3. (a) 4. (b) 5. (c)

REFERENCES

1. Abbo, C., Kinyanda, E., Kizza, R., Levin, J., Ndyanabangi, S., & Stein, D. (2013). *Prevalence, Comorbidity and Predictors of Anxiety Disorders in Children and Adolescents in Rural North-Eastern Uganda*. Springer Science and Business Media LLC. https://core.ac.uk/download/185398328.pdf (accessed on 28th July 2025).
2. Agathis, N., Greeley, C., & Raphael, J. L. (2019). *Improving the Health Care of Foster Children Throughout the US: Texas, A Case Example*. DigitalCommons@TMC. https://core.ac.uk/download/228022801.pdf (accessed on 28th July 2025).
3. Alkozei, A., Allen, J., Cooper, P., & Creswell, C. (2015). *Autonomic Arousal in Childhood Anxiety Disorders: Associations with State Anxiety and Social Anxiety Disorder*. Elsevier BV. https://core.ac.uk/download/42150578.pdf (accessed on 28th July 2025).
4. Altena, E., Baglioni, C., Espie, C. A., Ellis, J., Gavriloff, D., Holzinger, B., Schlarb, A., Frase, L., Jernelöv, S., & Riemann, D. (2020). Dealing with sleep problems during home confinement due to the COVID-19 outbreak: Practical recommendations from a task force of the European CBT-I Academy. *Journal of Sleep Research, 29*. https://doi.org/10.1111/jsr.13052 (accessed on 28th July 2025).
5. Hyman S. E. (2010). The diagnosis of mental disorders: the problem of reification. *Annual review of clinical psychology*, *6*, 155–179. https://doi.org/10.1146/annurev.clinpsy.3.022806.091532 (accessed on 28th July 2025).
6. Amrai, K., Ejei, J., Lavasani, M. G., Sharifian, M. S., & Taremian, F. (2011). *The Relationship Among Classroom Community, Attitude Toward Parents, Anxiety Disorders and Depression with Adolescent Suicide Probability*. Elsevier Ltd. https://core.ac.uk/download/pdf/82602660.pdf (accessed on 28th July 2025).
7. Andrade, A., Brennecke, A., Mallat, S., Brown, J., Gomez-Rivadeneira, J., Czepiel, N., & Londrigan, L. (2019). Genetic associations between voltage-gated calcium channels and psychiatric disorders. *20*, 3537. https://doi.org/10.3390/ijms20143537 (accessed on 28th July 2025).
8. Arruda, M., Cerutti, R., Faedda, N., Guidetti, V., Migliorini, D., & Verdecchia, P. (2016). *Behavioral Management of Headache in Children and Adolescents*. Springer Science and Business Media LLC. https://core.ac.uk/download/74325348.pdf (accessed on 28th July 2025).
9. Ayers, S., Chew-Graham, C., Ford, E., Farr, M., Hyde, J., Shakespeare, J., Mauthner, N., McCauley, J., Oates, S., & Lee, S. (2017). *Diagnosis and Management of Perinatal Depression and Anxiety in General Practice: A Meta-Synthesis of Qualitative Studies*. Royal College of General Practitioners. https://core.ac.uk/download/96598786.pdf (accessed on 28th July 2025).
10. Ayers, S., Copland, C., & Joekes, K. (2010). *Recognizing Anxiety and Post-Traumatic Stress Disorder in Cardiac Patients*. Mark Allen Group. https://core.ac.uk/download/9982809.pdf (accessed on 28th July 2025).
11. Baldwin, S., Donovan, C. L., Ford, M., March, S., & Spence, S. H. (2019). Using stepped-care approaches within internet-based interventions for youth anxiety: Three case studies. *Elsevier BV*. https://core.ac.uk/download/286371199.pdf (accessed on 28th July 2025).
12. Barlow, D. H., Boswell, J. F., Brooks, G. E., Dore, R., Espel-Huynh, H., Franklin, D. R., Goncalves, A., Ice, S., Lowe, M. R., Ortiz, S., Smith, M., & Thompson-Brenner, H. (2018). Evidence-based implementation practices applied to the intensive treatment of eating disorders: Summary

of research and illustration of principles using a case example. *Wiley*. https://core.ac.uk/download/286139395.pdf (accessed on 28th July 2025).

13. Białas, F., Cyboran, K., Kuc, M., Machaj, D., & Płaczek, A. (2022). *Generalized Anxiety Disorder, Panic Disorder–Diagnosis and Treatment*. Nicolaus Copernicus University, Toruń, Poland. https://core.ac.uk/download/587245714.pdf (accessed on 28th July 2025).
14. Wood, H. (2010). Integrating research with NHS clinical practice: Unwelcome intrusion or constructive triangulation? *Psychoanalytic Psychotherapy*, *24*(3), 252–261. https://doi.org/10.1080/02668734.2010.501571 (accessed on 28th July 2025).
15. Boecker, M., Döpfner, M., Erhart, M., Gilbert, M., Kaman, A., Ravens-Sieberer, U., Reiss, F., Schlack, R., & Westenhöfer, J. (2023). Gender and age differences in ADHD symptoms and cooccurring depression and anxiety symptoms among children and adolescents in the BELLA Study. *Robert Koch-Institut*. https://core.ac.uk/download/592047851.pdf (accessed on 28th July 2025).
16. Bond, R. L., Robinson, O. J., & Roiser, J. P. (2015). The impact of stress on financial decision-making varies as a function of depression and anxiety symptoms. https://core.ac.uk/download/29414538.pdf (accessed on 28th July 2025).
17. Brumbaugh, B. (2017). Interactions between BNST PACAP stress system and estrous cycling in non-ovariectomized female rats. *UVM ScholarWorks*. https://core.ac.uk/download/84397685.pdf (accessed on 28th July 2025).
18. Burns, D. D., Collins, K. A., Dozois, D. J. A., & Westra, H. A. (2004). Gaps in accessing treatment for anxiety and depression: Challenges for the delivery of care. *Elsevier BV*. https://core.ac.uk/download/571283863.pdf (accessed on 28th July 2025).
19. Chang, W. T., Cheng, C. T., Lung, F. W., & Shu, B. C. (2008). Anxiety and mood disorder in young males with mitral valve prolapse. *Dove Medical Press*. https://core.ac.uk/download/pdf/8500853.pdf (accessed on 28th July 2025).
20. Chen, C. W., Wei, L. C., & Chiu, H. J. (2024). Bridging gaps in shared decision-making for anxiety disorders: A commentary on Villena et al. https://www.semanticscholar.org/paper/40092c2cc3b497bdbf2c4f530b84653cb7283126 (accessed on 28th July 2025).
21. Chiappini, S., Corkery, J., De Berardis, D., Latini, R., Orsolini, L., Papanti, G. D., & Volpe, U. (2019). Use of medicinal cannabis and synthetic cannabinoids in posttraumatic stress disorder (PTSD): A systematic review. *MDPI AG*. https://core.ac.uk/download/287582001.pdf (accessed on 28th July 2025).
22. Compton, S. N., Franklin, M. E., Houghton, D. C., Maas, J., Neal-Barnett, A. M., Saunders, S. M., Twohig, M. P., & Woods, D. W. (2016). Comorbidity and quality of life in adults with hair pulling disorder. *e-Publications@Marquette*. https://core.ac.uk/download/213078703.pdf (accessed on 28th July 2025).
23. Contreras, J. (2019). Utilization of mind-body practices for adults with fibromyalgia: 2017 National Health Interview Survey. *DigitalCommons@TMC*. https://core.ac.uk/download/231832574.pdf (accessed on 28th July 2025).
24. Creswell, C., Harvey, K., O'Brien, D., Reardon, T., & Young, B. (2018). Barriers and facilitators to parents seeking and accessing professional support for anxiety disorders in children: Qualitative interview study. *Springer Science and Business Media LLC*. https://core.ac.uk/download/146486909.pdf (accessed on 28th July 2025).

25. d'Arqom, A., Sawitri, B., Nasution, Z., & Lazuardi, R. (2021). "Anti-COVID-19" medications, supplements, and mental health status in Indonesian mothers with school-age children. *13*, 699–709. https://www.semanticscholar.org/paper/8f26e0baea4ae5f1f804073f293dd87201 8db9e0 (accessed on 28th July 2025).

26. de Manincor, M. J. (2017). Yoga for mental health: Evaluation of yoga interventions for reducing depression and anxiety, and improving well-being. *American Psychological Association (APA)*. https://core.ac.uk/download/351786031.pdf (accessed on 28th July 2025).

27. Dietch, D. M., Kerr-Gaffney, J., Hockey, M., Marx, W., Ruusunen, A., Young, A., Berk, M., & Mondelli, V. (2023). Efficacy of low carbohydrate and ketogenic diets in treating mood and anxiety disorders: Systematic review and implications for clinical practice. *Frontiers in Nutrition, 9*. https://www.semanticscholar.org/paper/7cf1a3e49e6af9a94e63bc94bc647e64 ff35490e (accessed on 28th July 2025).

28. Farrand, P., Raue, P., Ward, E., Repper, D., & Areán, P. A. (2023). Use and engagement with low-intensity cognitive behavioral therapy techniques used within an app to support worry management: Content analysis of log data. *JMIR Mental Health, 12*. https://www.semanticscholar.org/paper/d5d29465c373fa8676ec878f26c5a4ff5c43fde6 (accessed on 28th July 2025).

29. Fernández-Aranda, F., Casas, M., Claes, L., Clark Bryan, D., Favaro, A., Granero, R., Gudiol, C., Jiménez-Múrcia, S., Karwautz, A., Le Grange, D., Menchón, J. M., Tchanturia, K., & Treasure, J. (2020). COVID-19 and implications for eating disorders. *European Eating Disorders Review, 28*, 239–245. https://doi.org/10.1002/erv.2738 (accessed on 28th July 2025).

30. Ferry, F., Bolton, D., Bunting, B., Murphy, S., O'Neill, S., & Devine, B. (2012). *Ageing, Health and Conflict: An Investigation of the Experience and Health Impact of "Troubles-Related" Trauma*. Northern Ireland Centre for Trauma & Transformation Trust. https://core.ac.uk/download/71357659.pdf (accessed on 28th July 2025).

31. Fleddermann, K., Molfenter, T., Vjorn, O. J., Horst, J., Hulsey, J. N., Kelly, B., Zawislak, K., Gustafson, D., & Gicquelais, R. (2023). Patient preferences for mobile health applications to support recovery. *JMIR Mental Health, 17*, 394–400. https://www.semanticscholar.org/pape r/711cbec94ebfb488ede1e8552063dc618f14cd7a (accessed on 28th July 2025).

32. Galán-Luque, T., Serrano-Ortiz, M., & Orgilés, M. (2023). Effectiveness of psychological interventions for child and adolescent specific anxiety disorders: A systematic review of systematic reviews and meta-analyses. *Revita de Psicología Clínica con Niños y Adolescentes, 10*(1), 31–41. https://www.revistapcna.com/sites/default/files/2261_2.pdf (accessed on 28th July 2025).

33. Ghebreyesus, T. A. (2020). Addressing mental health needs: An integral part of COVID-19 response. *World Psychiatry, 19*, 129, 130. https://doi.org/10.1002/wps.20768 (accessed on 28th July 2025).

34. Gómez Baya, D., Mendoza Berjano, R., Paíno Quesada, S., Salinas Pérez, J. A., & Sánchez López, Á. (2022). The role of developmental assets in gender differences in anxiety in Spanish youth. *Frontiers Media SA*. https://core.ac.uk/download/559262875.pdf (accessed on 28th July 2025).

35. Greiner, M., Hussong, J., Mattheus, H., Schiedermaier, U., & von Gontard, A. (2022). Anxiety disorders, depression and incontinence in preschool children: A population-based study.

Saarländische Universitäts- und Landesbibliothek. https://core.ac.uk/download/556183246.pdf (accessed on 28th July 2025).

36. Grezenko, H., Rodoshi, Z. N., Mimms, C. S., Ahmed, M., Sabani, A., Hlaing, M. S., Batu, B. J., Hundesa, M. I., Ayalew, B. D., Shehryar, A., Rehman, A., & Hassan, A. (2024). From Alzheimer's disease to anxiety, epilepsy to schizophrenia: A comprehensive dive into neuro-psychiatric disorders. *Cureus, 16*. https://www.semanticscholar.org/paper/ebfb1a0d96fb4d8caac799e76789a250e3601d0e (accessed on 28th July 2025).

37. Griffiths, M. D., Shonin, E., & Van Gordon, W. (2014). The emerging role of Buddhism in clinical psychology: Toward effective integration. *American Psychological Association (APA)*. https://core.ac.uk/download/30650561.pdf (accessed on 28th July 2025).

38. Gu, C., Ren, H., Jie, H., Wu, S., & Deng, X. (2024). Exploring the genetic and socioeconomic interplay between ADHD and anxiety disorders using Mendelian randomization. *Frontiers Media S.A.* https://core.ac.uk/download/621138035.pdf (accessed on 28th July 2025).

39. Hastuti, M. H., Dasuki, D., & Lidia. (2008). Hubungan antara kecemasan dengan aktivitas dan fungsi seksual pada wanita usia lanjut di Kabupaten Purworejo. *Gadjah Mada University*. https://media.neliti.com/media/publications/163714-ID-hubungan-antara-kecemasan-dengan-aktivit.pdf (accessed on 28th July 2025).

40. Hölzel, B. K., Metcalf, C. A., Hoge, E. A., Marques, L., Simon, N. M., Brach, N., & Lazar, S. W. (2020). Mindfulness and self-compassion in generalized anxiety disorder: Examining predictors of disability. https://core.ac.uk/download/357350557.pdf (accessed on 28th July 2025).

41. Hölzel, B. K., Metcalf, C. A., Hoge, E. A., Marques, L., Simon, N. M., Brach, N., & Lazar, S. W. (2013). Mindfulness and self-compassion in generalized anxiety disorder: Examining predictors of disability. *Hindawi Limited*. https://core.ac.uk/download/193415498.pdf (accessed on 28th July 2025).

42. Insel, T. R., Cuthbert, B. N., Garvey, M. A., Heinssen, R., Pine, D. S., Quinn, K. J., Sanislow, C. A., & Wang, P. (2010). Research Domain Criteria (RDoC): Toward a new classification framework for research on mental disorders. *American Journal of Psychiatry, 167*, 748–751. https://doi.org/10.1176/appi.ajp.2010.09091379 (accessed on 28th July 2025).

43. Kara, A. (2022). A review of childhood anxiety. *Mustafa Azizoğlu*. https://core.ac.uk/download/541041882.pdf (accessed on 28th July 2025).

44. Kays, D. (2018). Intimate partner violence, anxiety diagnosis, and binge drinking behavior among college students. *Digital Commons @ George Fox University*. https://digitalcommons.georgefox.edu/cgi/viewcontent.cgi?article=1242&context=psyd (accessed on 28th July 2025).

45. Kennedy-Moffat, J. (1997). The psychological impact of motor vehicle accidents: A New Zealand study. *Massey University*. http://hdl.handle.net/10179/13540. https://core.ac.uk/download/159449347.pdf (accessed on 28th July 2025).

46. Khare, S. K., March, S., Barua, P. D., Gadre, V. M., & Acharya, U. R. (2023). Application of data fusion for automated detection of children with developmental and mental disorders: A systematic review of the last decade. *Information Fusion, 99*, 101898–101898. https://doi.org/10.1016/j.inffus.2023.101898 (accessed on 28th July 2025).

47. Korany, W. M., Marzouk, D., El-hamid, A., & Allam, M. (2023). Development of practice guidelines for peripartum depression in primary healthcare. https://www.semanticscholar.org/paper/83afa9fa45b9d20bddb63ef812940625df891d1f (accessed on 28th July 2025).

48. Liu, J., Varghese, B. M., Hansen, A., Xiang, J., Zhang, Y., Dear, K., Gourley, M., Driscoll, T., Morgan, G., Capon, A., & Bi, P. (2021). Is there an association between hot weather and poor mental health outcomes? A systematic review and meta-analysis. *Environment International, 153*, 106533–106533. https://doi.org/10.1016/j.envint.2021.106533 (accessed on 28th July 2025).

49. Lomper, K., Ross, C., & Uchmanowicz, I. (2023). Anxiety and depressive symptoms, frailty and quality of life in atrial fibrillation. *International Journal of Environmental Research and Public Health, 20*. https://www.semanticscholar.org/paper/b7a6b86accc50dbefff2bc3be569cb4e2f53c4eb (accessed on 28th July 2025).

50. López-Fernández, F. J., Moreno-Amador, B., Falcó, R., Soto-Sanz, V., Marzo, J. C., Ibáñez, M. I., Cervin, M., & Piqueras, J. A. (2024). Suicidal behavior, mental health, and stressful life events among adolescents. *Psicothema, 36*(4), 351–360. https://doi.org/10.7334/psicothema2023.126 (accessed on 28th July 2025).

51. Lynn-Whaley, J., & Sugarmann, J. (2017). The relationship between community violence and trauma: How violence affects learning, health, and behavior. *Violence Policy Center*. https://core.ac.uk/download/87085562.pdf (accessed on 28th July 2025).

52. MacIsaac, H. (1952). A study of patients discharged improved who returned for further treatment to the Veterans Administration Mental Hygiene Clinic. *Boston University*. https://open.bu.edu/bitstream/2144/13468/1/MacIsaac_Hugh_1952_web.pdf (accessed on 28th July 2025).

53. Mahamid, F., Bdier, D., & Chou, P. (2021). Traumatic life events and psychological well-being among Palestinian adolescents: The mediating role of resilience. *CDS Press, Toronto, Canada*. https://concurrentdisorders.ca/ (accessed on 28th July 2025).

54. Malakcioglu, C. (2022). Validity and reliability of the Anxiety Assessment Scale: A new three-dimensional perspective. *Galenos Publishing House, 37*(2), 165–172. https://jag.journalagent.com/medeniyet/pdfs/MEDJ_37_2_165_172.pdf (accessed on 28th July 2025).

55. Mastnak, W. (2022). Chinese music therapy and clinical music education to treat anxiety disorders: The PLUS-model. *Gulf Publishers, 2*(1), 13–23. https://gulfpublishers.com/id/2024/01/MAMR202021GS-2022-01-24-05-03-46-000000.pdf (accessed on 28th July 2025).

56. Matsumoto, K., Hamatani, S., Shiga, K., Iiboshi, K., Kasai, M., Kimura, Y., Yokota, S., Watanabe, K., Kubo, Y., & Nakamura, M. (2023). Effectiveness of unguided internet-based cognitive behavioral therapy for subthreshold social anxiety disorder in adolescents and young adults: Multicenter randomized controlled trial. *JMIR Mental Health, 7*. https://www.semanticscholar.org/paper/6a039e9dcdea1c0634b91be9d68dddf51ef9f78d (accessed on 28th July 2025).

57. Merlo, L. J. (2016). A piece of my mind: Healing physicians. *JAMA, 316*(23), 2489–2490. https://www.semanticscholar.org/paper/6a94774b598385b8dcbbdcd793b5d689091fa849 (accessed on 28th July 2025).

58. Mills, C. (2018). From 'invisible problem' to global priority: The inclusion of mental health in the Sustainable Development Goals. *Wiley*. https://core.ac.uk/download/187115723.pdf (accessed on 28th July 2025).

59. Monaghesh, E., & Hajizadeh, A. (2020). The role of telehealth during COVID-19 outbreak: A systematic review based on current evidence. *BMC Public Health, 20*. https://doi.org/10.1186/s12889-020-09301-4 (accessed on 28th July 2025).

60. Morris-Rosendahl, D. J. (2022). Are there anxious genes? *Servier International*. https://core.ac.uk/download/549011125.pdf (accessed on 28th July 2025).

61. Muijs, M., & Stoeber, J. (2001). Patterns of situational appraisal in experiences of worry and anxiety. *Informa UK Limited*. https://core.ac.uk/download/90943.pdf (accessed on 28th July 2025).

62. Murthy, R. S. (2017). National mental health survey of India 2015–2016. *Indian Journal of Psychiatry, 59*, 21–21. https://doi.org/10.4103/psychiatry.indianjpsychiatry_102_17 (accessed on 28th July 2025).

63. Newman, L., Judd, F., Olsson, C. A., Castle, D., Bousman, C. A., Sheehan, P. M., Pantelis, C., Craig, J. M., Komiti, A., & Everall, I. (2016). Early origins of mental disorder–Risk factors in the perinatal and infant period. *BMC Psychiatry, 16*. https://doi.org/10.1186/s12888-016-0982-7 (accessed on 28th July 2025).

64. Nuruddaroini, M., Sulthan, M. A., & Zubaidillah, M. H. (2021). Strengthening resilience in children's psychological disorders of Abdullah Nashih Ulwan's perspective. *Sekolah Tinggi Ilmu Qur'an Amuntai*. https://core.ac.uk/download/478591590.pdf (accessed on 28th July 2025).

65. Oliver, M. (2020). Consider the ravens: An exploration of anxiety. *Western CEDAR*. https://core.ac.uk/download/346440961.pdf (accessed on 28th July 2025).

66. Peng, A., Lin, Z., & Zhu, C. (2022). Relationship of psychiatric disorders and sleep quality to physical symptoms in coronary artery disease. *210*, 541–546. https://www.semanticscholar.org/paper/e2ade63a91c99fb52cf79bf69a45351f1cdf18a3 (accessed on 28th July 2025).

67. PRAJESHA, T. M., & Veni, S. (2023). Hybrid feature selection model based on RFE and MRMR on anxiety disorder dataset. *Little Lion Scientific, 101*(10), 4023–4025. http://www.jatit.org/volumes/Vol101No10/31Vol101No10.pdf (accessed on 28th July 2025).

68. Pruessner, L., Timm, C., Kalmar, J., Bents, H., Barnow, S., & Mander, J. (2024). Emotion regulation as a mechanism of mindfulness in individual cognitive-behavioral therapy for depression and anxiety disorders. https://www.semanticscholar.org/paper/cb16c369f01e094423a45aaeccd3b911a4e47133 (accessed on 28th July 2025).

69. Reid, K. (2017). Prevalence and correlates of anxiety disorders in psychotic illness. *Department of Psychiatry and Mental Health*. https://core.ac.uk/download/185460514.pdf (accessed on 28th July 2025).

70. Rochefort, Z. S. (2019). Take control: A proposed mental health treatment program to be implemented in youth correctional facilities around Oregon based on the evidence-based TARGET program. https://www.semanticscholar.org/paper/a198dead742dbcaef76c3292cd7d060d711f6db2 (accessed on 28th July 2025).

71. Rothenberger, A., Coffey, B. J., Paszek, J., Leckman, J. F., Schlander, M., Bloch, M. H., Robertson, M. M., Hoekstra, P. J., Freeman, R. D., Banaschewski, T., & Roessner, V. (2010). *Tourette's Disorder and Other Tic Disorders in DSM-5: A Comment*. Springer-Verlag. https://core.ac.uk/download/pdf/8526233.pdf (accessed on 28th July 2025).

72. Sadock, B. J., Sadock, V. A., Ruiz, P., Pataki, C., & Sussman, N. (2015). *Kaplan & Sadock's Synopsis of Psychiatry: Behavioral Sciences/Clinical Psychiatry*.

73. Salloum, F., Farran, M., Shaib, H. S., Jurjus, A., Sleiman, R., & Khalil, M. (2024). The modulatory effect of Al-Assi river trout fish meal on OCD manifestations and molecular mechanisms in BALB/c mice. https://www.semanticscholar.org/paper/4f23549b964423230a81cbbd25b87fa25b9e7a59 (accessed on 28th July 2025).

74. Shaikh, A., Kamble, P., Daulatabad, V., Singhal, A., Madhusudhan, U., & John, N. (2024). Mental health challenges within the LGBTQ community: A societal imperative. *13*, 3529–3535. https://www.semanticscholar.org/paper/5a7d6c03efdfad1135fbeed5ddd8249c833277be (accessed on 28th July 2025).

75. Sharma, R., Kumarasamy, M., Parihar, V., Ravichandiran, V., & Kumar, N. (2023). Monoamine oxidase: A potential link in Papez circuit to generalized anxiety disorders. https://www.semanticscholar.org/paper/053e7a00960bc54892d67975390bf23c7e962c0d (accessed on 28th July 2025).

76. Sivertsen, H., Bjørkløf, G. H., Engedal, K., Selbæk, G., & Helvik, A. S. (2015). Depression and quality of life in older persons: A review. *Clinical Geriatrics Medicine, 40*, 311–339. https://doi.org/10.1159/000437299 (accessed on 28th July 2025).

77. Smith, M., & Storey, P. (2008). Methods and approaches to improving the emotional health and well-being of children: A briefing paper concerning interventions to prevent internalizing disorders. *Institute of Education, University of London*. https://core.ac.uk/download/pdf/82102.pdf (accessed on 28th July 2025).

78. Solmi, M., Raduà, J., Olivola, M., Croce, E., Soardo, L., Salazar de Pablo, G., Shin, J. I., Kirkbride, J. B., Jones, P. B., Kim, J. H., Kim, J. Y., Carvalho, A. F., Seeman, M. V., Correll, C. U., & Fusar-Poli, P. (2021). Age at onset of mental disorders worldwide: Large-scale meta-analysis of 192 epidemiological studies. *Molecular Psychiatry, 27*, 281–295. https://doi.org/10.1038/s41380-021-01161-7 (accessed on 28th July 2025).

79. Son, C., Hegde, S., Smith, A., Wang, X., & Sasangohar, F. (2020). Effects of COVID-19 on college students' mental health in the United States: Interview survey study. *JMIR, 22*, 21279–21279. https://doi.org/10.2196/21279 (accessed on 28th July 2025).

80. Starčević, V., & Aboujaoude, E. (2015). Cyberchondria, cyberbullying, cybersuicide, cybersex: "New" psychopathologies for the 21st century? *World Psychiatry, 14*, 97–100. https://doi.org/10.1002/wps.20195 (accessed on 28th July 2025).

81. Stein, D. J., Craske, M. G., Rothbaum, B. O., Chamberlain, S. R., Fineberg, N., Choi, K. W., de Jonge, P., Baldwin, D. S., & Maj, M. (2021). The clinical characterization of the adult patient with an anxiety or related disorder aimed at personalization of management. *World Psychiatry, 20*, 336–356. https://doi.org/10.1002/wps.20919 (accessed on 28th July 2025).

82. Stevens, J. S., Almli, L. M., Fani, N., Gutman, D. A., Bradley, B., Norrholm, S. D., Reiser, E., Ely, T. D., Dhanani, R., Glover, E. M., Jovanović, T., & Ressler, K. J. (2014). PACAP receptor gene polymorphism impacts fear responses in the amygdala and hippocampus. *Proceedings of the National Academy of Sciences, 111*, 3158–3163. https://doi.org/10.1073/pnas.1318954111 (accessed on 28th July 2025).

83. Sun, J. (2023). Treatment of mental anxiety disorders in students by combining cognitive behavioral therapy with college student management strategies. *International*

Journal of Health Sciences, 28, 65–65. https://www.semanticscholar.org/paper/edd91ce3f590e1e895f0b41e2b156eba0bacc529 (accessed on 28th July 2025).

84. Tatlı, Ç., & Türker, P. (2024). The roles of psychosocial factors and nutritional intervention on eating disorders. https://www.semanticscholar.org/paper/3af6e733eb1dfcc61795373ed354628d16ae32c8 (accessed on 28th July 2025).

85. Tondello, G. F., Nacke, L., Watson, D. K., & Wehbe, R. R. (2016). ABOVE WATER: Extending the play space for health. *Association for Computing Machinery (ACM)*. https://core.ac.uk/download/144150054.pdf (accessed on 28th July 2025).

86. Torbecke, J., Langhammer, T., Mewes, L., Lueken, U., & Fendel, J. (2024). Augmentation of cognitive-behavioral therapy for obsessive-compulsive and anxiety disorders: A protocol for a systematic review and meta-analysis. *BMC Psychology, 14*. https://www.semanticscholar.org/paper/df13649c0a54aa9c66751d8d667eeca2355c879f (accessed on 28th July 2025).

87. Tosti, B., Corrado, S., Mancone, S., Di Libero, T., Rodio, A., Andrade, A., & Diotaiuti, P. (2024). Integrated use of biofeedback and neurofeedback techniques in treating pathological conditions and improving performance: A narrative review. *18*. https://doi.org/10.3389/fnins.2024.1358481 (accessed on 28th July 2025).

88. Uluyol, B., & Meterelliyoz, K. S. (2023). *The Relationship Between Anxiety Symptoms, Anxiety Sensitivity, And Emotional Schemas in Patients Admitted to Psychiatry Outpatient Clinic*. Ivano-Frankivsk National Medical University. https://core.ac.uk/download/586746786.pdf (accessed on 28th July 2025).

89. Vineetha, S. (2019). A clinical study on the role of homoeopathy in managing anxiety disorders in school-going children of Kanniyakumari District. https://core.ac.uk/download/235670327.pdf (accessed on 28th July 2025).

90. Visco, V., Vitale, C., Rispoli, A., Izzo, C., Virtuoso, N., Ferruzzi, G., Santopietro, M., Melfi, A., Rusciano, M., Maglio, A., Di Pietro, P., Carrizzo, A., Galasso, G., Vatrella, A., Vecchione, C., & Ciccarelli, M. (2022). Post-COVID-19 syndrome: Involvement and interactions between respiratory, cardiovascular and nervous systems. *International Journal of Environmental Research and Public Health, 11*. https://www.semanticscholar.org/paper/22203458aff702aa75570577f7703ef300b8408c (accessed on 28th July 2025).

91. Wiederhold, B. K. (2020). Connecting through technology during the Coronavirus Disease 2019 pandemic: Avoiding "Zoom fatigue." *Cyberpsychology, Behavior, and Social Networking, 23*, 437–438. https://doi.org/10.1089/cyber.2020.29188.bkw (accessed on 28th July 2025).

92. Woodie, K. L. (2009). Childhood anxiety: How schools identify, assess, provide resources to and refer students with anxiety. https://core.ac.uk/download/5067576.pdf (accessed on 28th July 2025).

93. Zaami, S., Graziano, S., Tittarelli, R., Beck, R., & Marinelli, E. (2021). BDZs, designer BDZs, and Z-drugs: Pharmacology and misuse insights. https://www.semanticscholar.org/paper/a10ec8668ad96f9ac9c8fa054a8b90e4d7ccb2fd (accessed on 28th July 2025).

94. Zhu, J., Li, Z., Zhang, X., Zhang, Z., & Hu, B. (2023). Public attitudes toward anxiety disorder on Sina Weibo: Content analysis. *JMIR Mental Health, 25*. https://www.semanticscholar.org/paper/cc0a9299f14724b4e6c40a2c33ec514c02e4304b (accessed on 28th July 2025)

7

OBSESSIVE-COMPULSIVE AND RELATED DISORDERS

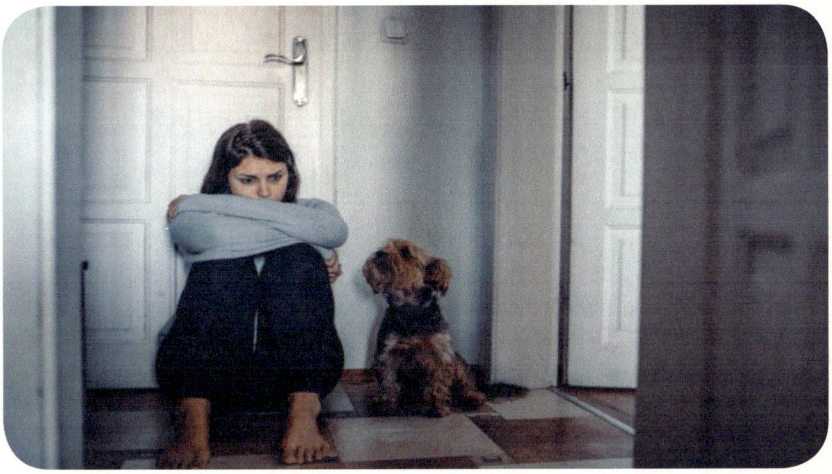

LEARNING OBJECTIVES

After studying this chapter, you will be able to:

1. Explain the types of obsessive-compulsive disorders;
2. Identify the symptoms and diagnosis;
3. List the causes and risk factors;
4. Describe the treatment options;
5. List the impact on daily life;
6. Focus on the current research and developments.

Introduction

Obsessive-compulsive and related disorders are characterized by their complex nature and present a special challenge to both sufferers and health care providers. These disorders, which are characterized as pervasive and intrusive thoughts (obsessions) and repetitive behaviors (compulsions), can have the power to ruin the quality and daily functioning of an affected person. For the majority of patients, routine first-line treatments , such as SSRIs and CBT may not be sufficient to alleviate symptoms. In fact, research has shown that a vast majority of patients continue to experience debilitating symptoms despite complying with treatment guidelines. Thus, awareness of possible adjunct treatments that can complement existing treatment techniques, such as vitamin and nutrient supplementation, is all the more necessary in combating the existing challenges presented by obsessive-compulsive disorders (Algin et al., 2025). Nutritional deficiencies have been quoted as a possible underlying reason for the continuation of obsessive-compulsive symptoms in those receiving treatment. Evidences suggest that decreased levels of necessary nutrients, particularly folic acid and vitamin B_{12}, can increase the severity of such disorders. The combination of these deficiencies with biochemical indicators of OCD provides a strong research path for investigating new treatment methods. Modern evidence indicates the statistically significant improvements in OCD patients' clinical performance following the combination of SSRIs with nutritional supplementation. These findings emphasize the importance of examining new approaches other than the conventional pharmacological treatments, as OCD, as well as related disorders, are multi-dimensional in nature (Algin et al., 2025). Aside from the pharmacological adjuncts, the role of non-pharmacological augmentation methods in enhancing CBT for obsessive-compulsive and anxiety disorders also needs to be seriously examined.

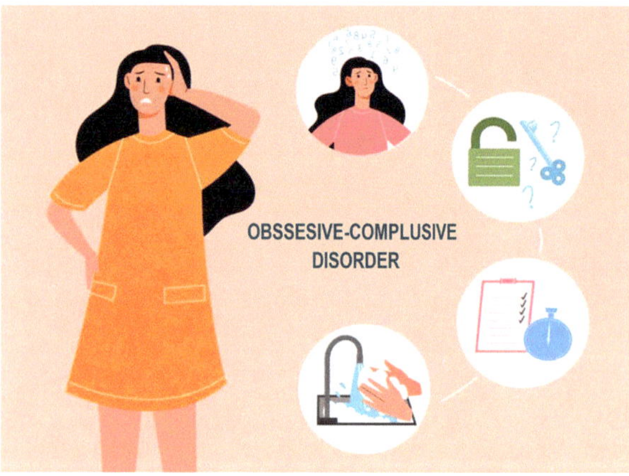

Figure 7.1. Obsessive compulsive disorder.

Source: https://external-content.duckduckgo.com/iu/?u=https%3A%2F%2Fnafsology.ae%2Fwp-content%2Fuploads%2F2023%2F03%2FObsessive-Compulsive-Disorder.jpg&f=1&nofb=1&ipt=acbc493202b384163c5051adc4c1f764f5364ec59fe51ca3fc4d108dd2406b9e.

Though CBT is a therapy stalwart, a high proportion of patients have suboptimal responses or face challenges in treatment adherence. Investigation for adjunct or alternative therapeutic modalities, including behavioral intervention and psychoeducation, has been extremely high in recent years. Systematic review and meta-analysis are continuing to assess the efficacy of such augmentation strategies in an orderly manner. This review aims to identify favorable impacts beyond first-line CBT, symptom reduction, response rates, and rates of dropout between the various patient groups. Such research is essential in updating treatment models and improving therapies for persons with obsessive-compulsive and spectrum disorders (Figure 7.1).

Definition of Obsessive-Compulsive Disorders

Obsessive-Compulsive Disorders (OCD) are a range of conditions that involve the presence of obsessions, compulsions, or both. Obsessions are recurring intrusive thoughts, images, or urges that create a lot of distress or anxiety and cause individuals to carry out compulsions—repetitive activities or mental acts to reduce this distress. The distinguishing feature of OCD is that the individual is aware of the unreasonable or excessive nature of these obsessions and compulsions, yet they are unable to fight off performing these rituals in a misguided attempt to prevent anxiety. This interplay between obsession and compulsion represents an arrest of decision-making and a self-sabotaging pattern that can severely impair daily functioning and quality of life. The complexity of OCD highlights its diagnosis as a mental disorder, which calls for a thorough understanding and empathetic approaches for effective management. The variability of OCD symptoms highlights the disorder's complexity in character, manifesting differently across individuals. One of the critical aspects involves the identification of specific compulsive behaviors associated with OCD subtypes. For instance, hoarding disorder, or abnormal cluttering with objects, and contamination fear with compulsive washing demonstrate the full spectrum of OCD symptoms. Research has established patterns between symptomatic presentations and cognitive processes underlying them, such as disgust sensitivity and danger expectancy. Of specific interest, one study analyzed the impact of these variables on washing behaviors and results indicated that disgust sensitivity was significantly related to compulsive behavior. These findings indicate not only the obsessions but also the cognitive appraisals underlying these actions to be accountable for the severity of OCD symptoms (Beck et al., 2010).

This highlights the significance of specially crafted interventions aimed at individual cognitive styles in OCD. An understanding of the definition of OCD also crosses over into shifting debate about behavioral addictions, other conditions that present with compulsive behavior without the presence of actual obsessions. Research currently suggests that those with activities , such as compulsive shopping or gambling exhibit comparable symptom profiles to those with substance use disorders. For example, a systematic review reported shared experiences of craving, dyscontrol, and impulsivity between alcohol addiction and behavioral addictions (McLachlan & Starkey, 2012). The results encourage redefining addiction criteria to encompass non-substance conditions. Such an interdisciplinary approach works towards advancing knowledge of OCD and associated disorders, providing more effective treatment approaches as well as putting forth the need for cross-disciplinary approaches in diagnosis and treatment within the mental health field.

Significance of Understanding These Disorders

The value of understanding obsessive-compulsive and comorbid disorders extends beyond the academic sphere; it is the foundation for intervention and treatment efficacy. Researchers understand that an understanding of the nuances of these disorders can significantly increase diagnostics and yield improved therapeutic outcomes for victims. The DSM-5 has expanded diagnostic criteria for obsessive-compulsive disorder (OCD) to facilitate a more individualized approach to the heterogeneity of the disorder. A key element of OCD comprehension is the definition of insight, which is one's perception of their symptoms and how they affect them. Research has shown that insight can have a notable effect on treatment success, meaning mental health practitioners should be able to measure their patients' level of insight in developing suitable treatment plans (Huang et al., 2023). Therefore, increased knowledge of these conditions is a precursor to more tailored and improved treatment. Apart from improving the therapeutic outcome, understanding obsessive-compulsive and related disorders is essential in managing the comorbidities that typically accompany these disorders.

Psychocutaneous disorders, anxiety disorders, and depressive disorders are among the conditions that tend to co-exist with OCD, creating complex treatment scenarios that necessitate a multidisciplinary team (Zagami et al., 2023). For dermatologists and psychiatrists alike, recognizing the interplay between physical symptoms and underlying psychiatric issues is vital for holistic patient care. Acknowledging these comorbidities not only fosters better patient-provider communication but also improves patients' overall well-being. Awareness of the intricate characteristics of these disorders allows clinicians to have holistic treatment strategies to address the psychological as well as physiological manifestations of a disorder and thereby ensure that the highest standards of care are offered to patients suffering from OCD and related disorders.

Finally, increased awareness and knowledge about obsessive-compulsive and related disorders go a long way in de-stigmatizing mental illnesses. Too often, such sufferers of these disorders must endure societal ignorance or condescension that exacerbates their anguish. By public and healthcare education regarding the facts surrounding OCD and related disorders, we foster a more understanding and supportive climate for such sufferers. In this way, in addition to enhancing patient care, we facilitate sufferers to seek assistance without dread of condemnation.

As stigma around mental illness remains on the wane, the paths to early intervention and support communities become more robust, thereby improving outcomes for those who labor with these complex disorders. Through widespread understanding and informed dialogue, society can reframe narrative on obsessive-compulsive and comorbid disorders and create a culture of healing and acceptance (Figure 7.2).

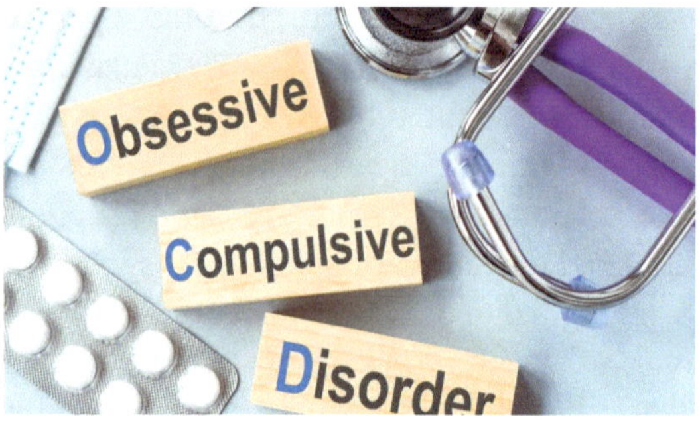

Figure 7.2. Effective intervention and treatment of obsessive-compulsive disorder.

Source: https://external-content.duckduckgo.com/iu/?u=https%3A%2F%2Fcounsellingcollective.net%2Fwp-content%2Fuploads%2F2025%2F01%2FMedication-Induced-Obsessive-Compulsive-and-Related-Disorder_20241116_185113_0022-1-1024x555.png&f=1&nofb=1&ipt=65654b75e37e7c14847a747485f2633200f5ef8583d5a51026c1e5ba654cd124.

7.1. Types of Obsessive-Compulsive Disorders

Learning Outcome

1. Obsessive-compulsive disorder (OCD).
2. Body dysmorphic disorder (BDD).
3. Hoarding disorder.

Obsessive-Compulsive Disorders (OCD) have a heterogeneous range of presentations with distinct challenges and clinical characteristics. Contamination OCD is perhaps the most recognized subtype, in which the person experiences obsessional anxieties about germs or dirt, thus performing compulsive washing or avoidance behaviors. Not only does this impact normal functioning, but it also causes substantial distress. Hoarding disorder, another feature, is marked by abnormal preoccupation with accumulating items, regardless of value, with eventually unsafe living conditions. Thus, this disorder can significantly disrupt social and occupational function. The interplay of avoidance behavior, compulsions, and extreme anxiety defines these types of OCD, noting the complexity of the disorder and the necessity for individualized therapeutic methods to manage symptoms effectively. In addition to the above categories, Obsessive-Compulsive and Related Disorders include disorders associated with compulsive behavior , such as Body Dysmorphic Disorder (BDD) and Trichotillomania. BDD is an occurrence that involves a preoccupation with perceived flaws in appearance, presenting typically with symptoms that are compulsive in nature, and may include recurrent grooming or persistent reassurance-seeking. In the meantime, Trichotillomania is the repeated compulsion to pull out one's hair, which leads to apparent hair loss and distress. Both of these conditions underscore the complexity of OCD-related disorders, where compulsive behavior is motivated by preoccupation with body image or appearance. It is important to understand such subtleties in the development of effective treatment modalities, a fact supported by current research efforts that aim to locate vulnerabilities and the best approach towards intervention for affected individuals. Fresh research has also begun to highlight the neurobiological substrates' role in various types of Obsessive-Compulsive Disorders and suggested that structural as well as functional brain alterations might be pivotal. Inferences from studies using neuroimaging techniques, especially within cooperative paradigms like the ENIGMA consortium, have been enlightening about the brain anatomy in OCD. These cortical thickness and subcortical anatomical studies offer vital clues to the neurodevelopmental processes of the disorder. Further research along such lines can yield more insight and help in the development of subtype-specific targeted treatments for OCD. The variation of modern findings holds promise for significant advancements in the use of treatment as researchers continue to unravel the complexities associated with obsessive-compulsive and comorbid disorders and identify both the biological and psychological mechanisms entailed with these disorders (Billieux et al., 2018; Arnold et al., 2020).

7.1.1. Obsessive-Compulsive Disorder (OCD)

Obsessive-Compulsive Disorder (OCD) is characterized by the presence of obsessions, intrusive ideas that cause anxiety, and compulsions, repetitive behaviors performed to alleviate such anxiety. OCD not only affects personal health but also disrupts social relationships and work life. The progression of OCD may be complex, with a majority of individuals experiencing a slow developmental onset, typically in childhood or early adolescence. Research has shown that the average age of onset of OCD is 14.5 years, suggesting that early recognition and treatment might be important for treatment response. It is essential to identify the development pattern of OCD in an effort to improve therapeutic measures and mental health promotion interventions since early intervention can significantly reduce the impact of the disorder in the long term (Solmi et al., 2021). The etiological underpinnings of OCD are clearer, with increasing evidence for a relationship between childhood trauma and the development of the disorder.

Neglect and emotional abuse, and other types of childhood adversity, have been found to be associated with increased symptom severity in OCD. A clinical sample study showed that individuals with previous histories of child maltreatment had higher OCD symptom severity than their counterparts without these backgrounds, underlining the need for mental health practitioners to take these traumatic histories into account when addressing treatment. The significance of this observation underscores the value of trauma-informed practice within OCD treatment protocols since unaddressed underlying trauma can increase symptom severity and impede recovery (Boger et al., 2020). In addition, treatment for OCD often involves cognitive-behavioral therapy (CBT), or more accurately, exposure and response prevention (ERP), which is known to significantly reduce symptoms.

The presence, however, of complicating factors, such as a past history of childhood maltreatment, can influence the outcome of treatment. Even though these kinds of factors can potentially cause difficulties, studies indicate that while childhood trauma experiences themselves don't appear to have an adverse effect on overall treatment results, they are associated with a higher baseline level of symptom severity. This emphasizes the need for personalized treatment plans that not only address the OCD symptoms but also introduce an overall dimension of knowing a person's psychological history to initiate recovery and provide better long-term results (Boger et al., 2020) (Figure 7.3).

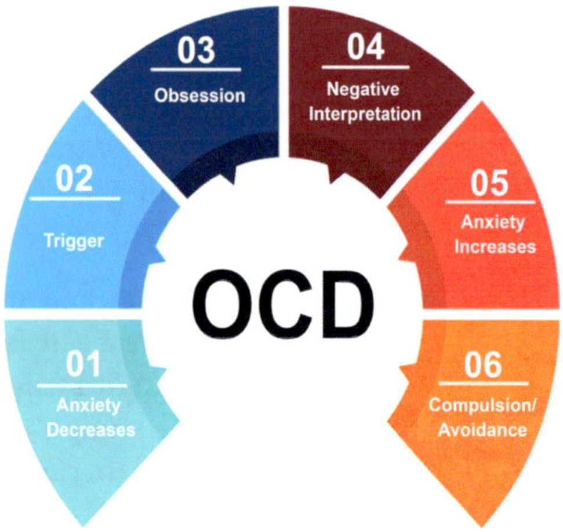
03
Obsession
04
Negative Interpretation
02
Trigger
05
Anxiety Increases
OCD
01
Anxiety Decreases
06
Compulsion/ Avoidance

Figure 7.3. Obsessive-compulsive disorders.

Source: https://external-content.duckduckgo.com/iu/?u=https%3A%2F%2Fcdn1.byjus.com%2Fwp-content%2Fuploads%2F2018%2F12%2FObsessive-Compulsive-Disorder.png&f=1&nofb=1&ipt=34da18805d1d281cac5f547f44a2d8d6910ce1fd76420a6d171618865527d171.

7.1.2. Body Dysmorphic Disorder (BDD)

Body Dysmorphic Disorder (BDD) is an unsettling phenomenon in the world of obsessive-compulsive and related disorders. Individuals afflicted with BDD have a strong preoccupation with perceived flaws or flaws in their body, often leading to extreme distress and impairment in daily functioning. BDD is not a short-lived episode of vanity or dissatisfaction; rather, it is an entrenched psychological disorder. Epidemiological studies have established that BDD is estimated to affect approximately 2% of the general population, though most of them remain untreated due to various barriers, including low awareness among mental health practitioners and low access to targeted therapies. The psychological processes underlying the BDDs also possess their own unique characteristics, including numerous times cognitive distortions and compulsive behaviors, as observed in other obsessive-compulsive disorders. The effects of BDD are not only confined to the mere appearance preoccupations of the person, as it also negatively impacts their overall quality of life.

The majority of individuals with BDD also have major comorbidities, most commonly anxiety and mood disorders, that further complicate their condition. In adolescents, studies have established that around 9.35% of teens who are treated for primary obsessive-compulsive disorder also have symptoms of BDD. This overlap demonstrates the way in which BDD can exacerbate the social and functional deficits of these patients, in that they are not only struggling with their appearance-related concerns but also with confusing symptoms of OCD. Notably, the severity of appearance anxiety is correlated with OCD-related impairment and maladaptive emotion regulation.

This overlap in disorders highlights the requirement for a broad therapeutic approach, taking into consideration the complexities of BDD within the overall framework of obsessive-compulsive disorders. Current treatments for BDD remain limited and largely yield modest gains, creating a need for the development of new therapeutic approaches. Both cognitive-behavioral therapy and pharmacotherapy have been found to be effective; yet, a significant number of patients report residual distress despite strict adherence to treatment recommendations.

Recent research indicates that mindfulness-based treatments may offer a complementary approach to existing treatments. Mindfulness exercises, with emphasis on non-judgment and heightened interoceptive awareness, already have demonstrated potential for diminished symptom severity of co-morbid illnesses, such as eating disorders and social anxiety disorder. Exploration of these practices as an adjunct to BDD treatment protocols could enhance outcomes by effectively resolving cognitive fixity and body image disturbance. As awareness of BDD grows, the use of such forward-thinking initiatives as part of treatment plans can translate to better and more available support for those suffering from this complex disorder (Racz et al., 2022; Iris et al., 2025) (Figure 7.4).

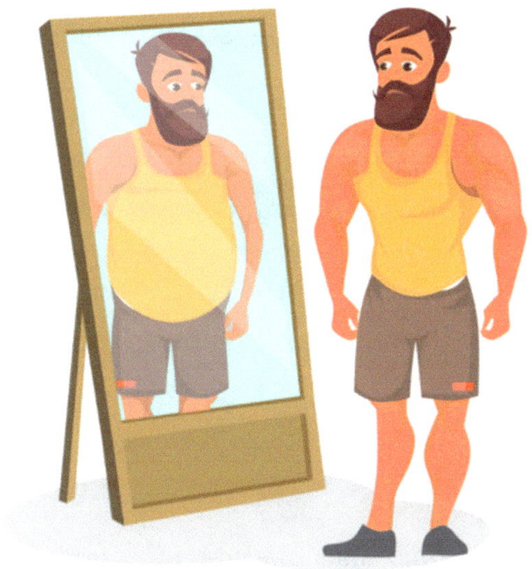

Figure 7.4. Body dysmorphic disorder (BDD).

Source: https://external-content.duckduckgo.com/iu/?u=https%3A%2F%2Fadaa.org%2Fsites%2Fdefault%2Ffiles%2F2022-10%2FBDD%2520men.png&f=1&nofb=1&ipt=7c25200d8290d84da30bb4a497ce90c68a718c54e7e8a6672c248243741746de.

7.1.3. Hoarding Disorder

With Hoarding Disorder increasingly recognized as part of the family of Obsessive-Compulsive and Related Disorders, it brings particular challenges not just for people with this condition but also for mental health professionals. The disorder is defined by repeated struggle to get rid of possessions, resulting in excessive clutter that severely impairs living areas and daily activities. Although traditionally viewed as a behavioral maladaptation, recent literature indicates that hoarding may be linked to the identical neurobiological processes seen in obsessive-compulsive disorder (OCD). The overlapping symptomatology suggests that at least some cases of hoarding are caused by the same cognitive distortions that cause OCD, such an inflated sense of responsibility and fear of loss. Understanding these connections is significant in that it can guide treatment approaches, potentially culminating in the development of specialized treatments that will address both hoarding and OCD elements of the patient population.

Compounding the clinical picture of Hoarding Disorder is that it has been discovered to be comorbid with other mental illnesses, including depression and anxiety. Research indicates that individuals with hoarding behaviors have greater distress and functional impairment, and these may complicate comorbid disorder symptoms. For instance, the entanglement of hoarding and anxiety creates a feedback mechanism in which the inability to throw away items provokes increased anxiety, further enhancing the phenomenon of hoarding.

This connection stresses the need for comprehensive evaluations of patients presenting with hoarding symptoms, as effective treatment hinges on an awareness of the overall clinical presentation, including comorbid psychiatric disorders. Interventions aimed solely at removing the clutter can prove unsuccessful, and a more comprehensive approach to therapy is necessary. Treatment of Hoarding Disorder is advancing, with cognitive-behavioral therapy (CBT) proving an encouraging first-line treatment. However, the availability of appropriate therapeutic modalities remains a significant barrier, most notably for younger people. The potential for internet-delivered CBT was highlighted by one study as a viable substitute for in-person therapy, showing noninferior efficacy in the treatment of obsessive-compulsive symptoms in children and adolescents. Access issues are particularly relevant given Hoarding Disorder, where stigma and resource availability may deter patients from reaching out. Against this background, innovative models of delivery that harmonize stepped-care principles and teletherapy could potentially provide vital support to those with hoarding behaviors, ultimately leading to enhanced mental health outcomes. While learning more about Hoarding Disorder evolves, identifying effective treatment frameworks well adapted to diverse needs remains a key area of concern in both research and clinical practice (Figure 7.5).

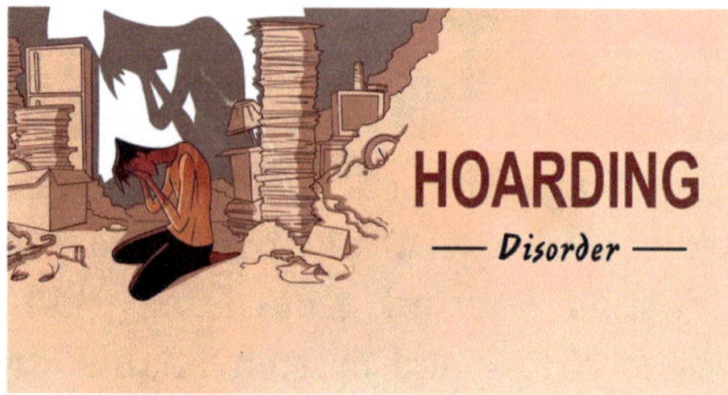

Figure 7.5. Hoarding disorder.

Source: https://mind.help/wp-content/uploads/2020/11/Hoarding-Disorder.jpg.

Test Your Knowledge

1. How do classic OCD, body dysmorphic disorder, and hoarding disorder differ in their core features?
2. What distinguishes obsessive-compulsive personality disorder (OCPD) from obsessive-compulsive disorder (OCD)?

7.2. Symptoms and Diagnosis

Learning Outcome

1. Common symptoms of OCD.
2. Diagnostic criteria for related disorders.
3. Challenges in diagnosing these disorders.

The symptoms of obsessive-compulsive disorder (OCD) are a particular challenge to diagnosis and treatment due to the intricacy of their nature. Bounding OCD at its center are obsessions—chronic, intrusive ideas or images that bring on extreme anxiety—and compulsions, repetitive behavior or mental behavior performed to alleviate such anxiety. The symptoms also operate in combination with one another in varying levels of severity, thus individualizing their expression. Moreover, the distress caused by obsessions and the compulsive behaviors employed to alleviate this distress can severely undermine daily functioning. According to Nielsen et al. (2025), emotion dysregulation plays a major role in the aetiology and continuation of OCD symptoms, often making it more challenging to diagnose by introducing additional emotional and behavioral features that must be considered. The intricacy of differential diagnosis also comes up when OCD presents with other psychiatric conditions, for instance, autism spectrum disorder (ASD). Both conditions share prominent common symptoms, such as cognitive inflexibility, worry, and abnormal social relations. Adolescents in particular can show symptoms of both OCD and ASD simultaneously, making it even more challenging for practitioners to make distinctions between such conditions. With the high degree of co-occurring gender-diverse clinical problems, such as attention-deficit/hyperactivity disorder and depression, there is a greater need for a robust diagnostic model. The symptom complexity requires an extensive, informed diagnostic procedure, highlighted by the literature in (Corey et al., 2024), which highlight the value of understanding converging symptoms and their implications for treatment. Due to the intricate symptoms of OCD, accurate diagnosis is dependent on comprehensive evaluation methods. Clinicians use standardized evaluation tools, such as the Yale-Brown Obsessive Compulsive Scale (Y-BOCS), whose aim is to measure the degree of symptoms of OCD. These tools can ascertain the exact nature of a patient's obsessions and compulsions, enabling an individualized treatment program. In addition, increased understanding of the functions of attachment styles has the potential to enhance diagnostic precision, as evidenced by research demonstrating relationships between insecure attachment and OCD symptoms through the mediating factor of emotion dysregulation. Investigation of these relationships, as presented in (Nielsen et al., 2025), emphasizes the merit of combining psychological theory and practice, setting the stage for treatments better focused on the emotional foundations of OCD.

7.2.1. Common Symptoms of OCD

Obsessive-Compulsive Disorder (OCD) is defined by several symptoms with the potential to significantly impair individuals' everyday functioning. Obsessions, which are intrusive and unwanted ideas, images, or urges that cause excessive anxiety or distress, form the core of the disorder. The obsessions can be concerning contamination, requiring symmetry, or something bad happening to the self or another. Compulsions are, however, repetitive behaviors or mental acts that an individual feels he or she has to perform in response to their obsessions or based on inflexible rules. For instance, a person can compulsively wash his or her hands to flee anxieties about germs, a practice that may provide short-term comfort from fear but long-term maintenance of the OCD cycle, as sustained relief from distress is usually not attained. Awareness of these root symptoms is essential within the framework of a diagnosis and treatment regimen for impacted individuals. Children and adolescents can be symptomatically very different from adults regarding OCD. Teenagers and children can have a hard time describing what they go through, so underdiagnosis and a delay in treatment are probable. The nature of obsessions in children's groups may be fears about the school running or family security, whereas compulsions may be rituals for the completion of homework or bedtime. From research, it has been found that OCD in this group may be established rapidly, possibly with depressive behaviors, which require intervention at an early age. The unique characteristics inherent to OCD in children can complicate diagnosis since it is normally mistaken for normal child behavior. Thus, experts involved in the treatment of children must be keen and proactive in identifying such symptoms (Khvatkov et al., 2024). Assessment measures of OCD symptoms play a significant role in clinical as well as research settings. Systematically constructed rating scales have been employed to measure the frequency and severity of obsessive and compulsive symptoms, enabling health practitioners to chart changes over time and ensure treatments are effective. Standardized tools clarify and define diagnosis and facilitate comparison of findings between studies as well as across treatment contexts. Notably, detailed assessments are able to yield improved treatment responses via the delivery of individualized therapeutic interventions that align with a person's own symptom profile. As the science progressively moved toward understanding OCD, the emphasis on structured observation and tested rating scales has grown, enabling symptom patterns and comorbidities to be recognized and alerting clinicians to create useful treatments for sufferers with this highly impairing disorder (Rajachandrasekar et al., 2023) (Figure 7.6).

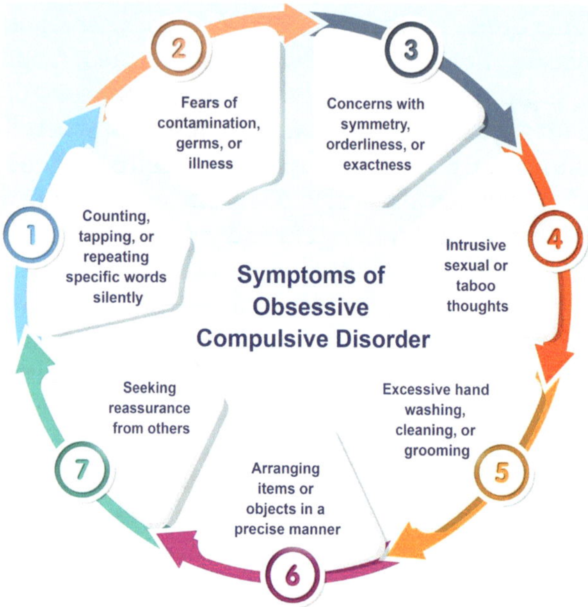

Figure 7.6. Common symptoms of OCD.

Source: https://continentalhospitals.com/uploads/mceu_75375279711701410649071.jpg.

7.2.2. Diagnostic Criteria for Related Disorders

Diagnostic criteria of obsessive-compulsive and related disorders in the Diagnostic and Statistical Manual of Mental Disorders (DSM-5) provide a systematic approach to thinking about such complex mental disorders. Possibly the most significant aspect of diagnosis is distinguishing among the various disorders under this category, such as Obsessive-Compulsive Disorder (OCD), Obsessive-Compulsive Personality Disorder (OCPD), and Body Dysmorphic Disorder (BDD). There are specific symptoms and Behavioral patterns for each of these conditions that must be carefully diagnosed. For instance, while OCD is largely characterized by intrusive thoughts and compulsive behavior, OCPD is characterized by perfectionism and excessive preoccupation with orderliness. It is critical to have a clear understanding of and correctly apply these criteria because differential diagnosis can have a large impact on treatment modalities and patient outcomes for patients with these disorders. In investigating OCPD specifically, more recent studies highlight the disorder's prevalence and how it influences daily functioning. One seminal study found that 51% of medical students screened who met the DSM-5 definition for OCPD had a stunningly high prevalence compared to the general population. The study highlighted the degree to which OCPD persons can experience greater anxiety and tension when there is academic pressure, such as exams. The subjects reported significant disruption in their sleep patterns, consonant with the fact that pressures of perfectionism can come to have disabling consequences, ultimately influencing academic performance. This incongruence between what the individual anticipates and what occurs to them can also give rise to a vicious circle of increasing harm to their mental health problems. It is therefore critical to recognize these diagnostic characteristics in making effective intervention strategies for these patients. Compassion for the state of the individual is a crucial consideration when dealing with OCD and measuring treatment efficacy. Those with declining or fluctuating insight will respond differently, since those with lower insight are often more challenging to treat in terms of symptom remission as well as adherence to treatment protocols. The DSM-5 accounts for this variation by widening the diagnostic criteria for the diagnosis of OCD to encompass such variability, thus establishing the need for individualized therapy modalities. Treatment of beliefs and insights related to their condition will lead to enhanced compliance with cognitive-behavioral therapies and, in the end, enhanced clinical outcomes. Increasing focus on insight does serve to underscore the work of extensive evaluation and intervention and thus push forward our understanding of obsessive-compulsive and related disorders as complex problems requiring cautious clinical strategies (Huang et al., 2023; Al-Na M'she et al., 2024) (Figure 7.7).

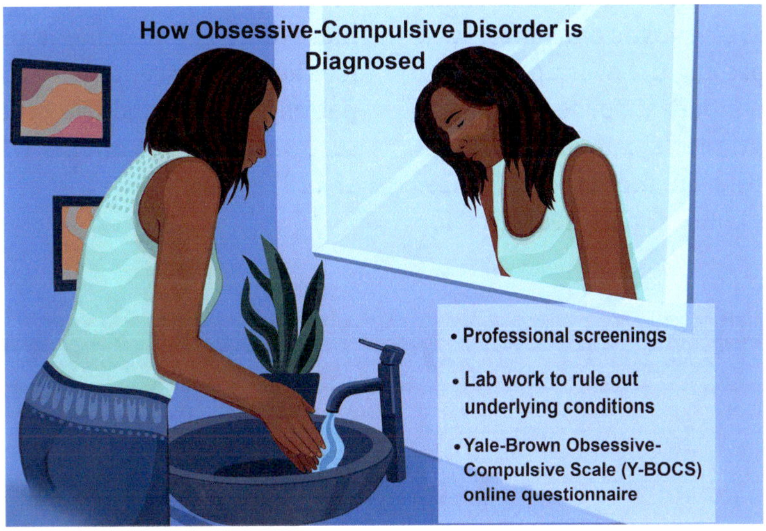

Figure 7.7. Diagnostic criteria for OCD.

Source: https://www.verywellhealth.com/thmb/JaOxQ15AgIZCpY7stGFipf60TGc=/1500x0/filters:no_upscale():max_bytes(150000):strip_icc()/zhansen_ocd-diagnosis-5105153_final-0095f5ed0ba64dc49ca3b6741ca6bcb1.jpg.

7.2.3. Challenges in Diagnosing These Disorders

Another group of difficulties in diagnosing OCRDs makes it even more difficult to treat and manage the disorder effectively. The greatest issue here is posed by co-morbid symptoms that are noticed in most anxiety disorders, and therefore, it is difficult to differentiate OCRDs from other psychiatric disorders. This gives rise to misdiagnosis or delayed treatment, which is even more problematic in susceptible populations, such as children. The inherent intricacies of diagnosing such disorders demand that one should have an absolute understanding of their symptomatology and their contexts of occurrence, for misidentification of the underlying disorder can result in improper treatment strategies, including the misuse of medications for other disorders. In the affected children with OCRDs, the identification brings a further facet of complexity in the diagnosis. For instance, the possibility of inducing mania had been indicated by one study with SSRIs, predominantly in young patients; therefore, in that case, the clinical presentation was obscured. For instance, a nine-year-old girl with a diagnosis of multiple OCRDs presented with mania of short duration following treatment with an SSRI, and such a case is illustrative of a diagnostic dilemma. This case points to the extreme care and vigilance that must be exercised during the diagnostic process, as well as the requirement for considering the long-term effects drugs might have on children as patients. This case describes the necessity of careful assessments to ensure proper, safe interventions are selected, considering the unique developmental circumstances of children. Also, the diagnostic challenges in OCRDs are served by the absence of homogeneous diagnostic criteria across different populations and age groups. This ambiguity can be the causative agent of varied interpretations and practices among clinicians, which leads to varied diagnostic outcomes. Lack of literature encompassing the overlap between OCRDs and other mood disorders further narrows the practitioner's knowledge base, further increasing the diagnostic difficulties. Furthermore, there is an urgent necessity for further studies on how such disorders come about in particular demographics, because it is by understanding these nuances that one can better be able to diagnose correctly. Improved diagnostic precision can ultimately allow for more efficient treatment programs optimized for the specific requirements of each individual patient, hence enhancing the general quality of care received by patients with OCRDs Sevda et al., 2024).

Test Your Knowledge

1. What are the hallmark symptoms of OCD, including obsessions and compulsions, and how are they assessed clinically?
2. How do diagnostic criteria in DSM-5-TR help differentiate OCD from related disorders such as anxiety or psychotic disorders?

7.3. Causes and Risk Factors

Learning Outcome

1. Genetic predisposition.
2. Environmental influences.
3. Neurobiological factors.

Pathogenesis of obsessive-compulsive disorder (OCD) and allied disorders is multifactorial, encompassing biological, psychological, and environmental factors. Genetic predisposition is a significant factor in the etiology of these disorders, as twin studies show a higher rate of concordance in identical twins compared with fraternal twins. This points towards the possibility of genetic factors playing a role in the emergence of symptoms of OCD. In addition, neurobiological data indicate that abnormalities exist in some areas of the brain, such as the orbitofrontal cortex and basal ganglia, involved in obsessive-compulsive behavior. The neuroanatomical abnormalities are consistent with the hypothesis that OCD could be the result of a malfunctioning cognitive control process, leading to intrusive thoughts recurring and repetitive actions becoming automatic. Knowledge of these biological foundations yields insight into possible interventions and therapeutic paths for those afflicted with these difficult disorders. Psychological mechanisms also contribute importantly to the origin and maintenance of OCD. Cognitive-behavioral conceptualizations propose that aberrant thinking styles, including exaggerated responsibility and catastrophic thoughts, play an important part in the disorder. People suffering from OCD are prone to cognitive distortions, which exaggerate danger and concerns they might have, and then seek ways to mitigate this perceived risk. For instance, a person with obsessive intrusive thoughts about getting contaminated tends to develop compulsive activities of washing, which might reduce anxiety for the moment but, over time, continually feed the obsession. This cycle of negative reinforcement continues the disorder, as well as the activities, and makes it difficult to eventually end the compulsion. Furthermore, stressful life experiences like loss or trauma can trigger the onset of OCD, implying the incorporation of psychological stressors into the treatment process. Comorbidity with OCD emphasizes the multifactorial nature of its risk factors.

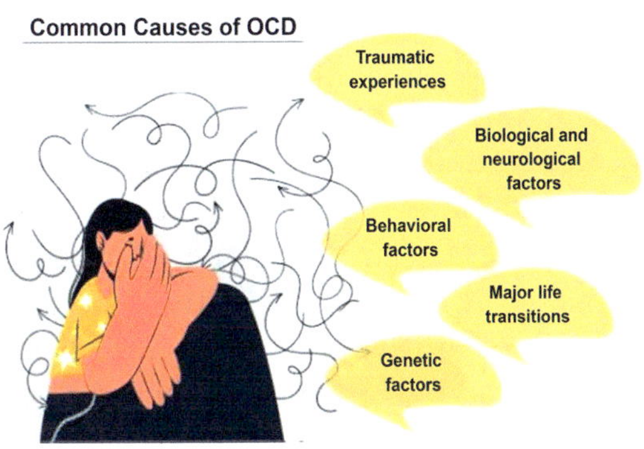

Figure 7.8. Causes of OCD.

Source: https://ezcareclinic.io/wp-content/uploads/2022/11/What-Can-Worsen-OCD-Symptoms-supporting-image-2-540x397.jpg.webp.

The majority of OCD-diagnosed individuals exhibit co-occurring symptoms of anxiety disorders, depression, or impulse control disorders, complicating both diagnosis and treatment. For instance, it has been noted that OCD and impulse control disorders have a high comorbidity, which indicates the interplay of these clinical phenotypes over time (Van Dael et al., 2011). Moreover, some demographic characteristics , such as age and gender, also contribute towards the expression and emergence of OCD symptoms. For instance, studies have shown that females are more likely to be affected by OCD than males, particularly in adolescence and early adulthood. Additionally, disorders , such as Parkinson's disease have been linked with higher counts of obsessive-compulsive traits, and therefore the need to continue examining interrelational patterns among neurological and psychological factors in the etiology of OCD and other similar disorders (Brown et al., 2013) (Figure 7.8).

7.3.1. Genetic Predisposition

The genetic liability lies at the heart of the aetiology of Obsessive-Compulsive Disorder (OCD) and co-morbid disorders. Clinical observations demonstrate that the participants with a family history of obsessions and compulsions and anxiety are at risk of developing these disorders themselves. For instance, children who develop anxiety disorders in early life have been found to exhibit a range of symptoms that appear later in life, like OCD, thus implicating an inheritance aspect associated with specific markers. Longitudinal research has suggested that these vulnerabilities will continue over the course of time, and thus, family patterns must be observed in clinical assessments. It is important to know genetic influences to make early diagnoses, particularly in children with symptoms of anxiety disorders, where intervention at an early point may prevent worse outcomes in adulthood, as indicated by findings for childhood anxiety disorders (Pop, 2019). Ongoing research into neurobiological pathways involved in genetic predisposition has identified pathways that may underlie OCD and anxiety disorders. Studies have shown that dysregulation of some neurotransmitter systems, led by serotonin, may be implicated in the manifestation of obsessive-compulsive symptoms. Variations in genes that influence serotonin transport and receptors may predispose certain persons to OCD. Further, the development of brain regions involved in emotional regulation and impulse control, like the prefrontal cortex and striatum, has been demonstrated to be influenced by genes. This relates genetic predisposition to not only behavioral traits, but to brain structural and functional changes that manifest as psychiatric illness in the form of OCD, and thereby suggests a biological origin for the gene-mental health outcome association (Barry et al., 2015). From the implications of genetic predisposition regarding diagnosis and treatment in obsessive-compulsive disorders, it is evident that a multidimensional strategy has to be employed. Genetic tests can also assist in the identification of persons at higher risk for developing OCD, allowing preventive measures to be directed. This is also a window of opportunity for the formulation of customized therapeutic regimens based on a patient's genetic makeup. In addition, the interaction between genetic susceptibility and environmental factors may improve the understanding of how OCD might develop or worsen under some conditions. Consequently, the precise knowledge of genetic and environmental interaction affirms the importance of multidisciplinary treatment approaches considering individual differences, ultimately improving the control of OCD and associated disorders (Pop, 2019).

7.3.2. Environmental Factors

The role of environmental factors is most important when examining obsessive-compulsive and other associated disorders, since they can be a determining factor in how the conditions develop and present. Family life, cultural rules, and trauma are just some of the elements that intertwine to allow obsessive-compulsive disorder (OCD) to form. Above all, individuals who have been exposed to dysfunctional family backgrounds with overcontrol or unpredictability are likely to produce maladaptive coping patterns. These can lead to the ritualistic aspects that characterize OCD as a means of regaining control over their lives. Furthermore, the complexity of such environmental factors is compounded further by genetic vulnerability interaction with psychological response to stressors, requiring multidimensionality in how the etiology of such disorders is conceived, as is the case with PMB changes as reported in the literature base, underscoring the need for holistic evaluations within the therapy context (Sharawy, 2023). Environmental factors also extend beyond family causes, as societal and cultural environments are extremely important in the lives of people in determining their psychological surroundings. Cultural beliefs may dictate the acceptability of certain obsessive thoughts or compulsive behaviors, as they may influence individuals' perception and reaction to their symptoms.

For instance, in cultures that emphasize perfectionism and high achievement, people will be scrutinized more closely for what they think and do, and there will be more anxiety and obsessive-compulsive behavior. The combination of environmental stressors and expression of OCD makes it even more critical to include culturally responsive strategies in treatment, which can lead individuals to navigate through their own socio-cultural expectations and address their mental health concerns.

These perspectives are what help explain the overall implications of environmental influences in OCD, adding further to the principle that psychological consequences must be separated from the social and relational contexts in which they develop (Sharawy, 2023). Further, the relationships between environmental influences and obsessive-compulsive disorder are observed in animal behavior, as a useful counterpoint to the significance of context in mental health. As with humans, animals can also suffer from behavioral disorders that have been found to coincide with conditions , such as OCD and anxiety disorders. Home environment modifications, lack of stimulation, or trauma are some of the causative factors that can trigger compulsive behavior in pets, showing the impact of environmental factors on mental health in animals as well. Understanding the behavioral manifestations in animals is crucial for better comprehension of human psychiatric illnesses because it could be that the same emotional and cognitive mechanisms are implicated. These lessons highlight the imperative of bringing together the affective and cognitive dimensions of environmental factors in treatments for obsessive-compulsive disorders to encourage holistic methods of thinking that account for both human and animal experience and the multifaceted nature of psychological pain (Figure 7.9).

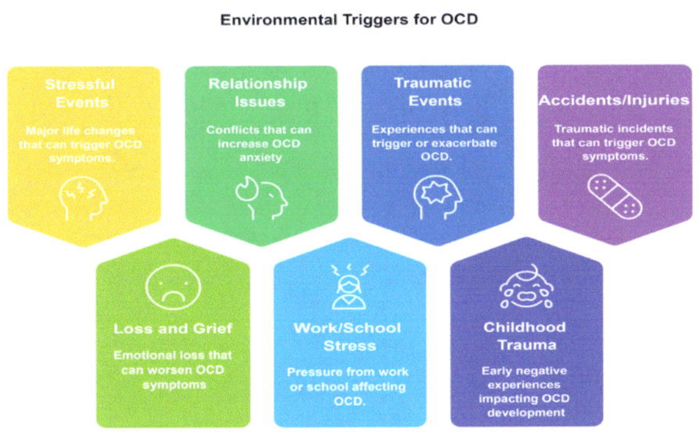

Figure 7.9. Environmental influences of OCD.

Source: https://relevancerecovery.com/wp-content/uploads/2025/03/Environmental-Triggers-That-Affect-OCD-visual-selection-1024x814.png.

7.3.3. Neurobiological Factors

The neurobiology of obsessive-compulsive disorder (OCD) and spectrum disorders has been among the subjects of intense research and has provided windows of insight into complicated relationships between specific brain elements and the occurrence of compulsive rituals. The corticostriatal circuitry involving the orbitofrontal cortex, caudate nucleus, and thalamus has been identified as especially significant in recent research. Dysfunction in this pathway is postulated to underlie the impaired decision-making and failure to inhibit intrusive thoughts that are hallmark features of OCD patients. Notably, imaging studies have revealed altered patterns of activity in these regions on tasks of inhibition of compulsive behavior. Through the identification of these neural correlates, scientists hope to delineate a more precise neurobiological model that will allow for the diagnosis and treatment of OCD and related disorders. In trichotillomania, a disorder that shares similar behavioral characteristics with OCD, neurobiological mechanisms play an equally significant role. Research shows that trichotillomania patients possess impaired response inhibition, which can be observed in self-control task performance impairments. Structural brain imaging also revealed significant gray matter density changes in regions implicated in inhibitory control, namely the frontal cortex.

These results point to the possibility of using alterations in brain morphology as biological markers for compulsive disorder involvement. This understanding of the convergence of neurobiological abnormalities and behavioral manifestations can finally culminate in intervention specifically directed at treating the mechanisms themselves and not merely symptom control, opening the way for innovative therapeutic approaches (Chamberlain et al., 2014). In addition, research into neurobiological dimensions of OCD is progressively bringing rich dividends with the emergence of more complex methodological paradigms.

Traditionally, psychiatric diagnoses have been symptom-oriented, with a tendency to induce diagnostic overlap and ambiguity. Recent developments aim towards a transdiagnostic approach, highlighting features like compulsivity related to specific neurobiological processes like goal-directed learning. Interfering with information from large population cohorts makes it easier for researchers to delineate further the psychiatric phenotypes and neurobiological substrates. These efforts have the potential to shed light on the genetic underpinnings of OCD, better define the validity of animal models, and ultimately guide more targeted therapeutic modalities (Gillan et al., 2017). This changing neurobiological perspective is a fundamental shift towards greater precision regarding OCD and other such disorders, with potential for a positive prognosis for therapies of the future (Figure 7.10).

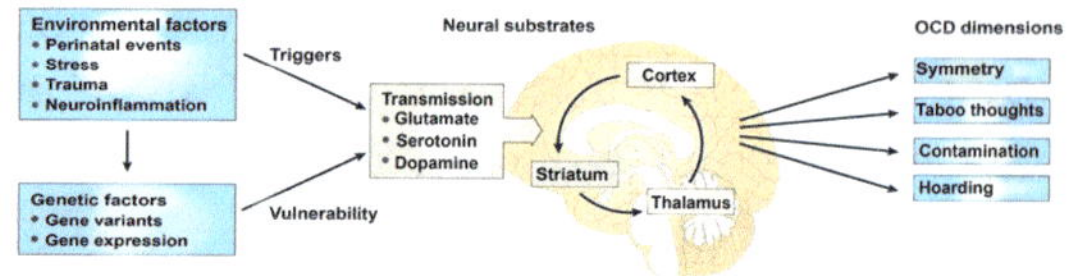

Figure 7.10. Neurobiological factors of OCD.

Source: https://media.springernature.com/lw1200/springer-static/image/art%3A10.1038%2Fnrn3746/MediaObjects/41583_2014_Article_BFnrn3746_Fig3_HTML.jpg.

Test Your Knowledge

1. What genetic, neurobiological, and cognitive factors are believed to contribute to the development of OCD?
2. How do environmental influences—such as stress, trauma, or learned behaviors—act as risk factors for obsessive-compulsive disorders?

7.4. Treatment Options

Learning Outcome

1. Cognitive behavioral therapy (CBT).
2. Medication management.
3. Alternative therapies and interventions.

When speaking of Treatment Options for Obsessive-Compulsive and Related Disorders, the significance of evidence-based treatments that have been shown to result in a significant reduction of symptoms should be mentioned. Cognitive Behavioral Therapy (CBT), or rather exposure and response prevention (ERP), has come to be the benchmark for the treatment of individuals suffering from obsessive-compulsive disorder (OCD). By raising the time exposure to the anxiety-provoking stimuli and the subsequent prevention of compulsive responses, patients become more resistant to their obsessions. Research has indicated that participants of ERP often experience a sudden drop in the frequency and intensity of their symptoms. Additionally, the combination of CBT with pharmacotherapy, such as the utilization of SSRIs, can even yield greater therapeutic rewards, particularly for patients who have moderately to severely symptomatic OCD. With ethics and practicality influencing treatment choices, understanding the complexity of these treatments is critical to attaining optimum patient outcomes. Aside from conventional methods of treatment, the incorporation of family-based strategies presents a new venue for intervention. Family members are usually at the center of OCD dynamics since their reactions towards a loved one's compulsions can influence the sufferer's recovery. Studies have indicated that family accommodation behaviors, which are activities performed by family members to reduce the distress linked to OCD, can actually reinforce the condition. Interventions , such as facilitated by Brief Family Consultation (BFC) have been developed to target family efforts away from accomplishing compulsive behaviors and toward developing healthier relationships. In studies assessing BFC, families evidenced reductions in accommodation without compromising overall quality of life. This pertains to an under-addressed aspect of OCD treatment, emphasizing the need to include family patterns within treatment interventions and, ultimately, in enhancing recovery outcomes for OCD patients (Conlon et al., 2015). Recent studies have also begun examining the co-occurrence between impulse control disorders and OCD, further illuminating the intricacies of comorbidities. There is a strong connection between some of the neurodegenerative illnesses, for example, Parkinson's Disease (PD), and impulse control disorders, with compulsive acting being taken into consideration. For instance, as studies show, there exists a subset of PD patients who acquire cravings similar to those seen in diagnosed impulse control disorders, suggesting that underlying dopaminergic mechanisms are at work (Brown et al., 2013). As such comprehension expands, treatment strategies need to be designed that address both the obsessive-compulsive and the comorbid impulse problems. The addition of detailed assessments incorporating comorbidity will further consolidate treatment strategies into multilayered, individually tailored interventions. Integrative thought is rapidly becoming the new center of current models of treatment for OCD and comorbid disorders, being centered on the necessity of ongoing research and intervention development.

7.4.1. Cognitive Behavioral Therapy (CBT)

Cognitive Behavioral Therapy (CBT) has become a mainstay of Obsessive-Compulsive Disorder (OCD) treatment, founded upon an organized approach that targets the maladaptive cognitive schemas responsible for the disorder. CBT is primarily the process of exposing the patients to their obsessive stimuli in a controlled manner while helping them master the ability to handle their anxiety by means of behavioral change. This is a procedure known as exposure and response prevention (ERP) used to deem power the compulsive behaviors people exhibit to lower their anxiety. Different research has demonstrated the utility of CBT to reduce symptoms of OCD and, therefore, it is a gold standard and one that is highly suggested by mental health professionals. For instance, a study confirms that CBT had a considerable role in reducing cognitive fusion and obsessive-compulsive symptoms among participants, confirming the strong efficacy of CBT in clinical scenarios (Hosseini et al., 2025). In addition to that, the adaptability of CBT allows it to be customized in accordance with individual patient needs, accommodating the particular presentations of OCD. This individualization is necessary since OCD often comes with various themes, such as contamination or intrusive thoughts, which must be addressed through a careful, specific plan of intervention. Secondly, assisted by cognitive restructuring techniques, CBT also enables clients to learn to dispute and modify cognitive distortions related to their obsessions. Patients are able to implement healthier thinking patterns in the long term with a greater awareness of cognitive distortions. Research has found that CBT and other therapies, such as brief psychodynamic therapy, have led to large effects on mental health conditions for patients with OCD, but CBT remains effective and again in reducing severe symptoms like anxiety and compulsivity (Hosseini et al., 2025). The duration of treatment and the number of sessions in CBT are also important, as there is evidence showing that even a limited number of sessions can be very effective. The majority of treatment programs consist of only 10 to 12 sessions, so it is more convenient and time-efficient for patients who desire to be cured from their incapacitating symptoms. Follow-up assessments have demonstrated that the therapeutic effects of CBT do not merely persist but even enhance with time, as coping skills learned are applied in the daily life of the patients. This long-term efficacy speaks for the therapy's capacity to affect enduring change in coping. With the evolution of CBT, there is a requirement for further exploration of its incorporation with other treatment modalities to achieve maximum treatment benefit in OCD and allied disorders, with the potential to benefit a larger group of patients (Hosseini et al., 2025) (Figure 7.11).

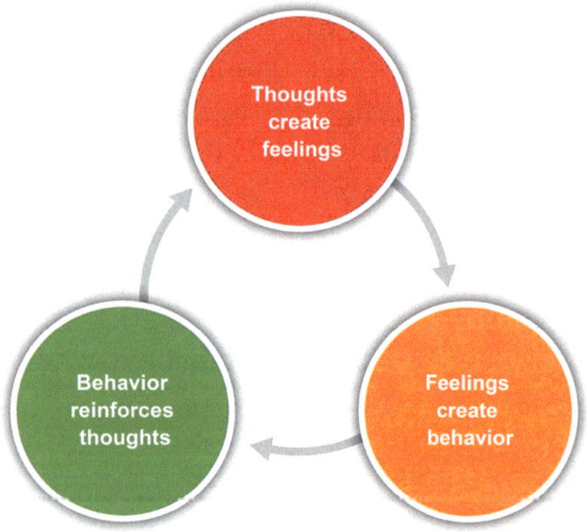

Figure 7.11. Cognitive behavioral therapy (CBT) for OCD.

Source: https://images.squarespace-cdn.com/content/v1/51e36ea9e4b0e2abc3eb9d10/1488845019714-ZX0S9L99JKR7593VCRGX/image-asset.jpeg.

7.4.2. Medication Management

Treatment of obsessive-compulsive disorder (OCD) and spectrum disorders often needs to be multifaceted, with medication management being a key part. Selective serotonin reuptake inhibitors (SSRIs) have emerged as the first-line pharmacologic intervention for OCD and have been demonstrated to have efficacy in the alleviation of symptoms involving both obsessions and compulsions. Even though these medications are extremely well-tolerated, their effectiveness can vary significantly among patients. It is crucial that healthcare workers monitor patients closely in the early stages of treatment to assess both efficacy and side effects, titrating dosages to maximize therapeutic effect. Personalized treatment is essential since some patients will have issues regarding comorbidities, which could complicate drug management and the general efficacy of treatment. Cognitive-behavioral therapy (CBT) remains a standard treatment for OCD and comorbid disorders, but faces numerous barriers to accessibility. Several such patients are reluctant to undergo CBT due to the stigmatization of value placed on the condition of OCD, as well as the severity of the therapy itself. This paves the way for the utilization of pharmacological treatment as a first-line response, which is a justification for drug management in such cases. New developments in neuroimaging techniques have indicated potential enhancement of response prediction to CBT and thus medication-therapy harmonization. As a whole, neurobiological processes may be employed to tailor treatment protocols such that therapists may predict patients who will benefit more from integrated therapeutic interventions or from initial prioritizing of medication management without therapy, thereby maximizing patient outcomes (O'Neill & Feusner, 2015). Even in disorders like body dysmorphic disorder (BDD), drug management also needs to be conducted with strategic planning. While CBT is the preferred treatment approach for BDD, its effectiveness varies depending on a variety of personal factors, including motivation and knowledge about the disorder. Research has identified that patients who are highly ready to change and highly optimistic about the therapy have the best chances of recovery from CBT, but this does not rule out SSRIs as an adjunctive treatment. For highly symptomatic or highly distressed patients, SSRIs may provide significant symptomatic relief and, thus, allow patients to engage more intensively in therapeutic efforts. By introducing medication management integratively, practitioners can foster the therapeutic relationship and establish a healing environment, knowing that some patients may be assisted through a two-way approach of treating the pharmacological and psychotherapeutic aspects of BDD treatment (Greenberg et al., 2019) (Figure 7.12).

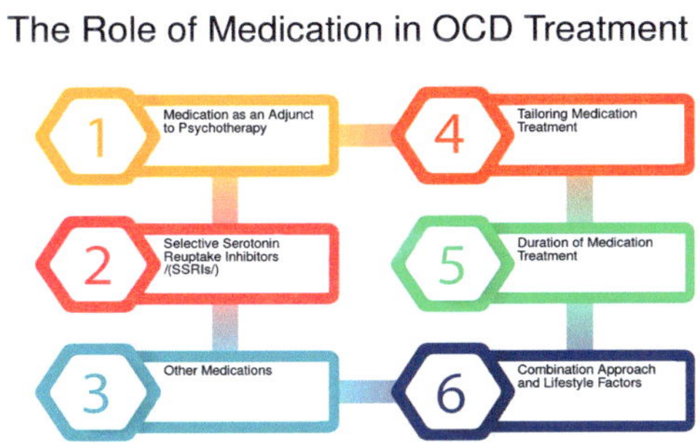

Figure 7.12. Medication management for OCD.

Source: https://fastercapital.co/i/Balancing-Act--Exploring-Medication-for-OCD-Management--The-Role-of-Medication-in-OCD-Treatment.webp.

7.4.3. Alternative Therapies and Interventions

In probing the application of alternative therapies and interventions for spectrum and obsessive-compulsive disorders, making an assessment of the incorporation of various complementary therapies with traditional treatment methods is very important. Although cognitive-behavioral therapy (CBT) is the gold standard for treatment of diseases , such as obsessive-compulsive disorder (OCD) and body dysmorphic disorder (BDD), not everybody is responsive to this evidence-based care. As discussed in current literature, the incidence of treatment resistance is considerable and underlines the need to create alternative interventions that are capable of enhancing outcomes. Therapies , such as mindfulness-based cognitive therapy and acceptance and commitment therapy have gained popularity since they allow people to develop greater self-knowledge and break the grip of compulsive ruminations and rituals. This second emphasis has the capacity to help patients build up resilience, offering a way of improving overall well-being and coping, especially for those with more severe symptoms as evidenced by the need to augment readiness to change (Greenberg et al., 2019). Furthermore, the combination of pharmacological treatments with other treatments has the capacity to cure obsessive-compulsive disorders. SSRIs are commonly prescribed to alleviate anxiety and compulsive behavior; their effectiveness, however, can be significantly enhanced by concomitant therapeutic strategies like exposure and response prevention in CBT. Even so, access to specialized therapists remains a concern, as indicated by problems faced by patients who suffer from stigma and pressure of rigorous therapy (O'Neill & Feusner, 2015). Therefore, alternative therapies , such as music or art therapy may be employed as adjuncts to conventional treatments and may provide patient expression with creative resources. These interventions can soothe anxiety and stabilize emotions, and they present an effective yet alternative means of addressing obsessive-compulsive behavior. Moreover, new technological innovations like computer applications and teletherapy present other pathways to effectively controlling obsessive-compulsive and related disorders. These platforms provide patients with round-the-clock access to therapeutic resources, education about their conditions, and self-help tools that can complement traditional interventions. By utilizing guided exposure exercises or mindfulness training via mobile apps, individuals may find that these tailored strategies enhance their sense of agency over their symptoms. Notably, research suggests that the long-term effectiveness of such treatment can be predicted, potentially guiding treatment adjustments before commencing CBT (O'Neill & Feusner, 2015). The more alternative therapies evolve and technology further becomes part of the treatment frameworks, the more necessary it is to evaluate their effectiveness using systematic research, eventually granting victims of their obsessive-compulsive disorders with combined, accessible, and tailored treatment methods specifically adapted to each of their individual needs.

Test Your Knowledge

1. How do cognitive-behavioral therapies, particularly exposure and response prevention (ERP), help in treating OCD?
2. What role do medications such as SSRIs and other pharmacological approaches play in managing OCD symptoms?

7.5. Impact on Daily Life

Learning Outcome

1. Effects on personal relationships.
2. Influence on academic and occupational functioning.
3. Coping mechanisms and strategies.

The impact of obsessive-compulsive disorder (OCD) on daily life is serious and extensive, often spilling over into other realms , such as interpersonal relationships, occupational environments, and general mental well-being. OCD individuals commonly experience compulsive behavior designed to prevent intrusive intrusions that lead to significant time consumption, possibly detracting from essential daily functioning. Such obsessions may include overwashing of the hands, ritualistic checking, or want for order, which can lead to frustration and inadequacy due to being handicapped by such rituals in everyday life. Such interference can result in widespread psychological discomfort, also adding to sensations of depression and anxiety, comorbidly experienced with OCD. As such, individuals become isolated from society and experience strained interpersonal relationships, thus affecting their quality of life and emotional well-being, which can resonate with the emotions identified in the studies of diseases like fibromyalgia and its psychological impacts (Carmen et al., 2019). The effects of OCD transcend the individual, and its influence is felt at the family and professional levels. Family members can become frustrated and confused by the compulsive actions of their family member, which may cause tension and conflict in the home. Excessive reassurance or understanding demanded by family members can strain relationships, as roles in the family shift while attempting to satisfy the needs of the individual with OCD. In the workplace, the individual might be unable to do tasks due to time spent on compulsions or anxiety precipitated by intrusive thoughts. This compromised functional capacity at work can lead to job insecurity or unhappiness, further contributing to distress for the individual. Therefore, the effect of OCD in working life and personal relationships is severe and widespread in nature and needs a comprehensive intervention plan with family and community support systems, as in the case of depression in the elderly (Avasthi & Grover, 2018).

Handling the daily conundrums of OCD necessitates a multimodal approach that involves psychologicalal intervention avenues , such as cognitive-behavioral therapy (CBT) and drug therapy. CBT, particularly exposure and response prevention (ERP), has been found to be beneficial in allowing individuals to confront their fears without performing the compulsive behavior, thereby reducing OCD's influence on daily life. Pharmacological treatments, including selective serotonin reuptake inhibitors (SSRIs), meanwhile, can help to reduce the accompanying depressive and anxiety symptoms, thereby helping to improve the overall functioning of affected individuals. Nevertheless, building an effective treatment strategy typically involves collaboration with healthcare professionals, family members, and peers in order to have access to all-around care. By addressing both the psychological and functional problems of having OCD, individuals can reassert control over their lives, enhance the quality of their lives and support positive social interactions, as encouraged by the strategy employed in the management of complexities of depressive disorders in the elderly (Avasthi & Grover, 2018).

7.5.1. Impact on Individual Relations

The interpersonal impact of obsessive-compulsive disorder (OCD) can be considerable and intricate. The individuals with OCD characteristically have intrusive ideas and compulsive acts that impact them negatively in terms of putting pressure on human relationships. Family members, partners, and friends get caught up with the person's obsessions and routines, thus leading to frustration and ignorance. For example, when an individual suffering from OCD requires repeated assurance or executes repeated actions, their loved one might unknowingly enable such a behavior, and this may culminate in increasing levels of stress and resentment between the two. By bringing to light the need for understanding the challenges brought about by OCD, accounts like Ethan and Ophelias in (Pattiselanno et al., 2025) emphasize that sensitization and compassion are needed in a bid to establish healthier relationships, referring to the destructive power that untreated OCD has on relationships among individuals. Additionally, the psychological load of OCD can lead to seclusion, hence making it harder for individual relationships. The majority of individuals with OCD find it difficult to cope with the stigmatization that accompanies the condition, thereby self-isolating themselves in case they are judged. Self-isolation normally creates a barrier that discourages an open discussion, and individuals around them feel isolated and do not know how to help them. As the individual tries to manage their symptoms, they unwittingly neglect others' emotional needs, increasing other family and friends' feelings of frustration and loneliness. The importance of interventions, such as Cognitive Behavioral Therapy, is highlighted in (Pattiselanno et al., 2025), as these treatments can empower individuals with the ability to not only control their OCD symptoms but also the relational tensions that arise from them and form improved relationships. Interventions grounded in mindfulness also present a very promising pathway for minimizing the negative effects of OCD on interpersonal relationships. Evidence shows that augmenting mindfulness has the ability to reduce symptom severity in patients suffering from comorbid OCD and MDD dramatically, thereby improving interpersonal relations and mental health. By rendering a person more sensitive to thoughts and emotions, mindfulness activities can potentially reduce the strength of obsessive thoughts and thereby improve relationships with people. Since the individuals learn emotional regulation and coping skills through being mindful, they can develop healthier relationships more effectively, breaking the pattern of dysfunction that usually follows OCD. Thus, implementing mindfulness in treatment programs not only improves one's own mental health but also serves as a necessary component to improve interpersonal relationships, leading ultimately to improving the overall level of relationships strained by OCD (Figure 7.13).

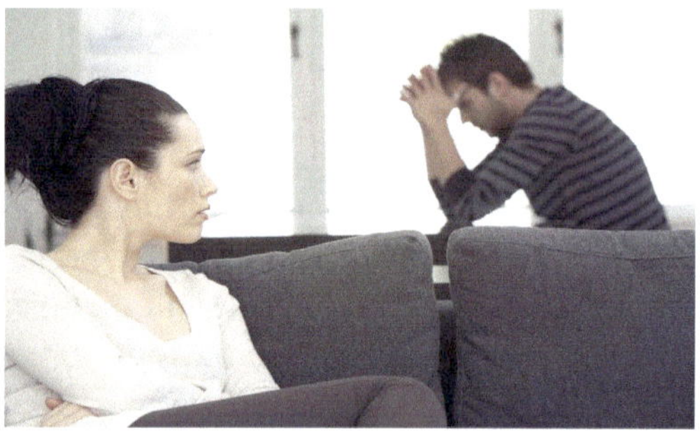

Figure 7.13. The impact of obsessive-compulsive disorder (OCD) on personal relationships.

Source: https://www.verywellmind.com/thmb/SywTupIXgN9fYm3VhUTE8EGgyVY=/2121x0/filters:no_upscale():max_bytes(150000):strip_icc()/GettyImages-745831421-0411a5826efc4121a2477f7a49c82350.jpg.

7.5.2. Influence on Academic and Occupational Functioning

The impacts of obsessive-compulsive and related disorders (OCRDs) on scholastic performance cannot be overestimated. Such students are prone to having intensified anxiety and compulsive symptomatology that mostly disrupts their capacity for focus and learning. This challenge is further exacerbated in rigorous academic environments, where the pressure to perform only acts to magnify symptoms of anxiety. For example, students may engage in repetitive off-task behavior, such as compulsive checking of work or constant studying of notes, which consumes valuable study time and disrupts the process of learning. Therefore, OCRDs can manifest as low academic achievement, truancy, and dropout, necessitating specialized interventions that aim to build academic resilience in the affected individuals. In professional environments, OCRDs also create huge barriers to employee productivity and overall job satisfaction. Workers with obsessive-compulsive tendencies may suffer from the hindrances of perfectionism and excessive preoccupation with their assignments, which can cause delays in completing projects and increase the stress factor. In highly stressful professions, such as medical or teaching, these characteristics may lead to burnout and impairment of job performance. Furthermore, the stigmatization of mental health can potentially isolate such individuals further and give rise to treatment evasion for their illness. Interestingly enough, research concludes that intervention by means of systemic support systems, such as accommodations to the workplace and mental health services, can work against these conditions. The intricate interaction between OCRDs and work functioning is essential in learning how to implement productive interventions in promoting mental health in the workplace. The COVID-19 pandemic has exacerbated the impact of OCRDs on academic and vocational functioning, and an urgent need for integrated strategies to counteract these issues. While institutions adapted to online learning and working, individuals encountered amplified stressors , such as loneliness, ambiguity, and disruptions in their structured lives. In this new setting, risks for academic failure and vocational malfunction escalated, as conventional coping resources became limited. The occurrence of maladaptive behaviors , such as excessive screen time or drug use, as coping strategies during lockdown has been proposed to be a concern (Oály et al., 2020). Furthermore, literature highlights that frontline healthcare professionals, and most importantly nurses, are more likely to experience poor mental health outcomes due to the co-occurring load of OCRDs and pandemic stressors (Johannes et al., 2021). This environment demands creative solutions that involve the use of digital aids and supporting mechanisms focused on enhancing resilience and psychological wellness.

7.5.3. Coping Mechanisms and Strategies

Coping skills and coping strategies are essential in the treatment of obsessive-compulsive and other disorders because of the interdependence of psychological states and compulsive behavior. Patients with these conditions are likely to exhibit maladaptive coping techniques, such as avoidance or ritualistic behaviors, whose purpose is anxiety reduction following intrusive thoughts. Deficient coping techniques have been shown to increase symptoms as well as enhance the disorder's severity. For instance, measures taken to relieve short-term distress could have long-term effects that lead to vicious cycles of compulsion and obsession. Adaptive coping strategies need to be created to enable individuals to cope with anxiety and thereby decrease the dependence on compulsive action towards universal welfare. Psychological therapies have helped equip humans with strategies to properly handle obsessive-compulsive and associated disorders. Cognitive Behavior Therapy (CBT) especially targets cognitive distortions and dysfunctional thinking, allowing patients to challenge their obsessional thoughts directly while reducing compulsive behaviors simultaneously. The therapy induces exposure and response prevention as integral parts of the treatment, allowing individuals to learn to expose themselves in small steps to feared objects or situations without performing compulsive rituals. Enhanced coping behaviors, including mindfulness and stress management competencies, allow individuals to deal with anxiety-provoking situations more effectively. Moreover, research results evidence that the use of such cognitive techniques with pharmacological interventions enhances overall treatment outcomes, resulting in an improved and multi-dimensional approach towards treating obsessive-compulsive disorders. The presence of psychological distress in patients suffering from conditions , such as noncardiac chest pain highlights the need to target both psychological and physiological dimensions in mind while considering coping approaches and mechanisms.

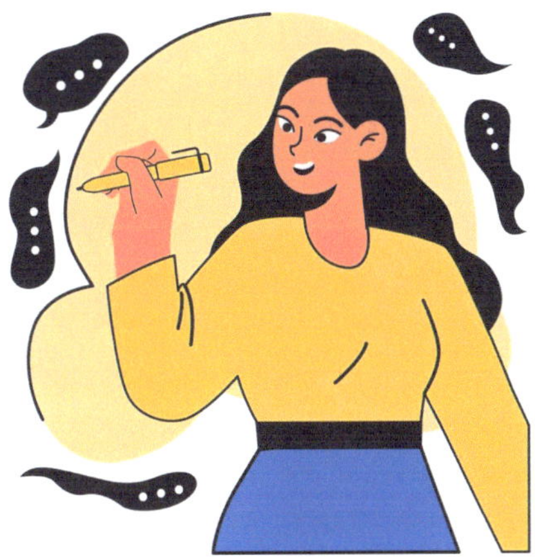

Figure 7.14. Coping mechanism.

Source: https://static.vecteezy.com/system/resources/previews/047/093/388/non_2x/coping-mechanism-emotional-intelligence-strategy-to-face-of-stress-vector.jpg.

Research suggests that disorders , such as depression and anxiety are often comorbid with disorders , such as obsessive-compulsive disorder in the patient, thus complicating coping mechanisms. Personalized strategies involving identification and change of maladaptive emotional processes can help improve coping substantially. Further, awareness of psychological phenomena , such as hypervigilance and altered perception of pain, allows for specially designed intervention. As pointed out by studies focusing on the interrelationship between psychological state and physical symptoms, understanding such dynamics is crucial in supporting the facilitation of effective coping strategies, consequently managing the broader spectrum of obsessive-compulsive and related disorders' symptoms (Gonzalez-Ibarra et al., 2024) (Figure 7.14).

Test Your Knowledge

1. How do obsessions and compulsions interfere with daily functioning, productivity, and interpersonal relationships?
2. What challenges do individuals with OCD face regarding time management, emotional distress, and social stigma?

7.6. Current Research and Developments

Learning Outcome

1. Advances in understanding the neurobiology.
2. Emerging treatment modalities.
3. The role of technology in therapy.

Emerging advances toward the understanding of obsessive-compulsive spectrum disorders (OCSDs) have enlightened the intricate relationships between sleep disturbance and OCSDs. Research highlights dysregulation of cortico-striatal-thalamo-cortical (CSTC) neurocircuitry as a unifying foundation for OCSDs, chronic tic disorders, and attention-deficit/hyperactivity disorder (ADHD). The significance of sleep research is serious, showing that patients with OCSDs subjectively complain of insomnia and other movement disorders of sleep. However, much of this research has yet to embrace polysomnographic methods, limiting the objectivity of sleep measurement. Closing these gaps by describing the neural pathways between OCSDs and sleep will allow for more accurate interventions, which will increase treatment effectiveness for both base disorders and sleep symptoms, both of which are often intertwined in individuals affected (Margaret et al., 2025). Further, the study of animal models has also come a long way, shedding greater light on the neurobiological substrate of obsessive-compulsive disorder (OCD). With the creation of transgenic models, researchers have begun to reveal the complex molecular profiles seen in OCD. The models enable the identification of the particular gene mutations for the disorder and correlating them with changes in affected brain regions and neural circuits. Despite the advances made, the research community still faces challenges due to the heterogeneity of model phenotypes, something that can obscure the development of personalized therapeutic strategies. Current approaches aim to refine these models so that they are more relevant and applicable, thus creating opportunities for new activities in treatment strategies. By the systematic alleviation of these limitations, researchers hope to further open up the pathophysiological mechanisms of OCD, ultimately allowing for more effective interventions (Huang et al., 2025). In addition to furthering knowledge in basic research, a greater emphasis is being put on integrating neuromodulation treatments and surgical treatments into the treatment approach to OCD. Frontline therapies today are medication and cognitive-behavioral therapy, but for many, they fail to work, and new research directions are sought. Neuromodulation techniques, such as deep brain stimulation, have been delineated for their ability to directly modulate pathological neural pathways. While more invasive, surgery may be a final option for treatment-refractory patients. As the research continues, it is also important to assess the long-term effects and safety profiles of these novel treatments. Through this holistic method, combining both novel research and careful clinical assessment, hope for significantly enhancing the quality of life of patients afflicted with OCD and other related disorders arises (Huang et al., 2025).

7.6.1. Advances in the Neurobiology

The research into the neurobiology of obsessive-compulsive and related disorders has advanced significantly in the last decade, providing new information on complex mechanisms behind such conditions. Technical improvements in neuroimaging, particularly functional magnetic resonance imaging (fMRI) and positron emission tomography (PET), have provided insight into dynamic cortico-subcortical interactions, crucial to the understanding of the pathophysiology of these conditions. These technologies allow scientists to chart activity in regions , such as the orbitofrontal cortex, striatum, and anterior cingulate cortex, which are involved in the activity of compulsive behavior and decision-making processes. Compiling these data with behavioral studies helps shed light on how aberrant neural activity might help lead to persistence of obsessions and compulsions, thus finding possible targets for better treatments. Modern developments also reveal the neurochemical elements that impact obsessive-compulsive disorders, particularly the neurotransmitter elements , such as serotonin and dopamine. These neurochemicals are instrumental in managing mood, behavior, and cognitive functions related to compulsions and impulses. It has been established that serotonergic dysfunction is largely responsible for the emergence of OCD symptoms and therefore, selective serotonin reuptake inhibitors (SSRIs) have been made the cornerstone of drug therapy. Second, the connection between the dopaminergic and the compulsive behavior characteristically found in OCD has been underscored as a potential causative explanation of the inability to cease the compulsions. An understanding of these connections between behavior and neurobiology is necessary for clinicians to be able to provide more personalized treatments so that they can better treat the mechanisms and symptoms of the disorder more comprehensively. In their work on the concepts of impulsivity and compulsivity, previous research has highlighted their commutative nature in the neurocognitive functioning model. Although these have been classically viewed as opposing traits, impulsivity as failing to think in advance and being risky, and compulsivity as an excessive drive towards averting harm, they are common in neuropsychological processes, particularly cortico-subcortical circuits. Recent studies identify the fact that thought and action inhibition impairment may lead to both impulsive and to compulsive behavior, attributing sophistication to both. These findings are essential to resolving the subtleties of behavior observed in obsessive-compulsive and spectrum disorders, guiding possible future investigation to identify common neural circuits and potential treatment regimes that can be used with patients showing evidence of both impulsivity and compulsivity in their behavioral presentation, as hypothesized by current advancements in cognitive and clinical neuroscience (Fineberg et al., 2014) (Figure 7.15).

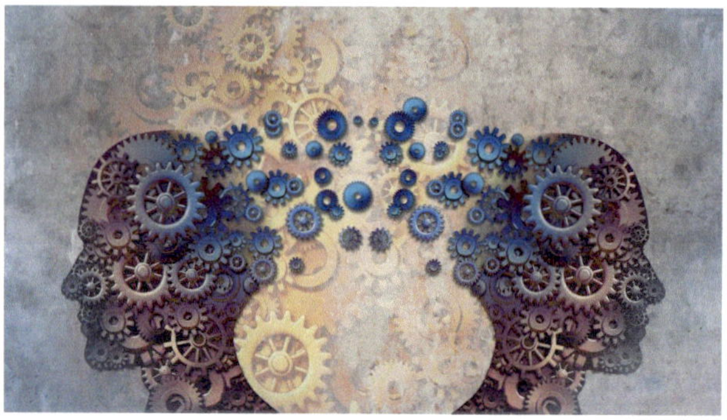

Figure 7.15. Advances in understanding the neurobiology underlying obsessive-compulsive disorder.

Source: https://cdn.sanity.io/images/0vv8moc6/psychtimes/2be82b531fe942d077671d1724e12808185e456d-1000x549.jpg?fit=crop&auto=format.

7.6.2. Emerging Treatment Modalities

The treatment scenario of Obsessive-Compulsive Disorder (OCD) and spectrum disorders has begun to shift significantly with the establishment of novel modalities complementing conventional protocols. Among them, Magnetic Resonance Imaging-guided Focused Ultrasound (MRgFUS) has presented a thought-provoking alternative. The procedure offers incisionless neurosurgical procedures, such as bilateral capsulotomy, which have shown promise in successfully targeting brain regions implicated in OCD and major depressive disorder. Initial reports indicate that MRgFUS is not only safe but also highly effective, and it is a cutting-edge treatment for patients whose ailments have proven to be unresponsive to traditional methods. Hence, care of parameters of effective lesioning, such as skull density ratio and angle of incidence, is essential to ensure maximum selection of patients for this novel treatment, possibly promoting the outcome for these disabling disorders (Davidson et al., 2020). In addition to MRgFUS, these new treatments also include internet-delivered Cognitive Behavioral Therapy (CBT) and Acceptance and Commitment Therapy (ACT), which have recently been identified for their effectiveness for the treatment of Body Dysmorphic Disorder (BDD) and related impulse-control disorders. Treatment via virtual platforms has provided the choice of treatment to individuals who may face challenges in attending in-person consultations, for example, stigma or mobility issues. These strategies leverage the convenience and flexibility technology provides to expose individuals to evidence-based methods in the comfort of their own homes.

Promising outcomes from research into the efficacy of online CBT when utilized alongside traditional modalities underscore the potential of such interventions in achieving an in-depth remission of the chronic and often disabling course of BDD, thereby improving the quality of life for patients involved (Sharma et al., 2019). More research on new treatment methods is the top priority as the science works to refine treatment measures for obsessive-compulsive and related disorders. Notably, treatment-resistant patients remain at the forefront of concerns; thus, treatments like repetitive Transcranial Magnetic Stimulation (rTMS) are becoming increasingly popular as possible alternatives. The non-invasive treatment aims to alleviate symptoms in those previously inadequately treated with pharmacotherapy or psychotherapy. Evidence indicates that rTMS, when added to conventional treatments, can lead to significant symptom reduction and significantly improve patient engagement. As clinicians continue to investigate the efficacy and safety profiles of these devices, as well as the neurobiological underpinnings on which they operate, the discipline is poised for advances that may, in the end, redefine treatment for obsessive-compulsive and related disorders (Sharma et al., 2019; Davidson et al., 2020).

7.6.3. The Role of Technology in Therapy

As mental health treatment evolves in the world, technology more and more starring role in the therapeutic intervention space, particularly for those who are seeking to break through the Obsessive-Compulsive and Related Disorders (OCRDs). Online communities, such as mobile apps and teletherapy treatment, have been valuable options for both treatment professionals and clients. The technology facilitates access to information and support previously unavailable. For example, self-help apps can give patients CBT skills specifically tailored for the treatment of obsessive-compulsive disorder, hence enabling them to apply coping skills on their own. Additionally, virtual reality is also being researched as a way of exposing people to their particular fear in a simulated environment where they can learn to confront their obsession safely, hence demonstrating how technology can complement conventional therapeutic interventions. The therapeutic potential of technology is considerably bolstered by data-driven approaches that render treatment more personalized. With the use of wearables and mobile sensors, clinicians can collect moment-by-moment data on a patient's habits and symptoms and thus design more tailored intervention plans. This personalization is particularly relevant in the context of OCRDs, where patient-specific compulsions and triggers could be profoundly dissimilar between patients. Technologies that enable symptom monitoring on a continuous basis enable treatments to be rapidly changed to meet the evolving needs of patients, ultimately enabling a greater likelihood of successful therapeutic outcomes. Additionally, the incorporation of artificial intelligence in therapy models holds the potential to further enhance treatment planning by allowing patient responses to be predicted based on prior experience, enhancing overall therapeutic experience. However, while technology offers numerous benefits in dealing with and treating OCRDs, it is imperative to critically evaluate its role in mental health treatment. As Brand et al. (2019) describes, the development of habitual behavior associated with cue-reactivity and decision-making is increasingly influenced by digital activity. This impact can present a two-edged challenge: technology can be used to enable treatment of OCD with personalized treatments, but it might also contribute in an indirect way to maladaptive behavioral plans in the event of being unchecked or unjustified. As Claudia et al. (2019) has further noted, special stress working in high-stakes environments imposes on people, including top athletes, necessitates understanding the intersection of physical performance and mental health. Consequently, mental health professionals are obligated to attempt, as best as they can, to weigh the technological opportunities for therapeutic benefit against the potential evils so that treatment for OCRDs is both effective and thorough.

Test Your Knowledge

1. What new insights from neuroimaging and genetics are shaping current understanding of OCD?
2. How are emerging treatments—such as deep brain stimulation, digital therapeutics, and precision medicine—advancing OCD management?

SUMMARY

The quest for obsessive-compulsive and comorbid disorders highlights the complexity of mental health diseases and points toward the necessity of holistic approaches to understanding and treatment. As has been demonstrated through research, processes like emotion regulation and attachment style are crucial in the development of disorders like Obsessive-Compulsive Disorder (OCD). The intercorrelation between attachment anxiety and avoidance, mediated through emotion regulation deficits, has implications that emotional well-being must be a key component of clinical assessment and intervention strategy. Prioritizing these elements enables practitioners to better address the resultant psychosocial disturbances underpinning the existence of OCD symptoms, thereby enhancing the efficacy of treatment programs (Nielsen et al., 2025). Also, personality disorder prevalence, particularly Obsessive-Compulsive Personality Disorder (OCPD), shows high correlations with stress-related mental illness , such as depression and burnout. The longitudinal study findings point toward the importance of recognizing OCPD traits , such as perfectionism, because they may exacerbate the stress response and further complicate attempts at recovery. Therefore, treatment plans should be specially designed by clinicians taking into consideration not only OCD symptoms but also addressing broader psychological structures related to personality disorders. Integrating awareness of OCPD in intervention may contribute to improved understanding of patients' lives and better long-term mental health results (Reinhardt et al., 2023). Finally, the interaction between individual differences, emotional processes, and more general psychological variables in obsessive-compulsive and comorbid disorders demands an interdisciplinary research and treatment strategy. As mechanisms underlying these disorders are increasingly understood, future research should endeavor to employ longitudinal designs in order to elucidate causal interactions between emotion dysregulation, attachment styles, and symptom development. Moreover, clinicians are encouraged to be sensitive to personality characteristics that make treatment trajectories more challenging. These factors will not only sharpen our theoretical model but also have significant practical implications, as interventions will be both focused and effective at alleviating the burdens of these debilitating disorders.

Obsessive-compulsive and spectrum disorders present a broad spectrum of clinical presentations that have a substantial effect on the daily functioning of individuals. Different clinical presentations of the disorders, including obsessive-compulsive disorder (OCD), body dysmorphic disorder (BDD), and hoarding disorder, have a shared underlying factor of intrusive thoughts and repetitive behavior designed to reduce anxiety. It is essential to know the prevalence and clinical features of these disorders in the development of appropriate treatments. There has been an increased frequency of mental illness issues, such as obsessive-compulsive disorder, particularly in stressful periods like the period of the COVID-19 pandemic, as revealed by recent studies. The higher prevalence indicates the necessity of adopting an integrative mode to cure the disorders appropriately and address the psychological distress experienced by the patients under extreme life stressors (Nochaiwong et al., 2021). The relationship between stress and worsening of obsessive-compulsive symptoms has been of interest in recent literature. According to research, environmental stimulation, including traumatic incidents or pandemics, has been determined as triggers to the onset or exacerbation of such disorders. Recent information on mental health within the COVID-19 pandemic revealed shocking increases in anxiety and stress symptoms, with profound implications for those at risk of obsessive-compulsive disorders. For example, OCD patients may have an exacerbation of their compulsions instigated by ambiguity and fear amidst adversity, affirming multifactorial causation of such illnesses. Such knowledge helps to illustrate the necessity of tailored treatments responsive to the evolving psychological landscape created by record-breaking global adversity (Rogers et al., 2020). In general, obsessive-compulsive and co-morbid disorders are complex disorders and require a complex understanding of their causal processes and determinants. Recent research not only sheds light on the extent and diversity of such disorders but also stresses the significance of contextual determinants, such as public health emergencies. As higher rates of mental illness are surfacing due to the COVID-19 pandemic, clinicians must concentrate on holistic treatment techniques that involve cognitive-behavioral therapy combined with medication management if necessary, patient-specifically. Moreover, the critical examination of social and economic determinants and their interaction with mental health during and outside emergencies will enhance the efficacy of interventions to reduce the burden of obsessive-compulsive and related disorders for affected people and society as a whole (Nochaiwong et al., 2021).

KEY TERMS FROM THIS CHAPTER

- Avoidance behavior
- Body dysmorphic disorder
- Checking behavior
- Cognitive distortions
- Compulsions
- Contamination fear
- Excoriation disorder
- Exposure and response prevention
- Habit reversal training
- Hoarding disorder
- Insight
- Intrusive thoughts
- Obsessions
- Obsessive-compulsive disorder (OCD)

CRITICAL THINKING QUESTIONS

1. **Obsessions in OCD are best defined as:**
   a. Repetitive behaviors that relieve stress
   b. Unwanted, intrusive thoughts or urges
   c. Flashbacks from traumatic events
   d. Memory problems due to anxiety
2. **Compulsions are:**
   a. Delusions of grandeur
   b. Sudden mood changes
   c. Repetitive actions aimed at reducing distress
   d. Hallucinations experienced during stress
3. **Which of the following is a common compulsion in OCD?**
   a. Visual hallucinations
   b. Excessive handwashing
   c. Recurrent nightmares
   d. Paranoia
4. **Body Dysmorphic Disorder is characterized by:**
   a. Fear of public places
   b. Repetitive hair pulling
   c. Preoccupation with a perceived physical defect
   d. Obsession with cleanliness
5. **The first-line pharmacological treatment for OCD is usually:**
   a. Antipsychotics
   b. Benzodiazepines
   c. Mood stabilizers
   d. Selective serotonin reuptake inhibitors (SSRIs)

Short Answer Questions

1. What is the key difference between an obsession and a compulsion?
2. Give two examples of common obsessions experienced by individuals with OCD.
3. What are typical compulsions, and how do they help the person with OCD?
4. Which brain region is often associated with obsessive-compulsive disorder in neuroimaging studies?
5. How does Body Dysmorphic Disorder (BDD) differ from OCD, even though it is in the same category?

Answer to Critical Thinking Questions

1. (b) 2. (c) 3. (b) 4. (c) 5. (d)

REFERENCES

1. Gillan, C. M., Fineberg, N. A., & Robbins, T. W. (2017). A trans-diagnostic perspective on obsessive-compulsive disorder. *Psychological medicine*, *47*(9), 1528–1548. https://doi.org/10.1017/S0033291716002786(accessed on 28th July 2025).
2. Al-Na'she, M., Massad, A., Al Khraisat, L., Al Rafai, M., Albashtawi, Y., Almohtasib, S., Alhayek, A., et al. (2024). Prevalence of obsessive-compulsive personality disorder in medical students. *Jordan Medical Journal.* https://www.semanticscholar.org/paper/53be28cccde25b907a41ad9c483b741b42105d5e (accessed on 28th July 2025).
3. Algin, S., Ahmed, T., Reza, M. M., Akter, A., Tanzilla, N. J., Haq, M. A., Ahmad, R., et al. (2025). Evaluating treatment outcomes of vitamin B12 and folic acid supplementation in obsessive-compulsive disorder patients with deficiencies: A comparative analysis. *Cureus, 17.* https://www.semanticscholar.org/paper/4d58f75ac73ac14062a1a3e2d93945683326c132 (accessed on 28th July 2025).
4. Arnold, P. D., Benedetti, F., Bertolin, S., Beucke, J. C., et al. (2020). An overview of the first 5 years of the ENIGMA obsessive–compulsive disorder working group: The power of worldwide collaboration. https://core.ac.uk/download/358463471.pdf (accessed on 28th July 2025).
5. Aspvall, K., Andersson, E., Melin, K., Norlin, L. M., Eriksson, V., Vigerland, S., Jolstedt, M., et al. (2021). Effect of an internet-delivered stepped-care program vs in-person cognitive behavioral therapy on obsessive-compulsive disorder symptoms in children and adolescents: A randomized clinical trial. *JAMA, 325*(18), 1863–1873. https://www.semanticscholar.org/paper/71d913ea25ddfaa26305e2f7cc33bd07bb6f6bff (accessed on 28th July 2025).
6. Van Dael, F., van Os, J., de Graaf, R., ten Have, M., Krabbendam, L., & Myin-Germeys, I. (2011). Can obsessions drive you mad? Longitudinal evidence that obsessive-compulsive symptoms worsen the outcome of early psychotic experiences. *Acta psychiatrica Scandinavica*, *123*(2), 136–146. https://doi.org/10.1111/j.1600-0447.2010.01609.x(accessed on 28th July 2025).
7. Avasthi, A., & Grover, S. (2018). Clinical practice guidelines for management of depression in elderly. *Indian Journal of Psychiatry, 60*, 341–341. https://doi.org/10.4103/0019-5545.224474 (accessed on 28th July 2025).
8. Beck, J., Barnett, K., Nottingham, K., Friend, K., Nunnally, K., Rachman, S., & Thorpe, S. J. (2010). The mediating roles of disgust sensitivity and danger expectancy in relation to hand washing behavior. https://core.ac.uk/download/9633104.pdf (accessed on 28th July 2025).
9. Billieux, J., Brand, M., Burkauskas, J., Carmi, L., et al. (2018). Manifesto for a European research network into problematic usage of the Internet. https://core.ac.uk/download/287581533.pdf (accessed on 28th July 2025).
10. Boger, S., Ehring, T., Berberich, G., & Werner, G. G. (2020). Impact of childhood maltreatment on obsessive-compulsive disorder symptom severity and treatment outcome. *European Journal of Psychotraumatology, 11.* https://doi.org/10.1080/20008198.2020.1753942 (accessed on 28th July 2025).
11. Brand, M., Wegmann, E., Stark, R., Müller, A., Wölfling, K., Robbins, T. W., & Potenza, M. N. (2019). The interaction of person-affect-cognition-execution (I-PACE) model for addictive behaviors: Update, generalization to addictive behaviors beyond internet-use disorders, and specification of the process character of addictive behaviors. *Neuroscience & Biobehavioral*

Reviews, 104, 1–10. https://doi.org/10.1016/j.neubiorev.2019.06.032 (accessed on 28th July 2025).

12. Brown, C. H. (2013). Expanding the spectrum of impulse control disorders in Parkinson's disease: The phenomenology of sweet craving. https://open.bu.edu/bitstream/2144/12061/6/Brown_Caitlin_2013_nosig_nocv.pdf (accessed on 28th July 2025).
13. Chamberlain, S. R., Derbyshire, K. L., Grant, J. E., Leppink, E. W., et al. (2014). Impaired response inhibition and excess cortical thickness as candidate endophenotypes for trichotillomania. https://core.ac.uk/download/77407772.pdf (accessed on 28th July 2025).
14. Chernoff, C., Belin-Rauscent, A., Puaud, M., Torrisi, S., Fouyssac, M., Németh, B., Yu, C. Z., et al. (2025). Compulsive coping behavior, which goal trackers do not develop, is exacerbated by chronic atomoxetine. *bioRxiv.* https://www.semanticscholar.org/paper/a345c528d61da7d8faf1b2b59f420bb0947f2758 (accessed on 28th July 2025).
15. Conlon, K. E., Harper, J., Pollard, C. A., VanDyke, M., et al. (2015). Brief consultation to families of treatment refusers with symptoms of obsessive-compulsive disorder: Does it impact family accommodation and quality of life? https://core.ac.uk/download/232208640.pdf (accessed on 28th July 2025).
16. Davidson, B., Mithani, K., Huang, Y., Jones, R., Goubran, M., Meng, Y., Snell, J., et al. (2020). Technical and radiographic considerations for magnetic resonance imaging-guided focused ultrasound capsulotomy. *Journal of Neurosurgery.* https://www.semanticscholar.org/paper/dac70712d2a0598a091fc1d0875f7f6ae645056d (accessed on 28th July 2025).
17. De Kock, J. H., Latham, H. A., Leslie, S. J., Grindle, M., Munoz, S. A., Ellis, L., Polson, R., et al. (2021). A rapid review of the impact of COVID-19 on the mental health of healthcare workers: Implications for supporting psychological well-being. *BMC Public Health, 21.* https://doi.org/10.1186/s12889-020-10070-3 (accessed on 28th July 2025).
18. Endres, D., Pollak, T., Bechter, K., Denzel, D., Pitsch, K., Nickel, K., Runge, K., et al. (2022). Immunological causes of obsessive-compulsive disorder: Is it time for the concept of an "autoimmune OCD" subtype? *Translational Psychiatry, 12.* https://www.semanticscholar.org/paper/31cab16ef096ebf7874acf899c177dc9f84e2f41 (accessed on 28th July 2025).
19. O'Neill, J., & Feusner, J. D. (2015). Cognitive-behavioral therapy for obsessive-compulsive disorder: access to treatment, prediction of long-term outcome with neuroimaging. *Psychology research and behavior management, 8*, 211–223. https://doi.org/10.2147/PRBM.S75106(accessed on 28th July 2025).
20. Fineberg, N., Chamberlain, S. R., Goudriaan, A. E., Stein, D. J., Vanderschuren, L. J. M. J., Gillan, C. M., Shekar, S., et al. (2014). New developments in human neurocognition: Clinical, genetic, and brain imaging correlates of impulsivity and compulsivity. *CNS Spectrums, 19*, 69–89. https://doi.org/10.1017/s1092852913000801 (accessed on 28th July 2025).
21. Furtado, G., Da Silva, D. B., & Sobral, F. (2022). Canine psychiatry: The importance of approaches to animal psychopathologies. *Environmental Smoke.* https://www.semanticscholar.org/paper/8ab6c0d876fcc47687476bda87b2b22ef7bda94a (accessed on 28th July 2025).
22. Galvez-Sánchez, C. M., Duschek, S., & Reyes del Paso, G. A. (2019). Psychological impact of fibromyalgia: Current perspectives. *Psychology Research and Behavior Management, 12*, 117–127. https://doi.org/10.2147/prbm.s178240 (accessed on 28th July 2025).

23. Gonzalez-Ibarra, F., Cruz-Ruiz, M., Murillo Llanes, J., Achem, S., & Fass, R. (2024). The role of psychological factors in noncardiac chest pain of esophageal origin. *Journal of Neurogastroenterology and Motility, 30*, 272–280. https://www.semanticscholar.org/paper/44119c47375cc371e1a83475cf43c32d9036d0ea (accessed on 28th July 2025).

24. Greenberg, J. L., Hoeppner, S. S., Phillips, K. A., Steketee, G., et al. (2019). Predictors of response to cognitive-behavioral therapy for body dysmorphic disorder. https://open.bu.edu/bitstream/2144/40196/3/Greenberg%20CBT%20BDD%20Predictors.pdf (accessed on 28th July 2025).

25. Hall, M. D., Gipson, K. S., Gipson, S., Colvin, M. K., Nguyen, S. T. T., & Greenberg, E. (2025). Disrupted cortico-striato-thalamo-cortical circuitry and sleep disturbances in obsessive-compulsive spectrum, chronic tic, and attention-deficit/hyperactivity disorders. *Harvard Review of Psychiatry, 33*, 114–126. https://www.semanticscholar.org/paper/142a971ba048cbea22c97de29292044c6808ea79 (accessed on 28th July 2025).

26. Härpfer, K., Carsten, H. P., Kausche, F. M., & Riesel, A. (2025). Enhanced performance monitoring as a transdiagnostic risk marker of the anxiety and obsessive–compulsive spectrum: The role of disorder category, clinical status, family risk, and anxiety dimensions. *Depression and Anxiety, 2025.* https://www.semanticscholar.org/paper/f4151008702414359a92b361e442be760ed56a09 (accessed on 28th July 2025).

27. He, I. R., Gaillard, A., & Rossell, S. L. (2025). Addressing body dysmorphic disorder through mindfulness: A new therapeutic frontier. *Australian & New Zealand Journal of Psychiatry, 59*, 405–412. https://www.semanticscholar.org/paper/aa73f18102a398734a286180c02842379a5dddd1 (accessed on 28th July 2025).

28. Hosseini, S. A. ., Nasri, M., & Dastgerdi , R. . (2025). Comparison of the Effectiveness of Cognitive-Behavioral Therapy and Short-Term Psychodynamic Therapy on Cognitive Fusion and Obsessive-Compulsive Symptoms in Individuals with Obsessive-Compulsive Disorder. Health Nexus, 3(1), 45-54. https://doi.org/10.61838/kman.hn.3.1.6(accessed on 28th July 2025).

29. Hosseini, S. A., Nasri, M., & Dastjerdi, R. (2025). Comparison of the effectiveness of cognitive behavioral therapy and short-term psychodynamic therapy in reducing alexithymia and impulsivity in individuals with obsessive-compulsive disorder. *KMAN Counseling and Psychology Nexus.* https://www.semanticscholar.org/paper/fff31dd2d85a47e7058c6fd02a19514ccd7ed05c (accessed on 28th July 2025).

30. Huang, X., Xiao, L. L., Wang, M., Wu, Y., Deng, H., & Wang, W. (2025). Advancing obsessive–compulsive disorder research: Insights from transgenic animal models and innovative therapies. *Brain Sciences, 15.* https://www.semanticscholar.org/paper/afb9d401206afdb2e20af4890cbc43499e89ffaf (accessed on 28th July 2025).

31. Huang, Y., Weng, Y., Lan, L., Zhu, C., Shen, T., Tang, W., & Lai, H. Y. (2023). Insight in obsessive-compulsive disorder: Conception, clinical characteristics, neuroimaging, and treatment. *Psychoradiology, 3.* https://www.semanticscholar.org/paper/aa459f661beb8d263e3dab1ef93b38f146283539 (accessed on 28th July 2025).

32. Khvatkov, A. A., & Medvedev, V. E. (2024). Features of the clinic and diagnosis of obsessive-compulsive disorder in children and adolescents. *Spravočnik vrača obŝej praktiki (Journal of Family Medicine).* https://www.semanticscholar.org/paper/24e3735c3d68f61ddcfc335504b926e9d92deaaa (accessed on 28th July 2025).

33. Király, O., Potenza, M. N., Stein, D. J., King, D. L., Hodgins, D. C., Saunders, J. B., Griffiths, M. D., et al. (2020). Preventing problematic internet use during the COVID-19 pandemic: Consensus guidance. *Comprehensive Psychiatry, 100*, 152180–152180. https://doi.org/10.1016/j.comppsych.2020.152180 (accessed on 28th July 2025).

34. Lieneman, C. C., Guastello, A. D., Munson, M., Barthle-Herrera, M., Bailey, B. A., Higham, M., Druskin, L. R., et al. (2024). Conceptualizing co-occurring autism spectrum disorder, obsessive-compulsive disorder, and gender diversity in adolescents: A narrative review. *Journal of Indian Association for Child and Adolescent Mental Health, 20*, 97–110. https://www.semanticscholar.org/paper/3b63414a8ab8fb5104f677bb633fe52ab7d96b38 (accessed on 28th July 2025).

35. McLaughlan, A. D., & Starkey, N. J. (2012). The classification of substance and behavioral addictions: A preliminary investigation. https://core.ac.uk/download/29200830.pdf (accessed on 28th July 2025).

36. Nielsen, S. K., Stuart, A. C., Winding, C., Pedersen, M. Ø., Daniel, S. I. F., Vangkilde, S., Rosenberg, N., et al. (2025). Adult attachment style, emotion regulation and obsessive-compulsive disorder – A preliminary cross-sectional mediational investigation of an attachment-based model. *Clinical Psychology & Psychotherapy, 32*(1), e70031. https://www.semanticscholar.org/paper/99724355f73b2ac8854e691b549e127e5d4279ee (accessed on 28th July 2025).

37. Nochaiwong, S., Ruengorn, C., Thavorn, K., Hutton, B., Awiphan, R., Phosuya, C., Ruanta, Y., et al. (2021). Global prevalence of mental health issues among the general population during the coronavirus disease-2019 pandemic: A systematic review and meta-analysis. *Scientific Reports, 11.* https://doi.org/10.1038/s41598-021-89700-8 (accessed on 28th July 2025).

38. Pattiselanno, P. P., & Basuki, R. (2025). Obsessions: A screenplay on obsessive compulsive disorder's impact on relationships. *k@ta kita.* https://www.semanticscholar.org/paper/d11782ac7a061121e87530c4f89fef9f8c1c2828 (accessed on 28th July 2025).

39. Pop-Jordanova, N. (2019). Different clinical expression of anxiety disorders in children and adolescents: Assessment and treatment. *PRILOZI, 40*, 5–40. https://doi.org/10.2478/prilozi-2019-0001 (accessed on 28th July 2025).

40. Racz, J. I., Mathieu, S. L., McKenzie, M., & Farrell, L. J. (2022). Pediatric obsessive–compulsive disorder and comorbid body dysmorphic disorder: Clinical expression and treatment response. *Child Psychiatry and Human Development, 54*, 1005–1014. https://www.semanticscholar.org/paper/d2a021c80c6b0ad54be8bd329b95e59869905bbd (accessed on 28th July 2025).

41. Rajachandrasekar, B., & Vaiyapuri, S. (2023). Rating scales in psychiatric disorders–why? *International Journal of Community Medicine and Public Health.* https://www.semanticscholar.org/paper/1d57fec455ac96d90081e650b2e4311845a2f317 (accessed on 28th July 2025).

42. Reardon, C. L., Hainline, B., Aron, C. M., Baron, D., Baum, A., Bindra, A., Budgett, R., et al. (2019). Mental health in elite athletes: International Olympic Committee consensus statement (2019). *British Journal of Sports Medicine, 53*, 667–699. https://doi.org/10.1136/bjsports-2019-100715 (accessed on 28th July 2025).

43. Reinhardt, P., Ellbin, S., Carlander, A., Hadžibajramović, E., Jonsdottir, I., & Lindqvist Bagge, A. (2023). Is the road to burnout paved with perfectionism? The prevalence of obsessive-compulsive personality disorder in a clinical longitudinal sample of female patients with stress-related exhaustion. *Journal of Clinical Psychology.* https://www.semanticscholar.org/paper/d51049b9c4bdd4e4edb2773efca49afb1a53932f (accessed on 28th July 2025).

44. Rogers, J., Chesney, E., Oliver, D., Pollak, T. A., McGuire, P., Fusar-Poli, P., Zandi, M. S., et al. (2020). Psychiatric and neuropsychiatric presentations associated with severe coronavirus infections: A systematic review and meta-analysis with comparison to the COVID-19 pandemic. *The Lancet Psychiatry, 7*, 611–627. https://doi.org/10.1016/s2215-0366(20)30203-0 (accessed on 28th July 2025).

45. Schurger, A., Hu, P., Pak, J., & Roskies, A. L. (2021). What is the readiness potential? *Trends in Cognitive Sciences, 25*, 558–570. https://doi.org/10.1016/j.tics.2021.04.001 (accessed on 28th July 2025).

46. Sevda, P., Rajpurohit, S. S., Suthar, N., Gupta, C., & Biyyala, D. (2024). Antidepressant-coincident manic episode in a prepubertal girl presenting with obsessive-compulsive or related disorders: A case report. *BJPsych Open, 10*, S287–S288. https://www.semanticscholar.org/paper/14d20165e7e77673d78afb51cf12d427d0e25b18 (accessed on 28th July 2025).

47. Sharawy, E. (2023). Do changes in personality, mood and behavior need to be incorporated in quality-of-life assessment? *AJOB Neuroscience, 14*, 315–317. https://www.semanticscholar.org/paper/32765b26e059275d1f6857acb18bf2e01791d90e (accessed on 28th July 2025).

48. Sharma, H., Sharma, B., & Patel, N. (2019). Body dysmorphic disorder in adolescents. *Adolescent Psychiatry.* https://www.semanticscholar.org/paper/c7a8e2c2fdd0802b596f8f0376fecf56bfe6864d (accessed on 28th July 2025).

49. Sheikh, M. A., & Alfonso, T. (2025). Mindfulness in treatment-seeking adults with comorbid obsessive-compulsive and major depressive disorders: Mediating effects of obsessive beliefs and mental well-being. *Indian Journal of Psychiatry, 67*, 513–521. https://www.semanticscholar.org/paper/b9f0a2bcbe6c9e6b939f1f3e2b3248204bac2937 (accessed on 28th July 2025).

50. Solmi, M., Raduà, J., Olivola, M., Croce, E., Soardo, L., Salazar de Pablo, G., Shin, J. I., et al. (2021). Age at onset of mental disorders worldwide: Large-scale meta-analysis of 192 epidemiological studies. *Molecular Psychiatry, 27*, 281–295. https://doi.org/10.1038/s41380-021-01161-7 (accessed on 28th July 2025).

51. Torbecke, J., Langhammer, T., Mewes, L., Lueken, U., & Fendel, J. (2024). Augmentation of cognitive-behavioral therapy for obsessive-compulsive and anxiety disorders: A protocol for a systematic review and meta-analysis. *BMJ Open, 14.* https://www.semanticscholar.org/paper/df13649c0a54aa9c66751d8d667eeca2355c879f (accessed on 28th July 2025).

52. Zagami, M., Klepper, E., Wienecke, E., Andrzejewski, M., Sikder, A., Ahmed, A., & Robinson, H. (2023). A review of psych cutaneous disorders from a psychotherapeutic perspective—Toolkit for the dermatologist. *Skin Health and Disease, 3.* https://www.semanticscholar.org/paper/462b9304379e97d3bad7ea77e51f0b698bbad9cb (accessed on 28th July 2025).

TRAUMA- AND STRESSOR-RELATED DISORDERS

8

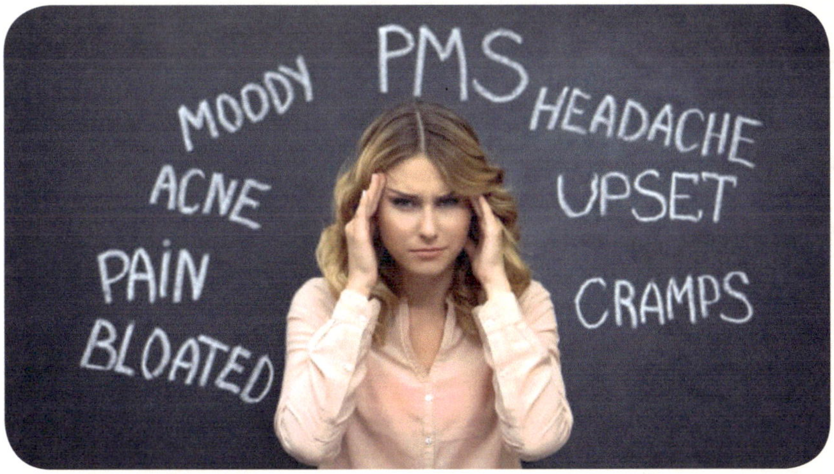

LEARNING OBJECTIVES

After studying this chapter, you will be able to:

1. List the types of trauma- and stressor-related disorders;
2. Describe the causes and risk factors;
3. Identify the symptoms and diagnosis;
4. Explain the impact on daily life;
5. Discuss the treatment options;
6. Explore the prevention and coping strategies.

Introduction

Trauma- and stressor-related disorder is a significant area of study in psychology since it has been established that traumatic experiences have a profound and lasting effect on one's mental health. Some of the disorders that fall under this category include post-traumatic stress disorder (PTSD), acute stress disorder, and adjustment disorders, among others, which are known to follow specific traumatic experiences. The heterogeneity of the disorders lies in the various mechanisms through which individuals react to stressors, influenced by a range of factors , such as personal history, cultural background, and biological vulnerabilities. It is crucial to learn about these mechanisms because they can provide insights into recovery pathways and effective treatments that are tailor-made to each individual. A defining characteristic of trauma- and stressor-related disorders is psychological resilience versus the nature of the experienced stressor. Current literature suggests that highly resilient people are likely to have effective coping mechanisms, which can significantly impact the impact of traumatic experience on mental functioning. For instance, Vietnam veteran studies indicate the significance of intrapersonal resources , such as hardiness and social support in preventing symptoms of PTSD. This trip into resilience underscores determinants of the emergence or exacerbation of trauma-related disorders, necessitating tailored interventions that augment resilience at an individual level and mitigate certain vulnerabilities, as suggested by Adams et al. (1998). Moreover, gender is similarly an important variable in the occurrence and manifestation of trauma-related disorders. Findings indicate that females are more likely to develop PTSD than men, a discrepancy that has stimulated interest in the biological and psychosocial processes underlying the phenomenon.

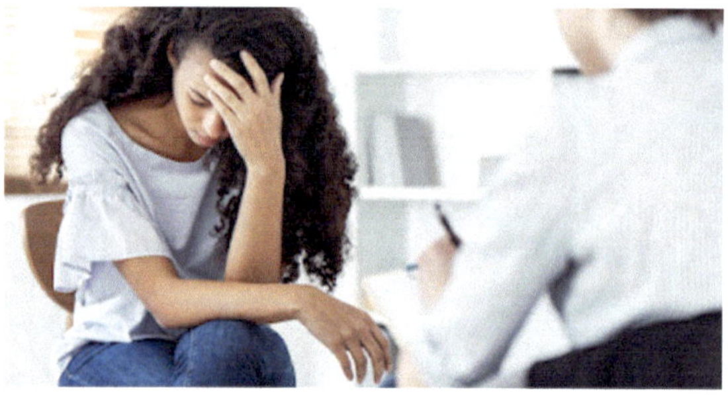

Figure 8.1. Trauma- and stressor-related disorders.

Source: https://external-content.duckduckgo.com/iu/?u=https%3A%2F%2Fblogger.googleusercontent.com%2Fimg%2Fb%2FR29vZ2xl%2FAVvXsEjea3vf53O83baUqZoEw9HK9M40CGnyVIciIFUjnrzE3jfF5KojlLhwmKzFhIJilGJIQ3QJay8YqqGAQB2zc8swYHAfBG0jMl51rjeNCAShb-HJDqq5C1dSkDRBfZ0Ljpvr_2EYFPhSiWbEjjCQe0Um4NJ9FSSIMC69A4I_0uFXKB6wxjVXVROPu45C%2Fw400-h259%2FKUJHU.png&f=1&nofb=1&ipt=bbc47fd779ab61ab500ab9cceb4c58d62a56cda0a5a3e858b0d729065cc860ac.

Research on hormonal influences on female animal model estrous cycles sheds light on the manner in which variables may be playing a contributory role in increased susceptibility to stressors. Findings suggest that interaction between stress response systems and hormonal changes may be to blame for accounting for mechanisms of gender differences in PTSD and hence, making it important to employ a gender-sensitive framework when researching trauma, as indicated by Brumbaugh (2017). Multidisciplinary practice ultimately aims to develop inclusive models of understanding and treating trauma- and stressor-related disorders (Figure 8.1).

Definition of Trauma and Stressor-Related Disorders

Trauma- and stressor-related disorders are different mental conditions that arise following exposure to traumatic events or significant stressors. These conditions are primarily defined according to the failure of an individual to cope with the emotional consequence brought about by ghastly experiences. The Diagnostic and Statistical Manual of Mental Disorders (DSM-5) categorizes these conditions into different categories, including Post-Traumatic Stress Disorder (PTSD), Acute Stress Disorder (ASD), and Adjustment Disorders. All categories reflect the complexity of the human traumatic response, emphasizing the fact that emotional and psychological reactions are extremely variable based on individual circumstances and the type of stressor. Symptom variability and experience highlight the demand for individually specific types of therapy addressing the particular details of the person affected, as cookie-cutter methods may not be sufficient for all patients. It requires a highly developed exploration of the conditions under which trauma- and stressor-related disorders arise to truly understand them. For instance, adjustment disorder (AD), which has long been considered an interim diagnosis, is an essential force in the clinical setting, especially where legal evaluations are required. Research has established that some demographic and clinical variables may influence the prevalence and expression of AD, such as the person's age, gender, and psychiatric illness history. Research on AD patients indicates that major stressors are work and family problems, such that there was a high level of correlation between the life stressors that result in the development of anxiety and mood disorders (Anastasia et al., 2016). The identification of this aspect serves as a significant awareness factor of what causes such disorders that may allow clinicians to come up with more efficacious therapies and care systems for patients. Furthermore, the impact of trauma and stressors is not limited to the individual who experiences them personally but also extends to caregivers and family members. Research has identified that diseases like cancer have the capability of inducing PTSD not only in patients but also in their family members, indicating a wider understanding of trauma (Paleczna, 2017). The multicomponent nature of trauma is emphasized through the need for integrated assessment techniques, recognizing the interdependence of people and social environments. The emphasis on a holistic approach could optimize comprehension and treatment of trauma- and stressor-related disorders. By recognizing the mutual effect of trauma on family and societal groups, health care workers can provide more inclusive care, ultimately enhancing the outcome for all concerned as they adapt to the issues after traumatic events.

Importance of Understanding These Disorders

Knowledge of trauma- and stressor-related disorders is necessary in developing effective treatment interventions and treatment plans. The disorders, such as post-traumatic stress disorder (PTSD), impact individuals in profound ways, resulting in chronic physical and psychological health issues. Effective diagnosis relies on the identification of risk factors for the disorders, as well as past psychological problems and degree of trauma. There is also evidence that implies victims of catastrophic auto accidents, for instance, are at higher risk of developing PTSD. The association between exposure to trauma and the onset of PTSD symptoms underscores the need for mindfulness in preparing mental health professionals with the ability to recognize such specific causes of PTSD so that they can intervene promptly and suitably (Kennedy-Moffat, 1997). Lastly, a greater understanding of these relationships allows clinicians to implement an intensive therapeutic strategy that treats the particular experiences and requirements of every patient. A wider knowledge base regarding trauma- and stressor-related disorders also has significant implications for public health and public safety initiatives. Knowledge about the impact of trauma on mental health can be applied to policy-making and resource planning for prevention. This is especially pertinent with regard to the wide prevalence of PTSD symptoms among specific groups, such as females, who are more statistically probable to be exposed to trauma-related symptoms. For example, it has been shown through research that chronic stress reactions, akin to anxiety disorders, can be induced by biological processes , such as hormonal alterations (Brumbaugh, 2017). As a result, integrating gender-specific research findings into trauma management strategies is instrumental in fostering resilience in at-risk populations. Using a prevention-focused and education-driven model, populations can empower individuals with resources and support systems that enable them to withstand the long-term effects of trauma. Full understanding of trauma- and stressor-related disorders also leads to a healthy perspective of mental well-being. It calls for the incorporation of cross-disciplinary practice among psychologists, social workers, physicians, and policymakers. That collaboration can generate more efficient interventions that address not only symptoms but also causes of trauma. By grasping the interaction between physical health, mental health, and societal forces, practitioners can develop integrative treatment plans that involve community assistance, therapy, and medication interventions. As illuminated by the patterns between trauma exposure, psychological disorder, and healthcare use, a complex comprehension is needed to develop healthy recovery environments for trauma-disordered individuals (Kennedy-Moffat, 1997). Not only does this multifaceted understanding benefit the affected, but it deepens the societal perspective of psychological recovery and resilience (Figure 8.2).

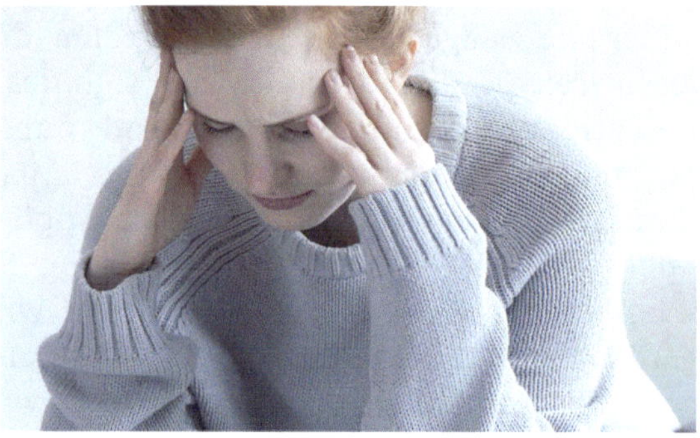

Figure 8.2. Trauma influences mental health.

Source: https://external-content.duckduckgo.com/iu/?u=https%3A%2F%2Fwww.talkingbrainscenter.com%2Fwp-content%2Fuploads%2F2021%2F07%2FTrauma-and-Stressor-Related-Disorders-PTSD-1536x1024.jpg&f=1&nofb=1&ipt=bd6b016a1178ebdc7a04115962a305abb6194823883f155edd37974b0ed04f0f.

8.1. Types of Trauma- and Stressor-Related Disorders

Learning Outcome

1. Post-traumatic stress disorder (PTSD).
2. Acute stress disorder (ASD).
3. Adjustment disorders.

The variety of trauma- and stressor-related disorders is extensive and encompasses disorders that evolve in response to psychologically distressing events. The most commonly recognized disorder is Post-Traumatic Stress Disorder (PTSD), with features , such as ongoing re-living of the traumatic event, avoidance of cues for the trauma, negative cognition and mood changes, and heightened arousal symptoms. The individual can experience flashbacks, nightmares, or extreme emotional distress when he or she is confronted with reminders of the trauma. Research indicates that individuals with a history of multiple exposures to various types of trauma are most likely to have the worst PTSD symptoms, which is due to the complex interplay between trauma exposure and mental health outcome (Brooks et al., 2015). This explains why efficacious therapeutic interventions managing both the trauma experience and psychological impact are highly necessary. There is also a significant class of disorders based on trauma known as Acute Stress Disorder (ASD), which shares many of the same signs as PTSD but occurs in the first month following a traumatic event. Individuals with ASD will have intrusive memories, dissociative reactions, and heightened anxiety, but for a lesser duration than those experiencing PTSD. The two are distinguished in clinical terms since early intervention can prevent the development of PTSD if treated properly. Treatments for ASD address coping skills and stabilization techniques that allow individuals to work through their trauma before symptom worsening, thus altering long-term outcomes (Baird et al., 2021). Thus, knowledge of the earliest signs of responses to trauma can inform treatment directions and enhance recovery interventions among the affected individuals. Some other conditions that are classed under trauma- and stressor-related categories include Adjustment Disorders, which result from particular stressors rather than from exposure to extreme trauma. The disorder is characterized by emotional or behavioral symptomatology that arises within three months of the start of the stressor and may involve symptoms of anxiety, depression, or conduct changes. The defining characteristic of Adjustment Disorders is that they are transient, and symptoms typically resolve as soon as the individual has adapted to the stressor or stressful situation. Evidence suggests that early treatment and diagnosis can significantly reduce the influence of the stressor on the functioning of the individual (Brooks et al., 2015). Understanding these diverse presentations of trauma-related disorders not only aids in diagnosis but also directs targeted therapeutic intervention to develop resilience and recovery (Figure 8.3).

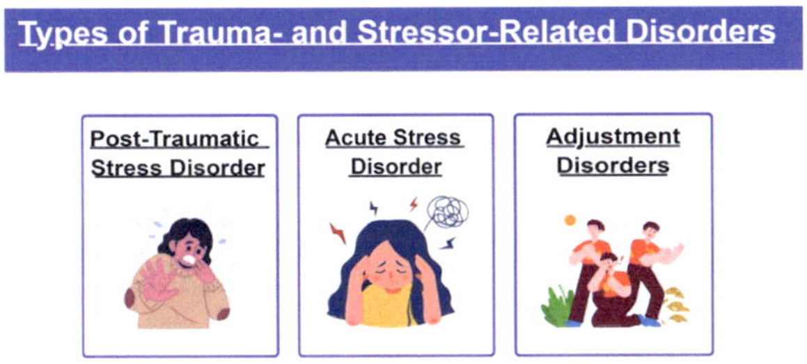

Figure 8.3. Types of trauma- and stressor-related disorders.

Source: https://external-content.duckduckgo.com/iu/?u=https%3A%2F%2Fimages.examples.com%2Fwp-content%2Fuploads%2F2024%2F07%2FTypes-of-Trauma-and-Stressor-Related-Disorders.png&f=1&nofb=1&ipt=6b0cee84dfae3427ddc6cd669edce624ea6e059103a4d6901da45a330a692313.

8.1.1. Post-Traumatic Stress Disorder (PTSD)

Post-Traumatic Stress Disorder (PTSD) is a severe mental illness that results from exposure to traumatic situations, for example, natural disasters, war, or severe accidents. The symptoms tend to result in severe debilitation, leading to hyper-arousal, flashbacks, and excessive anxiety. As previously hinted by more current research, these are the history of past psychological disorders or trauma, intensity of the traumatic event, and the extent of bodily trauma as precipitants to the development of PTSD after being exposed to extreme stressors (Kennedy-Moffat, 1997). Aside from this, the interpersonal setting under which one is subjected to trauma, including the victim's support networks and coping mechanisms, is important in moderating the severity of PTSD symptoms. It is important for the clinician to know these factors so that at-risk individuals can be identified early on and timely and appropriate intervention can be taken. Clinical diagnosis of PTSD has progressed leaps and bounds with growing research findings and clinical experience. Current practice emphasizes a multidimensional assessment approach with the understanding that traditional diagnostic criteria must be supplemented by information about the individual's life context and psychosocial stressors (Cooper et al., 2024). General physicians are most commonly the first point of contact for individuals suffering from PTSD and therefore, play an important role in recognizing symptoms early and giving initial treatment. GPs, as part of an overall treatment plan, can utilize evidence-based guidelines to assess patients' needs and prescribe psychological or pharmacological treatments. These treatments are not only crucial in the mitigation of the symptoms of PTSD but also in enhancing the quality of life in individuals suffering from it, hence the importance of early diagnosis and treatment. Beyond individual-level effects, PTSD has implications for both public health and that of communities. Victims of trauma have poorer physical as well as mental health, which translates to increased utilization of healthcare as well as its attendant costs. Specifically, sufferers from PTSD can experience prolonged episodes of restrictive sickness that highlight an extremely important link between health outcomes and trauma exposure (Kennedy-Moffat, 1997). This suggests integrated healthcare interventions that are directed not only towards the psychological aspects of PTSD but also towards the physical health effects. Addressing PTSD holistically involves recognizing the interconnectedness of physical and mental status, facilitating treatment guidelines that promote recovery and resilience among targeted populations. These strategies are critical in curbing the widespread effects of trauma as well as maintaining healthier communities (Figure 8.4).

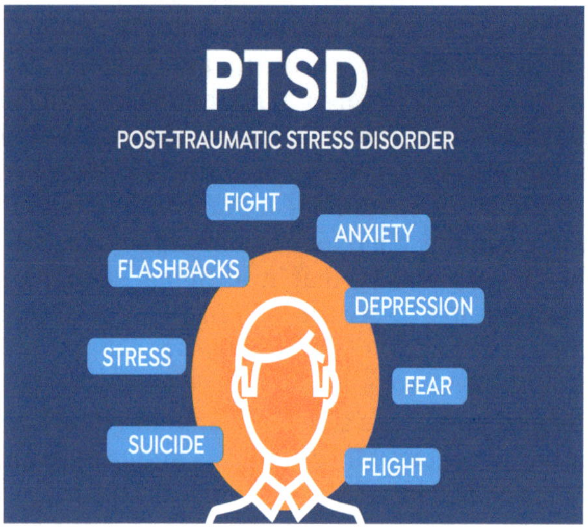

Figure 8.4. PTSD (post-traumatic stress disorder).

Source: https://external-content.duckduckgo.com/iu/?u=https%3A%2F%2Fmapupa.com%2Fwp-content%2Fuploads%2F2023%2F06%2FPTSD.webp&f=1&nofb=1&ipt=69ecbadc7db0115d881ad2b534e7fdea52d8d7bc615d6d8cc54b69b4b56120ef.

8.1.2. Acute Stress Disorder (ASD)

Acute Stress Disorder (ASD) diagnosis is crucial in the context of trauma- and stressor-related disorders since it is the instantaneous effect of traumatic experience. ASD happens between three days and a month following exposure to the traumatic experience, where victims may exhibit symptoms , including intrusive memories, negative mood, dissociation, avoidance behaviors, and heightened arousal. These symptoms may be concurrent with post-traumatic stress disorder (PTSD) but are chronologically differentiated insofar as individuals with ASD may not yet meet the criteria for PTSD. The occurrence of ASD differs by populations and forms of trauma; for example, accident victims, particularly motor vehicle victims, have been found to endure significant mental issues and a far higher incidence of ASD symptoms than non-victims, thus suggesting an extremely strong relationship between the level of trauma and the development of stress disorders (Kennedy-Moffat, 1997). The linkage between ASD and psychological outcomes is accentuated by some of the risk factors with the capacity to render people vulnerable to more severe and long-lasting psychological effects. Some studies indicate that prior psychiatric disorders, the intensity of the traumatic incident itself, and the extent of physical injury largely contribute to the production of symptoms of ASD. In fact, as the literature attests, traumatic life experiences and difficulties in emotional disclosure have been revealed to be associated with increased PTSD symptoms, and it highlights that psychological resilience can become impaired following the trauma (Kennedy-Moffat, 1997).

This highlights the importance of early treatment and intervention support for with ASD symptoms, as they risk developing chronic illnesses unless treated properly within the acute period following trauma. Moreover, the trauma of trauma extends beyond the immediate personal experience to affect people who are close to the traumatized individual, showing another psychosocial element of ASD. The carers and family members of individuals with life-threatening illnesses , such as cancer, for instance, may also experience trauma symptoms. Research has proven that PTSD may develop not only in the patients but also in their careers, demonstrating that trauma becomes evident in the social network. Hence, the comprehension of ASD calls for a universal perspective with regard to the indirect effects of trauma upon carers and relatives as well, with the evident need for comprehensive mental health services that take into consideration both direct victimization and support systems. This perspective is critical in informing the development of therapy interventions and fostering resilience after exposure to trauma (Figure 8.5).

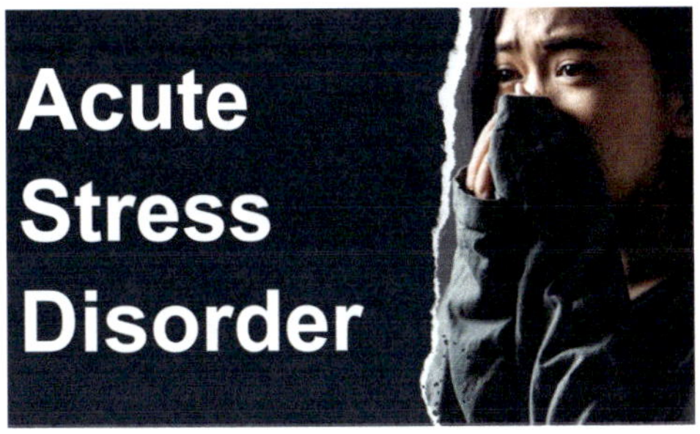

Figure 8.5. Acute stress disorder (ASD).

Source: https://external-content.duckduckgo.com/iu/?u=https%3A%2F%2Fi.ytimg.com%2Fvi%2FO570d-LKJRI%2Fmaxresdefault.jpg&f=1&nofb=1&ipt=a6896a791d3279cd6618d95a44c22d1e586317ba4ebaca788dfd7d17c5babffe.

8.1.3. Adjustment Disorders

Adjustment disorders (AD) are a complex response to particular stressors, distinguished from other trauma- and stressor-related disorders based on temporality and on the basis of reliance on discrete life events. The diagnosis emerges when, following a significant stressor, individuals exhibit symptoms that deviate from their usual functioning, for instance, loss of employment, divorce, or intense health anxiety. Research indicates that the disorders are capable of influencing the emotional life and daily living of the individuals with great seriousness, primarily contributing to depression, anxious mood, or both, as has been found in a study on AD patients that were predominantly typified by mixed depression and anxious mood (Anastasia et al., 2016). Notably, the clinical manifestations of adjustment disorders are often transient, vanishing once the individuals settle into their new situations or sources of stress are relieved. The demographic of individuals afflicted with adjustment disorders also contributes to the difficulty of comprehending such conditions. Clinical evidence indicates that stressors affecting individuals can have a strong correlation with their gender, age, and family circumstances. For example, in a study of 93 patients, work conflict or family conflict emerged as major stressors (Anastasia et al., 2016). This is important in the population finding that it would suggest a call for intervention with various groups in consideration, one that considers the unique stressor profiles for each.

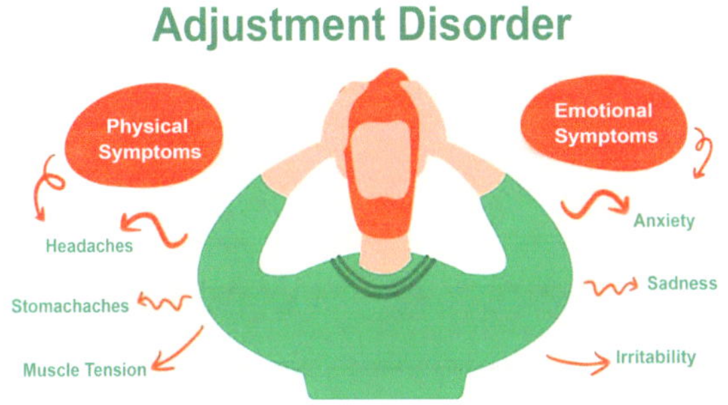

Figure 8.6. Adjustment disorder.

Source: https://external-content.duckduckgo.com/iu/?u=https%3A%2F%2Ftheforgerecovery.com%2F_next%2Fimage%2F%3Furl%3Dhttps%253A%252F%252Fimages.ctfassets.net%252Fveufu8dyuatc%252F2Sl0ibXKUjp9UdxwULf8sC%252F1ddaadffe16ea5fdc8268eb200cf065e%252FFORGE_Symptoms_of_Adjustment_Disorder_Infographic.webp%26w%3D3840%26q%3D95&f=1&nofb=1&ipt=b84dadf365c2cbfb274edef6a8e9c52ab4492ed8b522d0e9f5bab34a5f0f9472.

These variations notwithstanding, they recognize the necessity for the treatment modalities to adapt as well as emphasize the holistic approach in understanding the psychosocial variables that underlie the development of such disorders. In addition, resilience plays a major role in the way individuals cope with adjustment disorders, with implications for the course and severity of their symptoms. Investigative studies have emphasized the significance of resilience-recovery factors , such as social support systems and individual attributes , such as hardiness, in mitigating the effects of stressors. These findings underscore the interdependence of external support systems and internal capacity for coping and emphasize that there are people who do possess extraordinary adaptive potential to face adversity. Thus, understanding adjustment disorders is not only about a model for identifying stressors but also a consideration of resilience as a moderating variable in emotional outcomes with prospects for more targeted therapy (Figure 8.6).

Test Your Knowledge

1. How do PTSD, acute stress disorder, and adjustment disorders differ in terms of onset and symptom duration?
2. What distinguishes reactive attachment disorder and disinhibited social engagement disorder from other trauma-related conditions?

8.2. Causes and Risk Factors

Learning Outcome

1. Exposure to traumatic events.
2. Genetic predisposition.
3. Environmental influences.

An understanding of etiology and risk factors for trauma- and stressor-related disorders is essential for effective prevention and treatment. Traumatic exposure is a significant etiology, and it can be acute or chronic, such as accidents, assault, chronic illness, among others. For instance, cancer is a significant cause of trauma that impacts not only the patient but also his or her family members and caregivers. As noted, cancer-related PTSD can arise at any point in life, emphasizing the diversity in symptoms among children, adolescents, adults, and the elderly. Now that different manifestations have been identified, researchers are in a better position to address the specific psychological needs of the sufferers as well as secondary trauma victims , such as siblings and parents (Paleczna, 2017). In addition to the direct impact of traumatic events, several risk factors predispose a person to the development of trauma- and stressor-related disorders. Differences between individuals such as genetic susceptibilities, history of prior mental illness, and presence of strong social support systems, strongly influence resilience and susceptibility to these disorders. For instance, individuals with a history of depression or anxiety are more likely to develop PTSD following exposure to stressors. Besides, environmental factors, like socioeconomic status, community safety, and exposure to violence, can add their weight to traumatic events, potentially leading to increased rates of disorders. Researchers need to study these factors to develop targeted interventions dealing with these various risk factors, ultimately decreasing the occurrence of trauma disorders (Larauche et al., 2011). Another critical component in the understanding of trauma- and stressor-related disorders is the role of biological and psychological processes mediating the impact of stressors. Stressful events can bring about neurobiological changes that affect emotional regulation, which, in turn, could influence the development of such disorders as PTSD. Dysregulation of the hypothalamic-pituitary-adrenal (HPA) axis, for example, could manifest itself as stress sensitivity and lead to long-lasting psychological consequences. In addition, cognitive processes, that is, pathological coping or inappropriate styles of thinking, may perpetuate an individual's response to trauma. Recognition of such processes can guide future research and interventions in the prevention and treatment of trauma- and stressor-related disorders to allow complete comprehension of the modulation of internal and external processes on a subject's susceptibility (Paleczna, 2017) (Figure 8.7).

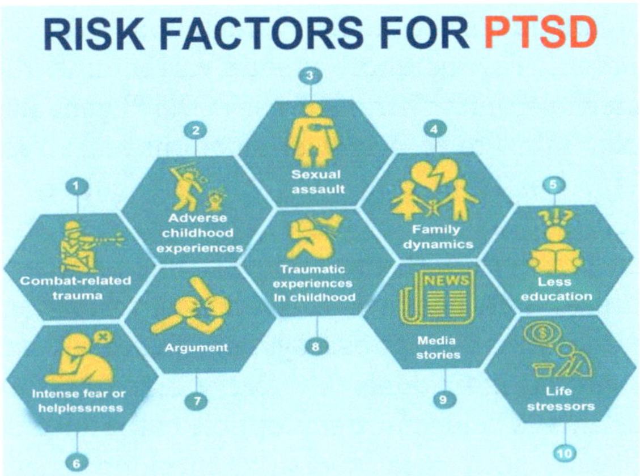

Figure 8.7. Causes and risk factors of trauma- and stressor-related disorders.

Source: https://external-content.duckduckgo.com/iu/?u=https%3A%2F%2Fi.pinimg.com%2Foriginals%2F3f%2F15%2Fc6%2F3f15c607deb0af53be06ea4d47fd2460.jpg&f=1&nofb=1&ipt=c10b3dcb07fd39beef43451d5a55da97c9412802c0cc052bf96210bf1b2bb264.

8.2.1. Exposure to Traumatic Events

The impact of traumatic exposure is extensive and intricate, significantly impacting one's psychological well-being. Traumatic exposure can lead to the development of numerous trauma- and stressor-related disorders, and the most important of these is post-traumatic stress disorder (PTSD). PTSD is best delineated by intrusive memories, heightened arousal, and avoidance behavior. These can emerge following a variety of traumatic exposures, including combat exposure, natural disasters, and severe accidents. Knowledge of the processes through which trauma acts is central to the development of effective treatments. Research indicates that there are particular factors, including social support and resilience, which mediate the effects of traumatic experience, and through which recovery and emotional adjustment may be promoted after trauma. Through consideration of such interpersonal resources, clinicians are in a stronger position to support those who are experiencing the sequelae of significant traumatic exposure. More detailed examination of personal traumatic incidents is noted to have distinctive patterns in reacting to traumatic events. For instance, research on Vietnam veterans illustrates how war-zone stressor factors are associated with PTSD symptomatology. The research applied structural equation modeling to establish trauma exposure-resilience-psychological outcome relations and showed that personal attributes like hardiness and social support are significant in minimizing PTSD symptoms. Such discoveries emphasize the significance of both individual and environmental elements in orchestrating the trauma reaction. Additionally, they emphasize that while traumatic experiences have a severe impact on mental health, the existence of resilience-recovery factors can strongly act as a buffer against detrimental outcomes. Such understanding is critical for practitioners seeking to customize interventions that can build resilience in individuals undergoing trauma-induced psychological difficulty (King et al., 1998). Moreover, some populations are at higher risk of developing trauma-related disorder due to exposure to high levels of traumatic experiences. For example, victims of serious MVAs are more likely to experience increased symptomatology of PTSD and other mental health difficulties. Studies on victims of MVA showed that psychological and severity of injury variables best predicted symptomatology of PTSD. Interestingly, while prior trauma exposure was supposed to be predictive of PTSD development, it did not share a direct, significant relationship. This distinction highlights the complexity of PTSD and also suggests that the actual process of being exposed to the trauma, rather than prior exposures, could be of most significance in psychological effect. Furthermore, the study indicated co-morbidity among health care usage and PTSD symptoms, emphasizing the reality that people who have been subjected to traumatic events require multi-faceted support mechanisms so that they may address their physical as well as psychological ailments (Kennedy-Moffat, 1997) (Figure 8.8).

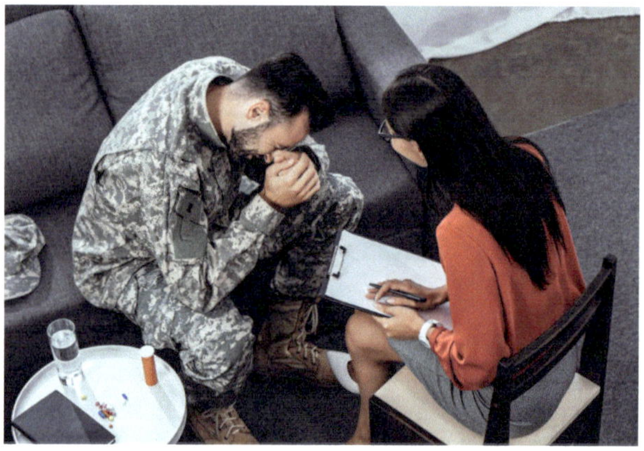

Figure 8.8. The impact of exposure to traumatic events.

Source: https://external-content.duckduckgo.com/iu/?u=http%3A%2F%2Fcoloradopaincare.com%2Fwp-content%2Fuploads%2F2019%2F10%2Fptsd-blog-photo.jpg&f=1&nofb=1&ipt=a43ae6102ee741bbb289cca5b499f0d76db139f63bd89a7db7afe6f17e9f923c.

8.2.2. Genetic Predisposition

The complex interaction between genetic vulnerability and environmental stressors is a major element in the pathogenesis of trauma- and stressor-related disorders. Genetic vulnerability refers to an individual's innate predisposition to specific conditions, which are then augmented through adverse life events. For instance, specific genetic variations can influence an individual's response to stress, perhaps leading to diseases , such as post-traumatic stress disorder (PTSD) or depression. Research has indicated that vulnerability for these conditions can't always be accounted for by genetics but is often the result of the interaction between genetic vulnerabilities and environmental factors, thereby creating a sophisticated model of risk and resilience to trauma. Genetic studies of stress-related disorders have highlighted the role of gene-environment interactions as central to the explanation of variation in vulnerability between persons. For instance, genetic variation in the catechol-O-methyltransferase (COMT) gene has been linked to control over emotions and stress response. Trauma in early life, particularly, is identified as one of the strong stressors that can interfere with the hypothalamic-pituitary-adrenal (HPA) axis, which is a critical component in the stress response system. Research has identified individuals who carry certain COMT variants as being more susceptible to the adverse effects of such early adversities, invoking genetic predisposition as a factor that can heighten the effects of traumatic experience (Cole et al., 2016). Such an intersection of genetic and environmental factors highlights the need for specific therapeutic interventions. Again, genetic predisposition is illustrated using animal models that quantify the effects of stressors on physiological and psychological reactions. Research employing animal models has been shown to demonstrate that stress-induced changes can affect stress-related disorder-related behaviors. For example, animal models exposed to stress during early life in the form of maternal separation exhibit behavioral profiles typical of increased anxiety and depression-like behaviors (Larauche et al., 2011). The findings suggest that genetic susceptibility, particularly with some of the stressors, increases the likelihood of developing the disorders known as irritable bowel syndrome and depression. It is critical to understand these mechanisms to create targeted interventions and preventive measures, taking into account both genetic predisposition and environmental experiences when treating trauma- and stressor-related disorders (Figure 8.9).

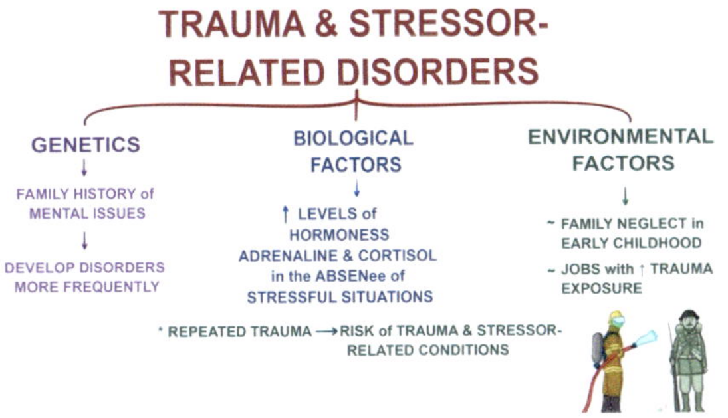

Figure 8.9. Genetic predisposition and environmental influences to trauma- and stressor-related disorders.

Source: https://smartypance.com/wp-content/uploads/2021/01/Trauma-and-stressor-related-disorders-overview.jpg.

8.2.3. Environmental Influences

Environmental variables play a key role in establishing the vulnerability of an individual to stressor- and trauma-related disorders. The dynamic interaction among environmental stressors and life experiences may impact mental health outcomes at varying stages of development. For instance, chronic exposure to environmental stressors, for example, economic instability, social isolation, or conflictual family environment, can exaggerate physiological reactivity and maladaptive coping. The stress theory, as presented, posits that stress must be recognized as an accumulative process, with both internal and contextual variables dynamically influencing one another over time. Through an integrative model for assessing environmental factors, researchers will be in a position to demonstrate how such influences contribute to psychological disorder development so that interventions may be specified to reverse their adverse effect on mental health (Crosswell et al., 2018). Child maltreatment (CM) is an exemplar of the potent environmental influence in the development of stressor-related disorders, illustrating how early trauma can predict the risk for mental disorders in later life. It has been documented that CM is greatly associated with many psychiatric disorders, including the neurodevelopmental disorders (NDDs). While the mechanisms mediating the associations between CM and increased prevalence of disorder remain multifaceted, evidence suggests that CM effects are moderated by shared environment and genetics. The implications are profound, reminding us of the importance of context in accounting for the emergence of disorders related to early adversity.

Medical professionals should be aware that maltreated children are not only at higher risk for single disorders but also present a multifaceted cluster of symptoms that require full assessment and planning for intervention based on their unique environmental histories (Dinkler et al., 2017). A consideration of environmental variables with regard to both stress exposure and coping involves knowing the nuances of trauma- and stressor-related disorders.

The intensity and type of stressors that are encountered can dictate the manner in which individuals traverse their contexts and respond psychologically. , such as, long-term financial struggles or living in unstable housing situations can reach an endpoint of chronic stress, which will accordingly impact physiological health and psychological resilience. Conversely, the availability of stable support structures and effective coping strategies may thwart such dangers, again emphasizing supportive environment construction. As stress researchers continue developing integrative models that account for both psychological and environmental determinants, it is evident that the regulation of these influences is essential in the treatment and prevention of trauma disorders. Apart from enhancing individual functioning, such interventions also promote a better society through good policy and community support interventions (Crosswell et al., 2018).

Test Your Knowledge

1. How do traumatic experiences such as abuse, violence, or disasters contribute to the development of trauma- and stressor-related disorders?
2. What biological, psychological, and social factors increase vulnerability to developing PTSD or related disorders?

8.3. Symptoms and Diagnosis

Learning Outcome

1. Emotional and psychological symptoms.
2. Physical symptoms.
3. Diagnostic criteria and assessment tools.

It is under the determination of a continuum of symptoms that would severely impact persons after being exposed to traumatic situations that post-traumatic stress disorder, or PTSD, and other trauma- and stressor-related disorders are diagnosed. Included, but not exhaustive, are intrusive recollections, avoidance behaviors, negative mood and cognitive changes, and changes in arousal and reactivity. These consequences are typically segregated into clusters that help to make accurate diagnosis, which makes clinicians move towards efficient treatment strategies. Recent advancements in clinical practice guidelines emphasize the importance of extensive screening and expert assessment. General practitioners are pivotal in this regard as the initial contact for individuals who are distressed following exposure to a traumatic event, hence being perfectly placed for early identification and intervention (Cooper et al., 2024). Moreover, trauma's impact goes beyond individualized symptoms and invades the family system and interpersonal relationships as well. Families of veterans can have unusually challenging times integrating soldiers returning from combat with PTSD. Normal symptoms , such as irritability and emotional numbing, cause stress in relationships, which can lead to issues like disruption of communication and emotional distance. Research further identifies that military families may possess unique stressors, including higher rates of substance abuse and intimate partner violence (Gourley, 2016). An awareness of these relational processes is important to inform interventions that not only address individual symptoms but also foster healthier family systems that facilitate recovery. Diagnosis is further facilitated by comorbidities that typically occur when trauma- and stressor-related disorders are present, which necessitate integrated evaluation. Individuals with PTSD frequently also experience co-morbid psychological disorders , such as depression, anxiety, or alcohol/substance abuse disorders, which complicate the clinical presentation and impact treatment outcomes. This contributes to the requirement of clinicians conducting integrative assessments that consider both the psychological and environmental forces operating. By creating an interdisciplinary collaborative therapeutic relationship, one can bring together a comprehensive treatment plan, combining psychological and pharmacological interventions as might apply best for the needs of the individual, further emphasizing the integral role of primary care professionals in the management of PTSD and associated disorders (Cooper et al., 2024) (Figure 8.10).

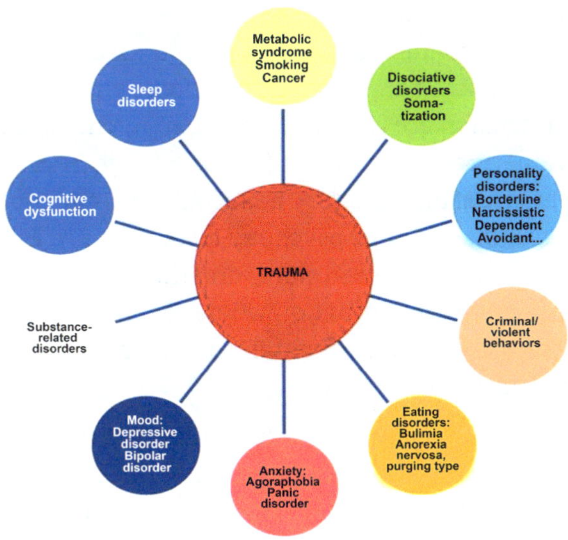

Figure 8.10. Symptoms and diagnosis of trauma- and stressor-related disorders.

Source: https://media.springernature.com/lw685/springer-static/image/chp%3A10.1007%2F978-3-031-47802-4_14/MediaObjects/429279_2_En_14_Fig2_HTML.png.

8.3.1. Emotional and Psychological Symptoms

Emotional and psychological symptoms usually become apparent clearly in the patients with trauma- and stressor-related disorders. These symptoms can include persistent nervousness, depression, and hopelessness, which overwhelm everyday functioning. Greater emotional distress usually comes with cognitive impairment, like Alzheimer 's-type memory problems or intrusions of posttraumatic memories, reminding the patient in vivid detail about the traumatic event. Individuals can struggle to regulate their emotions, leading to uncontrollable rage or excessive crying. This dysregulation is most evident in populations with high stressors, such as veterans. For instance, it has been discovered that intrapersonal factors , such as social support and resilience can mediate the severity of such symptoms, pointing to the role of intrapersonal resources and environmental factors in psychological recovery (King et al., 1998). The symptom inventory of psychology can also further exacerbate an individual's coping with trauma. Individuals would find it difficult to cope with helplessness, shame, or guilt, and these are additional burdens in terms of distress. Interaction between social relationships and emotional symptoms is central, as social withdrawal from fear of being judged can compound isolation and hopelessness. Research has revealed that additional negative life events during the post-trauma period may worsen outcomes for such patients. Moreover, the absence of sound support mechanisms tends to increase feelings of abandonment and hopelessness. Hence, such psychological symptoms have to be managed not just by therapies addressing the trauma itself but also by setting up a support system to facilitate recovery (King et al., 1998). Physiological impact of the emotional and psychological symptoms is also significant, having a tendency to coincide with the state of stress. Chronic emotional discomfort can lead to somatic complaints of a broad range, essentially turning the body into the site of the psychological discomfort. Evidence indicates that stressors from a wide range of sources, including psychological and physical stimuli, influence the causation and presentation of some conditions like irritable bowel syndrome. This is a major point of intersection for emotional distress and physiological health, demonstrating the complexity of trauma- and stressor-related disorders. Experimental models of stress highlight the importance of considering the intersection between psychological and physical components in trying to understand the comprehensive nature of these symptoms and their implications for treatment. Holistic approaches are thus critical to effective intervention (Figure 8.11).

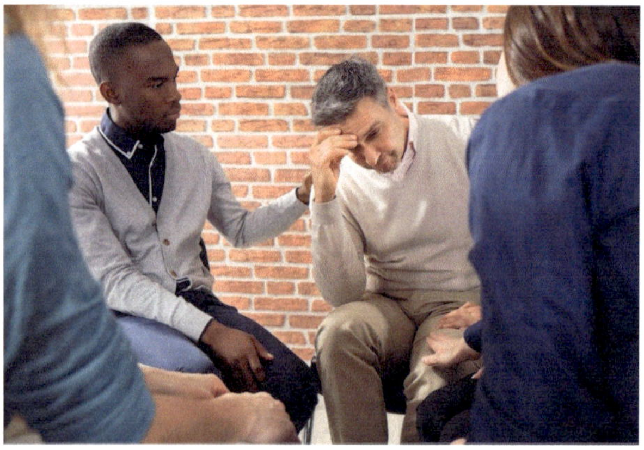

Figure 8.11. Emotional and psychological symptoms of trauma- and stressor-related disorders.

Source: https://footprintstorecovery.com/wp-content/uploads/AdobeStock_158942475.jpg.

8.3.2. Physical Symptoms

Trauma- and stressor-related disorders tend to manifest in a range of physical symptoms that can significantly impact the life of the patient. The symptoms could be as minor as chronic pain, fatigue, and gastrointestinal distress, which tend to be erroneously attributed to other unrelated illnesses. Physical manifestations of psychological distress demonstrate the intricate relationship between psychological and physical health, showing how emotional experience contributes to somatic complaints. Identification of these symptoms is essential in proper diagnosis and treatment since ignoring them may lead to improper interventions targeting the physical aspect only, leaving psychological considerations in the background. As studies evidence, physical symptom treatment of trauma may lead to improved health outcomes, and therefore, an integrated model of care must be adopted, recognizing the role of emotional distress in the management of physical conditions.

Furthermore, some types of trauma have been recognized as having resultant physical symptoms. For instance, individuals who have been exposed to significant traumatic experience, that is, war exposure, can have heightened risks for various stress-related physical disorders, including cardiovascular system-related ones. Notably, connections between trauma exposure and physical symptoms like heightened heart rate and tension are routinely drawn in psychological evaluations. It has been found through studies that visual and auditory hallucinations, common in trauma-induced psychotic disorders, are also linked with physical pain, creating a mutually interdependent situation where trauma enables both physical and mental pain to be present simultaneously.

The interplay between trauma and physical symptoms suggests that the therapeutic interventions must incorporate psychological treatment along with the treatment for somatic complaints to successfully minimize the effects of trauma. Finally, the management of traumatic physical symptoms is crucial to developing a trauma-informed model of care, which recognizes the pervasiveness of trauma on all aspects of health. A proper comprehension of how trauma impacts the physical dimensions of health can inform healthcare practice so that clinicians can recognize and respond to symptoms appropriately. Shame at having emotional distress and its somatic presentation can unhelpfully deter patients from seeking treatment, where the stigma of being identified as malingering is constantly present. Increased knowledge of the physiological impact of trauma can serve to validate patient presentation, thus encouraging treatment engagement.

Judicial hesitance to entertain emotional and physical injury claims, as has been seen in court arguments, only serves to underscore the necessity for supporting individuals experiencing physical symptoms of trauma through evidence-based clinical assessment (Grey et al., 2015). Lastly, addressing both the physical and psychological dimensions of trauma is required to move treatment protocols forward and promote overall health among trauma- and stressor-related disorder patients (Figure 8.12).

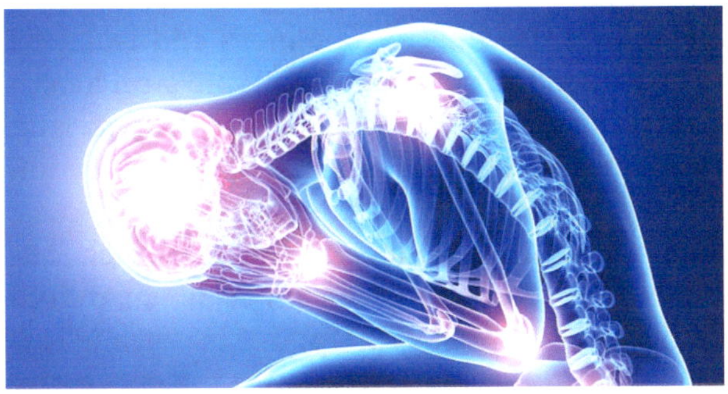

Figure 8.12. Physical symptoms of trauma- and stressor-related disorders.

Source: https://www.apa.org/images/body-stress-title-image_tcm7-230134.jpg.

8.3.3. Diagnostic Criteria and Assessment Tools

Diagnostic criteria for trauma- and stressor-related disorders are stated in conformity with prevailing models, primarily the Diagnostic and Statistical Manual of Mental Disorders (DSM-5). This manual provides specific signs and conduct criteria necessary for accurate diagnosis. Post-traumatic stress disorder (PTSD), for instance, is a significant class of this category that requires exposure to a traumatic event followed by intrusive memories, avoidance behaviors, negative cognition change, and heightened arousal. Assessing if an individual is eligible on these premises is dependent upon a clinician's thorough evaluation of symptoms and the number of months it has been since the incident, which should also extend to more than one month. Moreover, the frequency of symptoms will vary across individuals, thus making clinicians treat the risk of PTSD differently, which is a section specifically addressed in modern general practitioners' guidelines (Cooper et al., 2024). The use of valid assessment instruments is essential in making a diagnosis of trauma- and stressor-related disorders.

These may include structured interviews or standardized self-report questionnaires that quantify the severity and impact of symptoms. An example is the Clinician-Administered PTSD Scale (CAPS) which is widely utilized in research and clinical settings to assess PTSD symptomology systematically. These tools enable professionals to gather comprehensive data, which can be useful in improving comprehension of the disorder's impact on the patient's life and enhancing treatment planning. The use of these tools also facilitates the standardization of diagnoses across different populations and clinical settings, ultimately improving the quality of care provided to victims of trauma-related problems, emphasizing the importance of standardized methods in this area (Backholm, 2012).

Apart from clinical interviews and standardized questionnaires, individual and contextual information must be taken into account in diagnosing trauma- and stressor-related disorders. For instance, a patient's history of past trauma, life stressors at the moment, and social support networks may be crucial in symptom reporting. Furthermore, some groups, such as journalists who have been reporting on traumatic events in the field, may exhibit unique stress reactions and therefore, require specially developed assessment strategies (Backholm, 2012). This individualized approach not only raises the accuracy of diagnosis but also directs the crafting of targeted interventions. As highlighted in subsequent literature, awareness of the interaction between these variables and use of a broad range of assessment tools are essential for managing the complexities entailed in trauma and stressor-related disorders and, in the end, improving their therapeutic response (Cooper et al., 2024).

Test Your Knowledge

1. What are the key symptom clusters of PTSD, such as intrusion, avoidance, negative mood, and hyperarousal?
2. How do clinicians use DSM-5-TR criteria and structured interviews to differentiate between acute stress disorder and PTSD?

8.4. Impact on Daily Life

Learning Outcome

1. Effects on personal relationships.
2. Influence on occupational functioning.
3. Consequences for overall well-being.

The impact of trauma- and stressor-related disorders on daily living is grave and intricate, affecting people psychologically and physically. People who experience disorders , such as post-traumatic stress disorder (PTSD) typically have their day-to-day lives filled with intrusive thoughts or flashbacks regarding traumatic events. Intrusions might lead to heightened anxiety and emotional dysregulation that make social interactions complex and prevent professional responsibilities. For instance, a person will be unable to concentrate in the workplace, sacrificing their career advancement and job. Moreover, such disorders will strain relationships since relatives will be unable to understand the turmoil going on within their loved ones, leading to loneliness and isolation that worsen the condition. Even physical health is seriously compromised due to trauma and stress. Research has established a connection between PTSD and certain physical illnesses, such as chronic pain syndromes, which can diminish overall quality of life. When opioid analgesics are used by patients with PTSD for pain management, they unintentionally enhance their symptoms of trauma because extended use of opioids has been established to promote associative fear learning—a defining characteristic of PTSD expression. In such a case, individuals become engaged in a cycle of perpetuation, wherein attempts to minimize physical distress turn into the source of escalating psychological distress, complicating their daily lives. This interaction between physical and mental health imposes the need for integral treatment modalities that address both dimensions in unison. Moreover, the psychosocial impacts of these disorders filter their way into day-to-day functioning on job and social activity levels. People with trauma-related disorders can develop drastic changes in their behavior, which result in social withdrawal and less motivation to participate in hobbies or community activities previously enjoyed. Interruption of normal functioning can impair social skills and increase feelings of isolation, making it more difficult to form new relationships or sustain current ones. The effects of stressors in terms of occupational settings also support the feelings of inadequacy, and this creates a feedback cycle perpetuating the disorders' presence in daily life. This impact supports the essentiality of supportive environments and effectively operative interventions that can reduce the burdens of stressor- and trauma-related disorders, resulting in enhanced overall well-being (Figure 8.13).

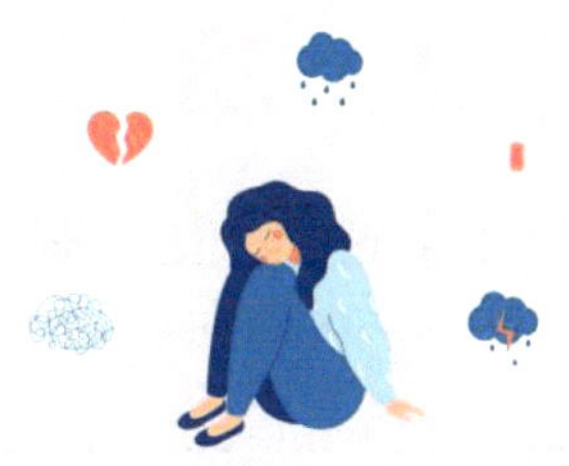

Figure 8.13. Trauma- and stressor-related disorders impact on daily life.

Source: https://www.thevillagefamily.org/sites/default/files/styles/events_blog/public/2022-05/adapting-after-trauma-and-stress.jpg.

8.4.1. Effects on Personal Relationships

The impact of trauma and stressor-related disorders can significantly strain personal relationships in most instances, resulting in their deterioration in interpersonal relationships and support systems. Victims of trauma may manifest withdrawal, irritability, and emotional deadness, which has can lead to isolation from relatives and friends. The nature of trauma makes victims feel isolated or misunderstood, which creates a vicious cycle where they end up ruining their relationships through ineffective communication. As highlighted in previous research, social support plays an integral role in de-emphasizing the effect of trauma; nevertheless, recovery might be compromised if interpersonal relationships are also affected (King et al., 1998). Thus, promoting communication openness and establishing stronger social ties becomes the utmost priority for patients suffering from these disorders, given that supportive relationships can serve as a protective shield against symptomatic presentation with a nexus to trauma. Moreover, personal relationships could be influenced by the perception that a partner is emotionally dependent or unavailable due to the experience of their trauma. For instance, the partners of individuals with post-traumatic stress disorder (PTSD) may struggle to cope with the intricacy of the emotional terrain generated by their loved one's experience. This cycle typically produces escalated tension and frustration in the relationship, with the one seeking closeness while the other withdraws. The avoidance and distress cycle perpetuates these feelings of helplessness and inadequacy because the victims of PTSD might view their own suffering as burdens to others (Kennedy-Moffat, 1997). Consequently, the dynamic between expectations for relationships and symptoms of trauma can plant resentment and affective distance, making it that much harder to seek healing and closeness in a relationship. Moreover, the impact of trauma seeps into wider social networks and communal connections beyond personal relationships. As those with trauma disorders struggle to cope with their experiences, they will find it increasingly difficult to engage in social interactions or communal activities, leading to social isolation. This withdrawal may erode earlier rich relationships and the sense of community membership on the part of the individual. The research places importance on the function of outside support systems in the healing process, theorizing that victims of high social isolation may find it more difficult to recover from trauma disorders (King et al., 1998). Communities must recognize these dynamics and construct such spaces that are inclusive of open communication regarding trauma so that individuals can reconnect with others and receive social support to facilitate healing and relationship repair.

8.4.2. Impact on Occupational Functioning

The influence of trauma- and stressor-related disorders on work functioning is an entrenched problem that hampers one's capacity to perform at the workplace. The disorders, particularly posttraumatic stress disorder (PTSD), have various symptoms , such as hyperarousal, intrusive memories, and emotional dysregulation that interfere directly with concentration and productivity (Ertelt, 2023). Its occupational performance impact is multidimensional: individuals could have more absenteeism, reduced job satisfaction, and interpersonal conflicts with colleagues, making it harder for them to work. Since trauma can also coexist with other mental disorders, the problems of such individuals are usually compounded, creating a vicious cycle of dysfunction that impedes their professional advancement and career longevity. Workplace bullying is another significant contributing factor that worsens the afflictions of those who already endure symptoms of PTSD. More current research has also indicated that observing bullying behaviors triggers short-term psychological disruptions, like the emergence of posttraumatic stress (PTS) symptoms, even among people without a history of prior trauma (Balducci et al., 2024). This shows that working spaces can turn into sources of additional tension that exacerbate existing conditions. The unpredictability of bullying incidents can also instigate workplace phobia, encouraging one to develop patterns of avoidance, further diminishing one's ability to engage actively in work-based activities. The interactional dynamics within the workplace, therefore, not only transmit individual vulnerabilities but also create a toxic environment leading to mental health deterioration. In order to effectively address these problems during occupational therapy, professionals must utilize the trauma-informed care model.

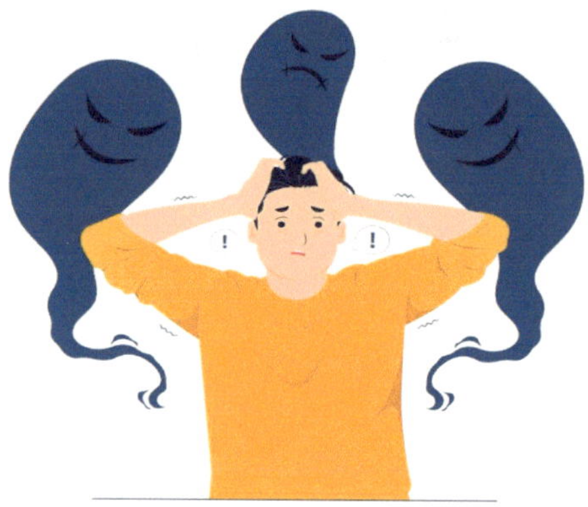

Figure 8.14. Trauma- and stressor-related disorders influence on occupational functioning.

Source: https://external-content.duckduckgo.com/iu/?u=https%3A%2F%2Fstatic.vecteezy.com%2Fsystem%2Fresources%2Fpreviews%2F010%2F549%2F836%2Fnon_2x%2Fschizophrenia-post-traumatic-stress-mental-disorder-concept-illustration-free-vector.jpg&f=1&nofb=1&ipt=4f4367a95635693169eb8ee8094590173cf2459c62a18195fc41f9d123f84692.

By learning about the prevalence of trauma and the comorbidities that may arise in client populations, occupational therapy practitioners are more effectively able to create their interventions to maximize occupational performance (Ertelt, 2023). Publishing resources , such as the Best Practice Occupational Therapy Interventions for Addressing Trauma and Posttraumatic Stress Disorder: A Practitioner Guide is a significant step toward preparing providers to integrate trauma-sensitive practices into practice. Thus, these strategies can potentially enhance resilience and functional status for individuals battling the dual burden of work demands and trauma, ultimately resulting in a healthier workplace culture fostering recovery and productivity (Figure 8.14).

8.4.3. Consequences for Overall Well-Being

Their impact on general well-being is serious and extensive, impacting both mental and physical well-being. Individuals with such disorders often experience higher rates of anxiety, depression, and social avoidance, significantly reducing their quality of life. The emotional toll includes the occurrence of intrusive thoughts, flashbacks, and heightened arousal symptoms, hindering daily functioning. Most significant, research indicates that serious motor vehicle accident victims are more likely to experience both mental and physical ill health. Specifically, such individuals report a greater prevalence of PTSD symptoms than non-victims and echo the cause-and-effect relationship between trauma and the presence of negative psychological outcomes. Understanding these interconnected consequences is crucial to the development of successful interventions for the alleviation of distress and enhancement of recovery for those thus affected (Kennedy-Moffat, 1997). In addition, the effect on global well-being carries over into numerous aspects of everyday life, including interpersonal relationships and job functioning. Inability to establish and maintain interpersonal relationships tends to arise as individuals navigate through their traumas and sense isolation. The continued stress that defines the trauma-related disorders may initiate other illnesses, thus complicating recovery. In essence, the relationship between psychiatric disorder and utilization of health care reveals a vicious cycle where mental disorders intensify physical disorders to an extent that one requires more health care. These findings support the necessity for an integrative treatment approach that transcends the treatment of psychopathology and promotes lifestyle choices and coping styles. It is this integrative approach that will facilitate improved outcomes and functioning among victims of abuse who have been traumatized (Kennedy-Moffat, 1997). Aside from these challenges, trauma disorder expression has been found to vary between men and women. Women, for instance, statistically are more likely to develop PTSD than men, with ramifications that biological and psychosocial factors have a role in variations in outcome. Evidence indicates that hormonal factors, notably those that are related to the menstrual cycle, have a significant role in what stress does to women's physiology. For example, PACAP and estrogen level fluctuations have been associated with changes in rat model anxiety-like behavior, offering some insight into the underlying mechanisms that underlie established gender differences in PTSD pathology. Through investigation of such biological factors, researchers hope to map why females are more stressor-sensitive and thus tailor therapeutic interventions. This gendered approach is essential in formulating advanced conceptualizations of trauma's effect on global health and constructing successful prevention and treatment interventions.

Test Your Knowledge

1. How do trauma-related symptoms affect functioning in work, relationships, sleep, and emotional regulation?
2. What challenges do individuals face with concentration, trust, and interpersonal communication following traumatic experiences?

8.5. Treatment Options

Learning Outcome

1. Psychotherapy approaches.
2. Pharmacological interventions.
3. Alternative and complementary therapies.

The treatment of trauma- and stressor-related disorders, particularly post-traumatic stress disorder (PTSD), entails a multidimensional approach that is a combination of pharmacological and psychological intervention. Both approaches are needed in treating the multi-dimensional aspect of PTSD, which can manifest in numerous symptoms like intrusive recollections, avoidance, and hyperarousal. General practitioners tend to be in a best-placed position to recognize the first signs of PTSD and are therefore instrumental to initiating treatment pathways. Updated clinical guidance gives evidence-based recommendations for GPs, with emphasis placed on the importance of tailored treatment plans based on the patient's unique experiences and needs. The GP does have a role to play beyond initial identification, as they also have a responsibility to provide ongoing care and to decide if referral to specialist mental health treatment is necessary, emphasizing the benefit of shared management in the treatment of PTSD (Cooper et al., 2024). Psychological treatments, namely cognitive behavioral therapy (CBT), have become firm mainstays in the treatment of PTSD. CBT aims at the modification of distressing thinking patterns that could continue to perpetuate traumatic responses, enabling individuals to interact with their trauma positively. Exposure therapy, which is part of CBT, has also been effective through the gradual exposure of patients to stimuli related to trauma in a controlled environment. Other areas of treatment are also available through innovations in other modalities , such as Eye Movement Desensitization and Reprocessing (EMDR). These psychotherapeutic interventions not only alleviate symptoms but also improve coping and resilience in trauma patients. With the expanding knowledge regarding PTSD, the conceptual framework of different therapeutic alternatives allows treatment pathways to be tailor-made that maximize the outcomes of recovery for the victimized individuals (Cooper et al., 2024).

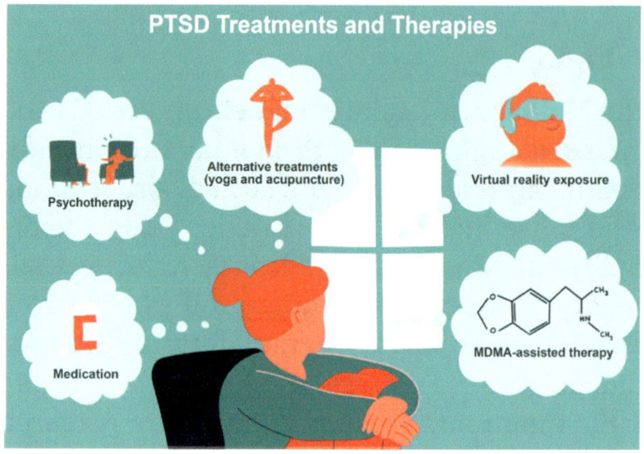

Figure 8.15. The treatment of trauma- and stressor-related disorders.

Source: https://external-content.duckduckgo.com/iu/?u=https%3A%2F%2Fwww.verywellmind.com%2Fthmb%2F1pRzfJBxjB_6z28KfflFa-xfIuo%3D%2F1500x1000%2Ffilters%3Ano_upscale()%3Amax_bytes(150000)%3Astrip_icc()%2Fptsd-treatment-2797659_FINAL-5c12be374cedfd00010f866a.png&f=1&nofb=1&ipt=4b504d2d254f0e8f16831e8e8c34b50fcf7ac1b6cfd32636b2e855892da4f8ab.

Apart from the traditional psychological interventions, new ones , such as horticultural therapy have also been discovered to be effective treatment interventions, particularly in some populations with stress disorders. Horticultural therapy uses gardening and plant-related activities as a treatment intervention to enhance emotional and mental health. It has been very effective in military veterans diagnosed with PTSD, offering sensory interaction, social interaction, and a sense of achievement.

Furthermore, these findings can be applied to refugee populations, who are known to have heightened levels of PTSD due to the trauma of being displaced. Horticultural therapy not only provides a healthy coping mechanism for distress but also promotes the community-building process, which can be a valuable factor in recovery for those who have been traumatized. These new modalities point to the need for increasing the treatment options for trauma- and stressor-related disorders (Figure 8.15).

8.5.1. Psychotherapy Approaches

There has been a succession of psychotherapy techniques formulated to treat the complex universe of trauma- and stressor-related disorders, all with their respective approaches and techniques. Psychodynamic therapy is one technique that focuses on understanding unconscious phenomena shaped by memories. This technique encourages a heightened sensitivity towards emotional conflicts stemming from trauma, hence the ability to heal through reflection and insight. Therapists help patients review their emotional responses, which oftentimes correlate with past life events or relationships between individuals. Through an analysis of such underlying cause conflicts, psychodynamic therapy aims to minimize trauma symptoms, emphasizing the interplay between internal narratives and external stresses. Empirical studies have demonstrated the success of this approach, which therefore makes it applicable in therapy environments, especially among those with the aftereffects of relational trauma (Cohen et al., 2018). Cognitive-behavioral therapy (CBT) is another but supplementary method of treating trauma that targets altering maladaptive cognition and behavior concerning painful memory. CBT integrates techniques used to challenge and rearrange adverse cognition schemas so that people come in command of their emotional responses. Exposure techniques and restructuring are used by therapists to help patients confront their fears in a secure setting in a systematic manner. Research has identified the effectiveness of CBT in reducing symptoms of PTSD and anxiety, particularly in people experiencing acute stressor-related reactions. This structured model not only enables clients to reconsider their traumatic experiences but also educates them on how to cope with later stressors, emphasizing the active model of recovery inherent in CBT (Cohen et al., 2018). The other dominant treatment approach is Eye Movement Desensitization and Reprocessing (EMDR), which targets specifically the distressing memories at the center of trauma- and stressor-related disorders. EMDR is bilaterally stimulating, typically through eye movement, when clients recall traumatic memories to facilitate adaptive reprocessing of the memories. The treatment is effective in reducing the intensity of traumatic memories and associated emotional responses within a short time frame, with substantial symptom decreases in PTSD. Clinical studies document the efficacy of EMDR, showing remarkable reductions in emotional regulation and psychological functioning. Moreover, the approach is also supplemented by findings from neuroscientific research, illuminating dissociation and body reactions in trauma therapy, and attaches strong importance to relational processes within therapy (Palmieri et al., 2015). Therefore, EMDR is an attractive option for therapists looking to tackle the complex interconnection between trauma and stress.

8.5.2. Pharmacological Interventions

Pharmacological interventions of trauma- and stressor-related disorders are all components of comprehensive treatment plans, particularly for the likes of post-traumatic stress disorder (PTSD). Several drugs , including selective serotonin reuptake inhibitors (SSRIs) and benzodiazepines, are commonly administered to alleviate symptoms concerning these disorders. SSRIs, for instance, are commonly prescribed as first-line treatments since they can very effectively manage anxiety and depressive symptoms concerning exposure to trauma. Heightened awareness of the disorders reinforces the importance of specific treatment programs incorporating pharmacotherapy in conjunction with psychological therapy. The dual approach is designed to manage not just symptoms but also neurobiological processes involved in the development and maintenance of trauma disorders, reaffirming the positioning of pharmacologic treatment confirmed in the current clinical practice guidelines as outlined in (Cooper et al., 2024). In addition to supporting the role of pharmacological therapy, newer evidence has also indicated that medication combinations may sometimes have added therapeutic benefit. For example, even though SSRIs are effective treatments, adding medications that affect other neurotransmitter systems can provide improved outcomes in symptom management. Also, new information emerges about the efficacy of newer medications, such as prazosin, which has been shown to be promising in reducing nightmares and hyperarousal symptoms of PTSD. Ongoing progress in the development of pharmacologic treatments reflects an acknowledgment of the dynamic interaction between trauma, stress, and neurobiology, thus necessitating ongoing exploration of novel therapeutic targets. Furthermore, the better understanding of the mechanisms of disorder comes, clinicians are in better positions to utilize such drugs for managing acute symptoms while encouraging patients' long-term recovery, as delineated in more current guidelines in an attempt to encourage practitioner support in treating such disorders (Larauche et al., 2011). What is important, however, is that the utilization of such pharmacological therapies must be accompanied by careful consideration of their limitations and potential side effects. While drugs can effectively alleviate distressing symptoms to a large extent, they can also create issues like dependency, particularly with benzodiazepines, that undermine patients' functioning when misused. Moreover, effective treatment includes regular reassessment of the effectiveness of pharmacotherapy and exploration of other interventions as needed. Active patient involvement in treatment decision-making enhances mutually supportive therapeutic relationships and allows them to be empowered participants in their recovery process. As research progresses to inform us on the interaction between exposure to trauma and neurobiologic consequences, ongoing development and refinement of pharmacologic treatments will be a critical component of best practice management of trauma- and stressor-related disorders so that patients receive multidisciplinary, patient-centered treatment as emphasized in the present practice guidelines (Cooper et al., 2024).

8.5.3. Alternative and Complementary Therapies

The evolution of complementary and alternative interventions has attracted significant attention in the case of trauma- and stressor-related disorders, particularly when conventional interventions are not effective. Techniques , such as horticultural therapy through gardening and plant-based activities have been noted to have positive effects in symptom reduction of post-traumatic stress disorder (PTSD). For instance, research on military veterans and combat soldiers diagnosed with stress disorders indicates that contact with nature and the practice of gardening can lead to important mental benefits. This therapy provides participants with a feeling of accomplishment and worth, which can in turn prove the tipping point for those recovering from the psychological effects of trauma. By integrating practices like horticultural therapy within treatment strategies, mental health professionals are better positioned to deal with the intricate experiences of individuals facing the long-term effects of trauma (Nadeau, 2019). Other than horticultural therapy, spiritually based practices are rich resources of alternatives for persons with trauma-related disorders. The case of the Tibetan refugee monks on PTSD illustrates the intricate dynamics between cultural heritage, spirituality, and mental health. These monks are faced with a unique challenge in the sense that their religious disciplines, which would otherwise promote emotional wellness, are interrupted by the srog-rLung imbalances that are fueled by trauma. Healing in this case must try to cure both the psychological symptoms of PTSD and yet respect and incorporate the patient's cultural and religious background. Therapies that blend Eastern spiritual practices with contemporary psychological techniques may provide a more comprehensive model for healing. These integrative methodologies hold the promise to foster resilience and enhance recovery in heterogeneous populations of trauma-exposed patients (Benedict et al., 2013). The success of alternatives and complements does not only reside in their holistic models but also in their ability to respond to unique individuals. Compared to traditional treatments that may have a more routinized protocol, alternatives allow for individualized care that is aligned with a patient's own experience and culture. This is particularly important for populations who may be resistant to conventional psychological treatment based on past bad experiences or cultural stigma surrounding mental illness. Being patient-focused and inclusive of their beliefs and values, alternative treatments offer a politicized space for healing. Overall, this growing inclusion of these interventions in mental health care is an indication of a more expansive and pluralistic definition of treating trauma and stressor-related disorders, culminating in greater efficiency in treatment effectiveness in those with these conditions (Figure 8.16).

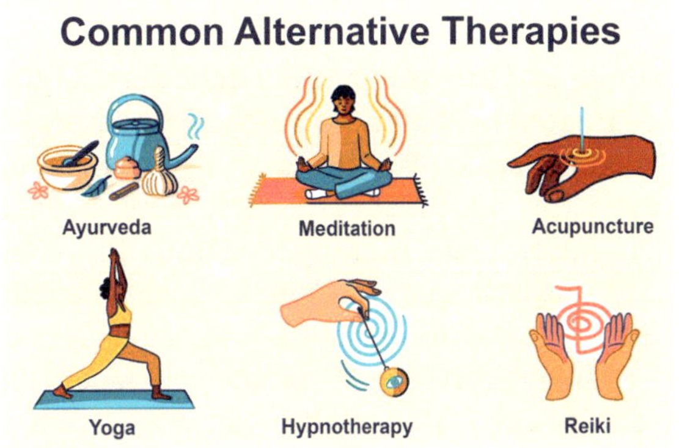

Figure 8.16. Alternative and complementary therapies.

Source: https://external-content.duckduckgo.com/iu/?u=https%3A%2F%2Fwww.verywellmind.com%2Fthmb%2FpuRzNEXvSspRLcSSf5sXgVTWEgU%3D%2F1500x0%2Ffilters%3Ano_upscale()%3Amax_bytes(150000)%3Astrip_icc()%2Falternative-therapies-types-and-uses-5207962_final-406a673fa76e41d9add8ce4771222dd0.png&f=1&nofb=1&ipt=374f49b99661b3c1fef93e4382f9ddec94202011ff0b34c3fecafc828b4e4ac3.

Test Your Knowledge

1. How do trauma-focused psychotherapies—such as CBT, EMDR, and prolonged exposure therapy—support recovery from trauma-related disorders?
2. What role do medications, such as SSRIs or anxiolytics, play in managing symptoms of PTSD and related conditions?

8.6. Prevention and Coping Strategies

Learning Outcome

1. Building resilience.
2. Community support systems.
3. Stress management techniques.

Trauma- and stressor-related disorders require to be treated with an all-encompassing approach that emphasizes prevention along with coping. Prevention is most effective where early intervention takes place, particularly in people at highest risk, such as veterans who develop PTSD or major depression. The identification of protective factors that create resilience, like psychological stability and purpose in life, is crucial to facilitate. Research indicates that nearly one-third of veterans who were originally rated as non-suicidal ended up growing suicidal ideation at a seven-year follow-up. Preventive interventions aimed at maximizing purpose and conscientiousness can more effectively lower such a threat, identifying preventive interventions as lowering the suicidal thought rate among high-risk groups (Norman et al., 2019). Coping strategies are also important in the mitigation of symptoms of trauma. These are divided into adaptive and maladaptive coping strategies, where the former promotes healthy emotional adjustment and the latter is likely to increase distress. Cognitive-behavioral treatment is most effective in causing the individual to change negative thoughts and learn healthier patterns of coping. Mindfulness exercises, social support, and habituation can be very helpful in assisting the individual to manage emotions. By actively teaching such skills, mental health clinicians can prepare individuals to successfully manage their stress, thus promoting a healthier psychological state and expanding the potential for prevention against subsequent trauma-related conditions. Moreover, understanding the link between exposure to trauma and revictimization highlights the unparalleled significance of tailored coping skills in the context of therapeutic intervention. Traumatized victims exhibit greater levels of emotional instability and psychological symptomology, which increase their likelihood of revictimization. Therefore, mental health services ought to be focused on resilience-building interventions that address previous trauma while encouraging emotional stability. One such intensive approach is to assess individual trauma histories and tailored coping mechanisms that enable victims to exit the revictimization cycle. Through the integration of these results into treatment programs, police and community collaboration can work together to build healthier environments for trauma survivors, effectively aiding in their recovery and reintegration into society (Brooks et al., 2015) (Figure 8.17).

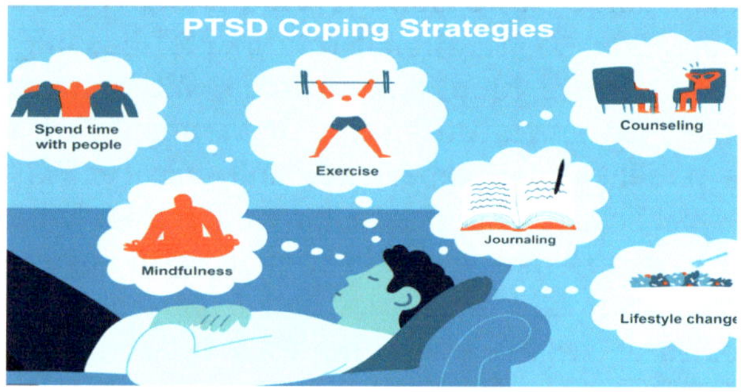
PTSD Coping Strategies
Spend time with people
Exercise
Counseling
Journaling
Mindfulness
Lifestyle change

Figure 8.17. Prevention and Coping Strategies for trauma- and stressor-related disorders.

Source: https://external-content.duckduckgo.com/iu/?u=https%3A%2F%2Fwww.verywellmind.com%2Fthmb%2F8NvmNEc42pk32pt8dX48p8IzBrA%3D%2F1333x1000%2Fsmart%2Ffilters%3Ano_upscale()%2Fcoping-with-ptsd-2797536_FINAL-5c12beae46e0fb00010177e7.png&f=1&nofb=1&ipt=eaee8659f5695fcb8eb68793a9cca934d1c498149ba664bd75c2a26b5c959382.

8.6.1. Building Resilience

Resilience is crucial in supporting individuals who navigate the complex landscape of trauma- and stressor-related disorders. Resilience is not a trait but a dynamic process that enables individuals to learn to adapt and recover following adversity. Resilience is constructed by forming protective factors that act as a buffer to ward off the negative impact of trauma and stress. Social support, coping skills, and community ties are all protective factors. The integration of trauma-informed care practices is paramount in the development of resilience, particularly in marginalized groups. By considering the experiences of Black, Indigenous, and People of Color (BIPOC) and other previously oppressed groups, practitioners are better placed to augment their understanding of resilience through culturally informed models. This is logical since healing practice in these communities works and is sensitive to their needs and values, thereby ultimately developing greater resilience to systemic barriers (Campbell & Khin, 2020). The nature of stress is complex and therefore hard to know and develop resilience from. Stressors are either acute or chronic and may differ in intensity as well as duration, therefore impacting individual response and coping. Specifically, cumulative stress over a lifetime can elicit a variety of physiological and psychological reactions to shape outcomes of health. Building resilience, therefore, requires an advanced understanding of the interaction between categories of stressors and individual and environmental factors. Researchers and clinicians must adopt full-framed models, for instance, by integrating epidemiological and psychophysiological frameworks, in order to advance the understanding of the richness of stress and resilience. By intervening in these interactions, we are able to develop more effective interventions that are individually adapted and foster resilience and enable individuals to thrive in the midst of trauma (Crosswell et al., 2018). Creating environments that foster resilience involves strategic intervention at multiple levels, ranging from the individual level to systemic intervention. These interventions must target the creation of social connections and enhanced emotional regulation as a precursor to resilience. Also, engaging community resources and networks can strengthen collective resilience capacity, offering collective spaces for healing and support. Developmental frameworks, drawing on theories , such as Bronfenbrenner's Ecological Systems Theory, can guide these efforts by highlighting the systemic forces influencing individual well-being. With the development of resilience in this multifaceted framework, people can be enabled not only to recover from stressor-related disorders but also to leverage their experience in furthering the prospects of growth and leadership within their communities. Resilience is therefore a key component of recovery, facilitating the transition towards healing and enduring health (Campbell & Khin, 2020).

8.6.2. Community Support Systems

Community support structures are central to the healing of trauma- and stressor-related disorders, particularly for the marginalized populations who may experience more entrenched issues as a result of systemic oppression. The reality of lives in those populations calls for an imperative of a trauma-informed and culturally competent form of support. Practitioners who bridge the fields of analysis not only share ideas but also strengthen tools that facilitate group healing. By embracing models , such as the Minority Stress Model and Bronfenbrenner's Ecological Systems Theory, clinicians are able to effectively address the unique needs of trauma-affected populations, consequently enhancing clinical outcomes and fostering resilience among at-risk populations (Campbell & Khin, 2020). The function of perceived social support within community systems cannot be overstated, with its potential effect of mitigating the influence of trauma. Research has indicated that individuals with strong social support networks have lower incidence levels of posttraumatic stress symptoms because the reassurance of such networks acts as a buffer against perceived stress. For veterans, for example, community attachment can be critical in managing the psychological aftermath of combat exposure. The relationship between social support and perceived stress is actualized as veterans with low support systems struggle more with PTSD symptoms, whereas those immersed within strong community relationships exhibit better health-related quality of life (Hart et al., 2006). Further, the development of effective community support systems is contingent upon an understanding of the variegated experiences of trauma across disparate populations. This awareness introduces the adaptive quality of interventions that address the cultural narratives of diverse populations. Certain populations, including veterans and minority ethnic groups, possess distinct experiences with trauma that must receive direct consideration and attention. The integration of resources within communities, including peer networks and culturally-responsive counseling agencies, plays an important role in the process of healing among individuals who suffer from trauma in their lives. As mental health practitioners develop such support networks, they not only facilitate the recovery of individuals but also community resilience, ultimately investing in the general well-being of communities (Campbell & Khin, 2020).

8.6.3. Stress Management Skills

Effective stress management techniques are crucial in patients who are experiencing trauma- and stressor-related disorders, particularly given the inclination of these disorders to increase psychological distress. Present-moment awareness and acceptance-based mindfulness strategies form a fundamental approach. Mindfulness meditation has been shown to reduce anxiety and enable emotional regulation, bringing relief from the deluge of feelings that come with trauma re-experiencing. Other studies validate these results, pointing out that not only does mindfulness make a person feel more connected to his/her thoughts and feelings, but also diminishes the intensity of stress response. By applying techniques of mindfulness in everyday existence, individuals can foster a firmer sense of self-awareness, thereby enhancing their resilience against disorder symptoms like PTSD. This liberal approach points to the integration of psychological resilience as a core component of the trauma healing process.

Besides mindfulness, physical activity has emerged as an essential stress coping strategy that can alleviate symptoms of trauma-related disorders. Exercise regularly stimulates the release of endorphins, which are popularly referred to as the body's natural mood elevators. Therefore, individuals who exercise regularly have lower anxiety and depression levels that are common in individuals who suffer from disorders related to trauma. Exercise can also assist in good sleeping habits and general body health, both of which are vital elements of stress management.

Finally, the addition of exercise , such as yoga, can be beneficial in that one integrates movement with consciousness in an effort to work on both the body and the psychological elements of stress. For health care workers, observing the value of exercise as part of treatment is invaluable, giving patients a balanced means of combating their stress.

Lastly, integration of support networks and interventions is also essential for individuals living with trauma- and stressor-related disorders. Having the capability to establish and maintain close relationships can be used as a protective factor in safeguarding individuals against the debilitating effects of stress. Social support provides emotional reassurance, provides a feeling of belonging, and urges individuals to share their experiences, which can quite readily diminish feelings of loneliness. Combined with psychological treatments, such as cognitive-behavioral therapy (CBT), the role of professional support cannot be exaggerated. Up-to-date clinical practice guidelines suggest that general practitioners who identify symptoms of PTSD explore not only medication possibilities but also refer to evidence-based psychotherapies like CBT to enhance coping and foster resilience (Cooper et al., 2024). With a multidimensional approach through acceptance from the community and professionals, people are well-positioned to navigate the intricacies of their trauma and stressor-related phenomena (Katzman et al., 2012).

Test Your Knowledge

1. How can early intervention, supportive counseling, and psychoeducation help prevent the progression of acute stress reactions into PTSD?
2. What self-care practices, resilience-building techniques, and community supports assist individuals in coping with trauma-related stress?

SUMMARY

Within the description of trauma- and stressor-related disorders, the significance of adjustment disorder (AD) is evident, as an area where there is a requirement for a conceptual framework for clinical use and for research purposes. Although often overlooked, AD is a vital component of mental health treatment, with the significance of its implications for legal constructions regarding stress and psychological distress being significant. Research has revealed that demographic and individual stressors are key to the presentation of AD, testifying to the influence of experience on clinical presentation. Of specific interest is the incidence of work-related problems, family distress, and health problems, as a result of their central position in being able to be treated within therapeutic settings, considering they directly correlate with patient outcome (Anastasia et al., 2016). An understanding of the unique stressor profiles inherent with AD can optimize diagnosis and inform targeted intervention programs. Furthermore, the interplay of trauma, stressors, and other mental health symptoms should not be overlooked. Outcomes in studies with veterans highlight that resilience and social support are mediators in the development of post-traumatic stress disorder (PTSD) symptoms. For example, hardiness and social relationships can act as buffers against the adverse consequences of traumatic incidents, which reflects a multifaceted interaction between internal traits and external environments. An examination of these associations implies that stimulating resilience and supporting helpful networks could reduce the impact of stressful events and enhance recovery from trauma. Consistently, findings on resilience-recovery factors are indispensable in explaining processes in trauma- and stressor-related disorders, translating into new interventions for affected populations (King et al., 1998). Research into trauma- and stressor-related disorders, that is, adjustment disorder and PTSD, is reflective of the intricate nature of psychological responses to adversity. The empirical evidence, conclusions and clinical experience emphasize additional specific criteria for diagnosis and the harmonization of individually tailored treatment approaches. By attributing attention to the appropriate patient experience and resilience factors that influence mental health, professionals can maximize their therapeutic impact. As the discipline continues to mature, ongoing study is essential to developing rich paradigms capable of addressing both the psychological and social dimensions of trauma. This combined knowledge will ultimately result in improved mental health results for individuals struggling with the challenges that accompany trauma and stressor-related disorders (Anastasia et al., 2016; King et al., 1998).

Trauma- and Stressor-Related Disorders are conditions of the mind that arise after exposure to traumatic events. One of the key considerations in research on these disorders is the strong correlation between the type of traumatic incident and the ensuing mental illness. Research with victims of motor vehicle accidents (MVA) reveals that victims of severe accidents experience physical and mental health complications, including PTSD. The study highlighted that several factors, including severity of the accident and level of injury, are critical in leading to symptoms of PTSD. Importantly, the study revealed that the victims reported higher ill-health and symptoms of PTSD than non-victims, establishing the significant impact of traumatic experiences on mental health and use of health care services (Kennedy-Moffat, 1997). But another important aspect of Trauma- and Stressor-Related Disorders is the neurobiology underlying the disorder. The neurobiological underpinning regarding the disorder involves the hypothalamic-pituitary-adrenal (HPA) axis as a key player in the response of the body to stress and trauma. HPA axis dysregulation is linked with a range of stress-related disorders, including PTSD and major depressive disorder. Understanding the healthy and pathological status of the HPA axis illustrates how chronic stress affects hormone regulation, particularly for corticotropin-releasing hormone (CRH) and adrenocorticotropic hormone (ACTH). Notably, the system's dynamics, for example, the timing and magnitude of traumatic experiences, can influence whether individuals acquire hallmark features of stress disorders, showing a complex interaction between biological response and psychological outcome (Chou et al., 2016). Additionally, the treatment implications of research findings in Trauma- and Stressor-Related Disorders are important. Knowledge of the HPA axis and regulation provides evidence for therapy that can be useful, such as exposure therapy. Modes of treatment can aim to balance out by treating dysregulation of the system, thereby lessening symptomatology of PTSD and the other disorders. The interaction between traumatic exposure, timing of stressful exposures, and consequent psychological responses necessitates that treatment interventions must be individually oriented in their strategy to challenge experience and biological response. Ongoing research is thus necessary to clarify our understanding of these disorders, eventually leading to more effective treatments and better outcomes for survivors of trauma (Chou et al., 2016).

KEY TERMS FROM THIS CHAPTER

- Acute stress disorder
- Adjustment disorder
- Avoidance behavior
- Cognitive restructuring
- Complex PTSD
- Dissociation
- Emotional numbing
- Flashbacks
- Hyperarousal
- Intrusive memories
- Nightmares
- Post-traumatic stress disorder (PTSD)
- Prolonged exposure therapy
- Re-experiencing

CRITICAL THINKING QUESTIONS

1. **Which of the following is a hallmark symptom of Post-Traumatic Stress Disorder (PTSD)?**
   a. Grandiose delusions
   b. Recurrent intrusive memories of the traumatic event
   c. Hypersomnia
   d. Disorganized speech
2. **Acute Stress Disorder differs from PTSD primarily in:**
   a. Type of symptoms
   b. Cause of the trauma
   c. Duration of symptoms
   d. Treatment approach
3. **A child exposed to chronic neglect and abuse may develop which trauma-related disorder?**
   a. Reactive Attachment Disorder (RAD)
   b. Separation Anxiety Disorder
   c. Oppositional Defiant Disorder
   d. Conduct Disorder
4. **Which of the following is NOT typically associated with PTSD?**
   a. Flashbacks
   b. Avoidance behaviors
   c. Mania
   d. Hyperarousal
5. **Adjustment disorder is diagnosed when:**
   a. Psychotic symptoms follow trauma
   b. Symptoms occur within 3 months of a major stressor and are excessive or impairing
   c. Symptoms are related to genetic factors only
   d. The individual has experienced hallucinations

Short Answer Questions

1. What is the defining feature of trauma- and stressor-related disorders according to the DSM-5?
2. Name the most well-known trauma-related disorder and briefly describe its core symptoms.
3. What is the difference between Acute Stress Disorder (ASD) and Post-Traumatic Stress Disorder (PTSD)?
4. What is a common trigger for Adjustment Disorder?
5. List two psychological symptoms and two physical symptoms that may occur in PTSD.

Answer to Critical Thinking Questions

1. (b) 2. (c) 3. (a) 4. (c) 5. (c)

REFERENCES

1. King, L. A., King, D. W., Fairbank, J. A., Keane, T. M., & Adams, G. A. (1998). Resilience-recovery factors in post-traumatic stress disorder among female and male Vietnam veterans: hardiness, postwar social support, and additional stressful life events. *Journal of personality and social psychology*, *74*(2), 420–434. https://doi.org/10.1037//0022-3514.74.2.420(accessed on 28th July 2025).
2. Akena, D., Alemayehu, M., Atwoli, L., Gelaye, B., et al. (2024). Relationships between trauma types and psychotic symptoms: A network analysis of patients with psychotic disorders in a large, multi-country study in East Africa. https://core.ac.uk/download/615460442.pdf (accessed on 28th July 2025).
3. Anastasia, A., Colletti, C., Cuoco, V., Quartini, A., Urso, S., Rinaldi, R., & Bersani, G. (2016). Demographic variables, clinical aspects, and medicolegal implications in a population of patients with adjustment disorder. *Neuropsychiatric disease and treatment*, *12*, 737–743. https://doi.org/10.2147/NDT.S92637 (accessed on 28th July 2025).
4. Backholm, K. (2012). Work-related crisis exposure: Psychological trauma and PTSD in news journalists. https://core.ac.uk/download/39949250.pdf (accessed on 28th July 2025).
5. Baird, G., Brewin, C. R., Briken, P., Burke, M., et al. (2021). An organization- and category-level comparison of diagnostic requirements for mental disorders in ICD-11 and DSM-5. https://core.ac.uk/download/374290613.pdf (accessed on 28th July 2025).
6. Balducci, C., Conway, P. M., & Vignoli, M. (2024). A weekly diary within-individual investigation of the relationship between exposure to bullying behavior, workplace phobia, and posttraumatic stress symptomatology. https://core.ac.uk/download/611902544.pdf (accessed on 28th July 2025).
7. Benedict, A. L., Grodin, M. A., & Mancini, L. (2013). Struggling to meditate: Contextualizing integrated treatment of traumatised Tibetan refugee monks. https://core.ac.uk/download/28945404.pdf (accessed on 28th July 2025).
8. Palmieri, Arianna & Kleinbub, Johann & Benelli, Enrico & Sambin, Marco & Broggio, Alice & Bianco, Simone. (2015). THE WORDS OF THE BODY: PSYCHOPHYSIOLOGICAL PATTERNS IN DISSOCIATIVE NARRATIVES. . https://core.ac.uk/download/80154470.pdf (accessed on 28th July 2025).
9. Brooks, M., Bryce, J., Graham-Kevan, N., Irving, A., et al. (2015). Repeat victimization, retraumatisation and victim vulnerability. https://core.ac.uk/download/42138066.pdf (accessed on 28th July 2025).
10. Campbell, C., & Khin, P. (2020). Building Resilience through Culturally Grounded Practices in Clinical Psychology and Higher Education. *The Vermont Connection, 41*(1). https://scholarworks.uvm.edu/tvc/vol41/iss1/7(accessed on 28th July 2025).
11. Chou, T., D'Orsogna, M. R., & Kim, L. U. (2016). Onset, timing, and exposure therapy of stress disorders: Mechanistic insight from a mathematical model of oscillating neuroendocrine dynamics. https://core.ac.uk/download/323078037.pdf (accessed on 28th July 2025).
12. Cohen, J., Cohen, S., Gilbert, P., Meads, C., Mogk, C., & Pennebaker, J. W. (2018). The impact of an emotionally expressive writing intervention on eating pathology in female students. https://core.ac.uk/download/287581774.pdf (accessed on 28th July 2025).

13. Cole, S. L. (2016). Effects of early life stress on anhedonia and striatal dopamine concentration depends on variation in catechol-O-methyltransferase (COMT) genotype. https://core.ac.uk/download/232614178.pdf (accessed on 28th July 2025).
14. Crosswell, A. D., Epel, E. S., Mayer, S. E., Mendes, W. B., et al. (2018). More than a feeling: A unified view of stress measurement for population science. https://core.ac.uk/download/305124133.pdf (accessed on 28th July 2025).
15. Dinkler, L., Lundström, S., Gajwani, R., Lichtenstein, P., Gillberg, C., & Minnis, H. (2017). Maltreatment-associated neurodevelopmental disorders: a co-twin control analysis. *Journal of child psychology and psychiatry, and allied disciplines*, *58*(6), 691–701. https://doi.org/10.1111/jcpp.12682(accessed on 28th July 2025).
16. Ertelt, M. K. (2023). Best practice occupational therapy interventions for addressing trauma and posttraumatic stress disorder: A practitioner guide. https://core.ac.uk/download/587997744.pdf (accessed on 28th July 2025).
17. Evans, C. J., Fanselow, M. S., Li, K., Pennington, Z. T., et al. (2020). Chronic opioid pretreatment potentiates the sensitization of fear learning by trauma. https://core.ac.uk/download/323082472.pdf (accessed on 28th July 2025).
18. Gourley, S. J. (2016). Possible causes of increased domestic violence among military veterans: PTSD or mefloquine toxicity? https://core.ac.uk/download/58827124.pdf (accessed on 28th July 2025).
19. Grey, B. J. (2015). The future of emotional harm. https://core.ac.uk/download/144230394.pdf (accessed on 28th July 2025).
20. Hart, C. L. (2006). Posttraumatic stress symptomatology in aging combat veterans: The direct and buffering effects of stress and social support. https://core.ac.uk/download/12207651.pdf (accessed on 28th July 2025).
21. Katzman, W. B., & Pastore, E. A. (2012). Recognizing myofascial pelvic pain in the female patient with chronic pelvic pain. https://core.ac.uk/download/305124272.pdf (accessed on 28th July 2025).
22. Kennedy-Moffat, J. (1997). *The Psychological Impact of Motor Vehicle Accidents: A New Zealand Study: A Thesis Presented in Partial Fulfilment of The Requirements for The Degree of Master of Science in Psychology at Massey University*. http://hdl.handle.net/10179/13540. https://core.ac.uk/download/159449347.pdf (accessed on 28th July 2025).
23. Larauche, M., Mulak, A., & Taché, Y. (2011). Stress-related alterations of visceral sensation: Animal models for irritable bowel syndrome study. https://core.ac.uk/download/323080393.pdf (accessed on 28th July 2025).
24. Nadeau, M. (2019). The role of horticultural therapy in the treatment of refugees with post-traumatic stress disorder. https://core.ac.uk/download/213463622.pdf (accessed on 28th July 2025).
25. Norman, S. B., Pietrzak, R. H., Pitts, M., Straus, E., et al. (2019). Purpose in life and conscientiousness protect against the development of suicidal ideation in U.S. military veterans with PTSD and MDD: Results from the National Health and Resilience in Veterans Study. https://core.ac.uk/download/323311016.pdf (accessed on 28th July 2025).

26. Paleczna, M. (2017). Cancer related PTSD symptoms in patients of all ages and their relatives, and general risk factors. Nowotwory. Journal of Oncology, 67(6), 359–364. https://doi.org/10.5603/NJO.2017.0058 (accessed on 28th July 2025).

27. Cooper, J., Metcalf, O., & Phelps, A. (2014). PTSD--an update for general practitioners. *Australian family physician*, *43*(11), 754–757.(accessed on 28th July 2025).

PERSONALITY DISORDERS

9

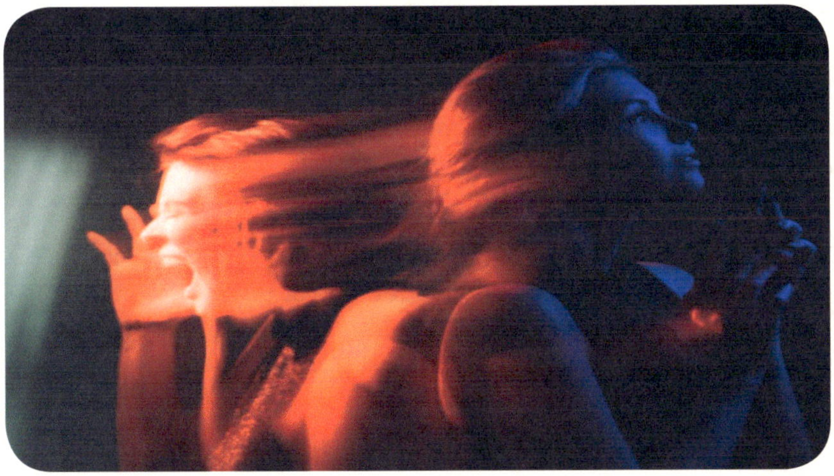

Introduction

An understanding of personality disorders is relevant to psychological treatment and testing because they significantly influence an individual's behavior, emotional status, and interpersonal relationships. Baffling schemes of thinking and behavior inconsistent with cultural norms, personality disorders often culminate in severe distress and impairment in functioning. The complexity of the problem necessitates a refined system of classification and diagnosis, which psychologists reflect in the comprehensiveness of their tests. Specifically, the intersection of varied diagnostic models, categorical and dimensional, indicates the importance of sound comprehension in optimizing therapy results. The occurrence of personality disorders within populations only serves to reiterate their relevance within clinical psychology, thereby indicating the importance of research as well as better intervention methods. In psychology, the diagnosis practiced by experts constitutes the foundation of study as well as a reaction to personality disorders. The psychological interviews generally reveal

LEARNING OBJECTIVES

After studying this chapter, you will be able to:

1. Explain the classification of personality disorders;
2. List the common types of personality disorders;
3. Describe the causes and risk factors;
4. Identify the symptoms and diagnosis;
5. Explore the treatment options;
6. Focus on the impact on individuals and relationships.

complexities of sophistication that demand psychological flexibility at the level of assessment. For instance, a mixed-method study indicated that psychologists assumed a dynamic approach to carrying out clinical interviews, constantly shifting between diagnostic hypotheses, client complaint assessments, and likely treatment options.

This flexibility of the assessment process demonstrates how crucial it is for practitioners to remain responsive to the dynamic presentational style of the client (Groenier et al., 2011). Through the recognition of substantive information that lies in clients' behaviors and histories, psychologists are made capable of better identifying the internal causes of suffering, and they become better at categorizing and personalizing treatments. Personality disorder study transcends individual assessment and raises critical evaluation of wide-ranging therapeutic models. Various modalities, such as classical psychotherapy and newer ones, try to address the unique challenges posed by personality disorders.

This involves examination of how various levels of functioning influence the treatment effectiveness and outcome. Also, models like the ones introduced in Bufford's work point to the central role of awareness and understanding in bringing about recovery from mental adversity (Bufford et al., 1988). Consequently, a well-balanced introduction to personality disorders demands an investigation into theoretical frameworks as well as practical implications so that a well-balanced comprehension may guide additional research into effective treatment strategies. Such, then, is this intricate debate that sets the stage for thorough comprehension of personality disorders and the necessity to enhance clinical psychology practice (Figure 9.1).

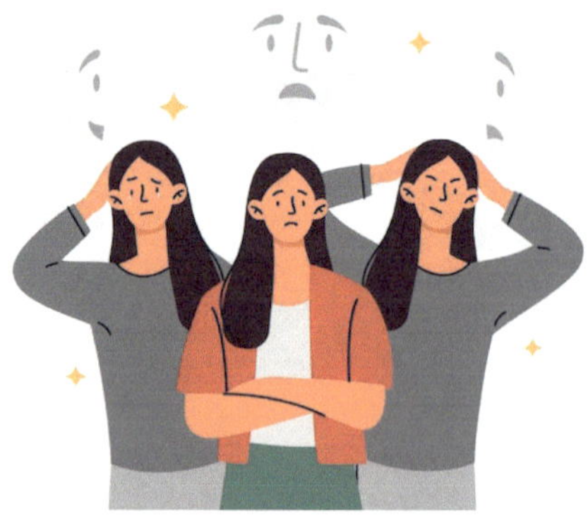

Figure 9.1. Personality disorder.

Source: https://external-content.duckduckgo.com/iu/?u=https%3A%2F%2Fimg.freepik.com%2Fpremium-vector%2Fpersonality-disorder-concept_118813-2879.jpg&f=1&nofb=1&ipt=531bc5cab9ea1a64e754c26f7a9bae78d27e9c2860b5bdc390cc42c70052afea.

Definition of Personality Disorders

A personality disorder is a group of mental disorders that are characterized by enduring patterns of behavior, cognition, and emotion that differ significantly from the expectations of the individual's culture. These patterns are generally inflexible and pervasive and often result in significant distress or impairment in social, occupational, or other significant areas of functioning. The Diagnostic and Statistical Manual of Mental Disorders (DSM-5) classifies personality disorders into three clusters, each of which provide descriptions of different maladaptive personality traits. For instance, Cluster A includes paranoid, schizoid, and schizotypal personality disorders that are more often described as having odd or eccentric behavior. Their definition has evolved with advances in psychological science and cultural attitudes, as challenged in much scholarly discourse over the role of culture in the presentation of psychological pathology. Additional research into personality disorders points to the intersection of biology, environment, and culture that influences their development and expression. The behaviors of such disorders tend to develop at a young age and are sustained by a host of cognitive as well as emotional mechanisms. For instance, those who exhibit negative affectivity tend to indulge in maladaptive thinking styles like rumination or hopelessness, especially in response to frustrated personal aspirations.

This tendency to evaluate differences between desired and obtained outcomes might enhance affective distress in the sense that such automatic cognitive patterns have been shown in literature to lead to cognitive vulnerabilities for disorders like depression and anxiety (Marchetti et al., 2016). The identification of the dynamics of these behaviors holds primary importance for effective diagnosis and therapeutic adaptation, proving the necessity of considering interpersonal frameworks in which these disorders manifest. Cultural background also makes personality disorders more complex to interpret, particularly in terms of how symptoms are expressed and perceived. Research indicates that culture has a significant impact on the experience of psychological pain, from symptomatology to patterns of help-seeking. For example, in certain cultures, emotional pain may be expressed somatically, such as depression in a broader sense throughout Chinese culture (Heine et al., 2002). This is a development that challenges the traditional Western paradigms of understanding mental health, and more sophisticated work is required that captures the cultural construction of action and identity. Lastly, a viable definition of personality disorders must incorporate these complex variables, admitting that personality is not simply a personal construct but also a product of the dynamic interplay between self and sociocultural environment.

Importance of Understanding Personality Disorders

Knowledge of personality disorders is not only significant for mental health practitioners but also for society in general. With complete comprehension of the characteristics and consequences of various personality disorders, practitioners can create more tailored therapeutic methods based on the unique needs of each individual. For instance, a detailed knowledge of the nuances of disorders like antisocial personality disorder can maximize the therapeutic bond between patient and practitioner. This awareness allows the practitioners to transcend the diagnostic labels and engage with patients in a more empathetic manner, eventually establishing a healing treatment setting. The importance of this process of relating is reflected by a study conducted on nursing students, in which one of the emerging themes was for the patient to be seen beyond the diagnosis, thus showing the healing power of understanding personality disorders in clinical practice (Alwin et al., 2025).

Moreover, the realization of personality disorders extends beyond the treatment room; it has implications for community life and social interactions. Awareness of the manifestation of personality disorders in behavior can dispel stigma and bring about greater understanding for individuals affected by personality disorders. When individuals in a community understand the causes of the behaviors of individuals with personality disorders, they can deal with them patiently and with empathy. This heightened understanding can aid more effective engagement with those affected in social contexts and the reduction of discriminatory occurrences, which are frequently fueled by misunderstanding. As a result, an understanding of personality disorders has a two-way function: it enhances therapeutic work simultaneously as it brings depth to relationships in the community. Further, the consequences of personality disorders are increasingly inseparably intertwined with the neurobiology of mental distress. Scientific research reveals that trauma, a common precipitating cause for all types of personality disorders, can potentially lead to dysregulation in psychological and physiological responses. Importantly, models , such as Damasio's somatic markers and Porges' polyvagal theory describe how these disorders can affect interpersonal processes and emotional regulation (Palmieri et al., 2015).

This complex interaction offers important implications for psychotherapy treatment. Once therapists are equipped with an understanding of the neurophysiological factors involved with personality disorders, they can design interventions that not only address psychological symptomology, but also maximize physiology. It is with such inclusion in models of treatment, therefore, that the multiform nature of personality disorders is rendered an ever-more salient consideration (Figure 9.2).

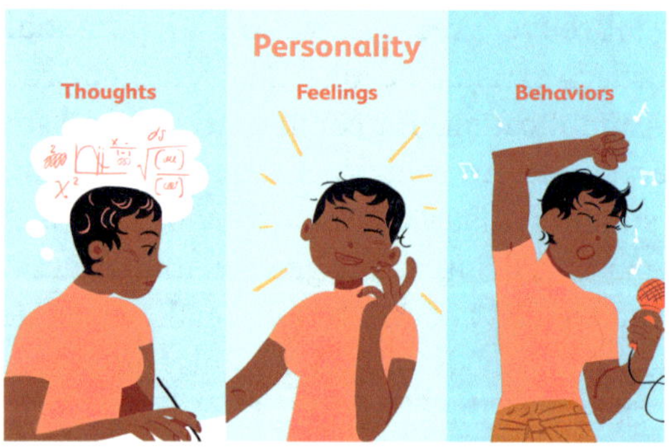

Figure 9.2. Importance of personality disorders.

Source: https://www.verywellmind.com/thmb/IlzUEm9032VX2ztyAO8uObamYX0=/6000x0/filters:no_upscale():max_bytes(150000):strip_icc()/what-is-personality-2795416_sketch-5b63480c46e0fb00250e38b2.png.

9.1. Classification of Personality Disorders

Learning Outcome

1. Overview of the DSM-5 criteria.
2. Categories of personality disorders.
3. Differences between personality disorders and other mental health disorders.

The DSM has been utilized for a long time in the diagnosis of personality disorders as an organized framework for searching and categorizing all the various types of disorders under the stated criteria. The latest of these, DSM-5, groups the personality disorders into three clusters: Cluster A (odd or eccentric), Cluster B (dramatic, emotional, or erratic), and Cluster C (anxious or fearful). This clustering highlights the complexity that is inherent to personality disorders because each of the clusters captures different presentations and underlying psychological processes. For instance, patients with Cluster A disorders, such as paranoid personality disorder, might exhibit pervasive distrust, while those in Cluster B, such as borderline personality disorder, exhibit mood and interpersonal instability. Such a multi-dimensional categorization not only enhances the accuracy of diagnosis but also directs the treatment plans made for the characteristic problems posed by each disorder. While the DSM categorization is a significant tool, it should be mentioned that there is still an argument concerning the validity and consistency of these categories. Research has established that personality disorders run together in the same individual, thus a demand for more sophisticated explanations that transcend fixed categories. The variability of the severity of the symptoms and the part played by the environment and sociocultural factors introduce complexity into the diagnosis. Further, the developing paradigms of psychological inquiry, such as the study of neuroticism as a universal risk factor for most mental disorders, imply that personality disorders may be studied better through a paradigm focusing on underlying tendencies rather than stringent categorizations. This paradigm shift leads clinicians to look towards the interconnectedness of personality traits and disorders so that they can plan better treatment programs. The sharedness of personality disorders among the general population further stresses the significance of correct classification and its connotations in mental health.

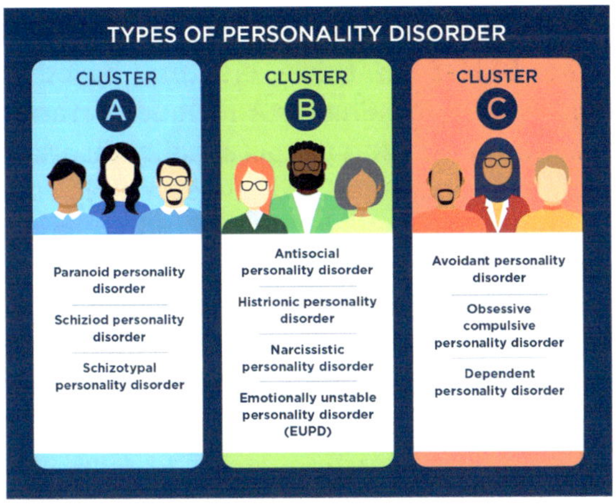

Figure 9.3. Classification of personality disorders.

Source: https://www.priorygroup.com/media/5j5dv4ff/personality-disorder-cluster-types.jpg.

Prevalence rates have been observed to differ widely in epidemiological studies, which is caused by the extensive variety of test instruments used in research. Findings indicate variation in prevalence from a low of 0.8% in Italy to a high of 26.7% in Hong Kong, demonstrating the effect of culture and differing conceptions of mental health on diagnoses. These variations point toward the necessity for standardization in classification and for critical examination of the measuring instruments used for these disorders. Also, since research has been focusing on the occurrence of personality disorders with comorbid conditions, there is an evident case for a convergence of research findings, including those related to Internet addiction, in the study of the underlying components of personality disorders. This would benefit the mental health profession in better facilitating the complexity in diagnosis and treatment of these disorders (Billieux et al., 2014; Barlow et al., 2017) (Figure 9.3).

9.1.1. Overview of the DSM-5 Criteria

The Diagnostic and Statistical Manual of Mental Disorders, Fifth Edition (DSM-5), is a critical device for the diagnosis of personality disorders, providing a set of standardized criteria that must be applied by clinicians. This system provides a systematic framework for the investigation of personality pathology, allowing for consistent and reliable diagnosis. The DSM-5 outlines the specific characteristics and behaviors that constitute a range of personality disorders, which are usually categorized into clusters A (odd or eccentric), B (dramatic, emotional, or erratic), and C (anxious or fearful). Each cluster contains unique disorders, such as paranoid personality disorder or borderline personality disorder, defining features, associated behaviors, and other clinical aspects that must be present to make a formal diagnosis. This structured approach not only assists the practitioner in diagnosing the mental health condition but also aids in improved communication among professionals dealing with complex issues. In its approach to personality disorders, one of the most salient features of DSM-5 is the focus on patterns of long-standing cognition, emotion, and behavior, greatly puzzling cultural expectations. Such patterns occur early in personality development as a pattern of persistent disorder rather than an acute situation. This is an important feature since it is what separates personality disorders from other mental disorders that may have worse symptoms. Also, the DSM-5 additionally specifies that the maladaptive patterns need to result in significant distress or impairment in personal, social, or occupational functioning, further highlighting the impact of the disorder on the individual's life. By encouraging a nuanced appreciation of psychopathology, the DSM-5 encourages more integrated assessment of the patient's experience, essential to effective intervention and treatment planning. By emphasizing the worth of developmental and contextual factors, current research underscores the significance of antecedent history in understanding personality disorders, a methodology that continues to evolve under the auspices of the DSM-5. More recent studies, however, show that behavioral styles in childhood and adolescence can indeed be predictors of adult personality pathology, thereby highlighting the necessity of early intervention and diagnosis.

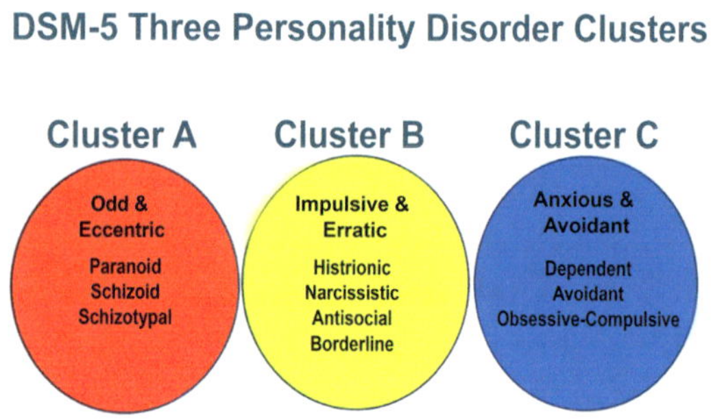

Figure 9.4. Categories of personality disorders.

Source: https://external-content.duckduckgo.com/iu/?u=https%3A%2F%2Fisompersonality154.weebly.com%2Fuploads%2F3%2F8%2F6%2F9%2F3869482%2Fpersonality-disorders-fa-11-2020-ca-bluegray_orig.jpg&f=1&nofb=1&ipt=52633ef3334af09e2c19f8e15e5e8587d9db8ae1ad8f31e1ffe37f1fc17f9272.

Furthermore, the necessity of incorporating typicality effects when conceptualizing psychiatric concepts also discredits traditional dichotomous categories typically included in diagnostic manuals. The new approach has been crafted to accommodate the subtlety of human behaviors, allowing less strict interpretation of DSM-5 criteria that can maximize the results of individuals suffering from these disorders. In this regard, the addition of developmental and historical factors increases the predictive validity of DSM-5 criteria, providing clinicians and patients with a more nuanced context (De Fruyt & De Clercq, 2014; Lieto et al., 2019) (Figure 9.4).

9.1.2. Categories of Personality Disorders

Personality disorders have largely been grouped based on the guidelines established in the DSM-5 in three clusters based on common features. Cluster A includes paranoid, schizoid, and schizotypal personality disorders, which are characterized by eccentric, odd, and unconventional behavior. Individuals in such groups tend to demonstrate an odd or complicated pattern of thinking that does not make it easy for them to socialize. For instance, a patient with schizotypal personality disorder may present with interpersonal deficits along with cognitive distortion, leading to enhanced social anxiety. Clustering allows clinicians to identify interventions tailored to address the precise needs of these patients and achieve better treatment outcomes, as well as a model for understanding the nuances inherent in these disorders (Tocarciuc, 2018). Entering Cluster B, these are antisocial, borderline, histrionic, and narcissistic personality disorders that are marked by dramatic, emotional, or unpredictable behavior. Individuals in this cluster tend to struggle with managing their behavior and their emotions. Bizarrely, borderline personality disorder is marked by unstable relationships and intense emotions, and the individual tends to exhibit a fear of abandonment. In contrast, people with antisocial personality disorder can display a habitual disregard for the rights of others, which often leads to criminal behavior. When such disorders are considered as belonging to Cluster B, therapeutic interventions can be offered that take cognizance of the emotional volatility and interpersonal conflicts that usually arise during treatment (Burrell-Hodgson et al., 2006). Finally, Cluster C comprises avoidant, dependent, and obsessive-compulsive personality disorders, which are heavily anchored in fear and anxiety responses. Avoidant personality disorder is normally found in individuals who are pathologically shy and have a persistent fear of criticism, which affects social interaction and self-esteem. Dependent personality disorder, on the other hand, is found in individuals who have excessive reliance on others, leading to submissive behavior and difficulty making independent decisions. Obsessive-compulsive personality disorder, which is distinct from obsessive-compulsive disorder, is characterized by a requirement for control and perfectionism. Understanding the intricacies of these personality disorders in Cluster C is imperative in developing effective treatment plans aimed at enhancing patients' coping mechanisms and the establishment of healthier relationships (Tocarciuc, 2018) (Figure 9.5).

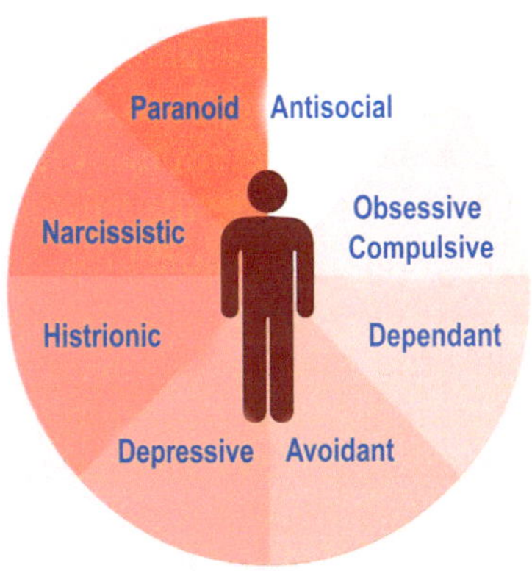

Figure 9.5. Most common personality disorders.

Source: https://external-content.duckduckgo.com/iu/?u=https%3A%2F%2Fstatic.wixstatic.com%2Fmedia%2Fca4d3c_964cff31141b4f97a240359e2edf9a80~mv2.png%2Fv1%2Ffill%2Fw_1000%2Ch_1000%2Cal_c%2Cq_90%2Cusm_0.66_1.00_0.01%2Fca4d3c_964cff31141b4f97a240359e2edf9a80~mv2.png&f=1&nofb=1&ipt=33438001af43d884f3eb82404b8ce0a444c5e9a79f0f9a42f10c50c974514660.

9.1.3. Differences Between Personality Disorders and Other Mental Health Disorders

The difference between personality disorders and other psychiatric illnesses is key to understanding the complexities of psychiatric diagnoses. Personality disorders encompass enduring patterns of inner experience, behavior, and cognition that deviate markedly from cultural norms, and typically emerge by early adulthood or adolescence. Other psychiatric illnesses, such as mood disorders or anxiety disorders, may develop later in life and tend to have more episodic courses. For instance, while an individual with generalized anxiety disorder may experience a persisting cycle of anxiety attacks, an individual with a personality disorder like borderline personality disorder will often evidence all-around instability in interpersonal relationships, self-image, and affect. The persistence of personality disorders makes them more resistant to treatment and recovery because specialized therapeutic approaches are required to effectively address their unique traits and impact on daily functioning. It is equally vital to know the underlying mechanisms that differentiate personality disorders from intermittent mental illness disorders. Personality disorders would be much more deeply rooted in a person's identity and influence the way they relate to others and perceive reality in the long run. Other mental illness disorders are usually marked by identifiable precipitants, like trauma or significant life events, that might trigger acute states. This division of time-dependent variables can influence the success of the treatment; for example, cognitive-behavioral therapy (CBT), commonly used in mood disorders, may only partly treat the generalized components of personality disorders. Measurement of the therapeutic process and outcome among personality disorder patients accounts for these discrepancies, for example, in research in which high levels of personality disorders were encountered among clinical populations, which suggests a complex relationship between treatment severity and disorder type. Moreover, therapeutic alliance and involvement are particularly challenging to establish when treating personality disorders compared to other mental disorders. The chronic nature of personality pathology has been shown to interfere with the establishment of trusting therapeutic alliances. In clinical practice, certain personality disorders, particularly the ones that are inwardly focused or emotionally limited in their behavior, have been discovered to be related to poor therapeutic alliance development, thereby interfering with the success of treatment (Palmeiri et al., 2015). Conversely, persons with episodic disorders may find it easier to engage since their issues are less embedded in their own self-construction. This dynamic implies that while personality disorders introduce relational challenges in a consistent way to therapy, those challenges are addressed by the interplay of disorder type and therapeutic modality. Appreciation of such complexity may enhance clinical practices and the quality of patient care, setting the stage for more effective strategies of treatment within the context of diverse psychological topographies (Palmeiri et al., 2015).

Test Your Knowledge

1. How does the DSM-5-TR categorize personality disorders into clusters A, B, and C based on shared traits?
2. What are the key differences between categorical and dimensional approaches to classifying personality disorders?

9.2. Common Types of Personality Disorders

Learning Outcome

1. Cluster A: Paranoid, Schizoid, and Schizotypal.
2. Cluster B: Antisocial, Borderline, Histrionic, and Narcissistic.
3. Cluster C: Avoidant, Dependent, and Obsessive-Compulsive.

Two of the most well-known categories used in personality disorders are the three identified by the Diagnostic and Statistical Manual of Mental Disorders (DSM-5) as Cluster A, Cluster B, and Cluster C. The disorders in Cluster A are those involving eccentric or unusual behavior, including Paranoid Personality Disorder, Schizoid Personality Disorder, and Schizotypal Personality Disorder. The patients in this cluster are likely to exhibit social withdrawal, cognition that distorts reality, and suspiciousness regarding others, describing the severe relational distress. The defining features of these disorders not only render interpersonal relationships impossible but could also provide the basis for pathological coping. Thus, the manifestation of Cluster A disorders highlights the necessity of certain treatment strategies to effectively manage their typical symptoms and promote general functioning within relationship contexts. Cluster B personality disorders, Antisocial, Borderline, Histrionic, and Narcissistic Personality Disorders, are dramatic and unstable behaviors that deviate significantly from cultural norms. As an example, individuals with Antisocial Personality Disorder are manipulative and aversive in their behavior with no respect for moral standards or other individuals' sentiments. In contrast, individuals with Borderline Personality Disorder display intense emotional instability and fear of abandonment, leading to volatile relationships.

Such disorders are capable of generating interpersonal difficulties and enhanced emotional distress, leading to a sheer need for new treatment modalities. Emerging trends in therapeutic models, such as Metacognitive Therapy (MCT), offer promise for addressing the needs of people with such disorders by solving the interpersonal conundrums inherent in them, enhancing their emotional control and interpersonal functioning and possibly minimizing bothersome symptoms hindering their well-being (Strand & Nordahl, 2024). Cluster C personality disorders, including Avoidant, Dependent, and Obsessive-Compulsive Personality Disorders, manifest diffuse anxiety and abnormal behavior. Individuals with Avoidant Personality Disorder are typically introverted, shy and feel inferior, potentially inhibiting their social lives and professional paths. In contrast, Dependent Personality Disorder patients usually reveal an overabundance of craving approval and direction from others, typically sacrificing their own needs at the cost of relationship maintenance. Obsessive-Compulsive Personality Disorder is characterized by inordinate preoccupation with orderliness, perfection, and control, leading to possible rigidity and interpersonal conflict. It is necessary to clarify these varied presentations of Cluster C disorders to produce effective interventions. With advancing science, the inclusion of techniques , such as augmented data-driven methods may be able to facilitate tailored treatment plans towards addressing the intricate needs of individuals marred by personality disorders (Kozhukhov et al., 2023).

9.2.1. Cluster A: Paranoid, Schizoid, and Schizotypal

Cluster A personality disorders, which consist of Paranoid, Schizoid, and Schizotypal disorders, are characterized by bizarre patterns of behavior, thought, and emotional reaction that lead to isolation from normal social relationships. Paranoid personality disorder is an excessive suspiciousness and mistrust of others so that benign actions are viewed as hostile. This ongoing vigilance can greatly limit interpersonal relationships and can create a self-fulfilling prophecy, because the distrust creates even more isolation. Schizoid personality disorder is defined by an enduring pattern of avoidance of social relationships and an inhibited range of emotional expressiveness. They like to be alone, which may start all sorts of misconceptions about their needs or wants in social situations. These traits identify the complexities and social challenges faced by those with disorders of this category. Schizotypal personality disorder, however, is characterized by anomalies in cognition, perception, and behavior, usually a milder form of schizophrenia. An individual may exhibit oddities , such as unconventional ideas or magical thinking, which perplex them as well as people around them. This disorder stands very much apart from the others in this cluster because it shares more extreme cognitive distortions, which can damage the ability to form and maintain close relationships. Recent studies examining personality trait development from childhood discovered that early identification and intervention of such personality disorders are critical. The knowledge of these conditions not only includes recognition of their expression but also a developmental orientation that feels how such patterns are likely to develop and solidify over time (Fortunato & Speranza, 2018). Psychotherapeutic interventions have emerged as potentially effective interventions for individuals with Cluster A personality disorders. Contrary to traditional notions of such illnesses as necessarily untreatable, subsequent evidence is more recent and implies that the patient may gain significant health benefits from structured psychotherapeutic treatment. Research carried out in various treatment environments has determined that intensive treatments, particularly those delivered in inpatient and day hospital environments, attain significant levels of psychiatric symptom reduction and quality of life (Andrea et al., 2011). These findings underlie the need for therapeutic interventions tailored to address the needs of the individuals within this cluster, re-telling the narrative of treatment of these vastly misinterpreted diseases. As research unfolds, a greater understanding of the therapeutic modalities that work will be key to maximizing the functionality and well-being of affected persons (Figure 9.6).

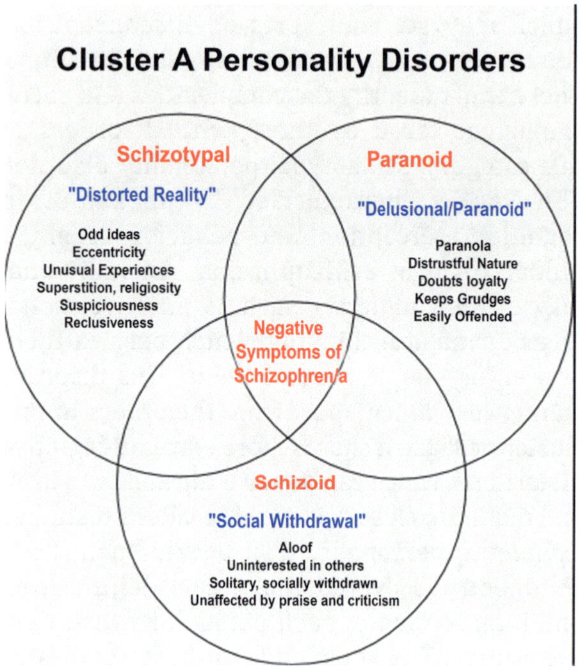

Figure 9.6. Cluster A: Paranoid, schizoid, and schizotypal.

Source: https://external-content.duckduckgo.com/iu/?u=https%3A%2F%2Fwww.tulasihealthcare.com%2Fwp-content%2Fuploads%2F2023%2F01%2FDifference-Between-Mood-Disorders-and-Personality-Disorders_Personality-Disorders.png&f=1&nofb=1&ipt=fd46ef0e87b666a94c8d6d6e93ec81d840da4d7ef33bf06a7cb5295aa2219bb3.

9.2.2. Cluster B: Antisocial, Borderline, Histrionic, and Narcissistic

The psychological landscape of personality disorders is dotted with distinct clusters that capture complex habits and mood swings. Cluster B personality disorders, specifically Antisocial, Borderline, Histrionic, and Narcissistic, are marked by erratic and flamboyant conduct that tends to upset interpersonal and social relationships. Antisocial Personality Disorder (ASPD) is a pervasive pattern of disregarding the rights of others, and this often leads to criminal behavior and a lack of empathy. Meanwhile, Borderline Personality Disorder (BPD) is defined by emotional, self-image, and interpersonal instability, typically accompanied by impulsivity and outbursts of extreme rage, depression, or anxiety. The drama surrounding such illnesses most commonly brings about monumental challenges to the lives of both the individuals suffering from them as well as the individuals within their environment, which require the adequate therapeutic interventions for addressing their complexities. Boselyn, further into Cluster B, Histrionic Personality Disorder (HPD) and Narcissistic Personality Disorder (NPD) also come into play with their special challenges. HPD is a pattern of excessive emotionality and hypersensitivity to interpersonal rejection with attention-seeking behavior that may be detected through dramatic acting out and excessive concern with physical appearance. HPD individuals may struggle with maintaining close relationships, perceiving things in terms of superficiality. On the contrary, NPD individuals possess an inflated sense of self and a strong need for admiration at the cost of empathy for others. The intricate interaction of the disorders is questioned in terms of diagnosis and treatment modalities, particularly in that cultural and gender biases may potentially exacerbate their symptoms. Research indicates that men are more frequently diagnosed with Antisocial PD while women are more frequently characterized by Histrionic and Borderline characteristics, underlining the urgent necessity for high-level understanding in clinical settings (Frantz, 2004). Moreover, the comorbidity of these disorders with other mental disorders is a complicating factor in diagnosis. For instance, customers with Borderline Personality Disorder will also be diagnosed with mood disorders, and this will lead to misinterpretation of their symptoms and challenges. This overlap will confuse the necessary traits that make up each personality disorder, thus setting a daunting challenge for clinicians in arriving at an accurate diagnosis. Studies have discovered that patients who present with complications of mood disorder and personality disorder tend to have a pathological borderline organization and thus a complicated approach to such interdependencies is vital for effective treatment (Ferraro et al., 2019). The practitioners should thus engage in diagnosis and treatment with an awareness of such complexities so that they can promote personalized treatment interventions that are guided by the intricate nature of Cluster B personality disorders (Figure 9.7).

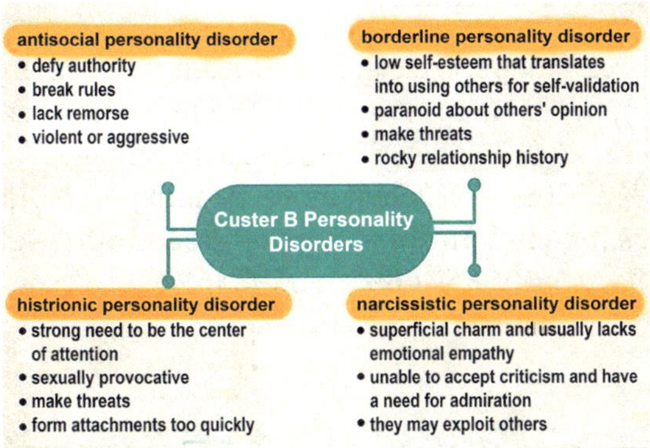

Figure 9.7. Cluster B: Antisocial, borderline, histrionic, and narcissistic.

Source: https://external-content.duckduckgo.com/iu/?u=https%3A%2F%2Fwww.wikihow.com%2Fimages%2Fthumb%2F5%2F5e%2FInteract-with-People-Who-Have-Cluster-B-Personality-Disorders-Step-1.jpg%2Faid9745109-v4-728px-Interact-with-People-Who-Have-Cluster-B-Personality-Disorders-Step-1.jpg&f=1&nofb=1&ipt=1aa9779c8e3a833cdf9e24397dff35457260ba5180a067ae281c0aa80f96094e.

9.2.3. Cluster C: Avoidant, Dependent, and Obsessive-Compulsive

Cluster C personality disorders, like Avoidant, Dependent, and Obsessive-Compulsive Personality Disorders, are characterized by pervasive fear and anxious patterns of behavior. Avoidant Personality Disorder patients are characterized by extensive social inhibition, inferiority of self-esteem, and hypersensitivity to critical rejection. The symptoms lead to an excessive desire to be accepted and a fearful response to potential rejection, which can severely restrict their relational and occupational engagement. Literature suggests that the traits may be early-onset in nature, and therefore, early intervention becomes crucial in managing the long-term effects of such personality traits. Understand how these characteristics evolve, mental health professionals will be better poised to help deal with coping strategies, highlighting the necessity for tailored therapies in working with individuals suffering from Cluster C disorders, particularly in early childhood environments, as seen in the existing controversy surrounding continuity of personality traits from childhood into adulthood (Fortunato & Speranza, 2018). Dependent Personality Disorder, found in Cluster C, has a pervasive and excessive preoccupation with being cared for, which results in submissive and clinging behavior and fear of separation. The disorder manifests itself through an extreme dependency upon others for support and decision-making, which typically results in an overwhelming sensation of helplessness when one is alone. This kind of dependence may sap personal and professional growth, bringing about a point where one will be in an unhealthy relationship because of their debilitating fear of being abandoned. The impacts of such dependence extend beyond intimate relationships since it might complicate the treatment process during therapy sessions. Research on the personality of individuals with personality disorders has documented a prevalence of dependency traits that complicate the therapeutic relationship and treatment, such that clinicians need to use strategic treatment practices that address these issues (Burrell-Hodgson et al., 2006). Obsessive-Compulsive Personality Disorder (OCPD) is another essential member of Cluster C, marked by a preoccupation with orderliness, perfectionism, and control at the expense of flexibility and efficiency. Individuals with OCPD show an inexorable demand for order and rules, which manifests itself as being ultra-detail-oriented, which can disrupt work and interpersonal relationships. Unlike the intrusive, unwanted ideas and compulsive behaviors of Obsessive-Compulsive Disorder (OCD), OCPD is the manifestation of a deep-seated conviction that everything has to be controlled in order to avoid chaos. Perfectionistic motivation can insert tremendous stress and disenchantment into the scene because individuals cannot meet their own unrealistically lofty expectations. These traits and how they affect therapy must be identified, especially since research indicates varying levels of personality traits between the therapeutic relationship and their effects on treatment dynamics and outcomes (Burrell-Hodgson et al., 2006). Through early identification and successful therapy, professionals can assist in improving the lives of victims of this disorder (Figure 9.8).

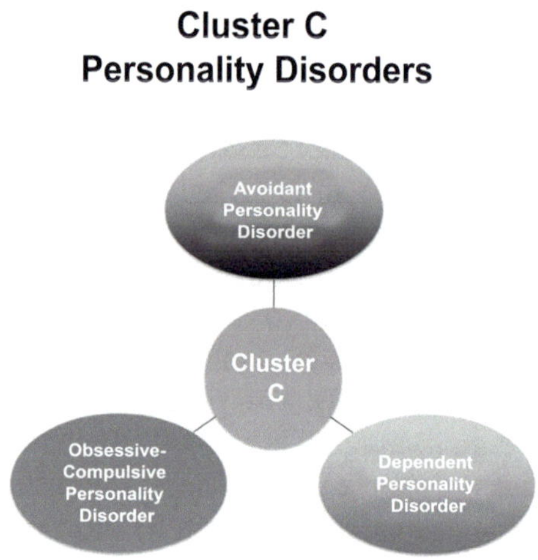

Figure 9.8. Cluster C: Avoidant, dependent, and obsessive-compulsive.

Source: https://external-content.duckduckgo.com/iu/?u=https%3A%2F%2Fslideplayer.com%2Fslide%2F8634551%2F26%2Fimages%2F25%2FCluster%2BC%2BPersonality%2BDisorders.jpg&f=1&nofb=1&ipt=408e8e260b34eb9460f94ce4068634697bae693a63f90a648b4131f901bc2b5d.

Test Your Knowledge

1. What disorders fall under Cluster A, Cluster B, and Cluster C, and what traits characterize each cluster?
2. How do borderline, antisocial, and avoidant personality disorders differ in terms of core behavioral patterns?

9.3. Causes and Risk Factors

Learning Outcome

1. Genetic predispositions.
2. Environmental influences and childhood experiences.
3. Neurobiological factors.

It is important to understand the causative factors and risk factors of personality disorders in order to develop effective interventions and treatment strategies. There are various theories suggesting that personality disorders are caused by multiple factors, with a complex interconnection between genetic susceptibility, environmental factors, and neurobiological factors. Research has also demonstrated that if one has a family history of personality disorders, then he or she is bound to develop them, which suggests a genetic vulnerability to personality disorders. Furthermore, childhood abuse, neglect, and trauma have been found to exponentially increase the risk of personality disorders in adulthood. These findings highlight the importance of early interventions among populations who are at risk to minimize the long-term consequences of such negative experiences, as underlined in a vast amount of mental health research on risk and protective factors concerning mental illness and well-being (Jenkins et al., 2008). The sociocultural context also plays a pivotal part in shaping the personality of an individual, as societal expectations and norms form individual growth perspectives. Adolescence is the period in which the identity of individuals is formed, and the reactions they receive from others and family members contribute significantly towards impacting their psychological health. For instance, attitudes toward mental health disorders can affect people's self-perspectives and vulnerabilities. Research has shown that various mental illness disorders, for example, eating disorders, are more stigmatized than other diseases, for instance as depression and diabetes. Such stigma generally leads to an absence of knowledge, thus further restriction and exacerbation of symptoms associated with disorders, which promotes maladaptive habits (McNamara et al., 2016). It is important to identify the social causes of personality disorders for the purpose of planning educational interventions to increase awareness and reduce stigma. Personality disorders also typically co-occur with other psychiatric disorders that complicate diagnosis and treatment. Such co-occurrence of anxiety or mood disorders leads to aggravation of symptoms of personality disorders in an individual, trigger a vicious cycle that is difficult to stop. Other risk behaviors like drug use and continued stress and other kinds of psychological susceptibility also often complicate the effectiveness of treatment. Awareness of these intersecting trajectories of mental health is highly important in creating integrative interventions that not only treat the personality disorder but also the entire mental health profile of a person. By an integrated treatment strategy consisting of individual and systemic issues, mental health professionals are in a better position to help patients with personality disorders obtain improved results and greater well-being (Jenkins et al., 2008) (Figure 9.9).

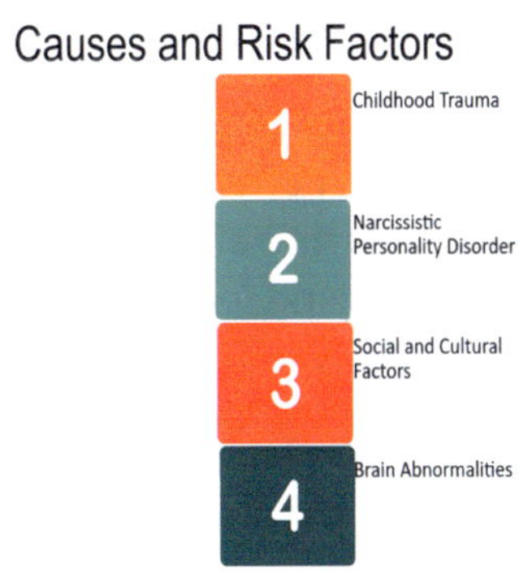

Figure 9.9. Causes and risk factors of personality disorders.

Source: https://fastercapital.co/i/Megalomania--The-Grandiose-Delusions-of-Hubristic-Minds--Causes-and-Risk-Factors.webp.

9.3.1. Genetic Predispositions

The genetic predisposition analysis defines prominent observations into the causation of personality disorders. Heredity significantly contributes to the expression of internalizing and externalizing behaviors, which suggests that the genetic makeup of an individual might shape the susceptibility to particular psychological disorders. Research focusing on these genetic bases shows that some genetic risk factors are associated with increased odds of occurrence for disorders , such as major depressive disorder and conduct disorder. It is imperative to understand how such genetic risks interact with environmental influences in developing better prevention and intervention measures. Interestingly, evocative gene-environmental correlation processes also suggest in more detail how genetic predispositions shape interpersonal interaction outcomes that impact personality development over time, particularly for adolescents (Bucholz et al., 2018). Furthermore, genetic predispositions imply more than susceptibility, as they can predetermine the expression of traits that are characteristic of personality disorders. For instance, there is evidence that indicates certain genetic patterns can lead to variation in personality traits , such as agreeableness, which can play a mediating role in the onset of psychopathological symptoms. This convergence of personality and genetics points toward the significance of an evolving understanding of how these traits might interact with environmental influences, for example, parental influence. A sample study of European American adolescents confirmed that genetic risk scores for depression were associated with lower parental knowledge, subsequently resulting in increased symptoms of depressive and conduct disorders. This is in line with the need for multi-determined approaches addressing both genetic and environmental components in personality disorders (Bucholz et al., 2018). Aside from psychological issues, genetic predispositions also have applicability to broader societal use, like the breeding of specific types of dogs with determined personality profiles. The case of the German Shepherd Dog (GSD) offers the same problem of interest for genetic predispositions and behavioral implications. Evidence indicates that demographic changes and health concerns related to GSDs have emerged, shedding light on the genetics that influence behavior, adjustability, and overall health. In veterinary clinical practice, collecting information about the health and behavioral disorders in breeds like the GSD raises the role of genetics not only in personality disorders in human beings but also in domesticated animals. These interspecies observations have the potential to enhance our knowledge of personality genetic architecture, with an overall perspective being offered of how tendencies manifest themselves under different circumstances.

9.3.2. Childhood Experiences and Environmental Influences

Personality disorder formation is significantly influenced by environmental and early experience. Research has consistently demonstrated that individuals who were exposed to childhood adversity, such as abuse or neglect, are significantly more likely to have multiple personality disorders as adults. Children raised in unstable or abusive home environments are more likely to acquire maladaptive coping strategies, which later form personality disorders in adult life. For example, individuals who have histories of sexual abuse during childhood have been found to score higher on neuroticism tests that are specifically linked to symptomatology of major depression as evidenced in twin studies where specific environmental difficulties shaped symptom patterns and experiences specific to each individual (Kendler & Aggen, 2017). As such, the interplay between genetic predispositions and negative childhood environments creates an intricate web that influences personality over time. Additionally, harmful dysfunction, as a theoretical construct put forward by Wakefield, provides a model through which to examine environmental contributions to the molding of mental health outcomes, particularly in children. According to this perspective, mental disorders result when psychological processes, as they are molded by nature and environment, fail to work normatively. In children, personality development is also plastic and amenable to significant change based on what they experience. This means that non-pathological manifestations of behaviors recognized as symptoms for personality disorders might stem from their normal response to stressful environments rather than purely pathological mechanisms (Hinshaw et al., 1999). Thus, comprehending personality disorders necessitates consideration of the overall environmental contexts under which children develop and mature, since these contexts powerfully affect their psychological resilience and vulnerability. In addition, the effects of these environmental forces reach beyond childhood into adulthood, disclosing the long-term effects of early experiences on personality structure. Extended exposure to negative circumstances throughout developmental years could lead to internalization of negative thoughts and inappropriate coping, establishing cycles of dysfunction. For instance, low parental warmth as determined by research linking childhood experience to personality in adulthood is a predominant symptom development factor (Kendler & Aggen, 2017). As such, individuals work through adult relationship development and stress, and their ensuing early life adverse experiences come to manifest as interpersonal relationship instability and emotional regulation difficulty, presenting as manifestations of several personality disorders. This renders it essential that the environmental contingencies are the focus of therapeutic interventions to optimize treatment effectiveness aimed at restructuring maladaptive personality styles forged through childhood adverse experiences.

9.3.3. Neurobiological Factors

The investigation of the neurobiological foundations of personality disorders is critical in understanding their etiology and manifestation. Research has increasingly discovered genes underlying personality traits and the involvement of some neurobiological pathways in shaping personality structures. Cloninger's system of personality trait categorization has provided a systematic approach to linking the traits with genetic markers and neurobiological processes. For instance, Cloninger's Temperament and Character Inventory permits the investigation of how certain patterns of neurobiology might be linked to personality styles , such as harm avoidance or novelty seeking. In profiles of substance use, for example, Alcohol Use Disorder (AUD), these associations are helpful, demonstrating that higher levels of craving can contribute to susceptibility to addiction behavior, thereby building a more detailed picture of personality disorders that are intertwined by biological propensities and environmental factors (Attilia et al., 2014). Further discrimination among personality disorders demonstrates that neurobiological processes operate not only at the genetic level but also exert influences on cognitive operations and emotion regulation. For example, spontaneous thinking, namely, mind-wandering and daydreaming, has been examined for cognitive vulnerabilities and emotional disturbances. The research demonstrates that intrusive spontaneous thought can lead to maladaptive cognitive styles, particularly in individuals who are prone to negative emotions. Such cognitive activities do involve balancing the difference between desired wishes and current experience, which is supposed to enhance vulnerability to mood disorders. It follows that in the case of personality disorders, the combination of cognitive processing and neurobiological predispositions is likely to create a high risk for depressive and anxiety-like symptoms (Marchetti et al., 2016). Addressing such cognitive processes is essential in understanding the full extent of neurobiological contributions to personality disorders. Integration of neurobiological elements into the treatment of personality disorders shows promising avenues for enhanced treatment efficacy. Traditionally applied psychotherapy methods have hitherto not tried to overcome physiological mechanisms that underlie psychological disorders. However, in line with advancing knowledge concerning neurobiological contributions, therapeutic interventions may be adjusted to apply to both cognitive restructuring and neurobiological interventions. For example, interventions acting on the targeted neurochemical mechanisms of craving can serve as an ancillary therapy for patients with personality disorders, particularly those that lead to substance abuse. In addition, the neurobiological model can direct clinicians in strategies for emotional regulation that aim at spontaneous thought processes. This two-level approach not only facilitates more effective treatment plans but also aligns therapeutic efforts with the biological realities of personality disorders and, thus, leads to a more integrated understanding of the interplay between biology, cognition, and behavior (Figure 9.10).

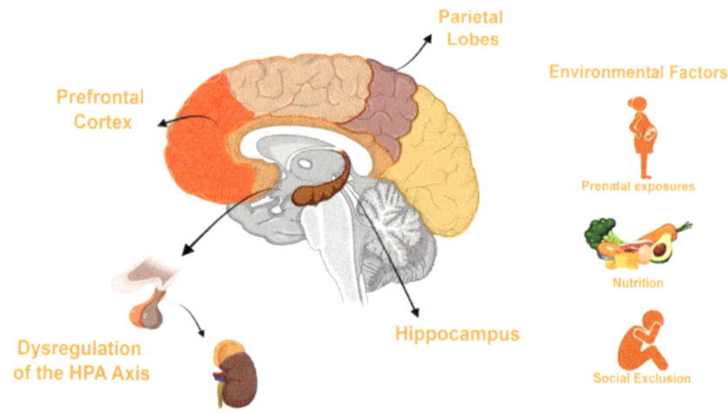

Figure 9.10. Neurobiological factors with personality disorders.

Source: https://pub.mdpi-res.com/brainsci/brainsci-15-00307/article_deploy/html/images/brainsci-15-00307-g005.png?1741931411.

Test Your Knowledge

1. How do genetic predispositions, early childhood experiences, and developmental factors influence the risk of developing personality disorders?
2. What role do family environment, trauma, and neurobiological factors play in shaping personality pathology?

9.4. Symptoms and Diagnosis

Learning Outcome

1. Common symptoms associated with personality disorders.
2. Diagnostic procedures and assessments.
3. Challenges in diagnosing personality disorders.

It is only by understanding the symptoms and diagnostic criteria of personality disorders that one can be effective in clinical intervention. Personality disorders are marked by enduring patterns of behavior, cognition, and inner experience that depart significantly from cultural expectations and lead to distress and impairment in functioning. Diagnosis is founded on careful assessment with standardized measures, one of which is the DSM-5, which enumerates specific criteria for each of the types of disorders, such as emotional instability, impulsivity, and interpersonal issues. These patterns of dysfunction are entrenched and prone to complicating diagnosis. Personality disorders must be distinguished from other mental disorders, especially because they tend to be comorbid. For instance, the presence of anxiety disorders alongside personality disorders may make it difficult to assess treatment procedures and outcomes, highlighting the need for comprehensive assessment to efficiently tailor therapeutic measures. Clinical presentation of personality disorders plays a major role in the severity of comorbid disorders, particularly anxiety disorders. Research indicates that patients with panic disorder often report comorbid personality disorders, leading to increased symptoms as well as lower functioning outcomes. For example, borderline and paranoid personality disorder patients exhibit heightened depressive and anxious symptoms that are crucial to note in the diagnostic process. The concomitance of these two conditions determines a pattern where the severity of panic disorder is significantly linked with some personality disorders, affecting not just the clinical course but also the quality of life in general. Symptoms, such as heightened agitation or mood shift, may require clinicians to reassess common treatment strategies since these call for a sophisticated plan of management. Hence, it is essential to know the role played by personality disorders in anxiety for the formulation of effective therapeutic interventions. Moreover, loneliness has emerged as an influencing factor among individuals suffering from personality disorders. This mood can compound the symptoms inherent within these disorders, making clinical presentation as well as patient-reported outcomes complicated. It has been shown that patients diagnosed with personality disorders report greater loneliness than patients presenting with other forms of mental illness, including psychotic illnesses. Loneliness tends to be concurrent with subjective social isolation and internalized stigma, which determines the general mental health picture. Attending to these psychosocial factors is most important to the comprehensive treatment of them, as it creates the foundation for more successful therapeutic intervention that addresses both symptomology and social life. By recognizing the profound impact of loneliness and how it correlates with personality disorders, clinicians can establish targeted interventions that address not only the symptomology but also the social challenges of these patients, ultimately resulting in better recovery.

9.4.1. Characteristic Symptoms for Personality Disorders

The manifestation of personality disorders is characterized by typical symptoms that significantly affect individuals' thoughts, feelings, and behaviors. Common symptoms across various personality disorders include long-standing patterns of thought that are significantly different from what is typical in society, leading to impairment in personal and professional life. For instance, in borderline personality disorder, there may be wide fluctuations of mood and unstable self-image, which may result in unstable relationships and impulsive behavior. Similarly, those with avoidant personality disorder are characterized by hypersensitivity to rejection and an intense fear of rejection that prevents them from forming any type of meaningful relationship. These symptoms, while varying by individual disorder, share the underlying theme of pathological functioning that underlies personality disorders and therefore compromises vital functions of everyday life. Furthermore, emotional dysregulation is an emergent symptom in the entire spectrum of personality disorders. Many people, particularly those with conditions , such as borderline or narcissistic personality disorder, struggle with controlling their emotional responses and, hence, display unstable behavior as well as relationship difficulties. In borderline personality disorder, for example, the overwhelming terror of abandonment may initiate extreme behaviors , such as self-injuring or angry battles with one's loved ones. This emotional instability not only leads to distress for the patient but also complicates their interactions with others, often leading to a pattern of miscommunication and conflict. The complexity of these symptoms demands a complete understanding of emotional management techniques in clinical settings, as they form a critical area of concern under treatment regimens. Cognitive distortions also accompany relational and emotional problems in individuals with personality disorders. The distortions manifest themselves through defective thought patterns that warp a person's perception of self and their world. In the case of paranoid personality disorder, for example, people may exhibit over-trustlessness and suspicion of other people, with a belief that everyone else has bad intentions. These types of distortions promote feelingss of isolation and inferiority, reinforcing maladaptive schemes. The recognition of these cognitive symptoms is imperative to successful diagnosis and treatment, as they may be responsible for the general psychopathology of personality disorders. Research indicates that their management by certain therapeutic interventions, as outlined in the literature, provokes improved outcomes in sufferers of various personality disorders and implicates the requirement for integrated treatment approaches (De Fruyt & De Clercq, 2014; Melrose, 2017 (Figure 9.11).

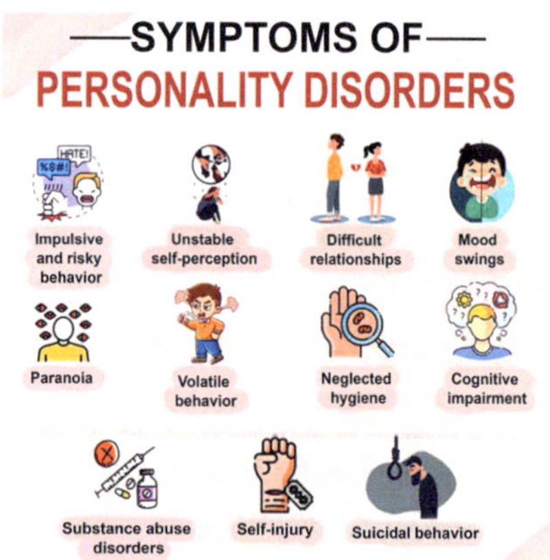
SYMPTOMS OF
PERSONALITY DISORDERS
Impulsive and risky behavior
Unstable self-perception
Difficult relationships
Mood swings
Paranoia
Volatile behavior
Neglected hygiene
Cognitive impairment
Substance abuse disorders
Self-injury
Suicidal behavior

Figure 9.11. Common symptoms associated with personality disorders.

Source: https://mind.help/wp-content/uploads/2022/08/Symptoms-Of-Personality-Disorders.jpg.

9.4.2. Diagnostic Procedures and Assessments

In the diagnosis of personality disorders, diagnostic procedures and assessment are of paramount significance in ascertaining and differentiating these multifaceted disorders. Clinicians make use of standardized assessment tools and interviews for the purpose of collecting a comprehensive knowledge of a person's personality characteristics and tendencies. One of the shared strategies involves structured diagnostic interviews , such as the Diagnostic and Statistical Manual of Mental Disorders (DSM-5) criteria which provides a systematic way of evaluating symptoms in all personality disorders. To supplement structured measures, self-report scales and observer-rated scales can also offer multidimensional evaluations of patients' personality functioning, particularly in the discrimination of co-occurring symptoms of disorders. This multi-faceted approach ensures a full evaluation, allowing for tailored intervention tactics to address the specific complexities of every disorder. Use of proven screening devices is of the most vital concern, particularly in settings , such as mental health facilities and prisons. For instance, writers have emphasized the need for developing more efficient screening measures, as evidence on disorders like ADHD within prison populations illustrates. To this end, the study applied the Barkley Adult ADHD Rating Scale (BAARS-IV) to evaluate its usefulness against a clinical diagnostic interview and emphasized the demand for accessible yet accurate diagnostic tools. The study emphasized the limitations of standard assessment tools while noting how modifications can be undertaken to enhance diagnostic accuracy. Through the utilization of a shorter screening measure, facilitators can more effectively identify those at risk for ADHD, opening earlier therapeutic interventions and mitigating the risk of co-morbid personality disorders in this at-risk group (Asherson et al., 2016). Furthermore, the integration of personality styles and therapeutic orientations has been a topic of significant recent interest in personality disorder assessment. Recent research examines the interaction of patient personality dimensions, dependent versus self-critical personality types—on response to differing psychotherapeutic modalities. By randomizing patients to treatment modalities based on these dimensions, clinicians can optimize outcomes with respect to therapeutic success, as noted in comparisons between cognitive behavioral therapy and psychodynamic psychotherapy. Stratified treatment allows for more individualized treatment concomitant with enhanced treatment engagement and adherence to the process. These findings can add to enhanced diagnostic procedures, which are not only interested in the identification of pathology but also in aligning treatment methods with the individual personality structure of the patient, thus playing a more effective and personalized treatment process (Baeken et al., 2017) (Figure 9.12).

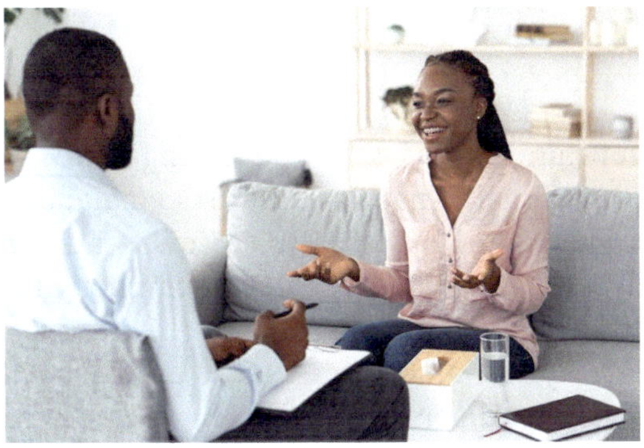

Figure 9.12. Diagnostic procedures and assessments of personality disorders.

Source: https://irishealing.com/wp-content/uploads/2024/08/iStock-1270403525-1-scaled-1.jpg.

9.4.3. Challenges in Diagnosing Personality Disorders

Personality disorders are a formidable challenge to mental health practitioners, primarily due to the intrinsic complexity and heterogeneity of the disorders. Unlike most psychiatric disorders, whose symptoms are distinct and definable, personality disorders are characterized by widespread and stable patterns of behavior and internal experience that manifest across situations. This intermixing of traits makes it hard to assess, as symptoms also have a tendency to overlap with other disorders and thus challenging differentiation. Furthermore, the subjective nature of psychological assessment further muddles proper diagnosis, as a reliance on self-reporting or clinical interviewing may lead to biases. The intricacies of personality disorders and the nuances of human behavior complicate efforts to establish a reliable diagnosis that, in turn, influences treatment modalities and outcomes for individuals suffering from the disorders. A further aspect of complexity in the diagnostic process stems from the stigma of personality disorders, both on patient disclosure and clinicians' attitudes. Sufferers of these conditions are also faced with societal prejudices that not only impede self-identification but can also result in avoidance of treatment. A fear of being labeled or stigmatized can discourage frank communication concerning symptoms, further hamstringing the diagnostic process. Clinicians can unconsciously contribute to this stigma and allow stereotypes to guide their evaluations. Consequently, the application of diagnostic tools and equipment could be biased, since clinicians may emphasize particular characteristics or tendencies and downplay others. The removal of this stigma is crucial in order to enhance diagnostic accuracy and create a more compassionate therapeutic context where people feel comfortable sharing their experiences and obtaining proper treatment. The use of normative values in diagnosis is critical for the clarity in diagnosing personality disorders. Studies show that existing models of mental illness are typically inadequate in that they do not satisfy the mandate of reconciling diagnostic classification and moral responsibility, such as in the case of various mental illnesses. Utilizing a model that weaves together normative consideration and practice, mental health professionals can more effectively address the needs of diagnosis. This model would encourage greater in-depth understanding of the individual's context and encourage the recognition of the complexity of personality disorders. In addition, application of instruments , such as the Wender Utah Rating Scale, as suggested by newer studies, can prove to be instrumental in developing effective tests for use in evaluating educational attainment and socio-economic status, leading to more personalized and fair treatment plans in the discipline (Asbjørnsen et al., 2015; Seely, 2019) (Figure 9.13).

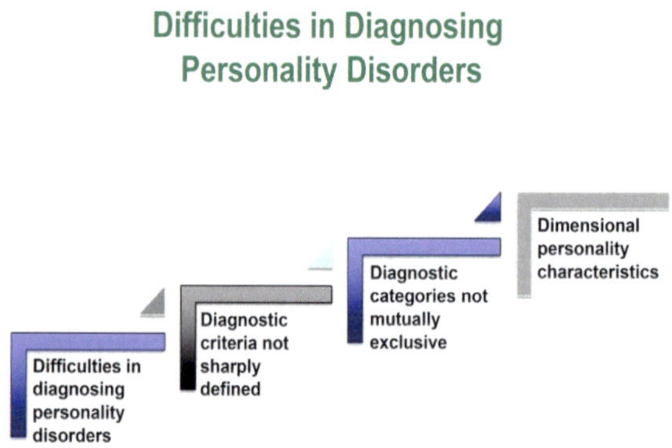

Figure 9.13. Challenges in diagnosing personality disorders.

Source: https://slideplayer.com/slide/10556552/36/images/7/Difficulties+in+Diagnosing+Personality+Disorders.jpg.

Test Your Knowledge

1. What diagnostic features help clinicians distinguish personality disorders from normal personality variations?
2. How are clinical interviews, behavioral observations, and standardized assessments used to diagnose personality disorders?

9.5. Treatment Options

Learning Outcome

1. Psychotherapy approaches.
2. Medication management.
3. Support and rehabilitation programs.

The treatment of personality disorders has advanced considerably in recent decades, with even more focus placed on treatment approaches designed to yield better patient outcomes. Once viewed as inherently resistant to therapy, personality disorders are now treated with multiple evidence-based treatments specifically designed to target specific symptoms and enhance overall functioning. Among these treatments, psychodynamic approaches have gained more acceptance due to the extent of understanding of the underlying emotional and relational dynamics that drive maladaptive behavior. Later systematic reviews and meta-analyses highlight the efficacy of psychodynamic psychotherapy as a first-line treatment for a variety of disorders, such as borderline personality disorder, for which patients have undergone dramatic alterations in emotional control and interpersonal relationships. Mentalization-Based Treatment (MBT) and Transference Focused Treatment (TFT) are two of the modalities under the treatment paradigm that have shown promising outcomes, and researchers have sought to learn more about their mechanisms and long-term outcomes (Rorie, 2016). The keys to the success of MBT and TFT are their structured but flexible designs, as they enable patients to critically explore their cognition and affect about their interpersonal encounters. MBT, for instance, is intended to help patients develop a better capacity to understand and interpret their own as well as other mental states, thereby advancing social relationships and decreasing impulsivity. In some studies, patients treated with MBT exhibited significant reductions in symptoms of borderline personality disorder-related anxiety and depression, and their quality of life was demonstrated to have increased. TFT, however, delves into the transference relationship that exists between the patient and therapist, pinpointing how historical struggles govern current concerns.

Both therapies have been effective in not only relieving symptoms but also allowing for deeper, richer interpersonal relationships, thereby addressing the core of personality disorders (Rorie, 2016). Aside from psychodynamic treatments, other modalities like dialectical behavior therapy (DBT) and cognitive-behavioral therapy (CBT) have also proven to be useful for those who are struggling with personality disorders. DBT, which was specifically developed for borderline personality disorder, blends standard cognitive-behavioral interventions with mindfulness skills to assist patients with extreme emotional states. By equipping individuals with coping skills and a balanced approach towards emotion regulation, DBT has also been shown to reduce self-injurious behavior and promote interpersonal functioning. Similar to the manner in which CBT offers interventions toward modifying distorted thinking patterns, patients can reinterpret their self-concepts and their conception of others. As the therapeutic landscape of personality disorders continues to change, it is increasingly necessary that clinicians tailor treatments based on individual patient needs, allowing for whole-person care that promotes long-term recovery and growth (Figure 9.14).

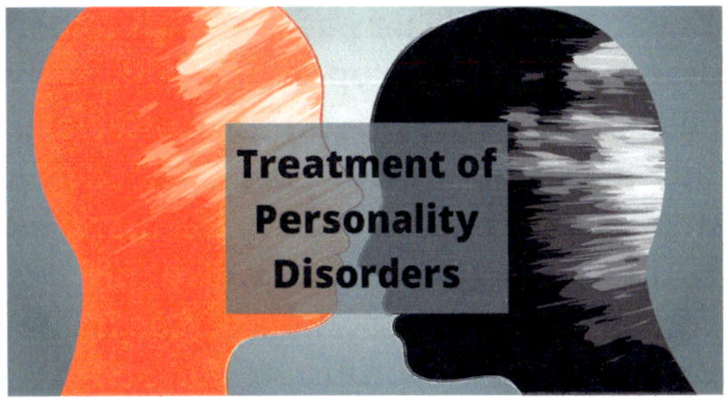

Figure 9.14. The treatment of personality disorders.

Source: https://external-content.duckduckgo.com/iu/?u=https%3A%2F%2Fmantracare.org%2Fwp-content%2Fuploads%2F2021%2F11%2FTreatment-of-Personality-Disorders.png&f=1&nofb=1&ipt=f19730f6b63d183c75775f02f885fb2a4395a351584f54e33788be8cf9bf4424.

9.5.1. Psychotherapy Approaches

The research on psychotherapy modalities is particularly helpful in the context of personality disorders, since the relationship between therapeutic style and patient traits is a critical element in treatment response. Cognitive-behavioral therapy and psychodynamic therapy are examples of many psychotherapy modalities that use systematic methods tailored to the needs of different patients. Cognitive-behavioral therapy, for instance, aims to change problematic patterns of thinking, making it suitable for patients showing rigid behaviors common in personality disorders. Conversely, psychodynamic therapy promotes deeper self-exploration, addressing unconscious forces driving personality. With current research showing that identifying the patient's personality traits can enhance the efficacy of the treatments, thus highlighting the need for a personalized intervention in treating personality disorder cases (Baeken et al., 2017), the decision to use a psychotherapy technique should not only consider the disorder but also the client's unique personality traits. The interface of the various psychotherapy modalities with patient personality styles is the success factor of treatment, especially for patients with comorbid conditions , such as depression and anxiety. For example, research on the interface of various therapeutic modalities concluded that organized therapies like CBT are more likely to yield favorable outcomes in patients with a dependent personality style, whereas inquiring therapies may be appropriate for self-critical patients (Baeken et al., 2017).

This contrast highlights the usefulness of aligning treatments to the underlying personality variables that may affect the course of therapy. Configuring the therapeutic approach so that it is consistent with the patient's personality traits can potentially facilitate greater engagement and treatment compliance, ultimately maximizing the overall effectiveness of psychotherapeutic interventions in the treatment of personality disorders. Furthermore, the role played by cognitive flexibility in psychotherapy outlines a crucial area in which personality-disordered patients can benefit from customized treatment.

Cognitive flexibility is a reflection of an individual's capability to adjust their behavior and thought patterns according to changing situations, something which is usually lacking in individuals with rigid personality features. Research suggests that increased cognitive flexibility is associated with better coping, which enables the patient to function more effectively with therapeutic procedures. By , including assessment of cognitive flexibility in treatment planning, therapists are better placed to respond to their clients' needs and deliver targeted interventions. This approach seeks to build up resilience and improve the patient's capacity to manage therapeutic challenges so that therapeutic effectiveness in treating personality disorders will be more affirmative (Figure 9.15).

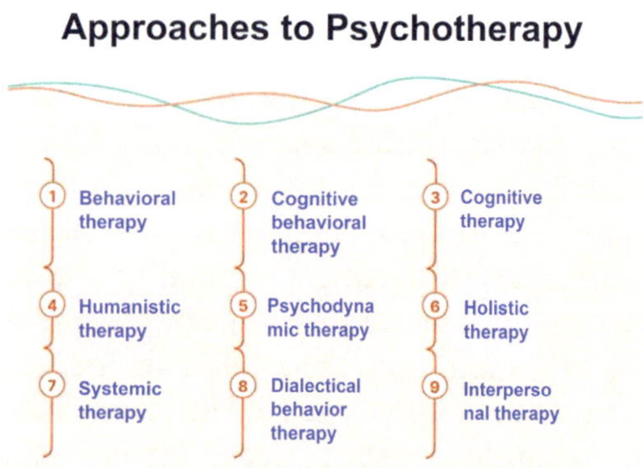
Approaches to Psychotherapy
1 Behavioral therapy
2 Cognitive behavioral therapy
3 Cognitive therapy
4 Humanistic therapy
5 Psychodyna mic therapy
6 Holistic therapy
7 Systemic therapy
8 Dialectical behavior therapy
9 Interperso nal therapy

Figure 9.15. Psychotherapy approaches.

Source: https://external-content.duckduckgo.com/iu/?u=https%3A%2F%2Fpsychologywriting.com%2Fwp-content%2Fuploads%2F2024%2F02%2FApproaches-to-psychotherapy-1024x866.jpg&f=1&nofb=1&ipt=0fb6d0f8de037f79c8d2d13abd74bcccd794cc4a988307d41c669e3206d3e87c.

9.5.2. Medication Management

Medication management of patients with personality disorders is necessary to address the complicated issues involved with these disorders. Although medication is not typically the first treatment option, it can be beneficial as an ancillary treatment to alleviate symptoms of anxiety, depression, and impulsivity that typically occur with personality disorders. For example, SSRIs may be prescribed for the management of mood swings or obsessive-compulsive symptoms in borderline or obsessive-compulsive personality disorder patients. But medication adherence and therapeutic collaboration should go together. Patients' awareness of their illness, along with their treatment-seeking behaviors, holds the key to successful pharmacological treatment, and therefore, comprehensive care strategies need to include psychotherapy alongside medication management. Medication management also involves the complexity of individual responses to treatment, particularly when there is comorbid illness. Research has shown that clients with personality disorders often experience overlapping mental illnesses, which can make treatment interventions and medication management more complicated. Surprisingly, the BDD patients, a personality disorder characterized by an over-sensitiveness regarding perceived appearance defects, can be treated with the help of cognitive-behavioral therapy (CBT) coupled with medications (Greenberg et al., 2019). This suggests that treatment schedules must be planned by clinicians based on the patient's individual symptoms and co-morbidities. Thus, ongoing assessment and readjustment of the medication can rectify side effects and optimize the therapeutic effects, improving the overall quality of life of the patients. Additionally, the evolving landscape of technology brings novel solutions to optimizing medication management in individuals with personality disorders. The fusion of smartphone and telecommunication technologies into psychiatric treatment has been found to improve compliance with treatment as well as monitoring.

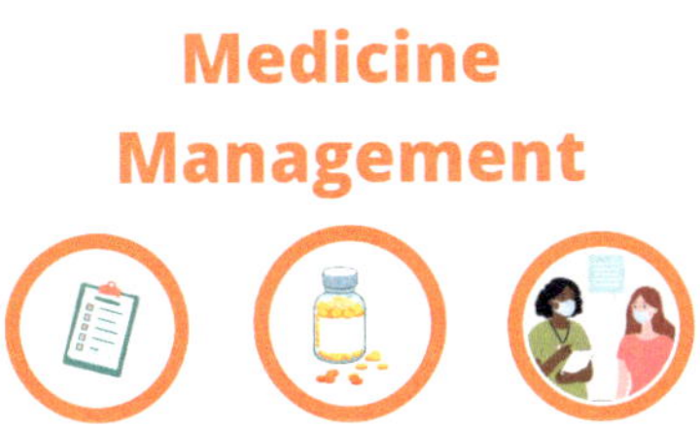

Figure 9.16. Medication management.

Source: https://external-content.duckduckgo.com/iu/?u=https%3A%2F%2Fwww.hiw.org.uk%2Fsites%2Fdefault%2Ffiles%2F2022-09%2Fmedicinemanagement-en_0.png&f=1&nofb=1&ipt=d2079f6eef1b07d0a7196752cf5c3e5a627206c9479015fc721f20d8a03ce877.

These patients can be reminded to take their medications and receive educational material that helps them manage their illness more effectively (Susick, 2011). Technological intervention does this easily and can simply reduce barriers to care, particularly among those who may find it hard with standard delivery of care. With these advancements, healthcare providers are able to provide real-time communication with patients, which facilitates better monitoring of drug efficacy and adjustment of treatment procedures. Eventually, the incorporation of technology in drug management not only addresses physiological needs but also optimizes the overall treatment of individuals who suffer from personality disorders (Figure 9.16).

9.5.3. Support and Rehabilitation Programs

Rehabilitation and treatment programs play a vital role in the treatment and management of personality disorders since they provide organized environments that are conducive to recovery and development. The programs, in most cases, use a combination of therapeutic approaches , such as cognitive-behavioral therapies, psychoeducation, and interpersonal skills training. Their goal is to make the individuals appreciate their conditions more, learn how to handle situations, and develop healthy interpersonal relationships. A holistic support program actively addresses both inner psychological needs and social readjustment, recognizing the role interpersonal relationships play in determining the process of recovery. Research highlights the necessity for such approaches, as effective rehabilitation has been shown to contribute to patients' functional and emotional status in significant ways, something that proves vital in the case of individuals fighting the multidimensionality of personality disorders (Becks et al., 1969). Implementation and effectiveness of such programs, however, also carry intricate operational and administrative concerns. Building a support system in clinical settings often requires forward thinking to ensure intervention mechanisms respond to the multifaceted needs of the patient population. A successful program will include specially trained professionals who are equipped to facilitate dynamic group interaction and offer individualized care depending on personality disorder types. Besides, the complexity of program success measurement demands solid methodology design, often requesting control groups and longitudinal examinations to aptly quantify outcomes over long time intervals. Proposals for such programs consequently need to prioritize most highly on such operational concerns in a bid to yield long-term benefit to participants as well as a positive impact on the overall healthcare system (Becks et al., 1969). The other key aspect of support and rehabilitation programs is the addition of both classical and modern therapeutic tools. No amount of commendation can express how much in-person human contact is cherished, given how ancient methodologies have centered upon the healing power of individual touch in mental therapy. But how such programs have picked up steam to embrace technological advancement, teletherapy and internet groups, for instance, suggests an emerging trend in psychological therapy. By employing both established communications media and emerging cyber locations, rehabilitation programs can optimize accessibility and maximize reach. This dual modality not only ensures complete support for individuals but also addresses varying preferences and circumstances that may affect attendance within traditional settings. The integration of these modalities ultimately creates a flexible and comprehensive approach to addressing the multifaceted issues presented by personality disorders.

Test Your Knowledge

1. How do psychotherapeutic approaches—such as DBT, CBT, and psychodynamic therapy—support individuals with personality disorders?
2. What challenges exist in treating personality disorders, and how do long-term therapy and multidisciplinary care help improve outcomes?

9.6. Impact on Individuals and Relationships

Learning Outcome

1. Effects on personal functioning and daily life.
2. Influence on interpersonal relationships.
3. Stigma and societal perceptions.

The impact of personality disorders on a patient is significant, at times resulting in significant problems in most aspects of daily life. Patients who have disorders , such as borderline or paranoid personality disorders may become sensitively emotionally dysregulated, impulsive, and have unstable relationships, which can prevent them from attempting to hold stable jobs or engage in healthy social relationships. The Recognition and Prevention (RAP) study highlighted that participants who were included in clinical high-risk (CHR) groups expressed a mix of personality and mood disorders, which revealed how these disorders influence one another. In this case, participants who were diagnosed with borderline personality disorder expressed symptoms that significantly hampered their role functioning, rendering them dissatisfied in various aspects of their lives. This means that the manifestation of personality disorders not only affects the diagnosed individuals but also has a ripple effect on their career and social relationships, consequently affecting their overall quality of life and mental health status (DaBreo-Otero, 2021). In addition to affecting individual functioning, personality disorders have ripple effects in interpersonal relationships. The relational dynamics get strained due to the behaviors and emotional patterns associated with these disorders. To illustrate, adults with insecure attachment, who are usually identified with cluster B personality disorders, tend to have unstable romantic relationships that are flavored with conflict and dissatisfaction. The integration of insecure attachment styles and personality pathology has the potential to create a relationship discord pattern that is difficult to break. Studies indicate that having an insecure attachment as a young child predisposes an individual to unhealthy adult relationships, leading to increased levels of conflict and distress in relationships (Bonnemort, 2020). This cycle of dysfunction highlights how personality disorders not only challenge the individual's experience but also cause significant barriers to the health and stability of their relationships. Understanding the impact of personality disorders is relevant in developing effective intervention strategies. Their intricateness necessitates an integrated understanding of both individual symptoms and relationship processes.

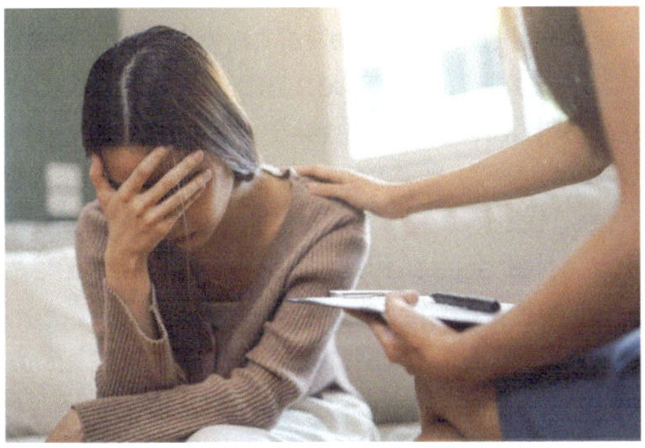

Figure 9.17. Personality disorders affect personal functioning and daily life.

Source: https://www.malvernbh.com/wp-content/uploads/2024/01/shutterstock_2291197001-1-min-1010x673.jpg.

Evidence-based treatment should aim at enhancing relational skills, secure attachment processes, and emotion regulation approaches to promote individual and relational adjustment. The need for intervention is further underscored by the high correlation between personality disorders and distressed relationships, as treatments that can facilitate secure attachment might be able to restrict the frequency of emotional distress and conflict. As a result, the integration of evidence shows that a dimensional approach to treatment can significantly improve people's mental health and interpersonal relationships and thus reflects the interconnected nature of such problems (Bonnemort, 2020) (Figure 9.17).

9.6.1. Effects on Personal Functioning and Daily Life

The complexities of personality disorders profoundly affect individual functioning and daily life, and symptoms tend to emerge in interpersonal relationships and emotion regulation. Borderline personality disorder (BPD) patients, for instance, show higher negative emotionality, which can impair their ability to manage relationships and cope with everyday stressors. Empirical evidence indicates that negative emotional reactivity, when compounded by aversive family environments, exacerbates the developmental severity of BPD symptoms during adolescence. This creates a problematic trajectory, as the symptoms serve to create instability in social and professional contexts, leading individuals to have ongoing issues with loneliness and frustration. Ultimately, the blend of emotional instability coupled with environmental stressors significantly compromises habitual functioning, which is reflective of the significance of understanding how these dynamics work for therapeutic applications that enhance the quality of life in those who are impacted by them (Stepp et al., 2015). The impact of personality disorders extends beyond emotional anguish to encompass significant disruption of psychological health and functioning. Sports participants, for example, can experience the detrimental consequences of maladaptive outcomes, including depression and burnout, when their psychological needs are thwarted. According to the theory of self-determination, thwarting autonomy can yield adverse consequences that propagate into other aspects of life, affecting performance and personal fulfillment. Such disruptions lead to physical symptoms and distress, making everyday life intolerable and leading to a cycle of decline in the state of life satisfaction. The need satisfaction and thwarting research thus sheds light on how personality disorders impair daily functioning, thereby indicating the necessity for supportive contexts that promote autonomy and emotional control in individuals with such issues (Bartholomew et al., 2011). Secondly, these patterns of maladaptive behavior repeatedly emerge in daily interpersonal transactions and responsibilities and produce a domino effect of negative consequences on the functioning of an individual. Personality disorder patients usually suffer from poor relationships that have catastrophic consequences for their social networks and support systems. As symptoms persist, these individuals are more likely to push away social opportunities, hence hampering their ability to form constructive relationships. Additionally, avoidance of stressors, if not possible to control, becomes a habitual response that supports separation and suppresses individual growth. External forces interacting with internal conflict are critical to understanding how personality disorders significantly contribute to the everyday lives of those afflicted with them. This disturbance not only affects individual well-being but also extends into family and social arenas, emphasizing the necessity for integrated models of treatment and care (Bartholomew et al., 2011; Stepp et al., 2015).

9.6.2. Impact on Interpersonal Relationships

The impact of personality disorders on interpersonal relationships is profound and multifaceted. Personality-disordered individuals can exhibit sets of maladaptive behavior patterns and affect patterns that can significantly disrupt social functioning. For example, personality disorder characteristics of unstable self-image and extreme emotional reactivity can lead to relationship misunderstandings and conflict. These same dysfunctional behaviors impact not only the subjects who are diagnosed with such disorders but also the significant others of the individuals, thereby creating a pattern of dysfunction that multiplies relational complexity. Friends and partners may also become bewildered or angered by the more erratic behaviors that individuals would then manifest, causing more relational stress and moving towards a pattern of avoidance or conflict, which maintains a state of isolation for both individuals. Empirical research supports the proposition that some personality traits have implications for relationship satisfaction. With the Actor–Partner Interdependence Model, empirical studies have confirmed the fact that self-reported relationship satisfaction is significantly influenced by personality traits , such as neuroticism and extraversion. Individuals who score high in neuroticism, which is common in individuals with personality disorder, struggle to control their emotions, leading to a high level of relationship dissatisfaction. Furthermore, the study indicates that relationship length is a moderator of these dynamics, and there are more pronounced connections between personality and satisfaction in short-term relationships. The longer the relationship gets, the more partners learn to accept each other's idiosyncrasies, which can soften the impact of one's personality-disordered behaviors, making the dynamics that influence levels of satisfaction in long-term relationships more complex (Durbin et al., 2010). The implications of these findings extend beyond mere academic interest, broaching the truth of relationship therapy and intervention strategies. Being aware of the interface of personality disorders and relationship satisfaction can inform therapy techniques such that practitioners are able to implement interventions congruent with individuals' styles and relational situations. For instance, therapies for emotional dysregulation can be particularly beneficial for couples dealing with one partner's personality disorder because these treatments correct the underlying issues of interpersonal distress. Additionally, the development of self-knowledge regarding one's personality traits can enable individuals to navigate their relationships. Through the detection of their behavioral patterns linked to their disorders, people can create better interpersonal relationships and minimize the devastating effects on their relationships (Verbeke et al., 2017).

9.6.3. Stigma and Societal Perceptions

The stigma of personality disorders exerts a huge influence on societal perception of people who possess them. Such stigma typically manifests itself in the form of negative stereotypes, which tend to raise misconceptions and establish a discriminatory environment. People with personality disorders are viewed, often falsely, as threatening or incapable of functioning normally, which results in social exclusion and psychological disturbance. These sentiments not only influence public opinion but also mental health care policy-making, thereby contributing to making access to such care even harder. In addition, broad ignorance regarding personality disorders leads to society's lack of compassion, thereby exacerbating the already strained self-acceptance and identity for those affected. Combating stigma is therefore imperative in creating a more tolerant society that can include those suffering from personality disorders. The convergence of stigma and mental health is most significantly found in vulnerable populations, where public perception can exacerbate an already troubled condition. As an example, studies reveal the role that stress experienced by those who identify as lesbian, gay, or bisexual (LGB) through stigma consciousness and internalized homonegativity has on how they view their mental health (Cox et al., 2008). This association identifies the point that stigma is not only a byproduct of misconceptions but is indeed associated with ramifications in the actual world, resulting in poor mental health conditions for the stigmatized group. In personality disorders, individuals get isolated and left behind by society due to biases in society, which later exacerbate symptoms and strengthen emotional issues. Social support counteracts some of these effects, but stigmatizing beliefs often deter individuals from presenting for care. Access to the appropriate care is also obfuscated by sociocultural factors, especially gender, race, and socioeconomic status. Research on ADHD, demonstrates disparities of access to services based on a variety of factors, including societal opinion (Chakrabarti et al., 2015). These inequalities extend to the realm of personality disorders, where stereotypes can prevent people from getting a diagnosis and treatment to improve their quality of life. Public awareness and education programs to eliminate myths around personality disorders can go a great distance in limiting stigma. By promoting an awareness of these complicated and sometimes misconceived disorders, society can build a more accommodating environment that allows people to pursue help without the stigmatization of judgment or discrimination, ultimately improving mental health outcomes and fostering societal acceptance.

Test Your Knowledge

1. How do personality disorders affect interpersonal functioning, emotional regulation, and daily decision-making?
2. What challenges do individuals with personality disorders face in maintaining stable relationships at home, work, and social settings?

SUMMARY

Personality disorder research entails a subtle interplay among clinical characteristics, diagnostic categories, and treatment strategies that reflect the complexity of human behavior. Personality disorders, defined as long-term patterns of thoughts, feelings, and behaviors that significantly deviate from norms in society, require delicate understanding and tolerance by the mental health community. The present understanding of disorders in the Obsessive–Compulsive and Related Disorders (OCRD) category, based on the ICD-11, indicates a sophisticated approach to classifying these disorders. It enhances diagnostic accuracy and treatment intervention by emphasizing the need for both clinical utility and worldwide applicability in practice. The common features, such as recurrent unwanted behaviors and ideas, facilitate collaboration among professionals to improve treatment success and quality of care for the affected (Atmaca et al., 2016). In addition, the effects of personality disorders extend beyond individual experiences to broader societal arenas, including the work and legal environments. An adjustment disorder (AD), long considered residual and overlooked, represents a textbook case of the effect of life stressors on personality development and mental illness. AD patients typically present demographic markers of specific stressors in the workplace and family that mirror the complexity of personality disorders. Emphasizing the social and environmental causation of such disorders encapsulates a pivotal aspect of prevention and treatment efforts. By recognizing the intricate interactions between personality pathology and life experience, clinicians and researchers can better customize interventions, paving the way for enhanced mental health services among diverse populations (Anastasia et al., 2016). Finally, continued investigation of personality disorders and their subtypes must seek to refine diagnostic characteristics and therapeutic models. It is important that the clinical community continue to address the changing context of personality disorders as new research develops. Further study of the prevalence, assessment, and treatment of these disorders is indicated to foster a balanced perspective of their complexity. The integration of the most recent scientific findings into clinical practice, on the one hand, enhances the validity of diagnoses and, on the other hand, aids in the development of effective treatment modalities based on individual needs. The intersection of research and clinical practice for the treatment of personality disorders will thus result in improved health outcomes among patients, enriching the whole field of mental health (Atmaca et al., 2016).

Understanding personality disorders involves a careful examination of various aspects, including their diagnostic features, their associated symptoms, and their impact on individuals' lives. Personality disorders are characterized by enduring patterns of behavior, cognition, and inner experience that differ significantly from cultural norms, significantly interfering with function, and causing distress in social relationships. Their occurrence demands effective interventions and treatments. Significantly, recent literature questions the traditional personality conceptualizations as being static, proposing that personality traits can evolve and shift over time (Allan et al., 2018). This emerging knowledge opens up the possibility of potentially coaching and therapy interventions explicitly designed to foster positive personality change, illustrating a hopeful route for individuals struggling with such problems. Loneliness is yet another crucial variable typically associated with personality disorders, significantly shaping people's mental health outcome. Research time and again demonstrates that personality disorder categories report greater levels of loneliness compared to other psychiatric diagnosis classes. For instance, patients suffering from common mental disorders and personality disorders report greater feelings of loneliness compared to psychotic disorder patients. This amplified sense of loneliness emphasizes the complex interplay between social and personality disorders. In addition, constructs , such as internalized stigma and perceived discrimination are highly correlated with loneliness, influencing overall well-being in personality-disordered individuals (Alasmawi et al., 2020). Elucidation of the complexities of personality disorders and associated loneliness is of critical concern for intervention design. Psychological and social treatment planning should involve combined treatment planning aimed at diminishing loneliness and promoting interpersonal relationships. Understanding the variation of loneliness by diagnostic category informs the planning of mental health services that address these pressing issues. As methods of treatment shift, consideration of the internal social dynamics of loneliness can enhance the impact of treatments for personality disorders. This many-faceted approach not only mitigates loneliness but also makes it possible for a more profound understanding of personality dynamics, providing individuals with an opportunity for transformation and enhancement of quality of life (Allan et al., 2018; Alasmawi et al., 2020).

KEY TERMS FROM THIS CHAPTER

- Antisocial personality disorder
- Avoidant personality disorder
- Borderline personality disorder
- Cluster A
- Cluster B
- Cluster C
- Dependent personality disorder
- Ego-syntonic
- Emotional dysregulation
- Histrionic personality disorder
- Identity disturbance
- Impulsivity
- Interpersonal dysfunction
- Narcissistic personality disorder
- Obsessive-compulsive personality disorder
- Paranoid personality disorder
- Personality disorder
- Schizoid personality disorder
- Schizotypal personality disorder
- Splitting

CRITICAL THINKING QUESTIONS

1. **Which of the following is characteristic of Borderline Personality Disorder (BPD)?**
   a. Excessive need for admiration
   b. Repeated disregard for the rights of others
   c. Intense fear of abandonment and unstable relationships
   d. Lack of interest in social relationships
2. **Antisocial Personality Disorder is most commonly associated with:**
   a. Hypersensitivity to criticism
   b. Disregard for societal norms and others' rights
   c. Excessive perfectionism
   d. Social withdrawal due to anxiety
3. **A person who is extremely dramatic, attention-seeking, and emotionally shallow may have:**
   a. Schizoid Personality Disorder
   b. Narcissistic Personality Disorder
   c. Histrionic Personality Disorder
   d. Avoidant Personality Disorder
4. **Paranoid Personality Disorder involves:**
   a. Lack of emotional expression
   b. Distrust and suspiciousness of others
   c. Disorganized thinking
   d. Grandiosity and delusions
5. **Which personality disorder is marked by extreme social inhibition and feelings of inadequacy?**
   a. Obsessive-Compulsive Personality Disorder
   b. Avoidant Personality Disorder
   c. Schizotypal Personality Disorder
   d. Dependent Personality Disorder

Short Answer Questions

1. What is a personality disorder, and how does it differ from other mental health disorders?
2. Which cluster of personality disorders includes paranoid, schizoid, and schizotypal types?
3. Name two characteristics commonly seen in Borderline Personality Disorder.
4. What is the main feature of Antisocial Personality Disorder?
5. Which personality disorder is associated with excessive emotionality and attention-seeking behavior?

Answer to Critical Thinking Questions

1. (c); 2. (b); 3. (c); 4. (b); 5. (b)

REFERENCES

1. Kendler, K. S., & Aggen, S. H. (2017). Symptoms of major depression: Their stability, familiality, and prediction by genetic, temperamental, and childhood environmental risk factors. *Depression and anxiety*, *34*(2), 171–177. https://doi.org/10.1002/da.22591(accessed on 28th July 2025).
2. O'Neill, D. G., Coulson, N. R., Church, D. B., & Brodbelt, D. C. (2017). Demography and disorders of German Shepherd Dogs under primary veterinary care in the UK. *Canine genetics and epidemiology*, *4*, 7. https://doi.org/10.1186/s40575-017-0046-4 (accessed on 28th July 2025).
3. Alasmawi, K., Lewis, G., Lloyd-Evans, B., Mann, F., et al. (2020). To what extent does severity of loneliness vary among different mental health diagnostic groups: A cross-sectional study. https://core.ac.uk/download/322366781.pdf (accessed on 28th July 2025).
4. Allan, J., De Fruyt, F., Leeson, P., Martin, B., et al. (2018). Application of a 10-week coaching program designed to facilitate volitional personality change: Overall effects on personality and the impact of targeting. https://core.ac.uk/download/186568682.pdf (accessed on 28th July 2025).
5. Marchetti, I., Koster, E. H. W., Klinger, E., & Alloy, L. B. (2016). Spontaneous Thought and Vulnerability to Mood Disorders: The Dark Side of the Wandering Mind. *Clinical psychological science : a journal of the Association for Psychological Science*, *4*(5), 835–857. https://doi.org/10.1177/2167702615622383(accessed on 28th July 2025).
6. Altindag, A., & Ozkan, M. (2003). Comorbid personality disorders in subjects with panic disorder: Which personality disorders increase clinical severity? https://core.ac.uk/download/pdf/26963153.pdf (accessed on 28th July 2025).
7. Alwin, N., American Psychiatric Association, Bolton, W., Bowers, L., Bradley, K., Burr, V., De Brito, S., et al. (2025). "They're really PD today": An exploration of mental health nursing students' perceptions of developing a therapeutic relationship with patients with a diagnosis of antisocial personality disorder. https://core.ac.uk/download/42138271.pdf (accessed on 28th July 2025).
8. Anastasia, A., Bersani, G., Colletti, C., Cuoco, S., et al. (2016). Demographic variables, clinical aspects, and medicolegal implications in a population of patients with adjustment disorder. https://core.ac.uk/download/54531098.pdf (accessed on 28th July 2025).
9. Andrea, H., Bartak, A., Bouvy, F., Busschbach, J., et al. (2011). Patients with Cluster A personality disorders in psychotherapy: An effectiveness study. https://core.ac.uk/download/19185906.pdf (accessed on 28th July 2025).
10. Asbjørnsen, A. E., Eikeland, O. J., & Manger, T. (2015). Symptoms of ADHD are related to education and work experience among incarcerated adults. https://core.ac.uk/download/215482749.pdf (accessed on 28th July 2025).
11. Asherson, P., Gonzalez, R. A., Gudjonsson, G., Hickey, N., et al. (2016). Diagnostic accuracy of a brief screening tool for attention deficit/hyperactivity disorder in UK prison inmates. https://core.ac.uk/download/77008141.pdf (accessed on 28th July 2025).
12. Atmaca, M., Fineberg, N. A., Fontenelle, L. F., Grant, J. E., et al. (2016). The classification of obsessive–compulsive and related disorders in the ICD-11. https://core.ac.uk/download/213085588.pdf (accessed on 28th July 2025).

13. Attilia, M. L., Battagliese, G., Berman, M. O., Blum, K., et al. (2014). Neurophysiological measures and alcohol use disorder (AUD): Hypothesizing links between clinical severity index and molecular neurobiological patterns. https://core.ac.uk/download/158327904.pdf (accessed on 28th July 2025).

14. Baeken, C., Bockting, C., De Geest, R., De Smet, S., et al. (2017). The Ghent Psychotherapy Study (GPS) on the differential efficacy of supportive-expressive and cognitive behavioral interventions in dependent and self-critical depressive patients: Study protocol for a randomized controlled trial. https://core.ac.uk/download/84044239.pdf (accessed on 28th July 2025).

15. Barlow, D. H., Sauer-Zavala, S., & Wilner, J. G. (2017). Addressing neuroticism in psychological treatment. https://open.bu.edu/bitstream/2144/40060/4/Addressing%20Neuroticism%20in%20Psychological%20Treatment%20FINAL-1.pdf (accessed on 28th July 2025).

16. Bartholomew, K., Bosch, J., Ntoumanis, N., Ryan, R. M., et al. (2011). Self-determination theory and diminished functioning: The role of interpersonal control and psychological need thwarting. https://core.ac.uk/download/pdf/1631248.pdf (accessed on 28th July 2025).

17. Jenkins, R; Meltzer, H; Jones, PB; Brugha, T; Bebbington, P; Farrell, M; Crepaz-Keay, D; + view all (2008) Mental health: Future challenges [Mental Capital and Wellbeing: Making the most of ourselves in the 21st century]. (Foresight Mental Capital and Wellbeing Project , pp. pp. 1-100). Government Office for Science: London, UK. (accessed on 28th July 2025).

18. Becks, W. (1969). A social rehabilitation program implementation and analysis: A demonstration-experimental proposal. https://core.ac.uk/download/143682999.pdf (accessed on 28th July 2025).

19. Groenier, M. , Beerthuis, V. , Pieters, J. , M Witteman, C. and Swinkels, J. (2011) Psychologists' Diagnostic Processes during a Diagnostic Interview. *Psychology*, **2**, 917-924. doi: 10.4236/psych.2011.29138.(accessed on 28th July 2025).

20. Palmieri, Arianna & Kleinbub, Johann & Benelli, Enrico & Sambin, Marco & Broggio, Alice & Bianco, Simone. (2015). THE WORDS OF THE BODY: PSYCHOPHYSIOLOGICAL PATTERNS IN DISSOCIATIVE NARRATIVES. https://core.ac.uk/download/80154470.pdf (accessed on 28th July 2025).

21. Billieux, J., Griffiths, M. D., Karila, L., Kuss, D. J., et al. (2014). Internet addiction: A systematic review of epidemiological research for the last decade. https://core.ac.uk/download/30640239.pdf (accessed on 28th July 2025).

22. Bonnemort, L. (2020). Exploring the impact of insecure attachment styles in couple adjustment through the lens of Cluster B pathology. https://core.ac.uk/download/327120910.pdf (accessed on 28th July 2025).

23. Bucholz, K. K., Dick, D. M., Edenberg, H. J., Kuo, I. C., et al. (2018). Understanding mechanisms of genetic risk for adolescent internalizing and externalizing problems: The mediating role of parenting and personality. https://core.ac.uk/download/212865887.pdf (accessed on 28th July 2025).

24. Bufford, R. K. (1988). Mental disorders–Chapter 6 of *Counseling and the Demonic*. https://digitalcommons.georgefox.edu/cgi/viewcontent.cgi?article=1009&context=counselingandthedemonic (accessed on 28th July 2025).

25. Burrell-Hodgson, G., Fowler, B., Jones, S. H., Tate, A., et al. (2006). Personality disorder in

primary care: Factors associated with therapy process and outcome. https://core.ac.uk/download/68622.pdf (accessed on 28th July 2025).

26. Chakrabarti, I., Coates, J., Daley, D., Kochhar, P., et al. (2015). Practitioner review: Pathways to care for ADHD–A systematic review of barriers and facilitators. https://core.ac.uk/download/30639389.pdf (accessed on 28th July 2025).
27. Cox, N., Dewaele, A., Van den Berghe, W., Vincke, J., et al. (2008). Minority-specific determinants of mental well-being among lesbian, gay and bisexual youth. https://core.ac.uk/download/55815155.pdf (accessed on 28th July 2025).
28. DaBreo-Otero, C. (2021). The course of Axis I and Axis II disorders in clinical high risk (CHR) adolescents. https://core.ac.uk/download/478555739.pdf (accessed on 28th July 2025).
29. De Fruyt, F., & De Clercq, B. (2014). Antecedents of personality disorder in childhood and adolescence: toward an integrative developmental model. *Annual review of clinical psychology*, *10*, 449–476. https://doi.org/10.1146/annurev-clinpsy-032813-153634(accessed on 28th July 2025).
30. Verbeke, L., De Clercq, B., Van der Heijden, P., Hutsebaut, J., & van Aken, M. A. (2017). The relevance of schizotypal traits for understanding interpersonal functioning in adolescents with psychiatric problems. *Personality disorders*, *8*(1), 54–63. https://doi.org/10.1037/per0000163 (accessed on 28th July 2025).
31. Durbin, C. E., Knobloch-Fedders, L. M., Saigal, S. D., Stroud, C. B., et al. (2010). Normal and abnormal personality traits are associated with marital satisfaction for both men and women: An actor–partner interdependence model analysis. https://core.ac.uk/download/213087478.pdf (accessed on 28th July 2025).
32. Ferraro, L., La Barbera, D., La Cascia, C., Lo Baido, R., Maniaci, G., Marrazzo, G., Sartorio, C., et al. (2019). Borderline personality in patients with poly-diagnoses treated for a bipolar disorder. https://core.ac.uk/download/287859112.pdf (accessed on 28th July 2025).
33. Fortunato, A., & Speranza, A. M. (2018). Personality traits and disorders in childhood: Clinical evaluation and diagnosis. Clinical Neuropsychiatry: Journal of Treatment Evaluation, 15(4), 222–235.(accessed on 28th July 2025).
34. Frantz, D. (2004). Gender and ethnic biases in personality disorder diagnostic criteria. https://core.ac.uk/download/154532640.pdf (accessed on 28th July 2025).
35. Greenberg, J. L., Hoeppner, S. S., Phillips, K. A., Steketee, G., et al. (2019). Predictors of response to cognitive-behavioral therapy for body dysmorphic disorder. https://open.bu.edu/bitstream/2144/40196/3/Greenberg%20CBT%20BDD%20Predictors.pdf (accessed on 28th July 2025).
36. Heine, S. J., Ryder, A. G., & Yang, J. (2002). Somatization vs. psychologization of emotional distress: A paradigmatic example for cultural psychopathology. https://core.ac.uk/download/10687096.pdf (accessed on 28th July 2025).
37. Hinshaw, S. P., & Richters, J. E. (1999). The abduction of disorder in psychiatry. https://core.ac.uk/download/pdf/84622.pdf (accessed on 28th July 2025).
38. Stepp, S. D., Scott, L. N., Jones, N. P., Whalen, D. J., & Hipwell, A. E. (2016). Negative emotional reactivity as a marker of vulnerability in the development of borderline personality disorder

symptoms. *Development and psychopathology*, *28*(1), 213–224. https://doi.org/10.1017/S0954579415000395 (accessed on 28th July 2025).

39. Kozhukhov, V., Neuman, Y., & Vilenchik, D. (2023). Data augmentation for modeling human personality: The Dexter Machine. http://arxiv.org/abs/2301.08606 (accessed on 28th July 2025).
40. Lieto, A., American Psychiatric Association, Boorse, C., Machery, E., Rosch, E., et al. (2019). Ontologies, mental disorders and prototypes. https://core.ac.uk/download/186331620.pdf (accessed on 28th July 2025).
41. (accessed on 28th July 2025).
42. McNamara, N., McNicholas, F., O'Connor, C., O'Hara, L., et al. (2016). Eating disorder literacy and stigmatizing attitudes towards anorexia, bulimia and binge eating disorder among adolescents. https://core.ac.uk/download/30650748.pdf (accessed on 28th July 2025).
43. Melrose, S. (2017). Persistent depressive disorder or dysthymia: An overview of assessment and treatment approaches. https://core.ac.uk/download/80298545.pdf (accessed on 28th July 2025).
44. Strand, E. R., & Nordahl, H. (2024). Do Patient's Interpersonal Problems Improve Following Metacognitive Therapy? A Systematic Review and Meta-Analysis. *Clinical psychology & psychotherapy*, *31*(2), e2973. https://doi.org/10.1002/cpp.2973 (accessed on 28th July 2025).
45. Rorie, K. (2016). Psychodynamic psychotherapy for personality disorders: A systematic review. https://core.ac.uk/download/217160320.pdf (accessed on 28th July 2025).
46. Seely, M. (2019). Managing madness: The ethics of identifying and treating mental illness. https://core.ac.uk/download/215444329.pdf (accessed on 28th July 2025).
47. Susick, M. (2011). Application of smartphone technology in the management and treatment of mental illnesses. https://core.ac.uk/download/12206606.pdf (accessed on 28th July 2025).
48. Tocarciuc, S. (2018). Efficiency analysis and determination of the need to implement the PID-5 international instrument in medical practice. Department of Human Physiology and Biophysics, Nicolae Testemitanu State University of Medicine and Pharmacy of the Republic of Moldova. https://core.ac.uk/download/335258160.pdf (accessed on 28th July 2025).

SUBSTANCE USE AND ADDICTION DISORDERS

10

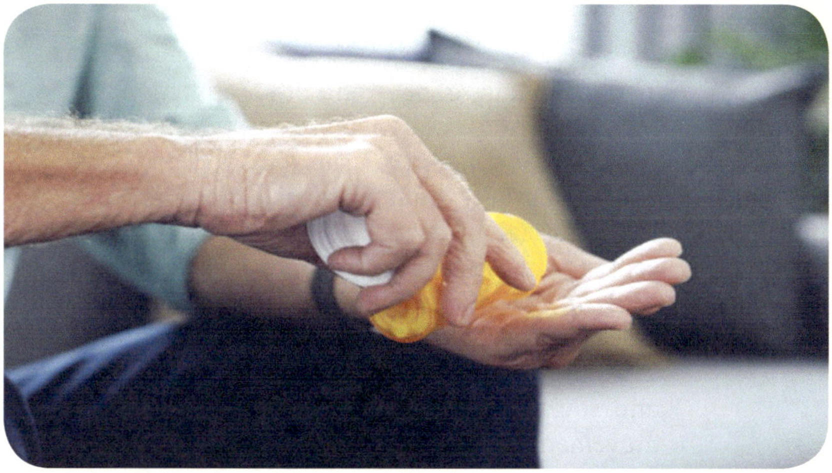

LEARNING OBJECTIVES

After studying this chapter, you will be able to:

1. Identify the types of substances;
2. List the causes of substance use disorders;
3. Explore the signs and symptoms of addiction;
4. Focus on the impact on individuals;
5. Explain the treatment options;
6. Describe the prevention strategies.

Introduction

The addiction and substance use disorder phenomenon has generated significant attention in the last couple of years and is a nascent challenge to public health and clinical psychology. These disorders are characterized by an individual's compulsive consumption of psychoactive substances despite ruinous effects. As concepts and definitions of such illnesses evolve, it has been increasingly necessary to recognize that addiction is not merely a result of the pharmacological effects of drugs, but also a product of the specific neurological and psychological make-up of the individual. Studies highlight the multidimensionality of addiction, necessitating a multidimensional approach to understand and treat such diseases. As mentioned in recent literature, enhanced knowledge of the neurobiological basis of addiction permits the development of more effective treatment interventions that are innovative and client-centered (Baconi et al., 2015). One of the key aspects of substance use disorders is how addiction and related co-morbid mental illnesses interact, particularly anxiety disorders. It is confirmed that individuals with substance use disorders typically face a double challenge because such disorders frequently overlap, rendering efforts at recovery more difficult. For example, studies reveal that most individuals with opioid use disorder are also diagnosable with anxiety disorders, further reflecting the complicated interrelationship between mental illness and drug use. This intersectional approach emphasizes the necessity of holistic treatment approaches that address both co-morbid psychological disorders and substance abuse. Identification of these dual diagnoses plays a critical role in establishing holistic interventions, thereby improving outcomes among subjects with substance use disorders (Barlow et al., 2017). As we explore the reality of substance use and addiction disorders, it is now necessary to adopt a vision beyond stigmatization and towards compassion.

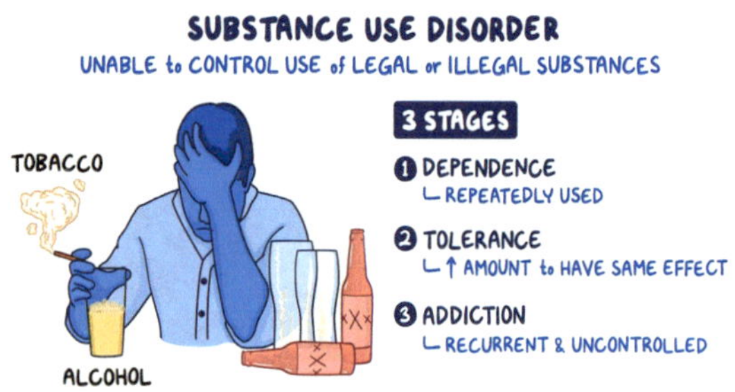
SUBSTANCE USE DISORDER
UNABLE to CONTROL USE of LEGAL or ILLEGAL SUBSTANCES
TOBACCO
ALCOHOL
3 STAGES
1 DEPENDENCE
REPEATEDLY USED
2 TOLERANCE
↑ AMOUNT to HAVE SAME EFFECT
3 ADDICTION
RECURRENT & UNCONTROLLED

Figure 10.1. Substance use disorder.

Source: https://www.osmosis.org/_next/image?url=https%3A%2F%2Fd16qt3wv6xm098.cloudfront.net%2FnNkHRDLGSi6CFI-9G-1TKT-0Q4qjL8pU%2F_.jpg&w=3840&q=75.

The labeling of addiction as a disease in all its complexity and not a question of moral frailty opens up the discourse on mental health and recovery from addiction in society at large. Moreover, the uptake of evidence-based treatment modalities that accommodate the reality of addiction's complexities necessitates the highest priority in clinical practice. A successful resolution of this public health problem necessitates greater awareness, education, and advocacy, not only for those who struggle with addiction but also for their families and communities. Thus, the creation of supportive environments, along with innovative treatment approaches, is a forward-looking solution to counteract the widespread consumption of substances and addiction disorders, ultimately building healthier societies (Figure 10.1).

Definition of Substance Use and Addiction Disorders

The vocabulary of drug and other addiction use includes a range of behaviors and physiological responses in relation to drug and other addictive use. Essentially, substance use disorders are characterized by compulsive substance use and seeking in the face of adverse consequences. One of the distinguishing features of such disorders is the impaired ability to control drug use, which often leads to chronic health and social problems. This loss of control is a movement from voluntary consumption of drugs to compulsive craving, mirroring mechanisms observed in behavioral addictions. Such definitions need to be understood by adopting an integrated perspective that not only identifies the pharmacological but also the psychological and social determinants of the development of substance use disorders. A wider perspective of addiction has recently emerged beyond the traditional concepts of substance dependence. For instance, behavioral addictions , such as gambling have some similarities with substance addictions, that is, tolerance development and withdrawal, suggesting the existence of similar underlying mechanisms. As quoted, gambling addiction is a new concern, specifically among adolescents, challenging the classical conceptions of addiction (Hasanović et al., 2021). Moreover, the recognition of these patterns in the arena of addiction is a testament to the multifaceted nature of compulsive behavior, rendering their treatment even more challenging. This advancement in understanding acts as proof for the necessity of dynamic definitions encompassing substance use disorders and behavioral compulsions alike, illustrating how addiction can be manifested in diverse forms other than substance intake. The complexity of addiction and substance use disorders is also illustrated in the neurobiological substrates underpinning their formation. Drug addiction has been proven not only as a result of the pharmacological effect of substances but also highly correlated with individual neurological and psychological processes, leading to characteristic patterns of dependence (Baconi et al., 2015). This perspective warrants more personalized treatment approaches, considering the contribution of genetic tendencies, environmental factors, and states of mind to individual cases of addiction. With changing treatment plans incorporating these discoveries, debates surrounding the definition and comprehension of substance use and addiction should also change, thereby allowing for more effective interventions directed at the causation and manifestation of these disorders in diverse populations.

Importance of Understanding These Disorders

It is essential to have a comprehensive understanding of substance use and addiction disorders to cope with the widespread impact these issues have on families, society, and the individual. Substance use disorders (SUDs) afflict millions of people, leading to deleterious individual and societal consequences, including illness-related issues, social stigma, and economic costs. The ability to recognize the indicators and subtleties of addiction enhances intervention and treatment provision, providing a more empathetic environment for those affected. Harm reduction and access to treatment initiatives demonstrate the significance of developing a deeper understanding of such conditions. Efforts outlined in initiatives against SUDs not only save lives but also improve the quality of care by employing evidence-based practices, which allow for affected individuals to once again take control of their lives and long-term health (Wallman-Stokes et al., 2015). Understanding addiction also involves comprehending the causes underlying its formation, such as genetic susceptibility, environmental influences, and psychological triggers. Comprehensive reviews prove that addiction most often arises from an interaction of such complicated risk factors, supporting the contention that treatment must be holistic. By the incorporation of upstream interventions, such as preventive treatment for at-risk populations, stakeholders can mitigate the perils of substance abuse before they escalate to full-blown addiction. Investment in early intervention is also crucial, particularly in those children who are at risk of future addiction. Utilization of existing structural resources, such as children's Medicaid, can assist in offering mental health screenings and preventive services so that at-risk populations can receive the assistance necessary to break cycles of addiction before they begin (Cannon et al., 2019). Lastly, the public consequences of addiction disorder and substance abuse call for a social knowledge transcending individual experience. The opioid epidemic, for instance, reveals the overall consequences of addiction, resulting in widespread economic and social impacts that hinder community productivity and health. Understanding the magnitude of these crises calls for multifaceted public health strategies dedicated to addressing the peculiar realities of addicted communities. By fostering a shared knowledge among public policymakers, health care professionals, and citizens, communities can prioritize prevention first, effective treatment, and well-educated policy initiatives that target resources to the most critical areas. In this manner, the battle against substance use disorders is no longer just a matter of individual treatment, but a societal moral obligation to keep all together (Cannon et al., 2019) (Figure 10.2).

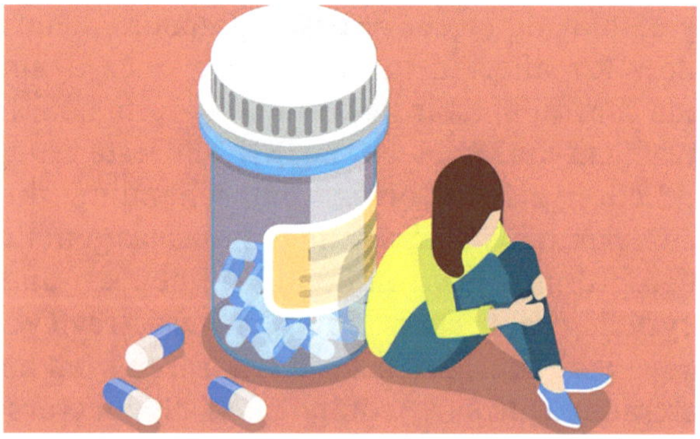

Figure 10.2. Importance of substance use and addiction disorders.

Source: https://external-content.duckduckgo.com/iu/?u=https%3A%2F%2Fwww.drugtargetreview.com%2Fwp-content%2Fuploads%2Fsubstance-abuse.jpg&f=1&nofb=1&ipt=e712ef79fa2b8aaab5c4250b76c0ebbb2ecbe0ef76f550e768e57429d4a94dad.

10.1. Types of Substances

Learning Outcome

1. Legal substances (e.g., alcohol, prescription medications).
2. Illegal substances (e.g., cocaine, heroin).
3. Emerging substances (e.g., synthetic drugs, designer drugs).

Classification of drugs that cause addiction disorders plays a crucial role in understanding the complexity of drug use and its effects on public health. In general, drugs can be classified as stimulants, depressants, opioids, and hallucinogens. Stimulants , such as cocaine and amphetamines enhance body and mind stimulation, which largely results in increased energy and euphoria. They can produce dangerous side effects, including cardiovascular problems and anxiety disorders. Depressants like benzodiazepines and alcohol, in contrast, depress the central nervous system and offer temporary relief for insomnia or anxiety, but with the risk of dependency and overdose. Knowledge of these differences is required for establishing effective treatment strategies and care services for victims of addiction. One of the most feared types of drugs is opioids, which have become the central topic in substance use disorder due to their epidemic rates. The opioid crisis has not only been associated with increased rates of addiction but also with dire socio-economic consequences, including an increase in foster care placements. As per the reports, 34% of the foster care admissions resulting from the factor of parental drug abuse are highlighted by the broader implications of opioid use on family functioning and child well-being. Additionally, prenatal exposure to drugs, in particular opioids, has been linked with developmental problems in newborns. Estimated 400,000 births affected by prenatal alcohol and illicit drug use makes stopping opioid use very important for health and safety assurance among high-risk groups, particularly infants that do not know the set of issues of maternal abuse of the drugs (American Academy of Pediatrics Council on Foster Care, Adoption, and Kinship Care, 2018). Hallucinogens, including drugs like LSD and psilocybin, are also defined by the unique impact that they have on perception and cognition. Once relegated to the periphery of substance use disorder discussion, recent evidence suggests that the drugs have therapeutic potential for the cure of mental illness, for example, the cure of post-traumatic stress disorder (PTSD) and other anxiety disorders. Nevertheless, non-medical use of hallucinogens can lead to unpredictable experiences that may exacerbate concomitant psychiatric disorders or provoke enduring perceptual changes. Also, the interaction between early interpersonal trauma and the onset of substance use disorders, as highlighted by current investigations, necessitates comprehensive prevention strategies addressing both the substance and exposure to trauma (Meulewaeter et al., 2019). Being aware of the subtleties of these various types of substances is imperative for ensuring successful intervention programs suited to the requirements of populations that have diversity (Figure 10.3).

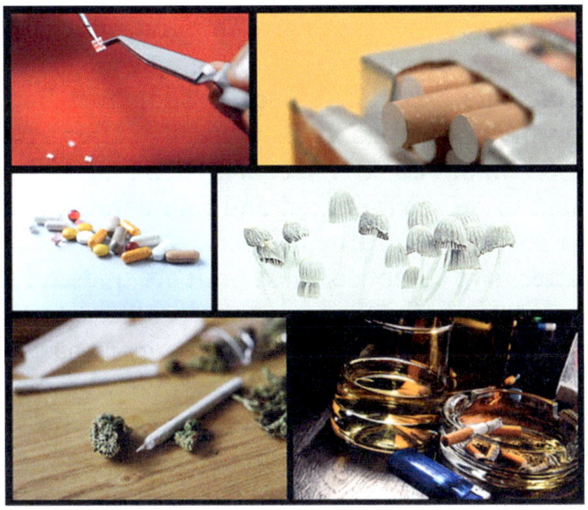

Figure 10.3. Types of substances.

Source: https://static.wixstatic.com/media/f6f10d_eb24bdcf82444b3fb8763d9a2335cb0c~mv2.png/v1/fill/w_568,h_476,al_c,q_85,usm_0.66_1.00_0.01,enc_avif,quality_auto/f6f10d_eb24bdcf82444b3fb8763d9a2335cb0c~mv2.png.

10.1.1. Legal Substances (e.g., Alcohol, Prescription Medications)

Lawful drug consumption , such as that of alcohol and prescription drugs, is high in the broader context of substance abuse and addiction disorders. Legal drugs are usually viewed as socially acceptable, but they carry significant health and social consequences when abused. For instance, alcohol, besides becoming a normal aspect of social life, has also turned into a cause of long-term illnesses, such is, liver disease and psychiatric illnesses. Research indicates that while the law is selling alcohol to adults, alcohol misuse leads to alcoholism, which adversely affects people, families, and society. In accordance with most research, public health systems are not able to restrict the influence of alcohol dependence, yet they emphasize large-scale preventative programs and education campaigns concerning moderate use. Pharmaceutically approved drugs, while primarily used to treat pain, possess the ability to open the doors of addiction if misused. These drugs are initially taken by individuals for the treatment of genuine health conditions, but through the act of over-prescription and not educating them, they become vulnerable to misuse. Opioids, benzodiazepines, and stimulants are some of the prescription drugs that are known to be very addictive. As can be seen in considering numerous different cases, the majority of individuals get addicted to these drugs and in the majority of cases, this goes tragically through overdose and in others through death. In addition, the situation is worsened in vulnerable groups , such as veterans, with post-traumatic stress disorder diagnosis leading them to self-medicate through prescription medication that has a tendency to be abused.

As evident from study outcomes, regulation of interventions of such trends necessitates accessible treatment aimed at education and recovery courses specifically geared towards those with substance dependence (Meulewaeter et al., 2019). As legal drug use continues to rise, public debate and policy debate have emerged in crafting effective interventions. Public debate regarding drug use can result in greater understanding and collaborative action towards resolving public health concerns. Engagement by organizations with diverse backgrounds, as noted in various guides, points to the importance of sharing personal experience to recognize the extent to which substance abuse impacts families and communities. Solutions involve exploring potential reforms in regulation, school systems, and intervention services that break the negative effects associated with alcohol and prescribed drug use. Interventions may include advocating harm reduction strategies, which seek to minimize drug harms more so than encouraging abstinence only. Lastly, creating informed community discourse may bridge the gap between awareness and action, eventually leading to more effective interventions in the case of substance use and addiction disorders (Aguiniga et al., 2015) (Figure 10.4).

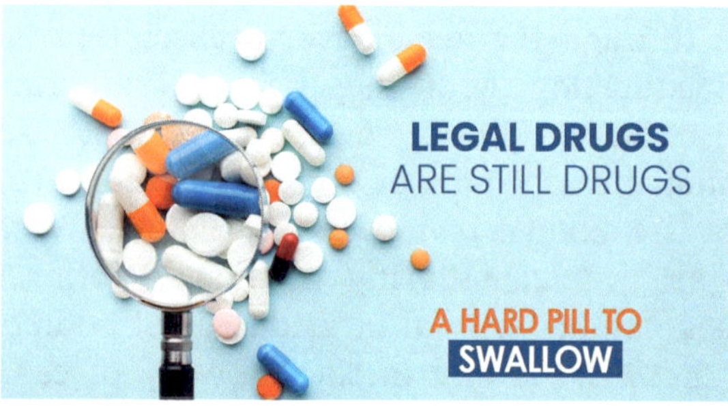

Figure 10.4. Legal substances.

Source: https://anchoredtidesrecovery.com/wp-content/uploads/2021/05/Hard-to-swallow.jpeg.

10.1.2. Illegal Substances (e.g., Cocaine, Heroin)

The charm of illegal drugs , such as heroin and cocaine is multifaceted, with both intrapsychic and sociocultural motivations involved. The initiation to such drugs can be an attempt at a longing for euphoria or escape from the vicissitudes of life. The development towards dependency is however, multifaceted. Cocaine, a very strong stimulant, produces feelings of euphoria and heightened energy, but also severe withdrawal effects with it that can create a cycle of dependency. Similarly, heroin's appeal lies in its quick action of creating pleasurable effects, but its tendency to create tolerance and physical dependence poses a gigantic issue for the users. Understanding these dynamics is crucial for making effective prevention and treatment interventions in the treatment of substance use and addiction disorders. The impact of these illicit drugs extends beyond individual health to have a significant impact on societal structures as well as economic burden. The economic burden of treating the resultant medical comorbidities of cocaine and heroin use by the healthcare systems is prohibitive, typically requiring cost-intensive care in emergency rooms and rehabilitation programs. Moreover, social implications , such as increased crime rate and family destruction depict the extreme impact of addiction. Both heroin and cocaine addicts usually suffer from discrimination and it becomes even tougher for them to be rehabilitated and reintegrated into the society. According to statistical research on patterns of co-abuse, most patients treated for opioid-related disorders have problems with alcohol as well, making recovery even harder (Backmund et al., 2003). An understanding of these broader implications is necessary in formulating inclusive policies aimed at reducing the prevalence of substance use disorders. Moreover, the interaction of marijuana and other illicit drugs poses legitimate issues regarding the onset of substance use disorders. Cannabis, which is usually considered a soft drug, has been linked to the onset of stronger substance use among adolescents.

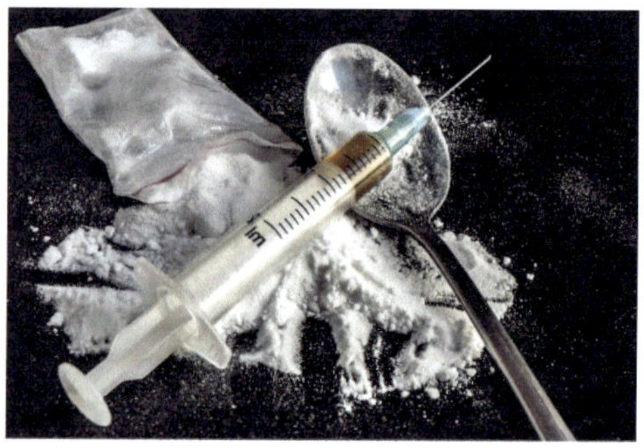

Figure 10.5. Illegal substances.

Source: https://www.drugfreekidscanada.org/wp-content/uploads/2016/08/heroin.jpg.

Its widespread availability and varied perceptions of risk are contributing factors to earlier patterns of use that lead users to try more varied quantities of drugs, such as heroin and cocaine (Cadoni et al., 2017). This trajectory poses basic questions to intervention development that aims for disruption of these patterns. Educational interventions for youth will have to emphasize the potential risks of youth cannabis use, particularly as a gateway drug. By addressing these aspects in an integrated manner, the field of substance abuse and addiction disorder can establish more effective prevention and intervention strategies based on the complicated network of substance interactions and diverse experiences (Figure 10.5).

10.1.3. Emerging Substances (e.g., Synthetic Drugs, Designer Drugs)

The landscape of drug use has changed dramatically with the advent of synthetic drugs and designer drugs, which pose new challenges to public safety and health. These drugs, introduced as legal alternatives to traditional illegal drugs, have unique pharmacological profiles that can elicit unexpected and alarming health consequences. Whereas naturally occurring analogs are limited by structural limitations at the molecular level, the availability of synthetic drugs for use facilitates manipulation at this level that bypasses existing drug controls, presenting a constant flow of new psychoactive substances (NPS) that can potentially enhance addiction risks. With increased popularity in use, especially among younger individuals seeking recreational highs, the threat posed by substance use disorders grows and necessitates a renewed evaluation of existing intervention strategies and treatment paradigms in addiction psychiatry. The distinction between the use of classical substance use disorders and NPS is important in treatment and management. New drugs have atypical psychopathological presentation, so diagnosis and intervention would be complicated. The association of synthetic cannabinoids with "new psychoses" underscores the importance of clinicians keeping abreast of the evolving nature of substance-related disorders. The distinctions within the clinical presentation of NPS-induced psychosis compared to the classic psychoses highlight the challenge that arises in treatment environments where the traditional approach is not sufficient. Therefore, a thorough understanding of the new substances and their typical effects will enable health care providers to formulate tailored therapeutic interventions and therefore, improve patient outcomes for this vulnerable population (Chiappini et al., 2019). Moreover, the greater frequency of newly emerging drugs is typically augmented by social attitudes that reduce their risks. For instance, the soft drug permissiveness of cannabis, despite evidence showing there to be some association between the use of cannabis and grave long-term cognitive and psychological loss, particularly among young users (Cadoni et al., 2017). Such a misconception can facilitate patterns of misuse, with initial experimentation on relatively harmless substances eventually leading to growing usage of increasingly dangerous NPS. Public health campaigns, therefore, must counteract as much the empirical evidence surrounding these drugs as the cultural explanations that underlie user behaviors. It can create an awareness about the potential for being addicted, as well as the realities of synthetic drug use, which can make the tide of substance use disorders linked with newer and synthetic drugs more manageable (Figure 10.6).

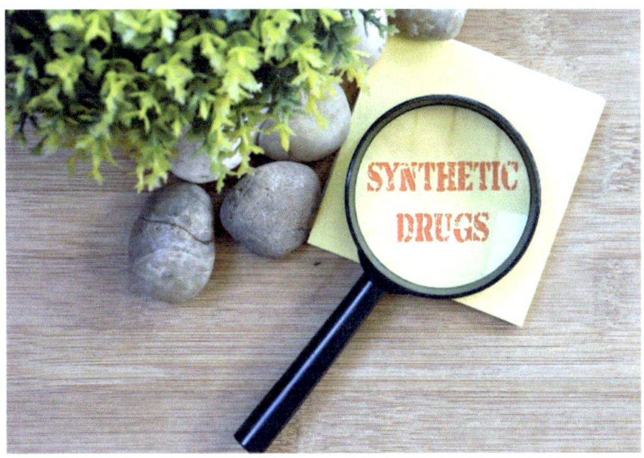

Figure 10.6. Synthetic drugs.

Test Your Knowledge

1. How do depressants, stimulants, and hallucinogens differ in their effects on the central nervous system and addiction potential?
2. What distinguishes legal substances (e.g., alcohol, prescription drugs) from illicit substances (e.g., heroin, cocaine) in terms of patterns of misuse?

10.2. Causes of Substance Use Disorders

Learning Outcome

1. Genetic predisposition and family history
2. Environmental factors (e.g., peer pressure, socio-economic status).
3. Psychological factors (e.g., trauma, mental health disorders).

Understanding the etiology of substance use disorders is a multifaceted endeavor that encompasses biological, psychological, and environmental determinants. On a biological level, genetic predisposition is a vital aspect with regard to how an individual responds to drugs in most situations, setting sensitivity or susceptibility to drug abuse. For instance, some genetic mutations have the potential to alter neurotransmitter processes, such as dopamine, which plays a crucial role in the reward system. Psychological problems, including underlying illness, also have a significant impact on the development of substance use disorders. Diseases , such as depression or anxiety will cause a person to turn to drugs as a way of medicating, hastening their reliance upon such drugs as a coping mechanism. Environmental influences, such as exposure to drug use within peer or family groups, complicate these psychological and biological factors further to create a complicated network of risk factors that predispose a person towards addiction. A longitudinal cohort study shows the direct association between substance abuse and psychiatric disorders, which offers valuable information about premature mortality among substance users. The study took a cohort of 561 users of drugs over several decades and found that male sex, opiate or barbiturate daily use, and the presence of neurosis predictably forecast early death from drugs (Baldacchino et al., 2011). Of note was the finding that risk for drug death at any single time was very elevated in the initial 15 years of follow-up, suggesting a window of risk when individuals with substance issues were especially vulnerable. In addition, this study points out that certain psychiatric disorders, here depression and anxiety, are excellent predictors of drug-related mortality. That is, treatment of mental illness is important in resolving the root causes of substance use disorders and hopefully averting negative long-term effects. In addition to biological and psychological factors, environmental and social processes are also at the center of the prevalence of substance use disorders. Socioeconomic status, the availability of drugs, and cultural views about drug consumption have a significant influence on drug attitudes and behavior at the personal level. Locations with poverty and limited access to mental health facilities tend to have higher rates of substance abuse because residents resort to drugs as a means of coping with their condition. Furthermore, social norms that legitimize or stigmatize drug use also have the ability to impact people's views and experiences of drugs. The dynamic interaction of external social components with personal conditions portrays the character of substance use disorders and highlights the need for holistic knowledge comprising different risk factors (Baconi et al., 2015). Treating these etiologies with multiple factors is essential in fostering the effectiveness of prevention and treatment interventions against substance use disorders (Figure 10.7).

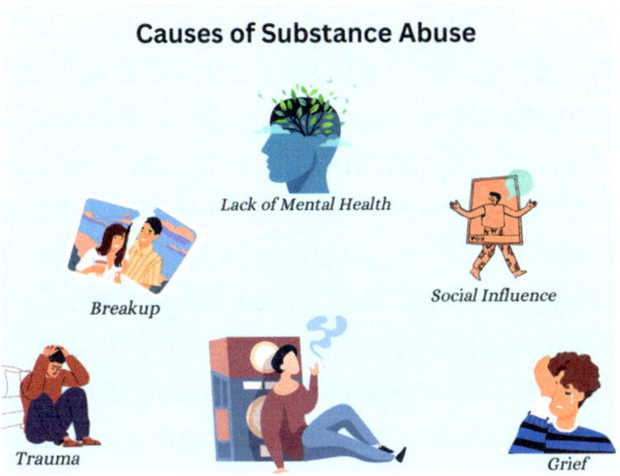

Figure 10.7. Causes of substance use disorders.

Source: https://lh7-rt.googleusercontent.com/docsz/AD_4nXdrBcqv3hfUVUYeXwpbCZ5bKjh7oSLzlxM-xvf1GPC29IhP3axiS4FZQ1LjoMtKMykd0vrZOmrYbi1x5Ml_djvQHlYrpp_0sknli1pPIq_TYG-W27p6xKfR1f4IETqg2HcptFFJKA?key=k-GgcV5JaeIRei8S7mYtObu7.

10.2.1. Genetic Predisposition and Family History

The role of genetic predisposition to drug abuse and addiction disorders has been a significant field of research, particularly concerning how family history influences these disorders. The complex interaction between genetics and environment dictates that an individual who hails from a family with a drug abuse background is likely to develop similar types of issues. This vulnerability is confirmed by studies that identify the mechanisms through which genes can account for up to 60% of the risk for substance use disorders. Genetic vulnerability is also compounded by traits like impulsivity and sensitivity variation towards substances, both of which increase individuals' vulnerability towards addiction (Schuckit, 2014). Hence, it is important to know that while genetics plays a dominant role, environmental contexts and personal experience also influence the trajectory of substance use in individuals with family histories of addiction. Family history is one of the significant determinants of the risk for the emergence of substance use disorders, as shown by data in genetic studies. Where drug use is prevalent in a household, younger families are likely to develop the same behavior as a mode of socialization or coping with stress. Family-based observational learning is a phase that makes some behavior normal, creating a feedback loop that enhances drug use generation after generation. Furthermore, the genetic predisposition that has been identified in research , such as the ABCD twin study, identifies the need for a more complex understanding of the role of family. Twin pair comparison studies not only teach us about the genetic and environmental dimensions of drug use but also identify that addiction is a complex phenomenon where family is one of the significant factors that affect an individual's likelihood of developing drug use issues (Banich et al., 2018). The current research into genetic susceptibility and family history of substance abuse disorders indicates that both can influence each other significantly and contribute to informing both prevention and intervention efforts. Knowing the genetic history of individuals will enable practitioners to determine their risk level more effectively, hence deploy individualized preventive strategies or therapies. For instance, individuals at increased family risk of drug use can be treated by early intervention programs with a focus on education and support aimed at countering risk before it escalates to addiction. This integrated model, informed by genetic research, can result in a wiser understanding of addiction as not necessarily an issue of choice or moral failing but as a disorder that arises out of complex genetic and environmental interaction. By acknowledging the contribution of both genetic vulnerability and family environment, public health programs may take on more effectiveness in attacking substance abuse and addiction disorders in vulnerable populations.

10.2.2. Environmental Factors (i.e., Socio-Economic Status, Peer Pressure)

Environmental factors are a crucial element in the prevalence of substance use and the establishment of addiction disorders. One of the main factors is peer pressure, particularly among youth and young adults. As research has pointed out, an overwhelming majority of substance abusers, that is, 81.6%, reported that friends played an important part in their first experience with drugs and alcohol. Such external pressure tends to reinforce a pattern of drug use among social groups, thus further complicating the process of resisting peer-initiated impulses. Through seeking approval and acceptance from their peers, the temptation to use drugs gains prominence, thus further advancing the likelihood of drug addiction. This knowledge is necessary for creating successful prevention and intervention programs for at-risk groups. Socio-economic status is a second key environmental determinant that involves substance use patterns. Most likely, those from lower socio-economic status are under higher stress, resource-poor environments, and are more apt to use substances as a coping strategy. From a poll among substance abusers, the breakdown was concluded to be that a significant majority were of socio-economic groups four and five, which confirms a high rate of correlation between socio-economic disadvantage and substance abuse. Poverty can prevent access to education and employment opportunities, hence creating patterns of despair which substance use becomes an escape strategy. Moreover, substance use disorders are equally prevalent among those facing economic hardship, since money can typically exacerbate mental illness. Addressing socio-economic disparity should be high on the agenda for effective public health policy in the reduction of the onset of addiction disorders. The stigma that relates to the use of substances severely hinders the process of recovery, making the addictions that already arise more difficult from external environmental influences. Those struggling with addiction often face social stigma, which can result in increased social isolation and relationship problems. Studies point to perceived stigma as a cause of relapse, with high correlations existing between stigma and several dimensions of relapse, such as peer pressure and emotional distress. This stigma is usually combined with socio-economic difficulties, thereby perpetuating the cycle where one feels stuck in their situation. Developing comprehensive strategies to target both stigma and socio-economic concerns is imperative in fostering recovery-promoting environments. By taking awareness and education as a priority, society can begin dismantling the stigma of substance use, ultimately achieving improved outcomes for people with addiction disorders.

10.2.3. Psychological Factors (e.g., Trauma, Mental Health Disorders)

The intersection between the psychological problems and substance use disorders (SUDs) is complex and significantly intertwined with the personal history of trauma. It has been determined through studies that interpersonal trauma experienced during childhood significantly increases the risk of SUDs in adulthood. The majority of substance abuser recovering mothers reflect on their experiences as parents, revealing how their own traumatic history as a child has affected parenting and parent-child relationships. This intergenerational cycle of trauma shows that the traumatic exposures at an early age might lead to unhealthy family relationships, thereby resulting in patterns of drug abuse. The prevention of such causative roots in treatment centers is thus significant to avoid perpetuating such cycles and foster healthier interpersonal relationships, which can lower the risk of addiction in subsequent generations (Meulewaeter et al., 2019). Gender disparities also have an important role to play in terms of how psychological factors lead to substance use disorder. Studies reveal that females with SUDs are more likely to have greater psychological disturbance and a higher traumatic history compared to their male counterparts. Despite boys displaying compromised cognitive performance in relation to drug use, girls show rapid-track progression from drug use to dependence due to their traumatic histories. This trend highlights the requirement of gender-specific treatment programs that recognize the unique psychological problems of both populations. For example, trauma-informed care to address the requirements of young women can be more effective by recognizing the implications of early abusive relationship experiences on their subsequent mental health and alcohol/drug use (Simonelli et al., 2017). Moreover, understanding the psychological underpinnings of addiction necessitates an extended model that encompasses mental health disorders. Individuals with a history of prior mental health disorders, such as depression or anxiety, are more likely to use substances as an unhealthy way of coping. The interaction among these mental health and substance use disorders complicates their treatment because the clinician needs to treat both if any recovery is going to be meaningful. Treatment models that treat mental health issues and drug dependence concurrently are essential for intervention to be successful. It is important to understand how psychological issues like trauma and psychiatric illness contribute to drug addiction so that healthcare providers can address them more holistically and specifically, ensuring that long-term recovery is promoted (Simonelli et al., 2017; Meulewaeter et al., 2019) (Figure 10.8).

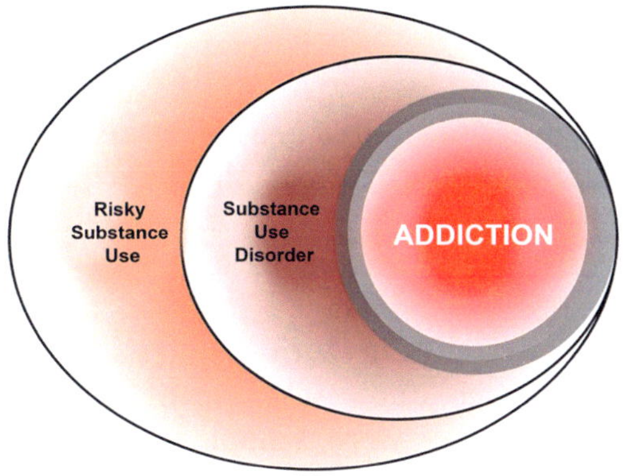

Figure 10.8. Psychological factors.

Source: https://media.springernature.com/full/springer-static/image/art%3A10.1038%2Fs41386-020-00950-y/MediaObjects/41386_2020_950_Fig1_HTML.png.

Test Your Knowledge

1. How do genetic vulnerability, brain chemistry, and family history contribute to the development of substance use disorders?
2. What environmental and psychosocial factors—such as peer influence, stress, trauma, and early exposure—serve as major causes of substance misuse?

10.3. Signs and Symptoms of Addiction

Learning Outcome

1. Behavioral changes (e.g., withdrawal from social activities).
2. Physical symptoms (e.g., changes in appearance, health issues).
3. Psychological symptoms (e.g., anxiety, depression).

The symptoms and signs of addiction are multifaceted and reflect the psychological and physical components of substance use disorders. The addicted patient may present with significant changes in behavior, such as a preoccupation with getting and using the substance and a significant decline in responsibility for work, school, or home. Social withdrawal is also noted as the relationships fail, leading to social isolation. Besides, addiction also usually manifests through an array of emotional symptoms in the form of anxiety, depression, or mood swings, as signs of the immense psychological toll of drug consumption. These emotional and behavioral symptoms may also serve as crucial warning signs for the onset of addiction, necessitating early treatment and therapy. Physical symptoms follow these psychological symptoms, giving additional proof of the depth of addiction. They can appear as physical alterations of appearance, for example, loss of weight or poor personal hygiene, which are directly related to the compulsive nature of drug intake. Withdrawal symptoms could also appear on reduction or stoppage of the drug, showing the biological dependence established. Individuals can complain of the growing tolerance, as they require larger quantities of the drug to achieve the same effect, which indicates a stage in the addiction process. Ultimately, these physical symptoms can profoundly compromise the quality of life, arguing the need for comprehensive assessment and treatment regimens that attempt to break the addictive cycle. Comorbid psychiatric illness severely complicates the identification and treatment of addictions. Evidence is available to argue a strong correlation between substance use disorders (SUDs) and several psychological disorders, including mood and anxiety disorders. For instance, participants in a study examining Dual Disorders reported that anxiety disorders were the most common comorbid with substance abuse, followed by bipolar disorder, and schizophrenia/schizoaffective disorder (Acquas et al., 2018). The difficulty of these dual conditions necessitates a multifaceted treatment plan that does not merely treat substance dependence but also psychological issues. As addiction becomes increasingly complicated with mental illness, medical professionals have the responsibility of being sensitive to such symptoms and signs, thus enabling early intervention and personalized treatment plans that can improve patient outcomes in the management of addiction and co-morbid diseases (Morse et al., 2006) (Figure 10.9).

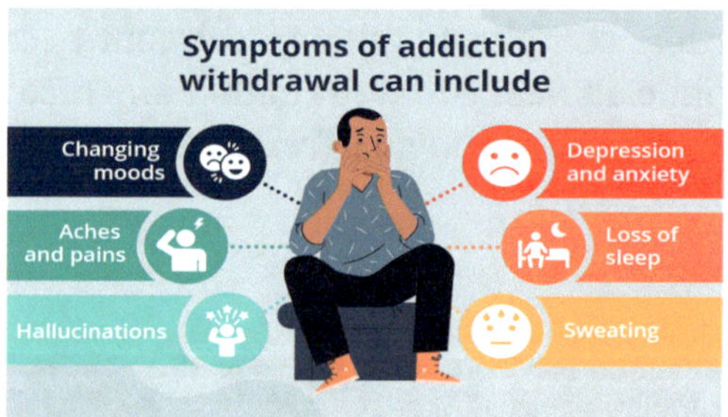
Symptoms of addiction withdrawal can include
Changing moods
Aches and pains
Hallucinations
Depression and anxiety
Loss of sleep
Sweating

Figure 10.9. The signs and symptoms of addiction.

Source: https://media.healthdirect.org.au/images/inline/original/addiction-withdrawal-symptoms_website_v09-04-25-f4eb0b.png.

10.3.1. Behavioral Changes (e.g., Withdrawal From Social Activities)

Substance use and addiction disorder development typically presage extreme behavior changes, among the most foreboding of which is social withdrawal. Individuals enthralled in addiction can begin withdrawing from friends and family as well as social activities, substituting these necessary contacts with substance consumption. Such withdrawal may stem from both shame at their addiction and the overwhelming desire to use and take drugs, which takes precedence over relationships and social responsibilities. In avoiding support groups and keeping themselves at arm's length, individuals may inadvertently exacerbate their conditions because social relationships are critical to healing and mental wellness. So the behavior change into isolation just perpetuates an addictive pattern and simultaneously denies the possibility of improvement or intervention. Additionally, the implications of substance use on social isolation can perpetuate a vicious circle of negative life consequences that further entrench patterns of addiction. As individuals become increasingly entrenched in substance use, other activities and pleasures , such as hobbies, family gatherings, and friendships, are given up. These changes can have the ability to foster both isolation and hopelessness, resulting in a breakdown of mental health that will become increasingly difficult to reverse. Social withdrawal minimizes opportunities for beneficial interaction and learning coping skills needed to bring about recovery. Fundamentally, the person's return to social settings is undermined, and so a cycle of addiction emerges that exploits loneliness and despair, keeping the person further removed from access to resources that can assist them in recovery. Compounding these behavior changes are also broader study paradigms on addiction that emphasize the neurological and psychological dimensions of the disorder. As in more recent studies, the addiction also alters the brain chemistry and brain processes, and it alters the response to social stimuli and relationships. The alterations can disrupt the ability to derive pleasure from social interaction, as described by most as anhedonia. Thus, the withdrawal from social activity is not only a conscious action but can also be a result of biological reactions inherent to the addiction itself. The convergence of social withdrawal with these neurological processes introduces essential questions to the treatment strategy and the integration of social support into the therapeutic setting. By breaking down the intricate interaction of these behavioral changes, scientists and practitioners can better comprehend the resulting challenges in patients who have substance use and addiction disorders, allowing for increased intervention and recovery procedures (Baconi et al., 2015; Griffiths et al., 2015).

10.3.2. Physical Symptoms (e.g., Changes in Appearance, Physical Issues)

Substance abuse and addiction disorders produce an array of physical symptoms that have the power to significantly alter the appearance and overall health of a person. Perhaps one of the most outward expressions of substance use is poor personal hygiene and grooming. As the addiction continues to progress, the absence of self-care is more apparent, appearing in overt changes , such as weight gain or loss, dermatological conditions, and oral status. These individuals can experience complexion alterations, typically pale or disheveled, caused most often by neglect or the physiological effects of drugs consumed. The alterations are not superficial; they indicate deeper health conditions that may vary from deficiencies in nutrients to organ injury, therefore making the bigger picture of addiction and its effects on physical health complex. In addition, certain substances are linked with certain health complications that may occur as a result of extended use. For example, alcohol misuse may result in liver diseases, mental impairments, and cardiovascular complications. Likewise, drug abuse involving drugs , such as methamphetamine is connected with serious dental complications usually referred to as meth mouth, which involves high levels of tooth loss and gum disease. The effects even extend into social relationships and the capacity for maintaining relationships or employment. As explained in the study, the older individual with substance use stands at risk for certain health threats and can be confronted with barriers to treatment due to these increasing health issues. This group is likely to already be experiencing comorbid medical illnesses that complicate the impact of substance use, thereby increasing the risk of adverse health outcomes (Forrester et al., 2011). Sport and exercise have become critical components in addressing the health consequences of substance use disorders. Engagement in regular physical activity has been shown to reverse some of the adverse health effects of addiction, aiding mental and physical rehabilitation. Participation in exercise has the power to contribute to overall well-being and recovery, enabling individuals to regain lost health and appearance. Further, heightening awareness about the connection between physical activity and disease promotes intervention, preventive and rehabilitative treatment for substance abuse. Crucially, there has been a focus on , including physical health strategies in holistic therapeutic interventions to achieve maximum benefits (Sabo et al., 2004). By recognizing the crucial role of bodily symptoms in substance abuse and addiction history, professionals can better equip themselves to modify their practice to better meet the varied and complex needs of those afflicted with such.

10.3.3. Psychological Symptoms (e.g., Anxiety, Depression)

Substance use disorders and the concomitant psychological signs and symptoms are an intricate interplay of several influences that can have a very significant impact on one's mental health. Increasing evidence suggests that patients with addiction have higher levels of anxiety and depression. For instance, alcohol dependence has been linked with more severe addiction symptomatology, including greater psychological distress. This connection suggests not only that use of drugs is possibly an unhealthy adaptation for underlying psychopathology but that it can become a kind of cause for compounding those very disorders with the passing of time. The accompanying stressors of addiction create a vicious cycle wherein unresolved psychological symptoms spur continued drug use, creating a spiraling trap that is difficult to break. It is significant to understand this association while developing successful treatment plans addressing both the addiction and its psychological aspects, thereby facilitating more holistic patient management (McLachlan & Starkey, 2012). Apart from alcohol dependence, other patterns of addictive behavior—, such as gambling or shopaholism-type behavior—have also been subjected to examination regarding their psychological impact. Early studies suggest that there are important similarities among behavioral addictions in symptoms like dyscontrol, craving, and impulsivity, all of which are shared by anxiety and depression. This would suggest a wider spectrum of addiction disorders that do not necessarily include substance use but share underlying psychological traits. The implications for treatment are also significant since therapists may potentially be required to consider convergent symptoms across different types of addiction in formulating treatments. Elaborating on diagnostic definitions of addiction enables healthcare workers to improve management of the intricate nature of mental suffering among addicts (McLachlan & Starkey, 2012). The growth in Internet addiction in recent years has served to further highlight the psychological signs and symptoms of substance abuse and other addictive behaviors. With global Internet usage spreading wider, scientists have begun to document negative consequences of overuse of the internet, including anxiety and depressive symptoms typical of individuals with compulsive internet use. Epidemiological studies indicate that such individuals report high levels of distress and daily functioning impairment comparable to classic substance use disorders.

The lack of a standardized diagnosis of Internet addiction further complicates the issue, resulting in varied prevalence rates and measures employed across studies. Thus, the victims of internet addiction may not receive adequate treatment or understanding of their sickness, and hence there is a requirement for a well-structured system that deals with modern-day behavioral addictions and their mental influences (Figure 10.10).

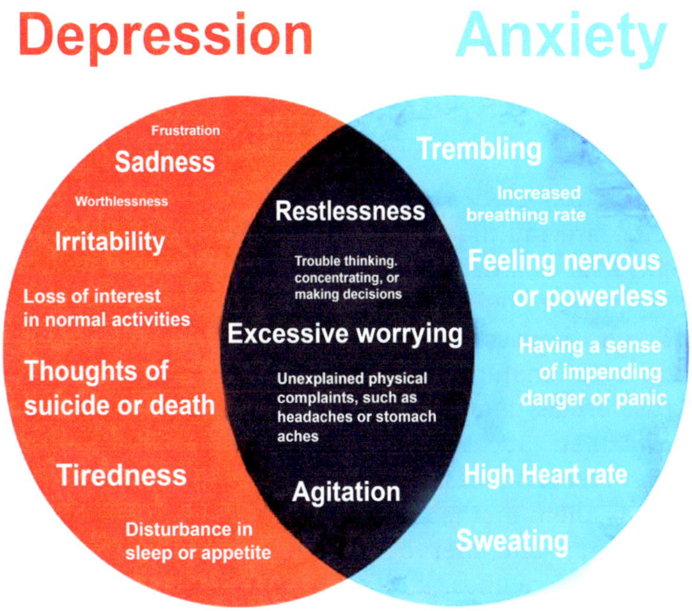

Figure 10.10. Psychological symptoms.

Source: https://mymsfamily.com/wp-content/uploads/2023/06/3-anxiety-depression-symptoms-overlap.png.

Test Your Knowledge

1. What behavioral, physical, and psychological signs indicate the presence of substance dependence or addiction?
2. How do tolerance, withdrawal, and loss of control play a role in identifying the severity of substance use disorders?

10.4. Impact on Individuals

Learning Outcome

1. Effects on physical health (e.g., organ damage, infectious diseases).
2. Effects on mental health (e.g., increased anxiety, depression).
3. Effects on personal relationships (e.g., family, friendships).

The impacts of drug addiction and abuse disorders on the individual are multifaceted, affecting not only the physical health of the person but also his or her psychological and social standing. The addictions that accompany drug abuse tend to ruin relationships with family and friends as trust erodes and social relationships become strained because of addiction. These individuals become increasingly isolated, using chemicals as their method of coping with their despondency, and thereby increasing the emotional pain of loneliness and despair. This vicious cycle can cause immense emotional pain, and in the extreme, a deep hopelessness. The consequences are not just individual; they ripple into families, affecting the emotional health of loved ones and straining social networks that support both the addict and the community around them. In addition, substance use disorders can have huge economic ramifications for individuals. The economic impact of addiction tends to be crushing, since the cost of maintaining a drug habit has been known to drive people into poverty, into debt, or into crimes like theft to continue using drugs. Another extreme consequence is job insecurity, where people end up losing employment and facing deteriorating professional prospects due to the stigmatization of addiction or due to the debilitating effects of drugs that impair them from efficiently operating in their working environments. Not only does this financial crisis adversely impact the individual's life, but it also leads to heightened reliance on social services, ushering in a spiraling cycle of maintaining the addiction-related issues. Implications to society are as far-reaching because the instability of the individual carries over into larger community settings, impacting resources, health care systems, and public safety. The imperative to respond to the role of substance use disorders is an appreciation of the complexity of needing full-treatment strategies that adapt to individuals' needs. Successful interventions must integrate mental health services because most persons addicted suffer from co-occurring mental illness, including depression or anxiety. The guidance of philanthropic funders highlights the importance of evidence-based treatment access, which holds immense promise in both preventing short-term harm and minimizing the long-term cost of drug use. Strategies aimed at saving lives, averting SUD illness, and improving overall care systems represent critical pathways to diminishing the harm imposed on individuals in this cycle. By focusing on fresh strategies that are focused on prevention and treatment of addiction, we can create healthier citizens who are less likely to fall victim to the catastrophic impacts of substance use disorders, hence contributing positively to society in general (Wallman-Stokes et al., 2015; Cannon et al., 2019).

10.4.1. Physical Health Consequences (e.g., Organ Damage, Infectious Disease)

Substance abuse and disorders of abuse usually lead to significant damage to the physical health, as it exists in the form of harm to various organs and vulnerability to infectious diseases. Body organs, for instance, the liver, the lungs, and the heart, can suffer irreparable damage due to the toxic effects of legal and illegal drugs. For instance, long-term alcohol consumption is well established to lead to liver disease, while the nicotine from tobacco can impair respiratory health, leading to COPD and increased susceptibility to respiratory infections. In addition, drugs compromise the immune system, making the drug user more susceptible to pathogens. These medical conditions of physical health can, however, exacerbate the cycle of addiction over time, as disease can push the patient towards drug consumption as a maladaptive coping strategy. It is important to understand these compounded consequences to develop an intervention that is specifically directed to reduce substance-related illness. Also, the combined action of drug consumption with infectious diseases can be best seen under the condition of a public health crisis, such as the COVID-19 pandemic. The convergence of addiction-induced damaged health and stress of a global health emergency can heighten risk among people with addiction disorders. It is indicated by studies that people with substance use behavior, such as khat chewing, are at higher risk in relation to the respiratory and cardiovascular systems and are thus more vulnerable to viruses like SARS-CoV-2. Individuals consuming khat, in addition to tobacco or alcohol, are at higher risk, as such compounds may worsen underlying disease and enhance the risk of severe COVID-19 (Abebe, 2022).

Such trends thus emphasize the need for health professionals to consider both patterns of addiction and general health while attending to patient demands during the time of a pandemic. Based on these limitations, it is essential that a multidimensional approach addressing both the physical health and addiction disorders is instituted (Abebe, 2022). Effective treatment not only needs to address the psychological dependency but must also offer intervention for the physiological consequences of substance use. This could include interdisciplinary collaboration among healthcare practitioners in the management of organ damage and the prevention of infectious complications involved. Strategies should involve screening for co-occurring health issues on substance users, as well as providing education on the potential health damage of substance use. Further, integrating preventative care and vaccines, particularly in the context of epidemic conditions, will be vital in safeguarding the health of vulnerable populations. By guaranteeing priority treatment for individuals with addiction disorders together, we can reduce the burden of the physical health consequences and enhance the well-being of these individuals (Clausen et al., 2023) (Figure 10.11).

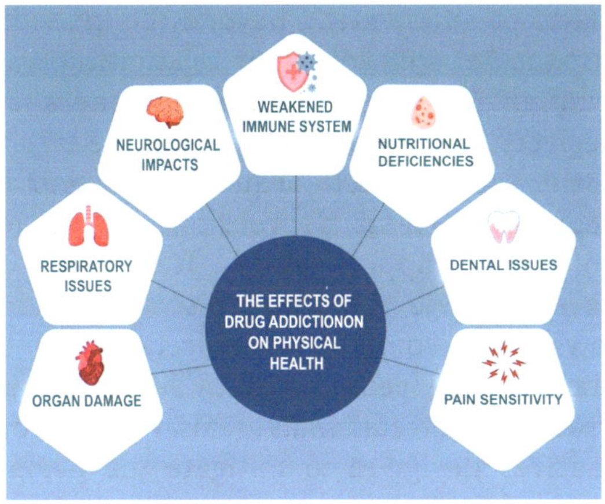

Figure 10.11. The impact of substance use and addiction disorders on physical health.

Source: https://valleyspringrecovery.com/wp-content/uploads/2024/05/the-effects-of-drug-addiction-on-physical-health-1536x1248.jpg.

10.4.2. Effects on Mental Health (e.g., Increased Anxiety, Depression)

The relationship between addiction and mental health is a complex and multidimensional issue, significantly influencing the course and severity of addiction disorders. It has been shown that SUD patients are commonly saddled with a high level of anxiety and depression that also amplifies the desire to use substances. For instance, alcohol-dependent patients demonstrate evidently heightened symptoms of depression and anxiety compared to their behavioral addiction counterparts. This similarity suggests that the disorders share a common psychological susceptibility since similar patterns of craving and impulsivity are found across various addictions, such as gambling and compulsive buying disorder, and expressed in initial evidence for expanding diagnostic criteria to encompass non-substance-use disorders (McLachlan & Starkey, 2012). The intertwining of these mental health disorders underscores the importance of combined treatment modalities that confront both addiction and related emotional distress. Additionally, the impacts of SUDs extend beyond the individual to frequently spill over into relationships and social environments. Family members and caregivers of addicted persons can be terribly emotionally impacted, acquiring co-occurring diseases , such as depression and anxiety among such support groups. It is significant to acknowledge the broader social factor; it allows for a complete interpretation of the addiction and a focus on healthy support groups surrounding affected individuals. Philanthropic initiatives designed to mitigate the harmful effects of SUDs not only enhance individual outcomes but can also assist in alleviating mass stress on communities and families. Through the provision of improved treatment, reduced stigma, and advocacy for institutional reform, funders can play a significant role in building a culture that encourages recovery and mental health for all stakeholders (Wallman-Stokes et al., 2015). Furthermore, prevention and intervention strategies have to be grounded on an understanding of the interplay of mental health and drug use. Continued research into psychosocial causes of addiction continues to play an essential role in designing prevention programs intended to reduce incidence rates of SUDs and establish mental health resilience. Building a successful treatment modality requires an understanding of the higher incidence of comorbid disorders. So, the treatment will not only work toward abstinence but also address the driving mental illnesses through the use of substances. And mounting evidence more and more points out that an integral approach in which mental health treatment is incorporated into the recovery models can significantly contribute to betterment in quality of life. By addressing both substance use and mental health problems at the same time, treatment specialists can achieve long-term recovery and instill well-being in patients who are coping with the double burden of addiction and psychological challenges (McLachlan & Starkey, 2012).

10.4.3. Effects on Personal Relationship (e.g., Family, Friendships)

The repercussions of drug abuse and addiction disorders on family relationships, particularly in domestic life, are immense and multifaceted. Families typically endure immense stress when one of their own is addicted, leading to a lack of communication and lost trust. The dynamics get altered with role reversal; a once responsible individual might turn irresponsible, driving away family members who feel compelled to become caretakers. This shift creates a tension-ridden atmosphere and emotional distance, wherein members of the family trade guilt with their loved one and anger with the situation. These stressors can even exaggerate pre-existing mental illness in the family, leading to an atmosphere filled with conflict and helplessness. Research identifies that such relationship tensions are capable of adding to more cases of dysfunctional families, which in turn may interfere with recovery processes and reenact drug use cycles (Garrido et al., 2019). Addiction affects not only the family but also friendships significantly due to drug consumption. Friends may initially rally around the defense of their addicted friend, minimizing the effects of the problem in the interest of loyalty. However, the situation may shift over time with declining trust. Friends would find themselves being more isolated, shouldering the impact of the behavior of the loved one, such as lying, volatility, or even financial exploitation. Thus, the beginnings of close friendships turn out to be shallow relationships with no depth and no support. This disintegration of friendships leads to betrayal and loneliness for the individual struggling with addiction as well as for the victims, highlighting how substance use destroys social networks and disables personal support systems (Cook et al., 2017). Calibrating the extent of substance abuse and its consequent effects demands social sensitivity to the forces underlying. The empirical literature emphasizes the importance of acknowledging the relational aspects of addiction in therapeutic practices, pointing out that effective treatment surpasses the limits of singular intervention. Methods involving the integration of the family matrix and restoring broken relationships can enhance healing to a considerable extent. By employing models based on a strengths-based continuum, clinicians can provide an atmosphere that allows for healing, ultimately leading to improved relationships between the patient and the family members. Combined models also empower families, giving them the tools necessary to support one another and minimizing the stigmatism associated with addiction. It is vital to establish this paradigm to achieve trust and resilience in relationships at risk of addiction disorder and substance misuse (Cook et al., 2017) (Figure 10.12).

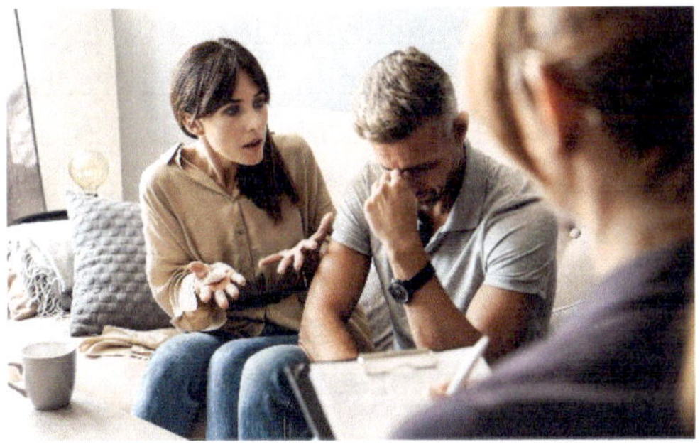

Figure 10.12. The impact of substance use and addiction disorders on personal relationships.

Source: https://www.peacevalleyrecovery.com/wp-content/uploads/2020/08/addiction-img1.jpg.

Test Your Knowledge

1. How do substance use disorders affect an individual's physical health, mental well-being, and cognitive functioning?
2. What challenges do individuals face in their personal relationships, employment, and daily responsibilities due to addiction?

10.5. Treatment Options

Learning Outcome

1. Behavioral therapies (e.g., cognitive-behavioral therapy, motivational interviewing).
2. Medication-assisted treatment (e.g., methadone, buprenorphine).
3. Support groups and community resources (e.g., AA, NA).

There should be an integrative treatment strategy to resolve substance use disorders (SUDs) with a focus on their complexity and community-level impact. Evidence-based treatments like behavior therapies and medication have been found to be successful in decreasing symptoms and guaranteeing recovery. Behavior therapies , such as Cognitive Behavioral Therapy (CBT) and Motivational Interviewing (MI) work toward altering maladaptive thinking patterns and building motivation toward change. These therapies are necessary to instill coping abilities and drug resistance in the patients. In addition, pharmacotherapy, in the form of drugs like buprenorphine and methadone for opioid addiction, can suppress cravings and withdrawal as well as overall improve the success of the treatment. This multi-modal therapy not only treats the individual's body dependency but also incorporates the psychological aspect, thus making the recovery process an even more robust one. The intersection between treatment delivery innovations and systemic reforms is paramount in improving the effectiveness of substance use treatments. Whole-of-treatment strategies should not only implement changes at the individual treatment level but also include modifications that increase access to care through policy transformation and activism. Increasing access to evidence-based treatment, according to Wallman-Stokes et al. (2015), is fundamental to successful management of SUD. In addition to that, communities must place emphasis on harm reduction strategies, which have been demonstrated to reduce the ill impacts of drug consumption.

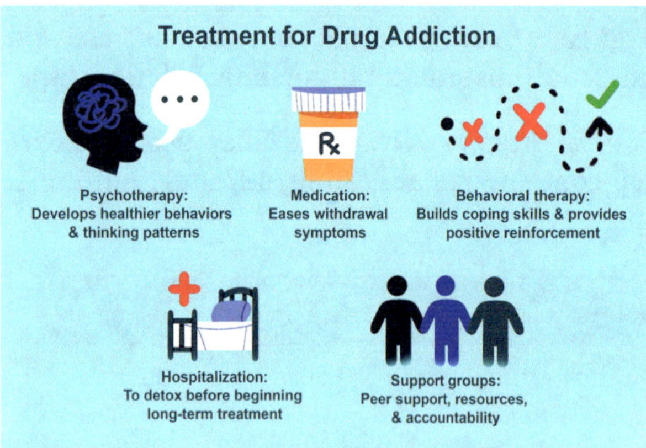

Figure 10.13. Treatment options for substance use and addiction disorders.

Source: https://www.verywellhealth.com/thmb/s-1nwHWIhWGGa41GOmxVUHVaDA4=/1500x0/filters:no_upscale():max_bytes(150000):strip_icc()/the-effects-of-drug-addiction-5214343-Final-63ee57687f0a4daa90b104897ad6579e.jpg.

By implementing policies that increase the provision of naloxone and overdose education, public health programs can hopefully salvage lives and minimize the general impact of addiction in society, marking the shift toward more holistic solutions. Finally, the future of SUD treatment lies in new methods that address both the individual and systemic barriers to care. Recommendations by experts, such as those provided in the study carried out by the Johns Hopkins Bloomberg School of Public Health, reflect the need for remodeled training in healthcare providers and appropriate prescribing practices (Alexander et al., 2015). With the support of philanthropic aid to build additional treatment opportunities, these proposals can lead to significant advancements in addiction treatment. With society grappling with the existing opioid epidemic, as well as other drug-related dilemmas, emphasis on individualized evidence-based treatment modalities, alongside community-based prevention, will have an integral role in supporting sustainable recovery and reducing the substance use disorder burden (Figure 10.13).

10.5.1. Behavioral Therapies (e.g., Cognitive-Behavioral Therapy, Motivational Interviewing)

Behavioral treatments, such as cognitive-behavioral therapy (CBT) and motivational interviewing (MI), play a critical role in the treatment of substance abuse and addiction disorders. Both treatments are focused on altering negative thought patterns and behaviors associated with substance abuse. CBT, in particular, enables an individual to identify and dispute irrational ideas regarding substance abuse, allowing them to develop healthier ways of coping. On the other hand, MI is aimed at enhancing a client's motivation to change. By using non-confrontational strategies, therapists make the client sensitive about their ambivalence towards quitting and thus promote intrinsic motivation. The practice of both of these strategies can lead to considerable positive alteration in treatment outcomes by enabling personal cues to be better understood, as well as creating mechanisms of effective handling of them within the context of their everyday lives. Evidence of the efficacy of motivational interviewing is convincingly established, especially in the treatment of alcohol and drug abuse. Its evidence base is especially significant as it confirms the necessity of using empirically supported treatments in treatment paradigms. As an example, one study proposed the need for proper training and supervision of therapists in order to implement MI effectively, showing the development of tools like the Motivational Interviewing Supervision and Training Scale (MISTS) to professionalize this training process (Madson et al., 2005).

By ensuring compliance with MI principles in therapists, the clients will be able to enjoy greater participation in the therapy process. These developments not only add to improved results in counseling but also point towards the necessity of continuous reviewing and refining therapeutic techniques in an attempt to best meet the intricate needs of addicted patients. Also, the addition of behavior therapies within correctional institutions has been fruitful in treating alcohol and drug use disorders among prisoners.

A significant portion of the prison population suffers from substance use disorders, which speaks to the critical intersection between addiction and criminality (Cline et al., 2018). The model suggests that the integration of models like Therapeutic Communities and CBT can give rise to an orderly platform for fostering sobriety about the psychological nature of addiction. These two-binned treatment approaches can provide adaptations to accommodate individual differences , such as the nature of the substance and demographic factors and contextual variables, thus enhancing overall functioning. Additionally, further research on implementing contextual adaptations from such approaches can demonstrate significant enhancement in rehabilitation outcomes in subjects within these systems, providing the key to a more effective strategy for treating substance abuse disorders in the criminal justice system.

10.5.2. Medication-Assisted Treatment (e.g., Methadone, Buprenorphine)

Medication-assisted treatment (MAT) is an emerging essential intervention for the treatment of addiction disorders and substance use, particularly opioid use disorder. MAT employs the use of pharmacologic agents, methadone and buprenorphine, alongside psychosocial treatment to enhance outcomes. Methadone is a long-acting opioid agonist that functions by suppressing withdrawal and decreasing craving, allowing for stabilization of the person's life as well as reduction in active illicit drug use. Buprenorphine, a partial agonist, offers similar benefits but reduced risk of abuse due to its ceiling effect. By safer withdrawal to recovery, MAT not only rebuilds the lives of individuals with addiction but can also have the potential to minimize the overall societally grounded costs of substance abuse, such as crime and health care. The effectiveness of MAT is exemplified across different settings with notable patient outcome improvements. For example, research confirms that patients on opioid agonist treatment (OAT) are more likely to exhibit higher heroin and other opioid abstinence rates than those in harm reduction treatment (HRT) strategies. This was illustrated in a comparison study where OAT patients had a higher percentage of urine tests that were negative for illegal drugs, showing the efficacy of methadone and buprenorphine maintenance treatment for promoting recovery and sustaining long-term abstinence (Bacciardi et al., 2016). In addition to its medical advantages, MAT can also enhance overall public health objectives through lower levels of overdose and greater overall stability within communities, particularly in those groups with strong exposure to opioid epidemics. Even with the established benefits, however, there are remaining challenges to accessing the MAT that continue to create difficulties towards broader acceptance and utilization of these treatments. Addiction stigma and regulatory constraints normally limit access to medications , such as methadone and buprenorphine. Moreover, the integration of MAT into existing health frameworks suggests a commitment to training healthcare providers in these modalities. Worth mentioning is the instance of high-risk groups, such as returning combatants with substance abuse disorders from mental illness, among which proposals for increased access to medication-assisted treatment (Wallman-Stokes et al., 2015) are included. Breaking through these barriers through policy reform and education can make MAT a central component of effective treatment approaches for substance use disorders, enhancing the potential for recovery for millions (Figure 10.14).

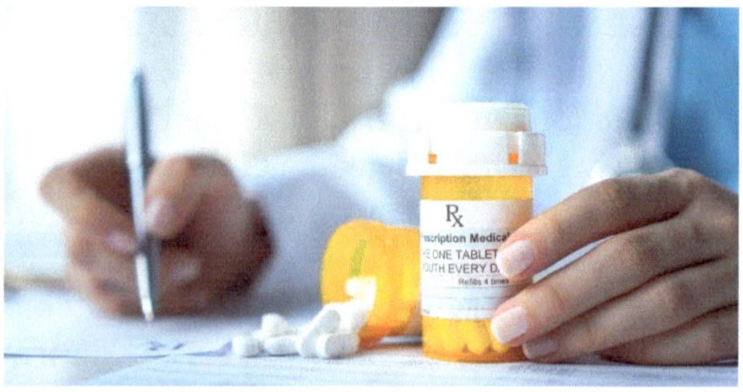

Figure 10.14. Medication-assisted treatment.

Source: https://www.bhgrecovery.com/hubfs/BHG-New-Medication-5.8.13.jpg.

10.5.3. Support Groups and Community Resources (e.g., AA, NA)

Support groups and communal resources play a strong role in the recovery situation among people who are fighting substance abuse and addiction disorders. Services , such as Alcoholics Anonymous (AA) and Narcotics Anonymous (NA) offer structured environments where members can share their experiences and struggles. These support groups are particularly important in an age where many afflicted with substance issues do not seek expert help due to stigma or lack of knowledge. This conclusion is aligned with a larger issue within healthcare environments, where clinicians themselves sometimes feel insufficient to treat addiction adequately. By creating a welcoming society, AA and NA also guarantee the existence of an open atmosphere that allows long-term engagement through consistent interaction, which is integral to long-term recovery. Addressing the particular requirements of individuals, such programs decrease feelings of isolation, thereby allowing collective work towards recovery from addiction, while supplementing the role of social bonds in recovery mechanisms (Meservey, 2017). Research shows that community-based resources like AA and NA significantly enhance an individual's possibility for maintaining sobriety. While these interventions do promote mutual support, they also constitute a philosophy that allows participants to exert control over recovery processes. Unlike the view that 12-Step interventions impose rigid structures that inhibit personal autonomy, research shows that members work actively to construct themselves as recovering people through these recovery structures. These results indicate that participants engage with the discourse offered by such support groups as active subjects and not passive ones. This interpretation, in addition to affirming their dedication to recovery, also chimed with professional values in healthcare, meaning that practitioners ought to rethink their understanding of 12-Step modalities (Duff-Gordon & Willig, 2020). The recognition that these models offer mechanisms for self-care erodes the stigma attached to traditional therapeutic approaches and opens a more nuanced discussion regarding the treatment of addiction. Further, integrating support groups and access to community resources into standard models of treatment has the great potential for optimizing general recovery outcomes for addiction. These organizations can enhance clinical interventions with sustained emotional support and practical coping skills. In addition, making referral pathways between healthcare providers and local recovery groups can close the gap between medical treatment and community-based recovery models. Both this cooperative process and empowering individuals to seek assistance also enable healthcare workers to resist the temptation to overlook viable community resources. Through building an integrated system of recovery, healthcare and community-based programs can synergistically work together to promote healthier social norms for addiction. Finally, the acceptance and promotion of such resources play a critical role in redefining the way society approaches substance use and addiction disorders, upholding the urgency for a holistic, integrated approach in recovery (Meservey, 2017).

Test Your Knowledge

1. How do detoxification, medication-assisted treatments (such as methadone, buprenorphine, or naltrexone), and therapy work together in managing addiction?
2. What roles do behavioral interventions—such as CBT, motivational interviewing, and relapse-prevention therapy—play in long-term recovery?

10.6. Prevention Strategies

Learning Outcome

1. Education and awareness programs.
2. Community-based interventions.
3. Policy and legislation changes.

Efficient prevention of addiction disorder and substance use is required to reduce the effect of the conditions on the health of people and society. The effort will require a multidimensional approach to saving lives and reducing the SUDs burden through various programs. An improvement of evidence-based treatment accessibility is one of the approaches, which could give people the power to break free from addiction by providing them with the necessary resources. Relieving the burden on healthcare systems involves not only curing the victims but also attempting to fix such system issues that hinder effective care. According to Wallman-Stokes et al (2015), it has been claimed that philanthropic donors can use their investment in funding programs that expand access and availability of such treatment methods, allowing communities to battle the rising SUD rates. Prevention also includes a necessary change in the general attitude towards addiction. Misinformation has a tendency to sustain stigma, lowering individuals' desire for help. Education campaigns that assist in reframing addiction as a disease, not a moral failing, are important. By evoking sympathy and pity in healthcare settings, an atmosphere of nonjudgment can be established that encourages individuals to access required care without fear of being judged. Increased knowledge of the drivers of substance abuse, including mental illness and social determinants, contributes to a more educated picture of addiction. As expressed in Wooton (2021), dismantling stigma regarding substances and developing humane care are at the center of developing effective prevention and treatment plans. Moreover, innovative programs that seek to reduce substance use must address education, community involvement, and policy reform. Intervention programs in youth can advance awareness of drug use hazards and the importance of healthy choice-making. Collaboration between schools, community organizations, and health professionals can facilitate increased outreach and establish healthy networks. A change in policy that targets the regulation of prescription patterns and access to drugs can further be a key prevention strategy. Building community opposition to addiction is an effort by many stakeholders working together to create and sustain effective prevention policies. Emphasized in Wallman-Stokes et al. (2015), investing in innovation and system reforms will address not only current challenges but also limit the future risk of substance use disorders (Figure 10.15).

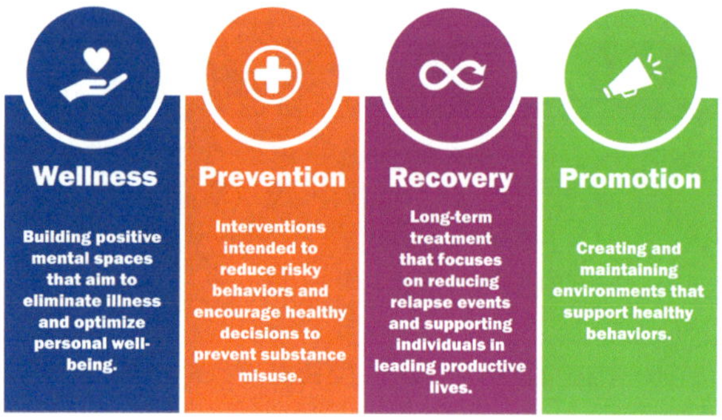
Wellness
Building positive mental spaces that aim to eliminate illness and optimize personal well-being.
Prevention
Interventions intended to reduce risky behaviors and encourage healthy decisions to prevent substance misuse.
Recovery
Long-term treatment that focuses on reducing relapse events and supporting individuals in leading productive lives.
Promotion
Creating and maintaining environments that support healthy behaviors.

Figure 10.15. Substance use disorder prevention.

Source: https://www.mmdhd.org/wp-content/uploads/2023/08/Website-Graphic-4-Prong.png.

10.6.1. Education and Awareness Programs

Educational and awareness programs are instrumental tools of prevention and treatment of substance use and addiction disorders. Through education provided to individuals about the hazards and implications of substance consumption, these programs can stop individuals from becoming addicts. Targeting only adolescents and young adults, such programs work towards dispelling myths surrounding drug use while promoting healthier lifestyles. Studies have shown that educated persons are better placed to seek assistance when faced with addiction pressure, thereby enhancing composite public health programs. The requirement is also likely to enhance understanding and involvement, with increased eventual provision of measures specifically tailored for most at-risk populations. With these menacing statistics of drug abuse, the use of education and awareness programs is not only good to implement but indeed a necessity in addressing such public health concerns. In addition to personal awareness, education programs should include healthcare workers and first responders to have a generalized response to addiction disorders. Medical students and professionals' education on proper prescribing habits, highlighted in recent reports, is crucial in averting the abuse of prescription drugs. The addition of overdose education and naloxone distribution programs can further empower first responders to effectively handle acute overdose situations, potentially leading to life preservation. The collaboration of the medical experts, patient advocates, and policy influencers plays a significant role in shaping the optimal practices applied in educational programs. By creating an educated healthcare environment, the stigma attached to substance use disorders can be decreased, opening the door for open discussions and compassionate treatment for victims. This strategy threads more robust support systems in the community, uniting against substance abuse. Apart from this, the effects of education and awareness campaigns can be magnified through collaborative efforts by philanthropic organizations, which can provide the resources necessary to implement innovative ideas. Through funding initiatives aimed at increasing access to evidence-based treatments and promoting public awareness campaigns, such organizations contribute toward a comprehensive system for addressing addiction. Focusing on long-term results, such as decreasing homelessness and improving health care access, is essential in taking away the lingering effects of substance use disorders from society as a whole. Education can empower communities to advocate for better policies and supportive systems aimed at good prevention and treatment strategies. It is thus a crucial step to integrate philanthropy into education and awareness campaigns to reduce the prevailing impact of substance use and encourage resilience in affected populations (Alexander et al., 2015; Wallman-Stokes et al., 2015).

10.6.2. Community-Based Interventions

Community-based programs are especially crucial when it comes to handling substance use and addiction disorders through the facilitation of local engagement and the provision of individualized support to impacted citizens. Such initiatives tend to depend on the idea that localized relationships and resources can facilitate better recovery results. By making use of local resources like local nonprofits, health organizations, and religious institutions, such initiatives are in a position to create recovery-conducive environments. For example, peer mentoring and support programs have been shown to reduce stigma and enhance relationships for individuals with addiction. There is evidence that not only do these kinds of community programs assist in getting individuals further along the recovery path, but that they help reduce the overall prevalence of substance use disorders in society, thereby addressing a significant public health problem (Wallman-Stokes et al., 2015). Furthermore, community-based programs also emphasize the need for comprehensive approaches that bring prevention, education, and treatment services together. Local programs have to be infused with evidence-based practices to realize their full potential and longevity. Efficacy is mostly found in programs focusing on reducing harms by distributing naloxone or syringe exchange programs, which provide immediate benefits , such as overdose death prevention and infectious disease transmission prevention. By addressing the complex issues of drug use, such interventions minimize the broader social and economic impacts of addiction, like homelessness and productivity loss. Long-term success requires sustained funding and creativity to facilitate these grassroots efforts and ensure that they remain responsive to the evolving needs of populations impacted (Wallman-Stokes et al., 2015). The involvement of community-based support networks and the application of neuroscience-informed approaches can render such interventions more effective. As research on the neurology of addiction continues to advance, scientific evidence must be transferred to community-based programs' practices. The merger of research and practice here can advance the understanding of the disease and enable tailor-made interventions. For instance, incorporating cognitive testing and neuromodulation interventions within community settings can create avenues for more specialized care. Not only does this incorporation address the individualized demands of those with addiction but also enhances community resilience and empowerment by allowing community-based intervention to positively address the issues of substance use and addiction disorders in the long term (Figure 10.16).

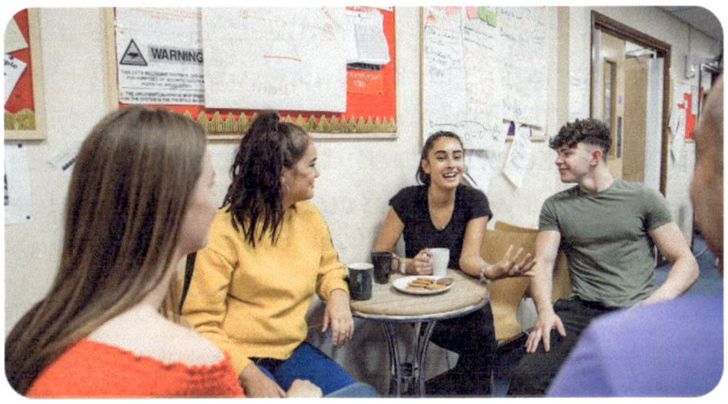

Figure 10.16. Community-based treatment for addiction.

Source: https://stairwayrecovery.com/wp-content/uploads/2022/02/community-4.png.

10.6.3. Policy and Legislation Changes

The landscape of substance use disorders and addiction has increasingly been shaped by broad policy and legislative measures aimed at addressing these pressing public health issues.

Drug use has varied between criminalization and public health approaches throughout history. The model that recognizes drug use is best responded to as an issue of health rather than crime has gained traction and led to the incorporation of harm reduction approaches. They seek to minimize the harmful health, social, and economic consequences of drug use without necessarily requiring abstinence. These shifts recognize a growing realization that structural factors—, such as access to medical care, economic opportunity, and social support—have significant roles in effective treatment and prevention of addiction. One of the most important demonstrations of policy reforms in the modern era is in the National Drug Policy 2015–2020 of New Zealand, which is a master response to substance use challenges. It stresses the necessity for a cross-agency response that integrates various social determinants , such as income, employment, housing, and education, into the response to the addiction problem. Through prioritizing collaboration among the local services, the communities, and the non-governmental organizations (NGOs), the policy will promote improved resource allocation and an assessment of the performance of interventions within the country. Through these concerted efforts, the policy will offer an agreed strategy for reducing the burden of substance use disorders and the well-being of those affected and the communities, and therefore prioritizing the application of equitable and sustainable solutions to curb addiction. The effect of stigma regarding addiction and substance use also significantly shapes public policy and legislative decisions. Stigma tends to contribute to service barriers, as people will fear judgment or discrimination if they try to seek help. Research demonstrates how stigma can enhance the opioid crisis, with research indicating that individuals are less likely to seek provided treatment due to fear about what other people think. Decreasing stigma, therefore, must be a priority of policy measures in order to enable interventions to be implemented and sustained. Public education and awareness campaigns are now being increasingly recognized by decision-makers as an essential component of integrated strategies for substance use. Through fostering a more educated and empathetic social perspective on addiction, policies are better enabled to support recovery and reduce the overall impact of substance use disorders on societies (Wallman-Stokes et al., 2015).

Test Your Knowledge

1. How can education, early intervention, and community programs reduce the risk of substance use disorders in vulnerable populations?
2. What role do policy measures, family support, and healthy coping skills play in preventing substance misuse and relapse?

SUMMARY

It is apparent that the relationship between these disorders and co-occurring mental disorders, namely major depression, is a multidimensional and intricate challenge in healthcare. The widespread prevalence of these comorbidities highlights the importance of integrated treatment to address simultaneously both substance abuse and mental illness. Specifically, study findings report a pooled prevalence of 3.2% among those with the concomitant conditions of substance use disorders and major depression, marking a serious public health concern that needs to be addressed with urgency. Effective management of the concurrent issues is crucial because it not only dampens individual distress but also averts broader societal consequences like increased disability and suicidal thoughts (Onaemo, 2019). Consequently, both clinicians and policy makers require a holistic understanding of these interlinked disorders. Of no less importance is the study of social processes that maintain substance use and addiction disorders. Noteworthy of mention has been the contribution of toxic relationships, particularly those in environments , such as night clubs, as a contributing factor towards the maintenance of substance use among those affected. Research illustrates how drug abuse is fostered by bad social relationships, thus complicating the process of recovery. Conversely, fostering good relationships as promoted under mental health programs has been shown to induce emotional resilience and aid in recovery (Iglesias et al., 2021). Therefore, treatment programs must target not only the drug abuse of the individual but also strive to enhance the quality of their social connections to ensure a multi-faceted rehabilitation process that can facilitate extended recovery. Finally, the finding achieved through this research emphasizes the necessity of adopting evidence-based integrated treatment models that target both substance use disorders and mental illnesses at the same time. Standard treatment models that isolate psychiatric or addictive etiologies are insufficient; instead, a paradigm shift to relational and community supportive models is needed. Collaborative models incorporating mental health treatment and substance use disorder treatment will more effectively prevent stigma and enhance patient outcomes. The findings of numerous studies highlight the reality that constructing supportive environments and healthy peer relationships significantly enhance the efficacy of treatment and overall recovery (Iglesias et al., 2021). With mental illness and addiction increasingly entangling, collaborative efforts among healthcare providers, patients, and community programs will be critical to preventing the impact of these disorders on people and society.

We need to understand the multifaceted nature of addiction and substance use disorders, which affect millions, to address the epidemic. The disorders are wide-ranging in substances , such as alcohol, opioids, and stimulants, each with its own set of problems and requiring tailored interventions. Substance use is not merely an individual issue but extends to family life as well as societal levels. It has been shown through research that approximately 20 million Americans, both youths and adults, are suffering from these issues, and with proper treatment and interventions, there is a dire need for it. While we explore the systems-related issues of drug abuse, note should be taken of the interrelationship between addiction, mental illness disorders, and socioeconomic status that greatly influences treatment access and outcome. Successful intervention of substance use and addiction involves a mix of short-term harm reduction and long-term prevention. Charitable donors fuel these initiatives through funding that is aimed at saving lives and reducing related diseases. Among the steps that are suggested to be implemented are enhancing access to evidence-based treatment, which has proven to successfully treat substance use disorder. Furthermore, an improvement of overall care for SUD-affected individuals requires systemic change, so that health policy and community support systems are in line accordingly. In addition to addressing the direct effects of addiction, this is instrumental to the environment in which recovery and resilience become possible within those afflicted by SUDs (Wallman-Stokes et al., 2015). Innovation is part of creating treatment methods, making research on substance use disorders of high importance. By funding new practices and programs, stakeholders are able to identify innovative forms of prevention and intervention, leading to a healthier population. Introducing evidence-based studies into care systems can also enhance the effectiveness of SUD treatment, making it possible for affected persons and families to navigate their recovery process. As communities organize to address substance use disorders, estimating the costs and benefits to society from a variety of interventions becomes of paramount concern. The multifaceted treatment not only reduces the burden on healthcare systems but also diminishes the emotional, financial, and social load these disorders have on individuals and families (Martinovic et al., 2014).

KEY TERMS FROM THIS CHAPTER

- 12-step program
- Abstinence
- Addiction
- Alcohol use disorder
- Cannabis use disorder
- Craving
- Dependence
- Detoxification
- Drug craving
- Dual diagnosis
- Harm reduction
- Medication-assisted treatment (MAT)
- Motivational interviewing
- Opioid use disorder
- Relapse
- Stimulant use disorder
- Substance use disorder
- Tolerance
- Triggers
- Withdrawal

CRITICAL THINKING QUESTIONS

1. **Which of the following best defines substance use disorder (SUD)?**
   a. Occasional recreational use of drugs
   b. Use of prescription medication as directed
   c. A pattern of use causing significant impairment or distress
   d. Use of caffeine and nicotine
2. **Which neurotransmitter is most commonly associated with the brain's reward system in addiction?**
   a. Serotonin
   b. Acetylcholine
   c. Dopamine
   d. GABA
3. **Tolerance refers to:**
   a. The body's allergic response to a drug
   b. Needing increased amounts of a substance to achieve the same effect
   c. The ability to stop using a drug at any time
   d. Experiencing no withdrawal symptoms
4. **Which of the following is a common symptom of opioid withdrawal?**
   a. Hallucinations
   b. Constipation
   c. Muscle aches and sweating
   d. Euphoria
5. **Which of the following treatments is a medication used in opioid addiction?**
   a. Sertraline
   b. Methadone
   c. Lorazepam
   d. Haloperidol

Short Answer Questions

1. What is the difference between substance use and substance use disorder?
2. Name three commonly abused substances included in DSM-5 classifications.
3. What are the four key criteria used to diagnose substance use disorders according to DSM-5?
4. What is tolerance, and how does it relate to substance dependence?
5. Define withdrawal and list two common withdrawal symptoms for alcohol.

Answer to Critical Thinking Questions

1. (c); 2. (c); 3. (b); 4. (c); 5. (b)

REFERENCES

1. Abebe, W. (2022). Use of khat and associated substances during COVID-19 pandemic: Potential adverse consequences. https://core.ac.uk/download/524768717.pdf (accessed on 28th July 2025).

2. Acquas, E., Akiskal, H., Archie, S., Bacopoulos, N., Blum, K., Bowirrat, A., et al. (2018). Patterns of management of patients with dual disorder (psychosis) in Italy: A survey of psychiatrists and other physicians focusing on clinical practice. https://core.ac.uk/download/287581518.pdf (accessed on 28th July 2025).

3. Aguiniga, D., Pratt, J., Shelby, K., Cox, M., & Thompson, M. (2015). Over the edge: What should we do when alcohol and drug use become a problem to society? https://core.ac.uk/download/75781210.pdf (accessed on 28th July 2025).

4. Alexander GC, Frattaroli S, Gielen AC, eds. The Opioid Epidemic: From Evidence to Impact. Johns Hopkins Bloomberg School of Public Health, Baltimore, Maryland: 2017.(accessed on 28th July 2025).

5. American Academy of Pediatrics Council on Foster Care, Adoption, and Kinship Care, D Waite, MV Greiner, Z Laris. (2018) "Putting Families First: How the Opioid Epidemic is Affecting Children and Families, and the Child Welfare Policy Options to Address It," Journal of Applied Research on Children: Informing Policy for Children at Risk: Vol. 9: Iss. 1, Article 4. DOI: https://doi.org/10.58464/2155-5834.1353(accessed on 28th July 2025).

6. Amr, M. A., Arockiasamy, A. P. R., & Sonbol, H. M. (2023). Relapse in substance use disorder and its relation to stigma: An outpatient based cross-sectional study. https://core.ac.uk/download/621451605.pdf (accessed on 28th July 2025).

7. Bacciardi, S., Bizzarri, J. V., Casetti, V., Conca, A., et al. (2016). The newer opioid agonist treatment with lower substitutive opiate doses is associated with better toxicology outcome than the older harm reduction treatment. https://core.ac.uk/download/127588245.pdf (accessed on 28th July 2025).

8. Backmund, M., Eichenlaub, D., Meyer, K., Schütz, C., et al. (2003). Alcohol consumption in heroin users, methadone-substituted and codeine-substituted patients: Frequency and correlates of use. https://core.ac.uk/download/16432718.pdf (accessed on 28th July 2025).

9. Baconi, Daniela Luiza; Ciobanu, Anne-Marie; Vlăsceanu, Ana Maria; Cobani, Oana Denisa; Negrei, Carolina; and Bălălău, Cristian (2015) "Current Concepts on Drug Abuse and Dependence," Journal of Mind and Medical Sciences: Vol. 2: Iss. 1, Article 4. DOI: https://doi.org/10.22543/2392-7674.1008(accessed on 28th July 2025).

10. Baldacchino, A., Bartu, A., Di Castelnuovo, A., Nyhlén, A., Oyefeso, A., Ghodse, A. H., Bargagli, A. M., et al. (2011). Substance abuse and psychiatric co-morbidity as predictors of premature mortality in Swedish drug abusers: A prospective longitudinal study 1970–2006. https://core.ac.uk/download/pdf/8610958.pdf (accessed on 28th July 2025).

11. Banich, M. T., Barch, D. M., Bjork, J. M., Heath, A. C., et al. (2018). The utility of twins in developmental cognitive neuroscience research: How twins strengthen the ABCD research design. https://core.ac.uk/download/212865813.pdf (accessed on 28th July 2025).

12. Barlow, D. H., Fitzmaurice, G. M., Greenfield, S. F., McHugh, R. K., et al. (2017). Development of an integrated cognitive behavioral therapy for anxiety and opioid use disorder: Study

protocol and methods. https://open.bu.edu/bitstream/2144/39158/3/nihms892592.pdf (accessed on 28th July 2025).

13. Madson, M. B., Campbell, T. C., Barrett, D. E., Brondino, M. J., & Melchert, T. P. (2005). Development of the Motivational Interviewing Supervision and Training Scale. *Psychology of addictive behaviors : journal of the Society of Psychologists in Addictive Behaviors*, *19*(3), 303–310. https://doi.org/10.1037/0893-164X.19.3.303 (accessed on 28th July 2025).
14. Barnett, M. L., Beletsky, L., Keyes, K. M., Kiang, M. V., et al. (2019). Stigma as a fundamental hindrance to the United States opioid overdose crisis response. https://core.ac.uk/download/323065349.pdf (accessed on 28th July 2025).
15. Billieux, J., Griffiths, M. D., Karila, L., Kuss, D. J., et al. (2014). Internet addiction: A systematic review of epidemiological research for the last decade. https://core.ac.uk/download/30640239.pdf (accessed on 28th July 2025).
16. Cadoni, C., Corkery, J., De Luca, M. A., Di Chiara, G., et al. (2017). Cannabis: Epidemiological, neurobiological and psychopathological issues: An update. https://core.ac.uk/download/287580833.pdf (accessed on 28th July 2025).
17. Cannon, Y. (2019). The kids are not alright: Leveraging existing health law to attack the opioid crisis upstream. https://core.ac.uk/download/225012727.pdf (accessed on 28th July 2025).
18. Castaño Garrido, C., & Valencia Ortiz, R. (2019). Uso y abuso de las redes sociales por parte de los adolescentes: Un estudio en México. https://core.ac.uk/download/288002409.pdf (accessed on 28th July 2025).
19. Chiappini, S., Corkery, J. M., De Berardis, D., Orsolini, L., et al. (2019). The bridge between classical and 'synthetic'/chemical psychoses: Towards a clinical, psychopathological and therapeutic perspective. https://core.ac.uk/download/287582435.pdf (accessed on 28th July 2025).
20. Martinovic, J., Jones, A., Christiansen, P., Rose, A. K., Hogarth, L., & Field, M. (2014). Electrophysiological responses to alcohol cues are not associated with Pavlovian-to-instrumental transfer in social drinkers. *PloS one*, *9*(4), e94605. https://doi.org/10.1371/journal.pone.0094605(accessed on 28th July 2025).
21. Clausen, T., Eide, D., Gabrhelík, R., Odsbu, I., et al. (2023). Gender differences in physical morbidity in opioid agonist treatment patients: Population-based cohort studies from the Czech Republic and Norway. https://core.ac.uk/download/653697439.pdf (accessed on 28th July 2025).
22. Cline, E. (2018). Substance abuse treatment in prison settings: A systematic review. https://core.ac.uk/download/212145875.pdf (accessed on 28th July 2025).
23. Cook, J., & Miller, A. (2017). The adolescent substance uses risk continuum: A cultural, strengths-based approach to case conceptualization. https://core.ac.uk/download/213072254.pdf (accessed on 28th July 2025).
24. Meulewaeter, F., De Pauw, S. S. W., & Vanderplasschen, W. (2019). Mothering, Substance Use Disorders and Intergenerational Trauma Transmission: An Attachment-Based Perspective. *Frontiers in psychiatry*, *10*, 728. https://doi.org/10.3389/fpsyt.2019.00728(accessed on 28th July 2025).
25. Duff Gordon, C., & Willig, C. (2021). Surrender to win: Constructions of 12-step recovery from

alcoholism and drug addiction. *Health (London, England : 1997)*, *25*(6), 651–668. https://doi.org/10.1177/1363459320912837(accessed on 28th July 2025).

26. Forrester, D., Galvani, S., Lapworth, K., Sullivan, S., et al. (2011). Working with older drinkers. https://core.ac.uk/download/30322076.pdf (accessed on 28th July 2025).
27. Griffiths, M. D., Kuss, D. J., & Pontes, H. M. (2015). Clinical psychology of internet addiction: A review of its conceptualization, prevalence, neuronal processes, and implications for treatment. https://core.ac.uk/download/30633161.pdf (accessed on 28th July 2025).
28. Hasanović, M., Hasanović, M., Jakovljević, M., Kuldija, B., et al. (2021). Gambling disorder as an addictive disorder and creative psychopharmacotherapy. https://core.ac.uk/download/512507761.pdf (accessed on 28th July 2025).
29. Khandhedia, S., Raval, C. M., & Thakor, N. (2017). Profile of substance abusers attending at de-addiction center of GMERS medical college, Dharpur-Patan, Gujarat, India: A cross-sectional study. https://core.ac.uk/download/544390948.pdf (accessed on 28th July 2025).
30. McLachlan, A. D., & Starkey, N. J. (2012). The classification of substance and behavioural addictions: A preliminary investigation. New Zealand Journal of Psychology, 41(1), 7–18.h(accessed on 28th July 2025).
31. Meservey, A. J. (2017). Addiction recovery support: Connecting primary care providers and community resources. https://core.ac.uk/download/84397660.pdf (accessed on 28th July 2025).
32. Ministry of Health (New Zealand). (2025). National drug policy 2015 to 2020. https://core.ac.uk/download/pdf/30671025.pdf (accessed on 28th July 2025).
33. Morales Iglesias, M., Piñero León, J. A., Racionero, S., Ugalde, L., et al. (2021). Toxic nightlife relationships, substance abuse, and mental health: Is there a link? A qualitative case study of two patients. https://core.ac.uk/download/419530741.pdf (accessed on 28th July 2025).
34. Morse, S. J. (2006). Addiction, genetics, and criminal responsibility. https://core.ac.uk/download/62553458.pdf (accessed on 28th July 2025).
35. Onaemo, V. N. (2019). Epidemiology of co-morbid substance use disorders and major depression. https://core.ac.uk/download/226151512.pdf (accessed on 28th July 2025).
36. Sabo, D., Miller, K. E., Heywood, L., & Melnick, M. J. (2004). Her life depends on it: Sport, physical activity and the health and well-being of American girls. https://core.ac.uk/download/71340387.pdf (accessed on 28th July 2025).
37. Schuckit, M. A. (2014). A brief history of research on the genetics of alcohol and other drug use disorders. https://core.ac.uk/download/323082635.pdf (accessed on 28th July 2025).
38. Simonelli, A., Parolin, M., Mapelli, D., Cristofalo, P., Cimino, S., & Cerniglia, L. (2017). Cognitive functioning, clinical profile and life events in young adults addicted to drugs. Does being a girl make a difference? Clinical Neuropsychiatry: Journal of Treatment Evaluation, 14(3), 226–238.(accessed on 28th July 2025).
39. Wallman-Stokes, C., Bechtolsheimer, G., Appel, J., Gable, J., Chiu, J., Rosqueta, K., & Hobble, R. (2015). Lifting the burden of addiction: Philanthropic opportunities to address substance use disorders in the United States. https://live-penn-impact.pantheon.io/wp-content/uploads/2016/2015/11/Lifting-the-Burden-of-Addiction.pdf. https://core.ac.uk/download/75783859.pdf (accessed on 28th July 2025).

CHILD AND ADOLESCENT PSYCHIATRY

11

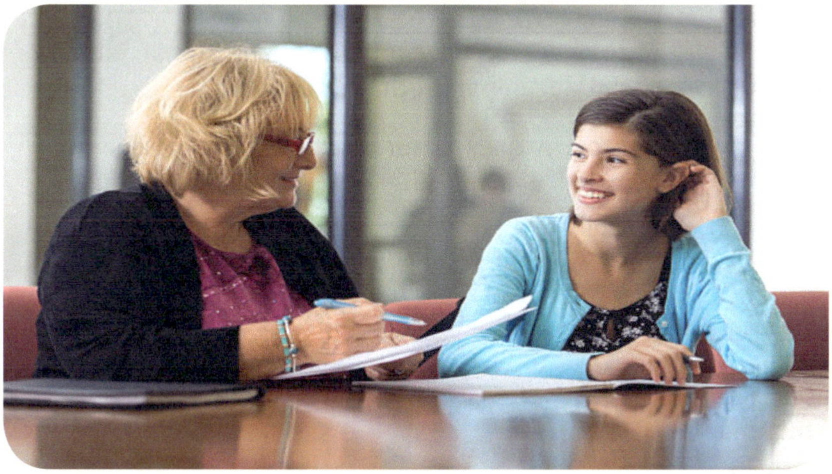

LEARNING OBJECTIVES

After studying this chapter, you will be able to:

1. List the common mental health disorders;
2. Discuss about assessment and diagnosis;
3. Explore the treatment approaches;
4. Describe the impact of social and environmental factors.

Introduction

Child and adolescent psychiatry is a clinical subspecialty that deals with the diagnosis, treatment, and prevention of mental health illnesses in children and adolescents. Children and adolescents' mental health conditions may be unique when compared with adults and are therefore recognized as requiring varied methods of assessment and intervention. Given the huge influence developmental stages exert on psychological well-being, practitioners must consider family relationships, social environments, and biology when working with issues of mental health. Recent epidemiological studies indicate the incredibly high rise in the prevalence of mental disorders in young people and demonstrate that there is a clear need for effective strategies and interventions. Whilst society is increasingly recognizing the indispensable role of mental health, child and adolescent psychiatry is at the forefront of cutting-edge practice that seeks to promote resilience, support healthy development, and help young people thrive in a rapidly changing world (Figure 11.1).

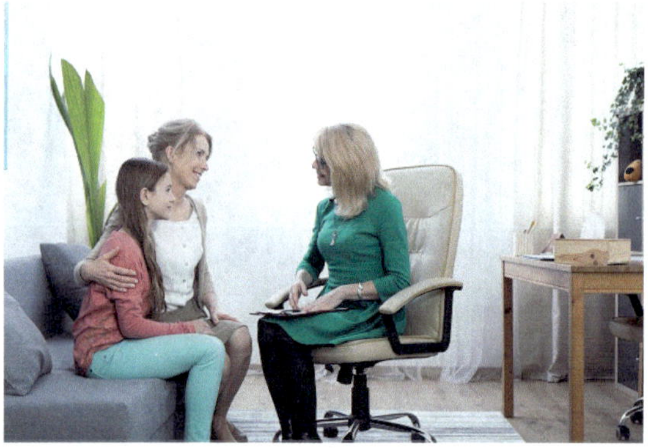

Figure 11.1. Child and adolescent psychiatry.

Source: https://harbormentalhealth.com/wp-content/uploads/2020/04/Child-and-Adolescent-Psychiatry.jpg.

Definition of Child and Adolescent Psychiatry

Child and adolescent psychiatry is a medical subspecialty concerned with the diagnosis, treatment, and prevention of mental illnesses in children ages 0 to 18 years. It recognizes that the psychological, emotional, and social development of children and adolescents is multifaceted and influenced by varied environmental and biological determinants. In particular, recent issues , such as the rapid uptake of digital technology by young people have come to the forefront as major determinants, with evidence indicating the potential risks that users are exposed to, from cyberbullying and exposure to offensive content (Livingstone & Smith, 2014). Besides, conditions like Attention Deficit Hyperactivity Disorder (ADHD) also reflect the complexity of psychiatric evaluation in which environmental, genetic, and psychosocial factors become interwoven to shape clinical understanding and treatment planning (Robaey & Schachar, 2007). Child and adolescent psychiatry thus not only directs attention towards symptom alleviation but involves an integrated strategy for providing developmental milestones and optimizing long-term functioning (Figure 11.2).

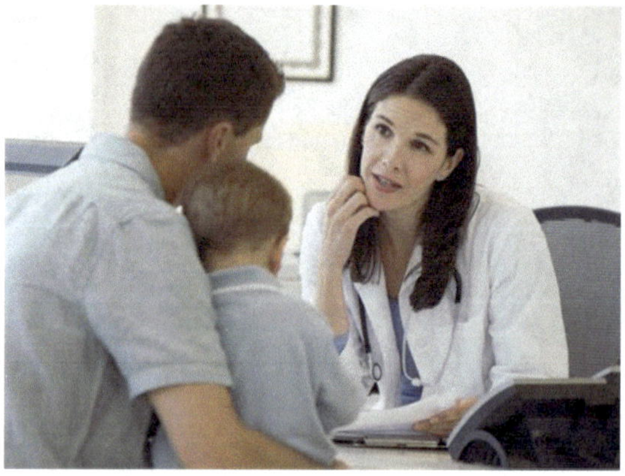

Figure 11.2. Psychological, emotional, and social development during childhood.

Source: https://external-content.duckduckgo.com/iu/?u=https%3A%2F%2Ftse3.mm.bing.net%2Fth%3Fid%3DOIP.2DFnnzI2cyO4_GKEBBNVDQHaFd%26pid%3DApi&f=1&ipt=09a44bbf800cb150f9171b405284e285d9492c953582c7a031ebe9445340040a&ipo=images.

Importance of Mental Health in Children and Adolescents

The mental health of children and adolescents is an integral component of their overall development and wellbeing and influences both their social performance and academic attainment. Research indicates that socioeconomic status, victimization or bullying, and social support are significant predictors of mental health for this group. For instance, a Norwegian study of 15,823 teens identified that poor family economy and low parental support were strong predictors of depressive symptoms and violent self-injury, validating the need for protective intervention in high-risk populations (Livingstone & Smith, 2014). Despite an increased demand for child and adolescent psychiatric care, the status quo is a disturbing lack of specialists in the field, particularly within underprivileged populations (Kim et al., 2003). This is an indication of the need to create mental health awareness and accessibility since early interventions can reduce enduring negative impacts, ensuring healthier life pathways for youth. It is crucial to tackle these obstacles to instill strong future generations.

Historical Context of the Field

The social history of child and adolescent psychiatry is intricate and one that has been shaped by societal attitudes towards mental illness and child rights. Children with psychiatric issues were first approached in a punitive framework akin to adult diagnostic frameworks that did not take into account developmental issues. This paradigm shifted fundamentally in the latter 20th century as researchers and practitioners began to advocate for more empathic and age-aware approaches to youth mental health. Pioneering developmental psychology research indicated the benefits of early intervention, along with the particular psychosocial influences on young individuals, thereby setting the stage for specialized practice that continues to evolve today. Besides, contemporary thinking focuses on the fusion of cultural contexts and the addition of coping with systemic injustices in mental health systems, as reflected in the reclaiming of psychiatric identities (Huxley et al., 2018). These changes throughout history underscore the evolution of the field in addressing children and adolescents' diverse needs (University of Nevada et al., 2013).

Overview of Common Psychiatric Disorders Among Teenagers

Familiarity with the kinds of mental health disorders that affect children is crucial for the best intervention and treatment. They are anxiety, depression, and neurodevelopmental disorders , such as ADHD. Evidence from research shows that neurotic, stress-related, and somatoform disorders are among the most prevalent diagnoses in child and adolescent inpatient environments, according to a study conducted in Pakistan. Consequently, United Arab Emirates studies focus on the impact of family and social stressors on mental illness and further point out that depression is more prevalent in women and often goes hand in hand with suicidal thoughts and self-injurious behaviors. This highlights the significance of early identification and tailored treatment of such disorders to minimize their long-term effects. In conclusion, a thorough understanding of these conditions lays a foundation for the development of effective child and adolescent psychiatric services, thus enhancing the overall mental health of adolescents (Figure 11.3).

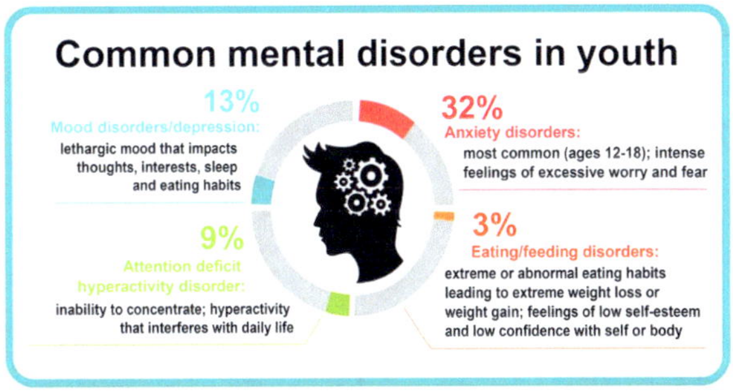

Figure 11.3. Common mental health disorders in youth.

Source: https://www.ndsu.edu/agriculture/sites/default/files/styles/large_non_crop/public/2024-08/common_mental_disorders.jpg.webp?itok=gvFmqR-3.

Role of Psychiatrists in Child and Adolescent Mental Health

Psychiatric contribution to mental health among children and adolescents is multifaceted and utterly important, particularly in addressing hard-to-treat conditions , such as attention deficit hyperactivity disorder (ADHD) and the psychological consequences of large-scale trauma. Evidence demonstrates that child psychiatrists lead interdisciplinary diagnostic groups when dealing with ADHD, as well as in the management of its treatment, as 82% of child psychiatrists prescribe pharmacological interventions compared to only 22% of pediatricians, demonstrating their central role here (Gavin et al., 2017). Moreover, the identification of children's special mental health needs is increasingly acknowledged across the world. It is crucial to recognize that unmet mental health issues can impact not only the individual child but also social stability and economic viability, thus emphasizing prioritizing mental health services in developing nations (Belfer, 2005). Psychiatrists, therefore, do not merely provide clinical treatment but also advocate for system changes to aid the well-being of vulnerable teenagers, thus achieving healthier trajectories of development (Figure 11.4).

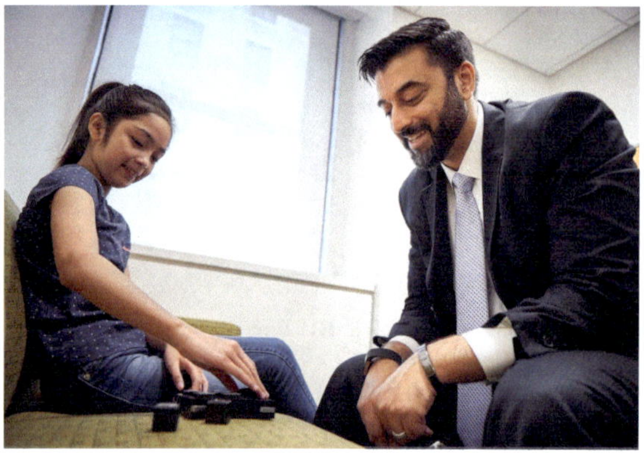

Figure 11.4. Role of psychiatrists in child and adolescent mental health.

Source: https://med.nyu.edu/departments-institutes/child-adolescent-psychiatry/sites/default/files/child-adolescent-psych-about-us-child-study-center-inline.jpg.

Significance of Early Intervention

Early intervention is particularly critical in child and adolescent psychiatry since it can significantly alter developmental patterns and minimize long-term psychological complications. Research has determined that the early treatment of conduct problems can be successful in preventing these problems from becoming a full-blown adolescent delinquency or adult antisociality. For example, Parent-Child Interaction Therapy (PCIT) has also been found to reduce disruptive behavior in children aged three and four years, with studies demonstrating large effect sizes for the reduction of conduct problems following treatment (Abrahamse et al., 2012). Also, findings from Clinical High-Risk for Psychosis (CHR-P) research report the possible benefits of early detection and treatment, with screening and tailored responses capable of fostering resilience and social adaptability in high-risk youths (Raballo et al., 2021). Consequently, the use of focused intervention strategies not only augments cognitive and emotional growth but also presents an arena for improved adult mental health outcomes, accentuating the need for early psychiatric intervention.

Challenges in the Field

The field of child and adolescent psychiatry is faced with an array of challenges that hinder the provision of effective mental health services. Among these is the lack of trained practitioners, particularly in low-resource settings, in which child and adolescent mental health care needs are largely not met (Negash et al., 2015). Such environments are where programs like the Collaborative International Exchange Programme between Ludwig-Maximilian University and Jimma

University aim to enhance capacity by promoting non-physician health workers in specialist mental health care. Practitioners, however, often encounter hard cases with both medical and psychiatric problems, thus making it more challenging to diagnose and treat (Negash et al., 2015). In addition, mental illness is stigmatized, preventing families from accessing services, which compounds the emotional distress of youth. Addressing such issues requires a multi-modal approach in terms of increasing training opportunities, increasing public awareness, and encouraging collaboration between health professionals to create resilient mental health interventions.

11.1. Common Mental Health Disorders

Learning Outcome

1. Attention-deficit/hyperactivity disorder (ADHD)
2. Anxiety disorders
3. Depression in children and adolescents
4. Autism spectrum disorders
5. Conduct disorder
6. Eating disorders
7. Bipolar disorder
8. Post-traumatic stress disorder (PTSD)
9. Substance use disorders

General mental health diseases in children and adolescents are of great concern and affect an estimated 9 to 21% of this population globally, according to recent studies (Özbek et al., 2010). Such diseases, such as depression, anxiety, and attention-deficit/hyperactivity disorder (ADHD), can have severe impacts not just on the persons but on families and educational systems as well. Problems in the identification and diagnosis of the disorders are largely methodological in the presence of epidemiological study flaws, including sampling bias and problems of case ascertainment, which make it difficult to formulate effective mental health policies (Özbek et al., 2010). Furthermore, the management of the disorders requires a paradigm shift toward alternative, project-based clinical practice beyond traditional classification of childhood and adolescent psychiatric disorders. This type of strategy builds cooperation among mental health agencies and encourages integrated care that is appropriate to each child's individual needs, which results in better outcomes in this at-risk population.

11.1.1. Attention-Deficit/ Hyperactivity Disorder (ADHD)

The complexity of Attention-Deficit/ Hyperactivity Disorder (ADHD) constitutes severe difficulties in the practice of child and adolescent psychiatry, necessitating a multidimensional approach to understanding and treatment. ADHD is one of the most prevalent neuropsychiatric conditions in children, with studies indicating that its effects can extend as far as into adulthood, affecting numerous aspects of life like education and interpersonal relationships (Tufan et al., 2011). Central to effective management is the understanding of the disorder's heritability, as genetic factors have an integral role in its presence and persistence. Recent studies have highlighted the significance of investigating the genetic underpinnings of ADHD, although the identification of specific genes is yet not feasible due to the disorder's heterogeneity (Tufan et al., 2011). Furthermore, the application of stimulant medication, of proven effectiveness in all age groups and both sexes, presents a compelling therapeutic choice, regardless of individual differences, putting more precise evaluation of their effectiveness under necessary investigation. Thus, ADHD remains a priority for the development of child and adolescent psychiatric treatment (Figure 11.5).

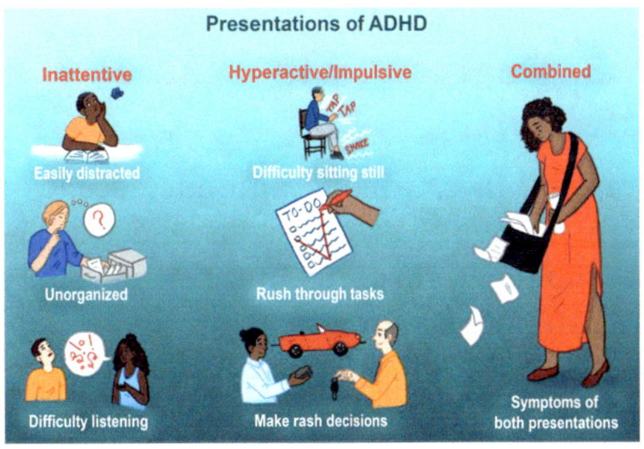

Figure 11.5. Attention deficit hyperactivity disorder (ADHD).

Source: https://counselingmatters.live/wp-content/uploads/2020/09/adhd-english.png?w=1400.

11.1.2. Anxiety Disorders

Anxiety disorders are among the most significant problems in child and adolescent psychiatry, exerting a significant burden on the daily lives of adolescents. Generalized anxiety disorder, social anxiety disorder, and specific phobias are some of the disorders that typically manifest with unwanted avoidance and fear behaviors. Their prevalence among adolescents is growing, and the evidence points towards the fact that disorders , such as SAD are markedly common, inducing considerable distress and contributing to long-term undesirable consequences if left untreated (Agersnap et al., 2022). Moreover, the comorbid condition of anxiety disorders and other mental conditions, that is, substance use disorders, is alarming; studies indicate that about 5% of adolescents with anxiety disorders also have issues of risky substance use (Orrin et al., 2024). This point in time underscores the necessity for targeted interventions, such as personalized cognitive behavioral therapy (CBT) methods for specific disorders like SAD, to more effectively address the particular problems faced by these adolescents and enhance their overall well-being.

11.1.3. Depression in Children and Adolescents

Depression in childhood and adolescence is a specific challenge to diagnosis and treatment, with mood disorders increasing globally. Underestimated for years, major depression is increasingly one of the most disabling conditions to afflict young individuals and imposes a huge burden on patients and families. Recent research underscores that chronic irritability is co-morbid with depressive symptoms in many instances, existing as a prominent indicator of mental pathology in this population (Busto-Garrido et al., 2017). The intricate relationship between depression and chronic irritability not only complicates the clinical presentation but also suggests a nuanced understanding of emotional regulation during formative years. In addition, identification and effective treatment of these mood disorders are essential, as failure to treat them in the initial phases may have long-term consequences for psychological wellbeing in addition to the ability to function daily (Caetano et al., 2013). Hence, ongoing studies and current treatment protocols are essential to improve outcomes for these affected children and adolescents (Figure 11.6).

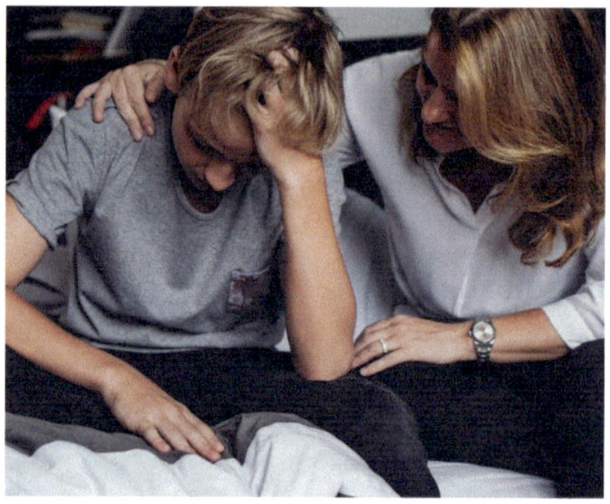

Figure 11.6. Depression in children and adolescents.

Source: https://cdnsm5-ss8.sharpschool.com/UserFiles/Servers/Server_1092603/Image/DMCC/Home/Mental%20Health%20Articles/03.01.2024%20Depression%20in%20Children%20and%20Adolescents.jpeg.

11.1.4. Autism Spectrum Disorders

Since autism spectrum disorders (ASD) continue to grow in importance in the domain of child and adolescent psychiatry, effective treatment modalities need to be understood. The recommended therapeutic approach, in particular for children and adolescents diagnosed with high-functioning ASD (HFASD), appears to be group-based SST. A recent study, conducted on 220 participants, has shown that the 12-week manualized SOSTA–FRA program can significantly enhance social responsiveness compared to the standard practices in treatment. Apart from enhancing social skills, the trial hypothesized that the intervention would contribute to the alleviation of depressive and anxiety symptoms in addition to enhanced pro-social behavior. Regardless of the clear advantages of these kinds of interventions, challenges remain in psychiatric training programs, where insufficient exposure to autism-focused clinical education has been found. Reports are that training directors acknowledge a need for more resources to treat ASD, which is an important cornerstone missing in current child and adolescent psychiatry training (Figure 11.7).

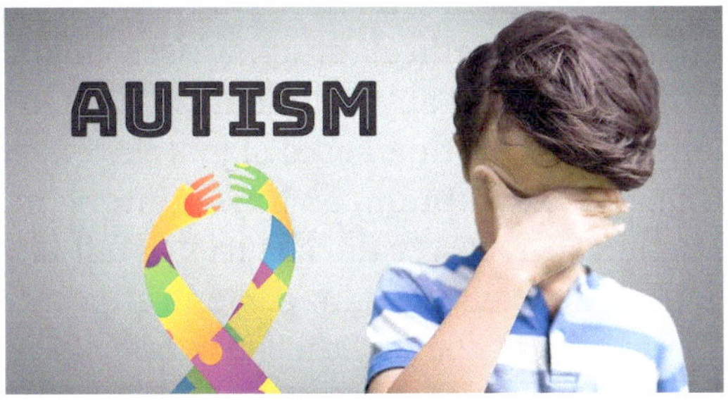

Figure 11.7. Autism spectrum disorders.

Source: https://astutecounseling.com/wp-content/uploads/2023/05/autism-.png.

11.1.5. Conduct Disorder

Conduct Disorder (CD) is a severe manifestation of behavioral and emotional difficulties, primarily observed among young individuals and adolescents. It is defined by a persistent pattern of violating societal rules and other individuals' rights. CD most often appears in the form of aggression, lying, and extreme rule violation. Knowledge of the underlying psychopathology is necessary for successful intervention; for example, a strong relationship exists between CD and co-morbid illness , including attention-deficit/hyperactivity disorder (ADHD) and mood disorders. These complications require the use of a multi-modal approach to treatment, preferably having the dual combination of pharmacotherapy and evidence-based psychotherapies. Studies have found that family-based and cognitive behavioral therapies are effective in controlling CD, promoting social skills, and improving negative behavior (Mani et al., 2005). In addition, proper diagnosis and individually tailored intervention can steer young people affected by CD in a different direction, underlining the significance of early intervention in child and adolescent psychiatry (Camilleri et al., 2009).

11.1.6. Eating Disorders

Childhood and adolescent eating disorders (EDs) have become an ever-growing concern in the field of child and adolescent psychiatry, requiring complete understanding and treatment. AN and BED are typically presenting conditions during these early years, and with studies reporting a prevalence of between 1% to 5% in adolescents with BED (Marzilli et al., 2018). The psychological impact of these diseases can also be severe and lead to emotional-behavioral challenges, social isolation, and even suicide ideation. AN, for instance, is typically accompanied by massive physiological impacts like menstrual irregularities and irreversible fertility issues due to hormonal imbalances (Ciobanu et al., 2020). As EDs impact this vulnerable population so strongly, identification at the outset and targeted psychological intervention are a must to decrease risk and support recovery. Therefore, awareness of the complexities surrounding EDs is vital in furthering youths' mental health and well-being.

11.1.7. Bipolar Disorder

Bipolar disorder, increasingly seen these days in child and adolescent psychiatry, is particularly challenging to diagnose and treat in its early stages. The disorder has also been discovered to manifest in symptoms that vary significantly from how it appears in adults and is also marked by intense irritability and swift mood swings, along with high co-morbidity of conditions like attention deficit hyperactivity disorder (ADHD).

All these complexities need to be treated with a comprehensive approach involving pharmacotherapy, namely the combination of mood stabilizers and atypical antipsychotics, which has proven effective (Caetano et al., 2013). Successful treatment is not limited to medication alone; the inclusion of evidence-based psychotherapies , such as cognitive behavioral therapy and family-based treatments, has helped the pediatric population (Caetano et al., 2013). With enhanced understanding about bipolar disorder, there is a requirement to continue exploring the particular psychopathology in young people in an effort to maximize diagnosis and establish individual treatment strategies that appreciate their own unique requirements (Caetano et al., 2013).

11.1.8. Post-Traumatic Stress Disorder (PTSD)

Post-Traumatic Stress Disorder (PTSD) is also highly prevalent among adolescents and children, often as a consequence of exposure to traumatic events , such as violence, abuse, or natural disasters. PTSD has serious consequences for psychological growth in that it does not only affect emotional regulation but also undermines social life as well as learning at school. Recent research, such as studies on trauma-focused cognitive behavior therapy (TF-CBT) and eye movement desensitization and reprocessing (EMDR), demonstrates the effectiveness of these interventions in symptom reduction for PTSD among children (Hoppen et al., 2024). More particularly, the standardized interventions provided in humanitarian settings have resulted in hopeful findings, highlighting the necessity of evidence-based interventions' accessibility for affected youth (Dozio et al., 2024). Given the lasting impact of PTSD on developmental trajectories, implementing specialized psychiatric interventions is required in an effort to block its long-term consequences and to build resilience among adolescents and children exposed to trauma.

11.1.9. Substance Use Disorders

Substance use disorders (SUDs) represent a critical dilemma in the practice of child and adolescent psychiatry, particularly because they have a multifactorial etiology with genetic, environmental, and developmental bases. Up to 23% of Brazilian adolescents have been reported to use drugs, and alcohol has been reported to be the most widely used substance (Del Prette et al., 2013). Identification and treatment of SUDs among this population necessitate a thorough understanding of co-occurring conditions, including mood and anxiety disorders, which tend to accompany substance abuse (Ayyildiz Didem, 2018). Medical practitioners ought to keep an eye out for any potential changes in the patient's behavior that could signal the onset of substance consumption, as timely intervention will significantly lower the chances of full-blown addiction. Successful management approaches ought to address not only the limitation of access to drugs but also promote social and academic interaction and thus increase the possibility of restoration of normal developmental patterns among affected youth (Figure 11.8).

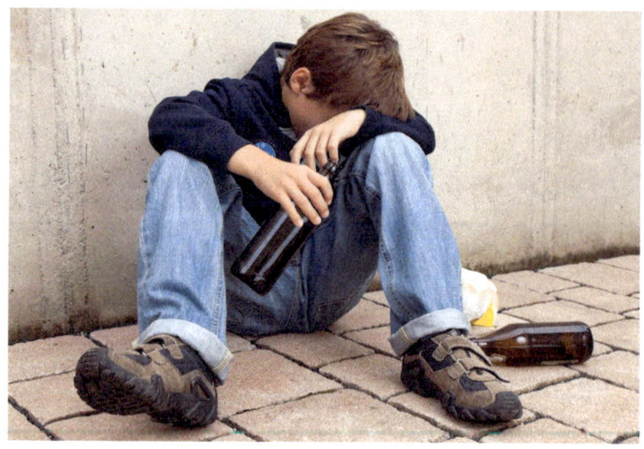

Figure 11.8. Substance use disorders in children and adolescents.

Source: https://mlfhdmqocr7f.i.optimole.com/w:1200/h:800/q:mauto/ig:avif/https://foothillsatredoak.com/wp-content/uploads/2024/08/childhood-trauma-and-substance-use.jpeg.

Test Your Knowledge

1. What are the key characteristics that differentiate anxiety disorders, mood disorders, and psychotic disorders from each other?
2. How do conditions such as depression, generalized anxiety disorder, and PTSD commonly present in clinical settings?

11.2. Assessment and Diagnosis

Learning Outcome

1. Importance of accurate diagnosis.
2. Clinical interviews and history taking.
3. Standardized assessment tools.
4. Role of parents and caregivers in assessment.
5. Cultural considerations in diagnosis.
6. Differential diagnosis challenges.
7. Multidisciplinary approach to assessment.
8. Ethical considerations in diagnosis.
9. Impact of misdiagnosis.

Assessment and diagnosis of child and adolescent psychiatry play vital roles in the identification of appropriate treatment regimens for young patients. Practitioners, through the application of a range of multidimensional approaches, conduct various forms of assessments , such as structured interviews, behavior ratings, and self-reporting measures, to gather comprehensive information about a child's mental status. Utilization of standardized scales like the Game Addiction Scale for Adolescents (GASA) and the NORC Diagnostic Screen for Gambling Problems (NODS-CLiP) highlights the need for detection of new problems like problem gaming and gambling among adolescents, such as has been reported by research to have high prevalence among adolescents seen in psychiatric clinics (André et al., 2022). Moreover, the full assessment should also consider psychosocial factors, comorbidities, and developmental history to adequately diagnose mental illness, optimizing the chance of early intervention and improved outcomes. A more nuanced understanding of such dynamics is necessary to advance child-focused care in psychiatry (Figure 11.9).

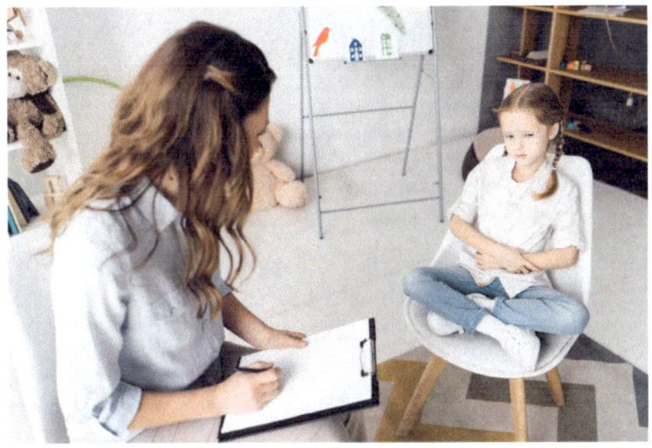

Figure 11.9. Assessment and diagnosis in child and adolescent psychiatry.

Source: https://www.socialworkportal.com/wp-content/uploads/2023/02/child-mental-health-assessment-jpeg.webp.

11.2.1. Importance of Accurate Diagnosis

Accurate diagnosis in child and adolescent psychiatry is essential to effective intervention and treatment plans. Misdiagnosis or delayed diagnosis might lead to inappropriate therapeutic interventions, which could aggravate a child's condition and hinder his or her development. The intrinsic complexities in diagnosing autism spectrum disorders (ASD), for instance, need cautious assessment. Research has indicated that the use of more advanced methodology, such as machine learning algorithms to maximize behavior testing, can enhance diagnosis efficiency among high-functioning adolescents and adults

(Hauck et al., 2020). Moreover, identification of distinct cognitive profiles in these populations highlights the necessity of interventions targeted at specific neuropsychological assets and challenges (Wagner et al., 2014). Thus, confirming a valid diagnosis not only directs the selection of suitable methods of treatment but also assists in gaining a profound understanding of every child's unique psychological landscape, finally resulting in more favorable development outcomes (Figure 11.10).

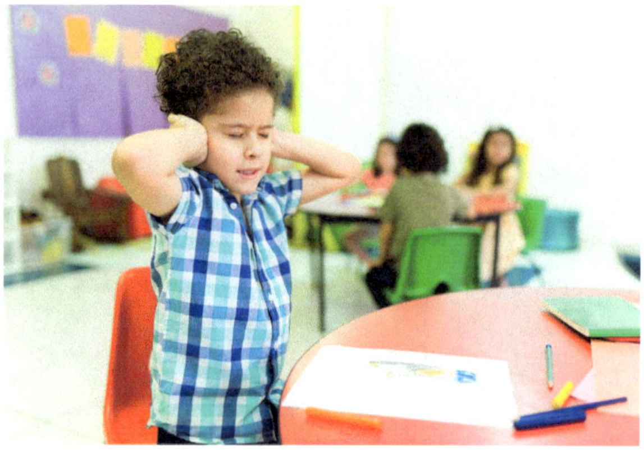

Figure 11.10. Accurate diagnosis in child and adolescent psychiatry.

Source: https://www.nurturingparenting.com/blog/wp-content/uploads/2023/01/young-boy-with-autism-1024x683.jpg.

11.2.2. Clinical Interviews and History Taking

Clinical interviewing and history taking take a pivotal role in child and adolescent psychiatry and guide the diagnostic and therapeutic process for children. It is not a matter of routine; it requires a complex understanding of developmental phases and psychosocial conditions. The clinician must employ communication modalities appropriate to the age of the patient to take comprehensive histories encompassing medical and psychosocial dimensions. Accurate history taking can reveal significant information concerning the emotional health of the child, interpersonal relationships, and environmental stressors for mental health status. Additionally, psychometric assessments , such as the Personality Inventory for DSM-5 (PID-5) can also enhance the assessment process, revealing important information on personality and psychopathology, particularly in inpatient settings (Ardizzone et al., 2016). Furthermore, poor transitions between child and adult mental health services leave adolescents at risk, necessitating thorough evaluation during clinical interviews for continuity of care (Appleton et al., 2020).

11.2.3. Standardized Assessment Tools

Standardized assessment tools are poised to play a pivotal role in the practice of child and adolescent psychiatry through the delivery of structured approaches to the evaluation of developmental and psychiatric disorders. Such tools, for instance, the Autism Diagnostic Observation Schedule (ADOS), give clinicians a reliable framework through which to diagnose such conditions as autism spectrum disorder (ASD), particularly in light of the challenge that accompanies evaluating older individuals (Hauck et al., 2020).

In addition, earlier studies emphasize the need to effectively identify developmental delays at early childhood, registering a high prevalence of under-detected cases in primary care clinics (Sices, 2007). Through the fortification of developmental monitoring and screening, the standardized tests not only enable accurate diagnoses but also provide space for early intervention approaches necessary to boost developmental outcomes. Therefore, as youth mental health issues continue to increase, the calibration and implementation of standardized measures remain critical to ensure that clinicians can make effective decisions and maximize treatment plans specific to children and adolescents.

11.2.4. Role of Parents and Carers in Assessment

Parents and caregivers are at the center of the assessment of child and adolescent mental health as they serve as key informants reporting information about a child's emotional and behavioral patterns. They are usually held accountable for the detection of emerging disorders and developing personality, according to the literature on early assessment processes. Properly involving parents ensures a holistic understanding of the child's world and dynamics, particularly in those cases when problems of behavior intersect with problems of socioeconomic status, such as being poor. Because caregivers are such an important part of the assessment process, their active participation can help to facilitate the early identification of issues, which can enable timely interventions that are tailored to the child's individualized needs. Finally, establishing the parents' and caregivers' roles not only enhances the validity of assessments but also encourages treatment collaboration in child and adolescent psychiatry practice (Figure 11.11).

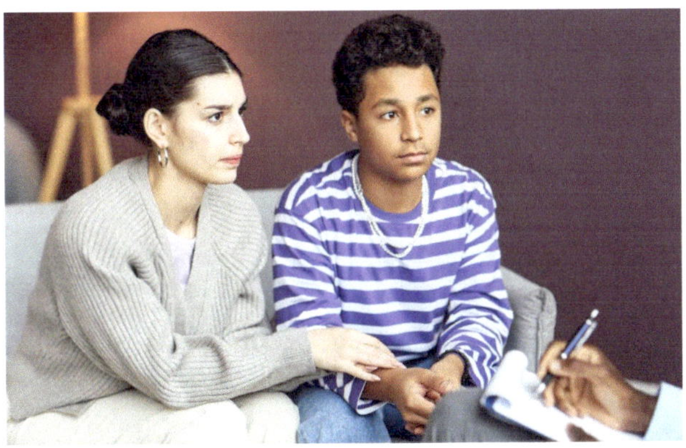

Figure 11.11. Role of parents and caregivers in assessment in child and adolescent psychiatry.

Source: https://dare2carepediatrics.com/wp-content/uploads/2023/07/mother-and-son-came-to-adolescent-psychologist-1.webp.

11.2.5. Cultural Considerations in Diagnosis

Cultural influences are an important consideration in the accurate diagnosis of mental illness among child and adolescent psychiatrists due to their ability to influence the presentation and interpretation of symptoms. Variations in cultural norms, values, and beliefs generally affect how adolescents and children present symptoms and how parents perceive these behaviors. For instance, the research that adapted the Child Mania Rating Scale to the Brazilian context highlights the importance of locally valid assessment tools that reflect local psychosocial dynamics (Meyer et al., 2024). Additionally, cultural sensitivity is also required in conditions , such as ADHD, since these may appear differently across various cultures; for example, hyperactivity in one culture might be normal playfulness in another (Sik Lee, 2019). Through the employment of appropriate diagnostic models in a culture, practitioners are thus better placed to handle such nuances, thus arriving at good and effective interventions for diverse populations.

11.2.6. Challenges in Differential Diagnosis

Differential diagnosis in pediatric and adolescent psychiatry is a difficult process due to the overlap of symptoms of various psychiatric disorders, thus confusing diagnosis. Several conditions commonly found among this population, such as Attention-Deficit/Hyperactivity Disorder (ADHD) and Bipolar Disorder, present with corresponding behavioral manifestations, which have similar symptomatology, thus complicating the identification and treatment. For instance, irritability, a symptom in pediatric bipolar disorder, is also common in children with ADHD and conduct disorders. The symptom overlap not only complicates the clinician's task but also can result in inappropriate treatment approaches if a proper diagnosis is not made sooner. Furthermore, studies highlight that children with greater ill awareness or family secrets are more emotionally challenging, thus complicating the clinical picture further (Shaffer et al., 2007). Hence, an interdisciplinary model of pharmacological and therapeutic interventions is required for enhancing diagnosis and optimizing outcomes (Mani et al., 2005).

11.2.7. Multidisciplinary Approach to Assessment

Multidisciplinary evaluation in child and adolescent psychiatry plays a crucial role in reaching details and personalized treatment plans. This involves the convergence of various professional opinions, including psychologists, pediatricians, social workers, and psychiatrists, for the comprehensive evaluation of the psychological, biological, and social dimensions of the child. With the utilization of structured and semi-structured evaluation tools, practitioners can obtain extensive developmental histories and observe interactions among the child and caregivers, which are crucial for proper diagnoses, particularly in conditions , such as autism spectrum disorder (ASD) (Johanna et al., 2024). In addition, this inter-disciplinary approach complements the biopsychosocial model, promoting enhanced communication between disciplines and an improved understanding of the child's needs (Mayall et al., 2022). Clinicians can identify strengths and weaknesses inherent in the child's development using this integrating process, which eventually yields more educated interventions and outcomes. Thus, a multidisciplinary approach becomes crucial in working with the intricacies of mental health in youth.

11.2.8. Ethical Concerns in Diagnosis

Ethical concerns in diagnosis within child and adolescent psychiatry are paramount based on the unique vulnerabilities of young populations. Ethical concerns most commonly occur for clinicians with regard to off-label medication usage, particularly for diseases for which there are no approved treatments, such as Disruptive Mood Dysregulation Disorder (DMDD). As illustrated in recent literature, although off-label prescribing, such as the prescription of amantadine, may produce beneficial outcomes, it has ethical implications in terms of informed consent and the sufficiency of risk assessment (Harinee et al., 2024). Further, diagnostic criteria for trauma-related conditions , such as PTSD, need to be implemented with caution, considering the differences in development in children and the influence of diverse traumatic experiences. Worldwide recognized tools, such as the Clinician-Administered PTSD Scale for DSM-5, secure an appropriate diagnosis while indicating sensitivity to the patients' context (Kouki et al., 2023). Therefore, resolution of such ethical challenges involves consideration of clinical efficacy as well as the potential consequences of misdiagnosis or inappropriateness in treatment for children undergoing psychiatric care (Figure 11.12).

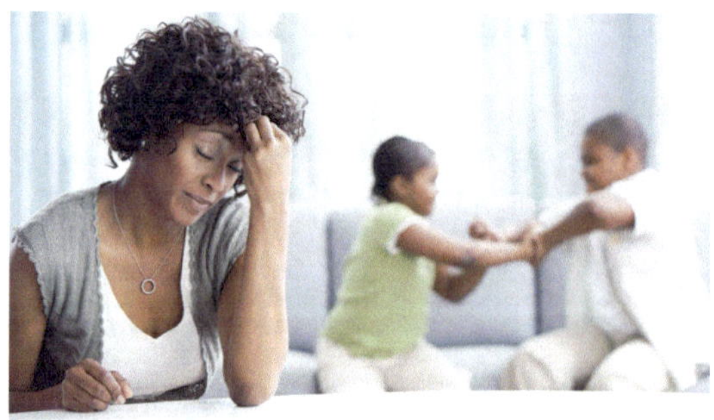

Figure 11.12. Ethical considerations in diagnosis.

Source: https://lirp.cdn-website.com/a173e1fd/dms3rep/multi/opt/77137496-56aa2e8b3df78cf772ad2844-020cf7d7-640w.jpg.

11.2.9. Impact of Misdiagnosis

Misdiagnosis within pediatric and adolescent psychiatry has serious implications, particularly when it involves challenging disorders like Borderline Personality Disorder (BPD) and pediatric bipolar disorder (PBD). Adolescents, in most cases, face unique challenges that make proper assessment and diagnosis more complex, thereby initiating stigma and potential inappropriate treatment (Sharp and Tackett, 2014). For instance, BPD symptoms might look exactly like symptoms of other disorders for mental illnesses, creating labeling that hinders timely intervention. The effects are dire, as understated or misdiagnosed adolescents have an increased incidence of self-harm and suicide attempts (Koehne et al., 2012). Furthermore, cognitive biases in clinical judgment exacerbate the issue, as demonstrated by recent studies on intervention programs aimed at correcting PBD estimation errors (Jenkins & Youngstrom, 2016). Therefore, an explicit understanding of these patterns of misdiagnosis is significant to enable early and effective treatment, ultimately leading to improved mental health outcomes for the children (Figure 11.13).

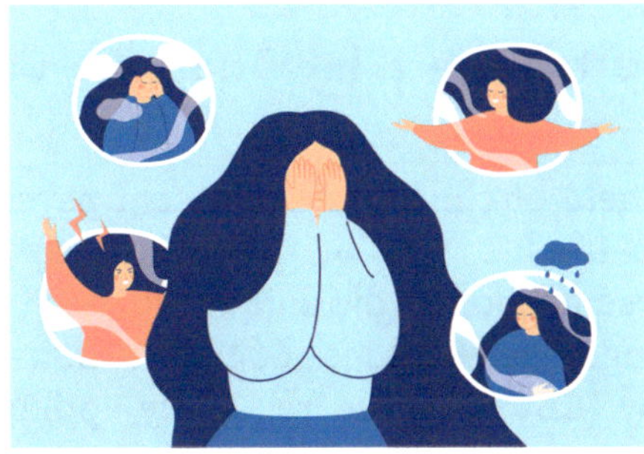

Figure 11.13. Impact of misdiagnosis.

Source: https://healthscopemag.com/wp-content/uploads/2021/04/BW.BoarderlinePersonalityDisorder.FI_.jpg.

Test Your Knowledge

1. How do clinicians use clinical interviews, psychological tests, and screening tools to assess mental health disorders?
2. What role do diagnostic systems like DSM-5-TR and ICD-11 play in ensuring accurate and consistent diagnosis?

11.3. Treatment Approaches

Learning Outcome

1. Psychotherapy options (CBT, play therapy, etc.).
2. Pharmacological treatments.
3. Family therapy and involvement.
4. School-based interventions.
5. Community resources and support.
6. Importance of individualized treatment plans.
7. Role of psychoeducation.
8. Monitoring and follow-up care.
9. Challenges in treatment adherence.

In psychiatry for children and adolescents, treatment procedures are increasingly specialized and evidence-based, specifically aimed at corresponding developmental requirements of young patients. Among such promising fields is , including sensory integration therapy, formulated in the 1960s by Jean Ayres, specifically emphasizing how children process sensory information and respond to environmental demands (Del Carmen et al., 2023). Along with this, machine learning predictive models have arrived alongside the paradigm shift towards patient-specific treatment protocols. Using these tools, diagnosis and treatment planning can be enhanced by accessing enormous digital information (Dominic et al., 2022). All these approaches underscore the importance of multidisciplinary treatment planning by occupational therapists trained in sensory approaches. As the discipline has evolved, bringing in established methods and emerging technologies might result in outcomes exponentially improved for adolescents and children with psychiatric issues.

11.3.1. Alternatives to Psychotherapy (Play Therapy, CBT, etc.)

In the field of child and adolescent psychiatry, the various types of psychotherapy are employed to address the unique mental illnesses of younger generations. Cognitive Behavioral Therapy (CBT) is most frequently applied due to its systematic approach to changing negative thought processes, thus enabling children to better manage anxiety and depression. Another effective method is play therapy, in which child patients can express feelings and experiences through the medium of play, which is often helpful to those unable to communicate verbally. Current advances in digital health technologies, such as virtual reality (VR) applications, also have potential for the therapy of some disorders, such as phobias and post-traumatic stress disorder (PTSD), using exposure therapy enhanced in controlled settings (Park et al., 2019). This set of therapeutic modalities forms a wide range of therapeutic tools for therapists to provide adaptability in treatment planning to match the individual development stages of the child and adolescent (Figure 11.14).

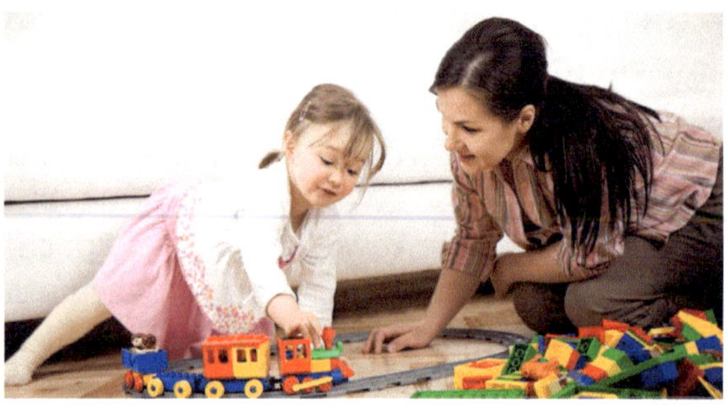

Figure 11.14. Play therapy.

Source: https://positive.b-cdn.net/wp-content/uploads/play-therapy.png.

11.3.2. Pharmacological Treatments

Pharmacological interventions are of absolutely vital significance in child and adolescent psychiatry, particularly in the management of disorders like Attention Deficit/Hyperactivity Disorder (ADHD) and tic disorders like Tourette syndrome. Research has established that drugs like methylphenidate and amphetamines have been shown to be effective across both genders and a wide range of ages, with preschool-aged children possibly receiving a less optimal response alongside increased side effects (Barke et al., 2010). Additionally, a comparative evaluation of behavioral therapy (BT) and pharmacotherapy (PT) for chronic tic disorders proved that both interventions reduced tic severity and improved quality of life significantly, with BT being a useful alternative to drug treatment when selecting therapy for children and adolescents (Cardona et al., 2018). Consequently, while drugs remain central to the extent possible, the growing recognition of behavioral therapies provides a balanced approach as an answer to the disparate requirements of child patients in psychiatric care.

11.3.3. Family Therapy and Involvement

Family therapy is central to the treatment and understanding of certain psychiatric issues in children and young people. By working with the entire family system, therapists can communicate more effectively, foster healthier relationships, and address underlying dynamics that are driving a child's mental health problems. Systemic intervention is particularly helpful when addressing issues of behavior, such as overuse of the screen or disordered sexuality, in which engaging the family is essential to effective intervention. Empirical studies reveal that children participating in family therapy programs are more effective at completing therapy, as revealed by recent evaluations of interventions that actively involve parents or caregivers in the intervention. Furthermore, successful interventions demonstrate the value added in developing coping skills in the family context and thereby strengthening social support and familial relationships as a whole. These programs assist both in the resolution of acute issues as well as in building long-term emotional resilience in young people.

11.3.4. School-Based Interventions

School-based interventions are a critical way of responding to children's and adolescents' mental health issues within school systems, as a pathway to early intervention and access to care. Research indicates that these interventions have the potential to positively affect students' grasp of mental illnesses while improving engagement and outcomes for those afflicted with conditions , such as depression (Jones et al., 2017). However, the effectiveness of programs like these is generally compromised by a number of barriers, including logistical challenges inherent within the school environment, training deficits for staff, and a need for technical assistance (Carroll et al., 2020). In order to ensure the maximum effectiveness of school-based mental health programs, the correct interventions should be selected that are suitable for the given scenario of a school with adequate training and support to the staff delivering them. Through addressing these complex problems, schools can facilitate a more supportive environment conducive to the mental well-being of students.

11.3.5. Community Resources and Support

Effective community resources and support networks are central to the practice of child and adolescent psychiatry, offering families struggling with mental illness invaluable support. These resources consist of local health services, schools, and non-profit organizations and offer a network of care that supplements and increases the treatment base. Notably, CAMHS has an important function in specialized care service delivery, oftentimes offered within specialized clinics for specific illnesses, like ADHD. Evidence indicates that 79% of CAMHS services operate these clinics, thereby highlighting their function in early intervention and complete management (Gavin et al., 2017). Further, initiatives like the proposed VCU Media Lab emphasize the synergy of new materials and tools capable of assisting in the education and treatment of these groups, emphasizing an integrative approach to addressing mental health among youth (Al-Mateen et al., 2001). Together, these systems form a support system operating beneath the surface to enhance resilience and recovery (Figure 11.15).

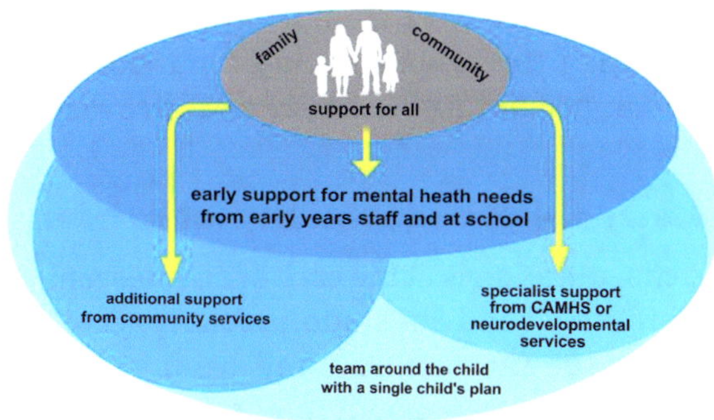

Figure 11.15. Child and adolescent mental health services.

Source: https://www.gov.scot/binaries/content/gallery/publications/publication/2020/02/child-adolescent-mental-health-services-camhs-nhs-scotland-national-service-specification/SCT01209444921_g01.gif.

11.3.6. Importance of Individualized Treatment Plans

The role of individualized treatment plans within child and adolescent psychiatry cannot be overstated, particularly in the face of psychological profile heterogeneity and developmental stages of this group. Children and adolescents are highly affected by psychiatric conditions , such as depression, characterized by heterogeneous clinical manifestations and comorbidities, whereby standardized approaches prove wanting (Hormi et al., 2024). Individualized treatment planning enables practitioners to tailor interventions according to the unique histories and needs of young patients, hence enhancing the effectiveness of treatment as well as encouraging a perceived greater involvement in the treatment process. The intricacies regarding medication management due to differential pharmacokinetic profiles and potentially unsavory side effects further illustrate the necessity for tailoring (Valentim, 2024). Through the integration of early intervention, individualized interventions, and collaborative models of care, professionals can have a profound impact on outcomes for young patients with mental health problems, reinforcing the essential role of individualized plans in promoting resilience and recovery.

11.3.7. Psychoeducation Role

Psychoeducation is at the core of an intervention within the child and adolescent psychiatry area to equip families and young people with information about mental illness and therapy processes. Psychoeducation enhances knowledge of diagnosis, treatment options, and the impact of various disorders, thereby making it possible for families to become active participants in treatment and decision-making. Research has identified that psychoeducative treatments lead to improved symptom management and greater treatment adherence among pediatric patients, particularly in the case of conditions like Pediatric Acute-onset Neuropsychiatric Syndrome (PANS), where anxiety and compulsive symptoms suddenly and severely emerge (Livingstone & Smith, 2014). Furthermore, initial psychoeducation fosters resilience and equips young patients with coping skills, significantly lowering family distress through treatment (Sholevar et al., 2017). By developing an educated support system, psychoeducation not only enhances clinical results but also improves the therapeutic relationship between caregivers, patients, and their families, leading to more successful and durable mental healthcare (Figure 11.16).

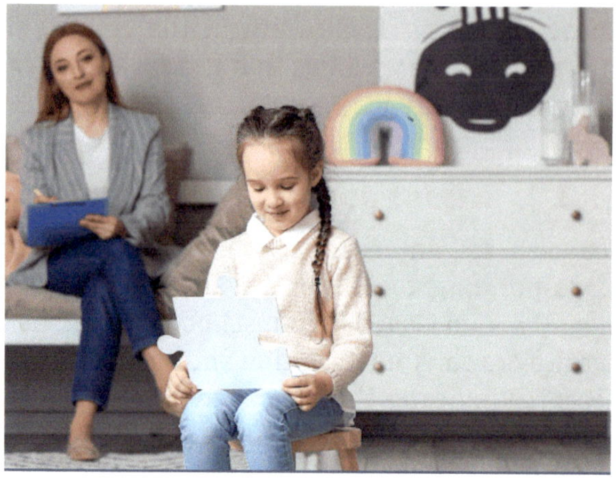

Figure 11.16. Psychoeducational assessment in schools.

Source: https://www.abbeyneuropsychologyclinic.com/wp-content/uploads/2024/08/2022-01-05.png.

11.3.8. Monitoring and Follow-Up Care

In the field of child and adolescent psychiatry, careful follow-up and monitoring are essential for ensuring the safety and health of adolescent patients. The necessity for close monitoring is further emphasized by Ireland's recent CAMHS audits, which found significant inconsistency in adhering to set standards of care, including baseline observations and regular monitoring (Halpin et al., 2024). Specific to worry was the finding that 98% of children had follow-up appointments scheduled, indicating a high level of commitment to continuity of care. However, studies also indicate that routine monitoring, especially for side effects of prescribed medication like antipsychotics, is typically suboptimal (Syed et al., 2023). This emphasizes the necessity for increased intensive training and routine procedures to enable sharp observation of patients' progress and reaction towards treatment, ultimately towards a more valid foundation for the provision of mental health care among this vulnerable population.

11.3.9. Challenges in Treatment Adherence

Adherence to treatment guidelines in child and adolescent psychiatry is also an issue that presents a myriad of challenges to optimal outcomes. One of the greatest challenges is the complex presentation of mental health diseases in children, where symptoms are very varied and inseparable from development and environmental factors. In addition to that, family functioning plays an important role in the sense that caregivers' understanding and acceptance of the treatment plan have a strong influence on levels of children's adherence. Modern therapies , such as sensory integration therapy, are good examples of new methods that may enhance levels of treatment engagement but require proper support and enactment in clinical settings in order to be effective (Del Carmen et al., 2023). Moreover, the emerging science of precision psychiatry attempts to personalize treatments, yet in actual application, it is limited by the standardization of outcome measures as well as by the translation of behavioral research into practice (John, 2024). Thus, the solution must be a multi-pronged strategy for addressing these challenges and enabling effective adherence.

Test Your Knowledge

1. How do pharmacological treatments and psychotherapies—such as CBT, DBT, or psychodynamic therapy—differ in managing common mental health disorders?
2. What factors determine whether an individual receives inpatient, outpatient, or community-based mental health care?

11.4. Impact of Social and Environmental Factors

Learning Outcome

1. Influence of family dynamics.
2. Socioeconomic status and mental health.
3. Impact of bullying and peer relationships.
4. Role of schools in mental health.
5. Media influence on youth mental health.
6. Cultural stigma surrounding mental illness.
7. Effects of trauma and adverse childhood experiences.
8. Importance of community support systems.
9. Strategies for promoting resilience.

The social and environmental determinants of child and adolescent mental health make a deep and multifaceted impact on pathways and developmental outcomes. Inequalities in mental health services and outcomes are most often found to correlate with socioeconomic status, race, and ethnicity and represent the existence of underlying systemic inequalities that determine the degree of access to services and assistance (Livingstone & Smith, 2014). For instance, children under poor conditions, for instance as poverty and broken family environments, are more prone to the development of disorders like Reactive Attachment Disorder (RAD), which is brought about by poor caretaking experiences (Pritchett et al., 2012). These risks under environmental conditions disrupt the formation of secure attachments and, consequently, result in extreme socio-behavioral issues in adult life. This renders the whole process needs an all-inclusive child and adolescent psychiatry, where the imperative importance of context in building resilience and the promotion of mental health equity in different populations is recognized. The treatment of these determinants renders it feasible for mental health professionals to better serve the affected youth.

11.4.1. Influence of Family Dynamics

Family processes lie at the core of the causation and maintenance of children's and adolescents' mental health disorders, with attendant implications for psychiatric practice. Empirical evidence has consistently pointed out that interpersonal dynamics within families can predispose people to the onset of various psychopathologies, including eating disorders and affective disturbances. For instance, empirical evidence indicates that the quality of parent-child attachment is inversely related to the adolescent's psychological well-being, considering that impaired interaction has a tendency to exacerbate distress symptoms (Battistella et al., 2015). Further, systemic approaches also point toward the importance of grasping family context, considering that interventions should be sensitive to such relational processes in order to facilitate better therapeutic gains (Marzilli et al., 2020). It is thus crucial for mental health professionals to identify the intricacy of family relationships to create effective treatment plans. Through resolving these underlying relationships, psychiatrists can best guide the emotional and psychological development of their adolescent patients.

11.4.2. Socioeconomic Status and Mental Health

Socioeconomic status (SES) is a significant determinant of children's and adolescents' mental health, influencing access to resources and opportunities for psychological well-being. Existing research has revealed vast differences in youth mental health and service use across SES, with lower socioeconomic groups being placed at elevated risk for emotional and behavioral disorders. These groups of people are often plagued by barriers of limited access to quality health care, mental illness stigma, and poor parental support because of economic pressure (Livingstone & Smith, 2014). Additionally, the interplays between temperament and socioeconomic disadvantage have not been adequately examined, notably how the factors could account for moderation between parent practices and child psychopathology (Flouri, 2008). Comprehending these dynamics is critical for the creation of specialized interventions that address the specific challenges posed by vulnerable youth, ideally leading to a more just mental health environment in our culture.

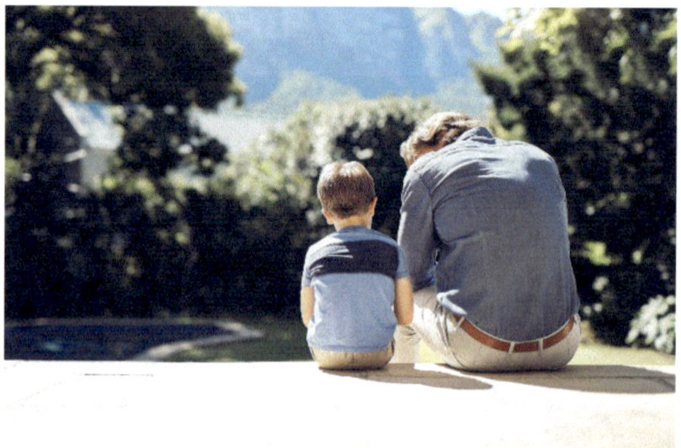

Figure 11.17. Socioeconomic status and mental health.

Source: https://assets.weforum.org/article/image/5-y0J9aKLq2gMxX4Jk60jgTmosZEwCTU9MSqGGNm0uA.jpg.

11.4.3. Impact of Bullying and Peer Relationships

Its impact on the mental well-being of children and adolescents is noteworthy, not only for individual bullying targets but also for the dynamics of peer relationships in schools. Victims of bullying often experience increased anxiety, depression, and decreased self-esteem that may persist even after the bullying has ceased, hence affecting peer relations and school performance. Studies indicate that school-level antibullying interventions do exist, but their potential to drastically decrease these internalizing symptoms is restricted and effect sizes exhibit at best symptomatic relief in anxiety and depression (Carolina et al., 2022). Even more difficult is this situation due to the nature of peer relationships because the mere existence of bullying leads to climates of fear and distrust, limiting social support, which might result in emotional resilience. Therefore, resolving these problems calls for a multi-faceted strategy, with interventions that are effective combined with promoting empathy and healthier peer relationships in order to reduce the long-term psychological impact of bullying (Goldberg et al., 2010).

11.4.4. School Role in Mental Health

In recent years, schools have come to realize their central positioning in nurturing the mental health of young people more and more, especially with mounting fears about the mental health crises among youth. Schools are key access points for the delivery of mental health services by way of early identification and intervention of psychological disturbances. School-based mental health literacy programs are some of the programs that have been set to enhance students' mental health knowledge, hence creating a favorable environment for assisting persons in need (McCaffrey & Cawthorpe, 2023). Furthermore, incorporating mental health services into schools can facilitate collaboration among school systems and healthcare systems to offer students comprehensive support. As a sign of the demanding character of school mental health care, improvement strategies like stability in funding and holistic training of staff are crucial in creating operational, durable mental health frameworks in school settings (Misty et al., 2023). This multi-component program is finally a testament to the role of schools in securing the children's mental well-being (Figure 11.18).

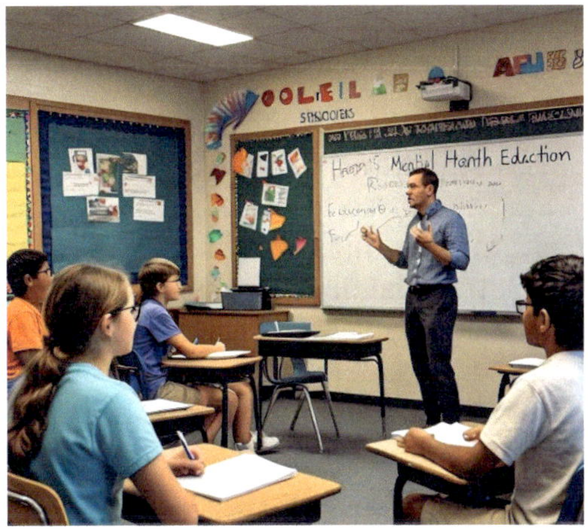

Figure 11.18. Role of schools in mental health.

Source: https://miro.medium.com/v2/resize:fit:1400/1*igjgHw8Ax4B7Up4EiY1RbQ.jpeg.

11.4.5. Media Influence on Youth Mental Health

The effect of the media on adolescents' mental health has become a high priority in the discipline of child and adolescent psychiatry, with both adverse and complex implications. With further expansion of the internet, adolescents are exposed to increasingly more social media that distorts body perceptions and amplifies feelings of isolation or inferiority, particularly among vulnerable subgroups , such as alternative youth cultures. Studies show that adolescents in such subcultures, like those that call themselves "Alternative" (e.g., Goth or Emo), report greater prevalence of self-harming behaviors, usually as a coping strategy for managing emotional pain and facilitating social membership (Hill et al., 2014). In addition, the disintegration of parent-child relationships, along with changes in social norms, has further rendered it impossible to measure the media's impact, and with heavy repercussions on the mental health of young people from various socioeconomic backgrounds (Collishaw et al., 2011). Such dynamics must be understood for pediatric mental health interventions to be effective.

11.4.6. Cultural Stigma Surrounding Mental Illness

Cultural stigma surrounding mental illness remains a significant barrier to the utilization of mental health services, particularly among various ethnic groups. For instance, research on South Asian family experiences in Scotland revealed that stigma surrounding mental illness previously dissuaded utilization of Child and Adolescent Mental Health Services (CAMHS) among such families (Bradby et al., 2007). The interviewees identified fear of gossip and the social stigma linking mental illness to madness as making it hard for them to receive help. The stigma extends beyond individuals with mental illnesses and even extends to their families, causing feelings of isolation and discrimination (Rhys Price-Robertson, 2015). The cultural context emphasizes the importance of developing services that are not only accessible but also culturally specific. This eradication of stigmas must be done collectively to establish understanding and acceptance among communities so that mental illness is seen as a true health issue that deserves attention and support (Figure 11.19).

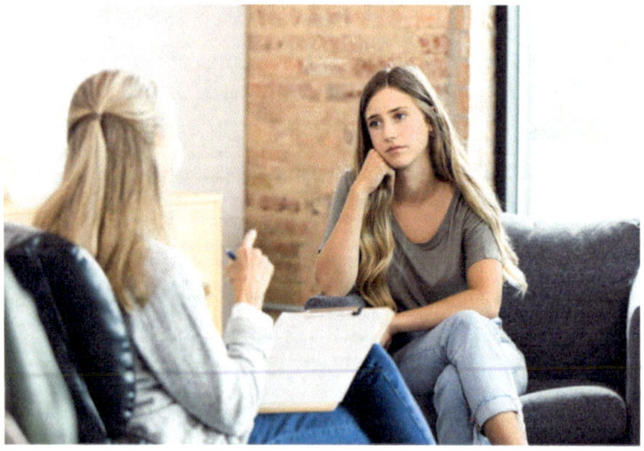

Figure 11.19. Cultural stigma surrounding mental illness.

Source: https://wp04-media.cdn.ihealthspot.com/wp-content/uploads/sites/193/2024/02/Adolescent-Mental-Health-Village-Pediatric-Group-768x512.jpg.

11.4.7. Effects of Trauma and Adverse Childhood Experiences

Trauma and adverse childhood experiences (ACEs) exert a major influence on mental health, particularly in the disciplines of child and adolescent psychiatry. Evidence indicates that children who have experienced multiple ACEs are at much greater risk of developing a range of psychopathologies, including anxiety, depression, and post-traumatic stress disorder (PTSD) (Lahiru Amarasena et al., 2021). Long-term trauma, whether witnessed aggression or parental psychopathology, not only affects neurodevelopment but also negatively influences emotional regulation and socialization (Lahiru Amarasena et al., 2021). These negative experiences are compounded when socio-economic factors, including family instability or systemic inequalities, are also present. This partnership highlights the need for early intervention in minimizing the effects of trauma and enhancing protective factors , such as supportive relationships and access to mental health services. At the end, it is very important to tackle these matters in order to develop resilience and enhance long-term functioning in such traumatized children and adolescents.

11.4.8. Importance of Community Support Systems

Support networks in the community form the core of child and adolescent mental health, and particularly child and adolescent psychiatry. Some of them are the network of relationships and resources that constitute families, schools, healthcare professionals, and social agencies coordinated as a single entity to produce an environment of support. They are required for the initial detection and treatment of mental issues, which typically arise in non-clinical settings like schools or community centers, indicating the demand for the integration of approaches beyond the realm of traditional mental health care (Annemans et al., 2011). Effective support systems not only allow children and youth to receive care but also promote resilience and healthy development, which are critical given the alarming rates of mental illness in young people (Belfer, 2005). Ultimately, the establishment of strong support systems will prevent mental health crises, with children and teenagers receiving comprehensive care that allows them to blossom and excel in the future.

11.4.9. Strategies for Promoting Resilience

Fostering resilience in children and youth is central to the creation of mental health and well-being, particularly where there is exposure to adversity. Successful strategies should include a multi-faceted approach addressing social and emotional learning through educational systems. Available evidence indicates that school-based mental health programs targeting resilience can significantly counteract the detrimental consequences of experiences of adversity, such as childhood victimization (Cavioni et al., 2020). It should also be noted that the protective factors , such as emotion regulation, social relationships, and community support, not only instigate good health outcomes but also protect the population against the effects of prior traumas (Banyard et al., 2017). By integrating these strategies into intervention and prevention, practitioners can create supportive environments that enhance emotional resilience, equipping children and adolescents with the ability to overcome adversity and thrive amidst challenges. These programs are the building blocks for the development of a resilient next generation that has what it takes to overcome the vicissitudes of life.

Test Your Knowledge

1. How do stress, trauma, family relationships, and socioeconomic conditions influence the development or severity of mental health disorders?
2. In what ways do stigma, access to care, and cultural beliefs affect treatment-seeking behavior and recovery outcomes?

SUMMARY

The specialty of child and adolescent psychiatry is most crucial in understanding and treating the particular mental health disorders of young populations. Newer research identified early intervention as its most critical priority, including the fact that most adolescents with diagnoses , such as PTSD have significant symptom remissions within the first few months following trauma, but may require some additional treatment to achieve optimum recovery (Fearon et al., 2016). Simultaneously, psychotherapeutic strategies, including psychoeducational interventions, are reported to be effective in preventing and treating adolescent depression, with variations between study designs calling for additional empirically valid assessments to establish best practice (Jones et al., 2017). Not only do these results inform clinical intervention, but also suggest the necessity of continued research focusing on simplifying existing paradigms of treatment as well as enhancing outcomes for the affected youth. Lastly, encouraging an overall awareness of these dynamics is imperative to policymakers and practitioners alike to further respond to the mental health needs of adolescents and children.

In child and adolescent psychiatric research, several findings surface that illustrate the complexities of psychiatric condition among children. An example is posttraumatic stress disorder (PTSD), and research has revealed that symptom rates and levels of diagnosis drop quite significantly in the first six months after exposure to trauma; about 50% in the early months. However, natural recovery in all these cases tends to need assistance, with ongoing symptoms lasting longer than this period if left unaddressed. Intervening too is early child development (ECD), especially in low- and middle-income contexts, as many of the intervening factors , such as caregiver activity and dietary diversity, were identified to play a significant role in influencing outcomes in development. Thus, an understanding of the interrelationship between trauma recovery and developmental health highlights the critical importance of interventions that possess the ability to promote resilience and well-being in affected youth, fostering a child and adolescent psychiatry framework.

KEY TERMS FROM THIS CHAPTER

- Adolescent depression
- Attachment disorders
- Autism spectrum disorder (ASD)
- Childhood-onset schizophrenia
- Conduct disorder
- Developmental delay
- Encopresis
- Enuresis
- Intellectual disability
- Learning disabilities
- Mood dysregulation
- Oppositional defiant disorder (ODD)
- Reactive attachment disorder (RAD)
- Risk behaviors
- Selective mutism
- Separation anxiety disorder
- Tic disorders
- Tourette syndrome

CRITICAL THINKING QUESTIONS

1. **Which of the following is a core symptom of Attention-Deficit/Hyperactivity Disorder (ADHD)?**
   a. Repetitive and restrictive behaviors
   b. Inattention and hyperactivity-impulsivity
   c. Hallucinations and delusions
   d. Excessive worry about multiple issues
2. **Autism Spectrum Disorder (ASD) is primarily characterized by:**
   a. Poor appetite and weight loss
   b. Impaired social interaction and communication with repetitive behaviors
   c. Sudden episodes of intense fear
   d. Aggressive outbursts only
3. **Separation Anxiety Disorder in children involves:**
   a. Fear of speaking in public
   b. Intense fear or distress when separated from attachment figures
   c. Recurrent intrusive thoughts
   d. Alternating periods of mania and depression
4. **Conduct Disorder is characterized by:**
   a. Excessive daydreaming and lack of focus
   b. Persistent patterns of violating social rules and the rights of others
   c. Difficulty with reading and writing
   d. Sudden mood swings
5. **Which disorder involves persistent difficulties in reading despite normal intelligence?**
   a. Dyslexia
   b. ADHD
   c. Conduct Disorder
   d. Oppositional Defiant Disorder

Short Answer Questions

1. What is child and adolescent psychiatry, and how does it differ from adult psychiatry?
2. List three common psychiatric disorders in children and adolescents.
3. What are the core symptoms of Attention-Deficit/Hyperactivity Disorder (ADHD)?
4. How does Autism Spectrum Disorder (ASD) typically present in early childhood?
5. What are risk factors for developing mood disorders during adolescence?

Answer to Critical Thinking Questions

1. (b); 2. (b); 3. (b); 4. (b); 5. (a)

REFERENCES

1. Negash, A., Abera, M., Gruber-Frank, C., & Frank, R. (2015). An adolescent with significant emotional and medically unexplained complaints: case report and proposal of an intervention. Child and adolescent psychiatry and mental health, 9, 48. https://doi.org/10.1186/s13034-015-0080-5 (accessed on 28th July 2025).
2. Abrahamse, M. E., Boer, F., Chavannes, E. L., Coelman, F. J. G., Junger, M., & Lindauer, R. J. (2012). Parent-child interaction therapy for preschool children with disruptive behavior problems in the Netherlands. *BioMed Central*. https://core.ac.uk/download/pdf/11484250.pdf (accessed on 28th July 2025).
3. Bor, W., McGee, T. R., & Fagan, A. A. (2004). Early risk factors for adolescent antisocial behaviour: an Australian longitudinal study. *The Australian and New Zealand journal of psychiatry*, *38*(5), 365–372. https://doi.org/10.1080/j.1440-1614.2004.01365.x(accessed on 28th July 2025).
4. Agersnap, T. N., Hougaard, E., Jensen, M. B., & Thastum, M. (2022). Diagnosis-specific group CBT treating social anxiety in adolescents: A feasibility study, 10, 89–101. https://www.semanticscholar.org/paper/32d92b320efa52aa66d456a138ff04dc7f930f53 (accessed on 28th July 2025).
5. Al-Mateen, C., Carney, M., Diehl, S., & Moriarty, L. J. (2001). VCU Media Lab. *VCU Scholars Compass*. https://core.ac.uk/download/215486731.pdf (accessed on 28th July 2025).
6. American Psychiatric Association, Bagner, G., Baker, B. L., Behan, K., Brenner, S., Campbell, S. B., Crawley, S. A., Einfeld, S., Eyberg, S., Feldman, M., Fox, N. A., Gavidia-Payne, S., Greene, R. W., Hofstra, M. B., Kaufman, J., McIntyre, L. L., Mendez, J. L., Nicholson, J., Nock, M. K., Patterson, G. R., Reid, J. B., Roberts, C., Sanders, M. R., Sigafoos, J., Snell-Johns, J., US Department of Education, Webster-Stratton, C., & Weis, R. (2009). Treatment outcomes for toddlers with behavior problems from families in poverty. *e-Publications@Marquette*. https://core.ac.uk/download/213076118.pdf (accessed on 28th July 2025).
7. André, F., Håkansson, A., Johansson, B. A., & Claesdotter-Knutsson, E. (2022). The prevalence of gaming and gambling in a child and adolescent psychiatry unit, 11. https://www.semanticscholar.org/paper/9a21bca4ceedef065cf2ebbad49b05f657a25e22 (accessed on 28th July 2025).
8. Annemans, L., Eyssen, M., Mommerency, G., Schoentjes, E., Swartenbroekx, N., Van den Heede, K., & Verhaeghe, N. (2011). Organisatie van geestelijke gezondheidszorg voor kinderen en jongeren: Literatuurstudie en internationaal overzicht. *Federaal Kenniscentrum voor de Gezondheidszorg (KCE)*. https://core.ac.uk/download/55771707.pdf (accessed on 28th July 2025).
9. Appleton, R., Canaway, A., Elahi, F., Singh, S. P., & Tuomainen, H. (2020). "I'm just a long history of people rejecting referrals": Experiences of young people who fell through the gap between child and adult mental health services. *Springer Science and Business Media LLC*. https://core.ac.uk/download/305119827.pdf (accessed on 28th July 2025).
10. Ardizzone, I., Borroni, S., Fantini, F., Ferrara, M., Fossati, A., Krueger, R. F., Markon, K. E., Somma, A., Terrinoni, A., & Williams, R. (2016). Reliability and clinical usefulness of the personality inventory for DSM-5 in clinically referred adolescents: A preliminary report in a sample of Italian inpatients. *Elsevier BV*. https://core.ac.uk/download/74320718.pdf (accessed on 28th July 2025).

11. Ayyildiz, D. (2018). Kleptomania and attention deficit hyperactivity disorder: Case report. *Association of Medical Doctors Sanamed*. https://core.ac.uk/download/201577473.pdf (accessed on 28th July 2025).

12. Banyard, V., Grych, J. H., & Hamby, S. L. (2017). Health effects of adverse childhood events: Identifying promising protective factors at the intersection of mental and physical well-being. *e-Publications@Marquette*. https://core.ac.uk/download/213087241.pdf (accessed on 28th July 2025).

13. Barbato, M., AlHumairi, S., Nafie, S., Dhuhair, B. A., & Dabbagh, N. (2020). T31. Time to talk mental health in Dubai: Describing a sample of adolescent help-seekers accessing mental health services, 46, 243–243. https://www.semanticscholar.org/paper/a626de07d21e99ddcc126c3256ff87ac97bef9e3 (accessed on 28th July 2025).

14. Barke, E., Coghill, D., & Cornforth, C. (2010). Stimulant drug effects on attention deficit/hyperactivity disorder: A review of the effects of age and sex of patients. https://core.ac.uk/download/55797029.pdf (accessed on 28th July 2025).

15. Battistella, P. A., Comis, I., Gatta, M., Simonelli, A., Sisti, M., Sudati, L., & Svanellini, L. (2015). Intergenerational transmission of attachment: Family interactive dynamics and psychopathology—What kind of relationship in adolescence? *Sciencedomain International*. https://core.ac.uk/download/53361572.pdf (accessed on 28th July 2025).

16. Belfer, M. L. (2005). Child and adolescent mental health around the world: Challenges for progress. *Indian Association for Child and Adolescent Mental Health*. JIACAM Vol. 1, No. 1, Article 3. https://core.ac.uk/download/pdf/86268.pdf (accessed on 28th July 2025).

17. Bender, S., Cholemkery, H., Elsuni, L., Freitag, C. M., Kieser, M., Kroeger, A. K., & Kunz, C. U. (2013). The group-based social skills training SOSTA-FRA in children and adolescents with high functioning autism spectrum disorder—Study protocol of the randomized, multi-center controlled SOSTA-net trial. https://core.ac.uk/download/14528049.pdf (accessed on 28th July 2025).

18. Berbenyuk, A., Alameeri, A., Bin Ismail, A., Zary, N., & Sultan, M. (2024). Empowering primary care physicians in child and adolescent psychiatry: A needs assessment on collaborative care in Dubai. *11*. https://www.semanticscholar.org/paper/0f495f7db89e3933f486da3b9d32e279c94afd10 (accessed on 28th July 2025).

19. Bevan Jones, R., Thapar, A., Stone, Z., Thapar, A., Jones, I., Smith, D., & Simpson, S. (2018). Psychoeducational interventions in adolescent depression: A systematic review. *Patient education and counseling*, *101*(5), 804–816. https://doi.org/10.1016/j.pec.2017.10.015(accessed on 28th July 2025).

20. Pritchett, R., Rochat, T. J., Tomlinson, M., & Minnis, H. (2013). Risk factors for vulnerable youth in urban townships in South Africa: The potential contribution of reactive attachment disorder. *Vulnerable children and youth studies*, *8*(4), 310–320. https://doi.org/10.1080/17450128.2012.756569 (accessed on 28th July 2025).

21. Bradby, H., Varyani, M., Oglethorpe, R., Raine, W., White, I., & Helen, M. (2007). British Asian families and the use of child and adolescent mental health services: a qualitative study of a hard to reach group. *Social science & medicine (1982)*, *65*(12), 2413–2424. https://doi.org/10.1016/j.socscimed.2007.07.025 (accessed on 28th July 2025).

22. Brown, J., Croudace, T., Deighton, J., Fonagy, P., Patalay, P., & Wolpert, M. (2014). Measuring mental health and wellbeing outcomes for children and adolescents to inform practice and policy: A review of child self-report measures. Springer Science and Business Media LLC. https://core.ac.uk/download/30663528.pdf (accessed on 28th July 2025).

23. Busto-Garrido, M., Gutierrez-Bedmar, M., Gutierrez-Casares, J. R., Gutierrez-Castillo, D., Martin-Lunar, M. T., Navas-Gonzalez, J. R., Pena-Andreu, J. M., & Rodriguez-Rosado-Martinez-Echevarria, A. M. (2017). Association between chronic irritability and depressive symptoms in children and adolescents. https://core.ac.uk/download/214839514.pdf (accessed on 28th July 2025).

24. Caetano, S. C., Kieling, C., Rocha, T. B. M., & Zeni, C. P. (2013). Mood disorders in childhood and adolescence. FapUNIFESP (SciELO). https://core.ac.uk/download/37710914.pdf (accessed on 28th July 2025).

25. Camilleri, N., Cassar Parnis, A., & Cassar, J. R. (2009). Problems associated with the diagnosis and the prescribing of anti-psychotic medication in children and adolescents for psychiatric conditions, by non-psychiatric specialists. Malta Medical Journal. https://core.ac.uk/download/46602212.pdf (accessed on 28th July 2025).

26. Cardona, F., Chiarotti, F., Pellico, A., Rizzo, R., & Silvestri, P. R. (2018). A randomized controlled trial comparing behavioral, educational, and pharmacological treatments in youths with chronic tic disorder or Tourette syndrome. Frontiers Media SA. https://core.ac.uk/download/188827600.pdf (accessed on 28th July 2025).

27. Carlisle, L. L., Cook, E. H., Hellings, J. A., King, B. H., Marrus, N., Pruett, J. R., Stigler, K. A., Szymanski, L., AACAP Autism and Intellectual Disability Committee, & Veenstra-VanderWeele, J. (2014). Training of child and adolescent psychiatry fellows in autism and intellectual disability. SAGE Publications. https://core.ac.uk/download/157829004.pdf (accessed on 28th July 2025).

28. Carroll, B., Clarke, T., Farthing, S., Fonagy, P., Gee, B., Jackson, C., King, K., Murdoch, J., Notley, C., & Wilson, J. (2020). Review: Delivering mental health support within schools and colleges–A thematic synthesis of barriers and facilitators to implementation of indicated psychological interventions for adolescents. Wiley. https://core.ac.uk/download/305118502.pdf (accessed on 28th July 2025).

29. Cavioni, V., Grazzani, I., & Ornaghi, V. (2020). Mental health promotion in schools: A comprehensive theoretical framework. University of Malta. Centre for Resilience & Socio-Emotional Health. https://core.ac.uk/download/322748597.pdf (accessed on 28th July 2025).

30. Marzilli, E., Cerniglia, L., & Cimino, S. (2018). A narrative review of binge eating disorder in adolescence: prevalence, impact, and psychological treatment strategies. *Adolescent health, medicine and therapeutics*, *9*, 17–30. https://doi.org/10.2147/AHMT.S148050(accessed on 28th July 2025).

31. Cerniglia, L., Erriu, M., & Cimino, S. (2020). The role of family relationships in eating disorders in adolescents: A narrative review. MDPI AG. https://core.ac.uk/download/296244843.pdf (accessed on 28th July 2025).

32. Ciobanu, C., Fica, S., Poterasu, M., & Rowland, D. L. (2020). Anorexia nervosa and reproduction: Connecting brain to gonads. ValpoScholar. https://core.ac.uk/download/304672903.pdf (accessed on 28th July 2025).

33. Collishaw, S., Gardner, F., Maughan, B., Pickles, A., & Scott, J. (2011). Do historical changes in parent-child relationships explain increases in youth conduct problems? J Abnorm Child Psychol. https://core.ac.uk/download/2734219.pdf (accessed on 28th July 2025).

34. Del Prette, G., Lopes, G. M., Nobrega, B. A., & Scivoletto, S. (2013). Use of psychoactive substances by adolescents: Current panorama. FapUNIFESP (SciELO). https://core.ac.uk/download/37710896.pdf (accessed on 28th July 2025).

35. Dozio, E., Bizouerne, C., Wamba, V., & Atienza, N. (2024). Comparing the effectiveness of narrative therapy and EMDR-GTEP protocols in the treatment of post-traumatic stress in children exposed to humanitarian crises. https://www.semanticscholar.org/paper/f132a719e63b9ac8b418d955798b7230f5f94ce1 (accessed on 28th July 2025).

36. Elzamzamy, K., Naveed, S., & Dell, M. (2024). Religion, spirituality, and pediatric mental health: A scoping review of research on religion and spirituality in the Journal of the American Academy of Child and Adolescent Psychiatry from 2000 to 2023, 15. https://www.semanticscholar.org/paper/91be32021694a75f89c08a2481280eea46efb8e5 (accessed on 28th July 2025).

37. Fearon, P., Fraser, A., Halligan, S. L., Hiller, R. M., Lobo, S., McKinnon, A., & Meiser-Stedman, R. (2016). Research review: Changes in the prevalence and symptom severity of child posttraumatic stress disorder in the year following trauma–A meta-analytic study. Wiley. https://core.ac.uk/download/41993811.pdf (accessed on 28th July 2025).

38. Flouri, E. (2008). Temperament influences on parenting and child psychopathology: Socio-economic disadvantage as moderator. https://core.ac.uk/download/pdf/82610.pdf (accessed on 28th July 2025).

39. Gavin, B., Neto, F. H., McNicholas, F., Mulligan, A., & Tatlow-Golden, M. (2017). Attitudes and reported practice of pediatricians and child psychiatrists regarding the assessment and treatment of ADHD in Ireland. Cambridge University Press (CUP). https://core.ac.uk/download/159108018.pdf (accessed on 28th July 2025).

40. Goldberg, D., Ghodse, A., & Cordeiro, C. (2010). The best and worst of academic psychiatry—Part II Chairmen. https://www.semanticscholar.org/paper/66e3e455697e0632000edc2fff7a212319dc07a9 (accessed on 28th July 2025).

41. Green, J. G., McLaughlin, K. A., Alegria, M., & Loder, S. (2015). Disparities in child and adolescent mental health and mental health services in the U.S. William T. Grant Foundation. https://core.ac.uk/download/75780891.pdf (accessed on 28th July 2025).

42. Gupta, A., Zorzi, J., Ho, W. J., Baretti, M., Azad, N., Griffith, P., Dao, D. Y., Kim, A. K., Philosophe, B., Georgiades, C., Kamel, I., Burkhart, R., Liddell, R., Hong, K., Shubert, C., Lafaro, K., Meyer, J., Anders, R., Burns, W., & Yarchoan, M. (2023). Real world impact of hepatocellular carcinoma stage and hepatic function on health-related quality of life. https://www.semanticscholar.org/paper/d41e47a79fb4fb2c2bc854a13ab074f60bb6450d (accessed on 28th July 2025).

43. Guzman-Holst, C., Zaneva, M., Chessell, C., Creswell, C., & Bowes, L. (2022). Research review: Do antibullying interventions reduce internalizing symptoms? A systematic review, meta-analysis, and meta-regression exploring intervention components, moderators, and mechanisms. 63, 1454–1465. https://www.semanticscholar.org/paper/00b12fed270571ffeab6ede990a2a4037560dbbc (accessed on 28th July 2025).

44. C Halpin, D O'Driscoll, I Whyte, A Herlihy, S McCarthy, A national audit of prescribing in Child and Adolescent Mental Health Services (CAMHS), International Journal of Pharmacy Practice,

Volume 32, Issue Supplement_1, April 2024, Pages i43–i44, https://doi.org/10.1093/ijpp/riae013.054(accessed on 28th July 2025).

45. Hauck, F., Kamp-Becker, I., Kliewer, N., Küpper, C., Poustka, L., Roepke, S., Roessner, V., Schad-Hansjosten, T., Schultebraucks, K., Stroth, S., & Wolff, N. (2020). Identifying predictive features of autism spectrum disorders in a clinical sample of adolescents and adults using machine learning. https://core.ac.uk/download/288845804.pdf (accessed on 28th July 2025).

46. Hoppen, T., Wessarges, L., Jehn, M., Mutz, J., Kip, A., Schlechter, P., Meiser-Stedman, R., & Morina, N. (2024). The efficacy of psychological interventions for child and adolescent PTSD: A network meta-analysis. https://www.semanticscholar.org/paper/a063c9816129dbe2ac6f4b7fb0615cf9c0887c72 (accessed on 28th July 2025).

47. Hormi, S. E., Rachidi, L., Laslami, Z., Oualidi, H. E., Nemrany, H., Benkirane, S., Sakhi, A., & Benjelloun, G. (2024). Depressive disorders in child and adolescent psychiatry: Epidemiology, risk factors, and clinical manifestations in Moroccan children and adolescents. https://www.semanticscholar.org/paper/f36559770a6379a712afb341089320a14d222890 (accessed on 28th July 2025).

48. Imran, N., Bodla, Z., Asif, A., Shoukat, R., & Azeem, M. (2021). Pakistan's first child & adolescent psychiatry inpatient unit: Characteristics of admitted patients and response to treatment over a 7-year period, 37, 305–311. https://www.semanticscholar.org/paper/6652801cf9bdd73ea778270a86691611b88c00dc (accessed on 28th July 2025).

49. Javaid, S. F., Afzal, A., & Ahmed, Z. Y. (2023). Serum prolactin level monitoring in children and adolescents on antipsychotic treatment: Evaluating the current practice in Al Ain, United Arab Emirates, 9, 135–135. https://www.semanticscholar.org/paper/77dff702f7b2361560d31ea8123afdcbb1e4c793 (accessed on 28th July 2025).

50. Jenkins, M. M., & Youngstrom, E. A. (2016). A randomized controlled trial of cognitive debiasing improves assessment and treatment selection for pediatric bipolar disorder. *Journal of consulting and clinical psychology*, *84*(4), 323–333. https://doi.org/10.1037/ccp0000070(accessed on 28th July 2025).

51. Kim, J. I., & Yoo, H. (2024). Diagnosis and assessment of autism spectrum disorder in South Korea, 35, 15–21. https://www.semanticscholar.org/paper/c16b14a8edd3ae9b705115829cb291e1ce1af839 (accessed on 28th July 2025).

52. Kim, W., & The American Academy of Child and Adolescent Psychiatry. (2003). Child and adolescent psychiatry workforce: A critical shortage and national challenge, 27, 277–282. https://www.semanticscholar.org/paper/bcb9755fdb3b81c47d09441a2f305241eb2df3a9 (accessed on 28th July 2025).

53. Kouki, N., Bourgou, S., Rezgui, H., Naffet, A., Hamdoun, M., & Belhadj, A. (2023). Clinician-administered PTSD scale for DSM-5, child and adolescent version: Clinical characteristics of pediatrics population, 66, 737–738. https://www.semanticscholar.org/paper/0646e57d107278763d8cc3e2adb60599d74d1104 (accessed on 28th July 2025).

54. Lee, Y. S. (2019). The past four years research work of the Adult Attention-Deficit/Hyperactivity Disorder Special Interest Group in the Korean Academy of Child and Adolescent Psychiatry, 31, 3, 4. https://www.semanticscholar.org/paper/65612e8f216f08a0249e3d07d552404c5c9767b3 (accessed on 28th July 2025).

55. Leikauf, J. E. (2024). Precision psychiatry implementation in child and adolescent psychiatric clinical practice: Opportunities and challenges. https://www.semanticscholar.org/paper/a93cb12b1ed5d77fbd5e8ef572f9049149fa7892 (accessed on 28th July 2025).

56. Livingstone, S., & Smith, P. K. (2014). Annual research review: Harms experienced by child users of online and mobile technologies: The nature, prevalence and management of sexual and aggressive risks in the digital age, 55(6), 635–654. https://www.semanticscholar.org/paper/4e87ea756df003df06eb62bea01235ccfcc106bc (accessed on 28th July 2025).

57. Maiyuran, H. J., Saylor, C., Appel, J., & Rice, T. R. (2024). Ethical considerations of off-label prescribing in disruptive mood dysregulation disorder, 35(4), 288–295. https://www.semanticscholar.org/paper/ffb638c2a2eff1baba6cdfac7af5ca6b93d9a433 (accessed on 28th July 2025).

58. Mani, N., & Pavuluri, S. K. (2005). Integrating pharmacotherapy and psychotherapy for pediatrics bipolar disorder: Translating science to service. Indian Association for Child and Adolescent Mental Health. https://core.ac.uk/download/pdf/86380.pdf (accessed on 28th July 2025).

59. Maria Del Carmen, M. L., Nadia, B. B., & Irene, C. I. (2023). Sensory integration in a department of child and adolescent psychiatry, 66, 392–392. https://www.semanticscholar.org/paper/b464c36dc9e4a1d39bfef589971fd312d82ca06a (accessed on 28th July 2025).

60. Mattei, G. (2019). Fashion industry as a source of inspiration for the 'Mental Health Department 4.0': An overview. https://core.ac.uk/download/287850256.pdf (accessed on 28th July 2025).

61. Mayall, M., Teoh, Y., McDermott, B., Sadhu, R., & Bosanquet, M. (2022). Child and adolescent mental health multiaxial classification: A useful biopsychosocial framework for pediatrics? 58. https://www.semanticscholar.org/paper/85df9ac30bcb1914896fe8deef72b300daaf6fc0 (accessed on 28th July 2025).

62. Eden McCaffrey, David Cawthorpe. (2023). Modelling the Clinical and Economic Impacts of Foundation-Funded versus Staff-Driven Quality Improvement Mental Health Strategies. Qeios. doi:10.32388/0DKU2V. (accessed on 28th July 2025).

63. Meyer, T. D., de Figueiredo, V. L. M., Youngstrom, E. A., Araújo, J. M. G., & de Mattos Souza, L. D. (2024). Psychometric evidence of the adaptation to the Brazilian context of the Childhood Mania Rating Scale–Parent/Guardian Version (CMRS-P). https://www.semanticscholar.org/paper/fea199f0fd7479c3e4d39a234dc6e931c8f48a26 (accessed on 28th July 2025).

64. Ng, W. Y. K. (2024). Editorial: Equity, diversity and inclusion in child and adolescent mental health–A perspective from the American Academy of Child and Adolescent Psychiatry (AACAP), 29(2), 192, 193. https://www.semanticscholar.org/paper/d1d0c696d62927dcb87df6ffcac8c30351b44487 (accessed on 28th July 2025).

65. Özbek, A., Dursun, O. B., & Güvenir, T. (2010). Epidemiologic studies in child and adolescent psychiatry: A review of methodology. *Psikiyatride Güncel Yaklaşımlar*. https://core.ac.uk/download/pdf/27165470.pdf (accessed on 28th July 2025).

66. Park, M. J., Kim, D. J., Lee, U., Na, E. J., & Jeon, H. J. (2019). A literature overview of virtual reality (VR) in treatment of psychiatric disorders: Recent advances and limitations, 10. https://doi.org/10.3389/fpsyt.2019.00505 (accessed on 28th July 2025).

67. Pitre, C., Daignault, I. V., Chouinard Thivierge, S., & Tourigny, M. (2024). Factors associated with therapy non-completion for children with problematic sexual behaviors. https://www.

semanticscholar.org/paper/925c80996538d9b98b1cb00fab927afccfc0018c (accessed on 28th July 2025).

68. Raballo, A., Poletti, M., & Preti, A. (2022). Editorial Perspective: Psychosis risk in adolescence - outcomes, comorbidity, and antipsychotics. *Journal of child psychology and psychiatry, and allied disciplines*, *63*(2), 241–244. https://doi.org/10.1111/jcpp.13438 (accessed on 28th July 2025).
69. Price-Robertson, R. Fatherhood and mental illness: A review of key issues. Australian Institute of Family Studies. CFCA PAPER NO. 30 2015 https://core.ac.uk/download/pdf/30672738.pdf (accessed on 28th July 2025).
70. Richards, M. C., Benson, N. M., Kozloff, N., & Franklin, M. (2023). Remodeling broken systems: Addressing the national emergency in child and adolescent mental health. pp. 20220283. https://www.semanticscholar.org/paper/119e63342b8d7402115a446f41a0776730754eb5 (accessed on 28th July 2025).
71. Robaey, P., & Schachar, R. (2007). Emergent perspectives on ADHD: Sharing knowledge and extending care, 16(2), 49, 50. https://www.semanticscholar.org/paper/0f6ff08ca3d99c7c96927ff84087560c6ece5141 (accessed on 28th July 2025).
72. Sholevar, F., Butryn, T., Bryant, L., & Marchionni, C. (2017). The shortage of psychiatrists and other mental health providers: Causes, current state, and potential solutions, 3, 5–5. https://doi.org/10.4103/ijam.ijam_49_17 (accessed on 28th July 2025).
73. Sices, L. (2007). Developmental screening in primary care: The effectiveness of current practice and recommendations for improvement. The Commonwealth Fund (CMWF). https://core.ac.uk/download/71350769.pdf (accessed on 28th July 2025).
74. Swedo, S. E., Frankovich, J., & Murphy, T. K. (2017). Overview of treatment of pediatric acute-onset neuropsychiatric syndrome, 27, 562–565. https://doi.org/10.1089/cap.2017.0042 (accessed on 28th July 2025).
75. Torous, J., Bucci, S., Bell, I., Kessing, L. V., Faurholt-Jepsen, M., Whelan, P., Carvalho, A. F., Keshavan, M. S., Linardon, J., & Firth, J. (2021). The growing field of digital psychiatry: Current evidence and the future of apps, social media, chatbots, and virtual reality, 20, 318–335. https://doi.org/10.1002/wps.20883 (accessed on 28th July 2025).
76. Tyborowski, B. T. (2020). Adolescent Borderline Personality Disorder: A Diagnosis More Hopeful Than Harmful. Bard Digital Commons. https://core.ac.uk/download/346432154.pdf (accessed on 28th July 2025).
77. University of Nevada, Las Vegas–William S. Boyd School of Law. (2013). Conference Bibliography: Juvenile Justice 1999–2013. Scholarly Commons @ UNLV Boyd Law. http://scholars.law.unlv.edu/jjc2013/1 (accessed on 28th July 2025).
78. Valentim, J. (2024). Comprehensive management of antidepressant therapy in pediatric psychiatry. https://www.semanticscholar.org/paper/3d6c6e0668beff3efdac541f2eaddf56e128d506 (accessed on 28th July 2025).
79. Wagner, A. E. (2014). Neurocognitive Profiles in Autism Spectrum Disorder. https://core.ac.uk/download/211347908.pdf (accessed on 28th July 2025).
80. Ware, O. D., Zerden, L. D., Duron, J. F., Xu, Y., McCarthy, L., Verbiest, S., Afkinich, J., Brown, Q., Williams, D. Y., & Goings, T. (2024). Prevalence of co-occurring conditions among youths

receiving treatment with primary anxiety, ADHD, or depressive disorder diagnoses. https://www.semanticscholar.org/paper/efca258142bcc63eaac41061f36099115d436efd (accessed on 28th July 2025).

81. Werner, M., Kapetanovic, S., & Claesdotter-Knutsson, E. (2024). Family-centered treatment program for problematic gaming and excessive screen use in a clinical child and youth population (FAME): Protocol for a feasibility pilot mixed method study, 13. https://www.semanticscholar.org/paper/179f95ac89391d9575e2c1177c30f65368a1cf41 (accessed on 28th July 2025).

82. Ylli, T., Stea, U., Kristiansand, N., University of Applied Sciences Inland, & Vrije University, Department of Developmental and Neuro-Psychology. (2023). Pressure, bullying and low social support predict depressive symptoms and self-directed violence, 33. https://www.semanticscholar.org/paper/3deac1de34c5d879fd93a28b626a365bfdeb6d97 (accessed on 28th July 2025).

GERIATRIC PSYCHIATRY

12

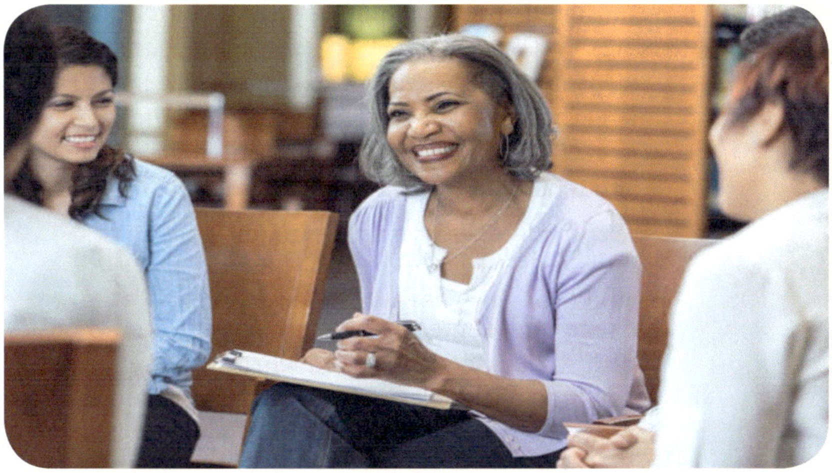

LEARNING OBJECTIVES

After studying this chapter, you will be able to:

1. Discuss aging and mental health;
2. Explain assessment and diagnosis;
3. Describe the treatment approaches;
4. Define the role of caregivers;
5. Focus on the ethical considerations;
6. List the current research and trends.

Introduction

Geriatric psychiatry is the field that positions itself at the intersection of old age and mental illness, confronting the unique problems of the aged as they contend with psychiatric illnesses and the complications of medical intervention. As the countries of the world age, the prevalence of mental illness among aging populations becomes more apparent. Incidentally, older patients experience drug side effects (ADRs) and a chain of complications because of the concurrent use of multiple drugs, referred to as polypharmacy in the majority of instances. Particularly in the field of geriatric psychiatry, high rates of potentially inappropriate medications (PIPs) are exemplified, which impede the best pharmacological control. These points emphasize the dire need for healthcare professionals to become more advanced in their prescribing patterns, whereby treatment pathways are individualized based on the specific needs and vulnerabilities of the geriatric population (Pfister et al., 2024). One such area of concern in geriatric patient management is the growing incidence of infectious diseases and their control using antibiotics. The prevalence of such infections, such as urinary tract infections, pulmonary infections, and cutaneous infections, deserves serious consideration of the appropriateness of antibiotic prescribing. A recent report states that almost 46.7% of antibiotic prescriptions in this population scored at least one of the criteria for PIP, which highlights the need for improved prescribing habits among the elderly (Pfister et al., 2024). Additionally, longer antibiotic courses lasting over seven days were identified as a common PIP, challenging the value of lengthy treatment in the elderly patient population.

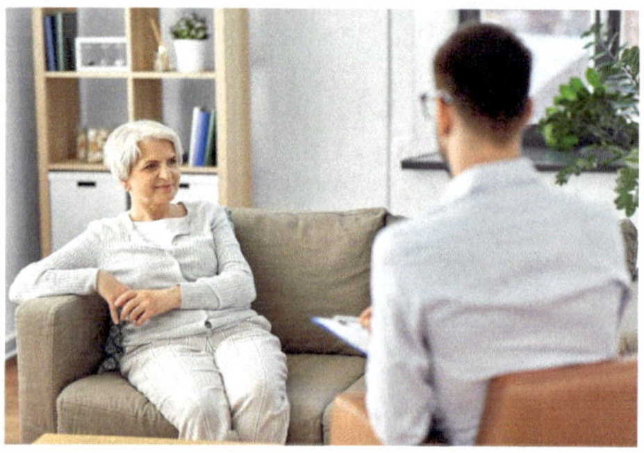

Figure 12.1. Geriatric psychiatry.

Source: https://familypsychnj.com/wp-content/uploads/2019/09/geriatric-psy.jpg.

Therefore, antibiotic stewardship is particularly appropriate in geriatric psychiatry, in which side effects from medications can play a significant role in affecting treatment outcomes as well as quality of life. In addition to medication management, geriatric psychiatry also entails the management of the behavioral and psychological symptoms of dementia that may present with significant barriers to care and overall quality of life. Interventions , such as the utilization of the arts and music have been demonstrated to support social integration and reduce neuropsychiatric symptoms in patients with dementia. The effectiveness of such therapeutic interventions suggests that a comprehensive and multidimensional approach is required in the management of older adults with complex needs. Opening communication among caregivers, families, and clinicians becomes pivotal in order to be able to offer holistic care. Last but not least, integrating mental health care into the entire geriatric care will require sustained research, innovative approaches, and commitment to overcome the unique challenges that arise in this critical field of study (Figure 12.1).

Definition of Geriatric Psychiatry

A thorough understanding of geriatric psychiatry relies on its definition as a psychiatric subspecialty that deals with the mental health and emotional well-being of elderly individuals. It treats the relationship between the mental conditions and other physical conditions common to the elderly population. Geriatric psychiatry is the diagnosis, treatment, and prevention of mental illnesses , such as depression, anxiety, and dementia, usually complicated by physiological changes and chronic diseases associated with aging. The need for specialized care in the population has grown as the world ages, making it imperative that psychiatrists be highly knowledgeable in psychiatric as well as medical issues. About health care systems, geriatric psychiatry plays a crucial role in integrating care in older patients with the long-term goal of enhancing their quality of life and functional capacity in the community (Gautam et al., 2022). One of the primary principles of geriatric psychiatry is interdependence between physical and mental health. Recognition that the mental state plays a significant role in chronic physical condition care is vital in promoting full patient care. For instance, mental illnesses might manifest physically or complicate existing medical conditions to result in suboptimal health outcomes. Also, pharmacological therapy for psychiatric illness must be carefully evaluated in older people since they might react with physical illness drugs. This has rendered careful evaluation based on the total medical history and psychosocial context of the patient more critical, hence ensuring a general approach for managing mental health in geriatric populations. The collaboration between health care professions is essential for developing strong treatment plans that address the requirements of mental and physical health (Scheffer et al., 2018). Development of geriatric psychiatry has been marked by increased respect for its contribution to dealing with the special concerns of older persons. Public health initiatives have placed stress on the need for mental illness services, particularly for elderly people and raised awareness of the prevalence of mental illness among them. Improved training in geriatric psychiatry among physicians, including primary care physicians, is also necessary for early diagnosis and treatment. These efforts are important in reducing the stigma traditionally associated with mental illness in older individuals and allowing them to be provided with compassionate care that is dependent on their particular circumstances. In addition, ongoing research in this field continues to identify novel therapeutic approaches and best practices, further enhancing the capability of being able to properly address issues in mental health. Collectively, geriatric psychiatry's changing definition reflects a larger devotion to enhancing health care outcomes among aging populations (Gautam et al., 2022).

Importance of Mental Health in Older Adults

The significance of mental health among the elderly cannot be exaggerated since it has a direct implication on their general well-being and quality of life. With the United States' aging population projected to reach approximately 95 million by 2060, the requirement for long-term sustainable mental care among the elderly demands equal importance. Mental disorders like depression and anxiety are prevalent among the elderly, and they significantly influence their physical wellbeing, mental functioning, and interpersonal relationships. Unaddressed mental disorders can speed up a decline in independence and raise the dependency level on caregivers, hence placing increased emotional pressure and financial burden on both the older individual and families. Moreover, mental care is required in an effort to improve the dignity and quality of life of the older population, leading to better health and an increased support system at the community level (Livingstone & Smith, 2014). Furthermore, the COVID-19 pandemic has hastened existing mental illness among the older population, with unprecedented gaps in psychiatric service and resources (Livingstone & Smith, 2014). The social distancing enforced by the pandemic, in terms of engaging with other individuals, has produced heightened loneliness, anxiety, and depression levels in this specific group. Research studies have established that such bad mental health conditions often spill over, having a further magnifying effect on cognitive loss as well as higher death rates among the elderly. The need for new mental health treatments has been illuminated in the face of this crisis as health infrastructures seek to transition towards the mounting geriatric psychiatry needs. Prioritizing telehealth and virtual care, coupled with community-based interventions, has been a shift in preventing loneliness while building social relationships among elderly individuals (Ipsit, 2020). Lastly, the interface between physical and mental health is especially relevant in geriatric psychiatry and underscores the need for an integrated practice of care. Physical illnesses , such as heart disease or diabetes can underlie psychological distress and, in turn, exacerbate physical health outcomes. In contrast, mental illnesses can complicate medical treatment adherence, creating a vicious cycle. Successful mental health interventions, including psychotherapy and medication management, have been found to decrease symptoms and improve functional capacity, and thus overall health in older adults. With the public becoming increasingly aware of the intricate interconnectedness of mental and physical health, there is a growing demand for clinicians to develop combined, whole-person models of care that foster mental well-being alongside traditional medical models (Livingstone & Smith, 2014) (Figure 12.2).

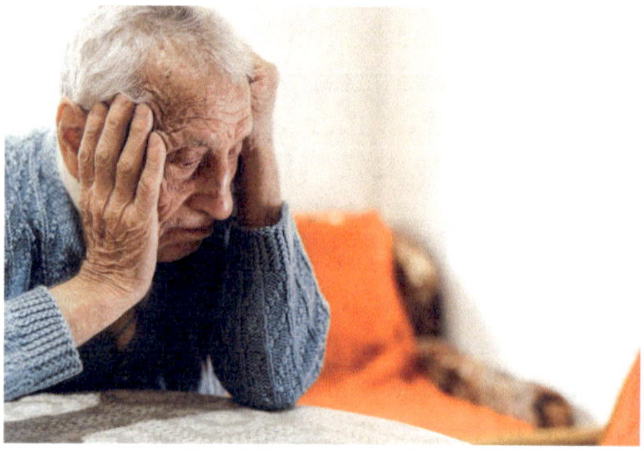

Figure 12.2. Mental health in older adults.

Source: https://thearborsassistedliving.com/wp-content/uploads/2019/09/9.26-arbors.jpg.

12.1. Aging and Mental Health

Learning Outcome

1. Common mental health disorders in the elderly.
2. Impact of aging on cognitive function.
3. The role of physical health in mental well-being.

The intersection of mental health and aging is increasingly significant in the field of geriatric psychiatry, as elderly patients often suffer from special psychological problems that have a critical impact on their general well-being. Most mental disorders in older people comprise depression, anxiety, and cognitive impairment, which are brought about by a variety of factors , such as chronic illnesses, social isolation, and loss of close relationships. Furthermore, these conditions are frequently compounded by the physiological changes associated with aging that affect mental health outcomes, further making diagnosis and treatment challenging. Meeting these demands necessitates a profound grasp of the complex aging-mental health interface, thus calling for expert-level interventions aimed at the geriatric population. Increased awareness is observed that mental health treatment needs to be a part of comprehensive geriatric care models to enhance quality of life and enable dignity in old age. Substance use disorders (SUDs) among older adults are a silent epidemic that necessitates urgent action in the field of geriatric psychiatry. As per the latest research findings, various forms of substance abuse, including alcohol, marijuana, and prescription medication, are on the rise among the aged. The reasons for such a rise could be treating chronic pain, isolation, and uncompensated mental illness, which can lead to self-medication tendencies. Further, with aging, the metabolic processes in the body predispose toward higher risks of side effects as well as render it more difficult to treat. The unawareness and stigma about SUDs lead to underdiagnosis and inappropriate treatment among elderly individuals. Therefore, intervention and rehabilitation can be effectively achieved only by embracing a multidisciplinary model that includes medical, psychological, and social support (Prasad et al., 2024). Furthermore, the implications of non-substance addiction in the elderly demand attention in the discipline of geriatric psychiatry. Behavioural addictions, such as gambling or internet addiction, are more common but less studied in the elderly. The population is more susceptible to adverse effects from such addiction due to the availability of concomitant physical and psychiatric conditions, worsening their general vulnerability and lowering their standard of living. Changing technology and social norms also play an important part in shaping the behavior patterns of seniors, both presenting challenges and opportunities for support. To address these addiction problems, geriatric psychiatry ought to develop specific assessment tools and intervention strategies based on the specific needs and circumstances of older adults, hence promoting a comprehensive mental health approach incorporating substance use and behavior disorders (Prasad et al., 2024) (Figure 12.3).

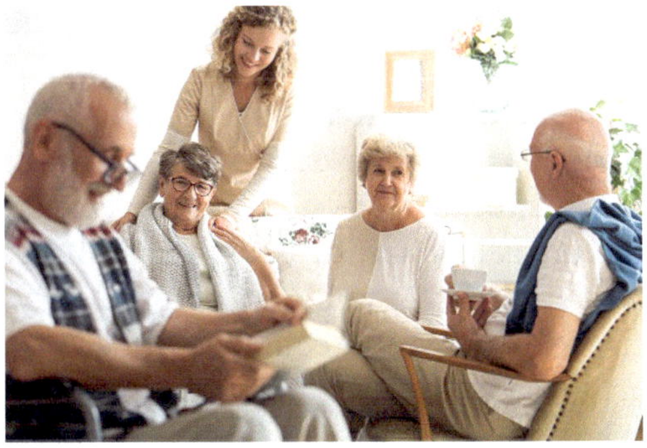

Figure 12.3. Aging and mental health.

Source: https://www.homecareassistancetampabay.com /wp-content/uploads/Senior-with-Friends-1.jpg.

12.1.1. Common Mental Health Disorders in the Elderly

The prevalence of frequent mental disorders among the older population certainly challenges geriatric psychiatry with numerous challenges. Depression and anxiety are two of the most prevalent disorders that can be observed among older groups, which not only affect their mental state but also their overall quality of life. Depression rates in this population have been reported as high as 53.4%, as evidenced by a study conducted in Northwest Ethiopia, whereby female gender, retirement, and social support as perceived were significantly associated with depressive symptoms (Shiferaw et al., 2024). Furthermore, anxiety often gets intertwined with such depressive disorders, hence complicating treatment. The intricate mechanisms of such mental disorders emphasize the need for universal screening and intervention strategies tailored to the unique needs of the elderly patients. A knowledge of various risk factors associated with mental illnesses in the elderly is essential to ensure that their needs are catered to effectively. For instance, the socioeconomic factors are of paramount significance; older adults who live in rural areas, who have received less than excellent education, and those who do not have a steady income are far more susceptible to depression (Shiferaw et al., 2024). In addition to that, the connection between the physical body and mental health cannot be overstated. Older individuals tend to have long-term physical issues that exacerbate their psychological misery, setting up a cycle of hopelessness and isolation.

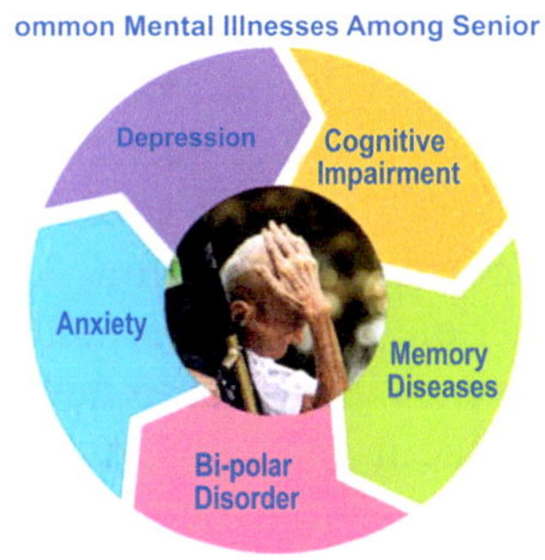
ommon Mental Illnesses Among Senior
Depression
Cognitive Impairment
Anxiety
Memory Diseases
Bi-polar Disorder

Figure 12.4. Common mental health disorders in the elderly.

Source: https://assistinghandscincinnati.com/wp-content/uploads/2020/10/8-Symptoms-of-Mental-Illness-350x350-1.png.

This complex interaction of contacts emphasizes the necessity for a multidisciplinary approach to geriatric care, in which management of physical health, social support, and mental health concurrently can lead to improved patient outcomes. Effective management and treatment of mental disorders among older adults highly rely on timely detection and a good healthcare system. Both depression and anxiety being highly prevalent, it is a necessity for early detection of these symptoms by healthcare workers and caregivers to evaluate and employ proven screening tools , such as the Geriatric Depression Scale and the Geriatric Anxiety Scale to improve diagnosis (Maraqa et al., 2024). Treatment should not only focus on drugs but should be complemented with psychosocial interventions to promote resilience and reduce loneliness. Training of health professionals, public education, and increasing access to mental health care are critical components of a national strategy to meet the rising tide of mental illness among older people and in the process offer them the comprehensive care they require (Figure 12.4).

12.1.2. Impact of Aging on Cognitive Function

With age, cognitive impairment is a serious problem in the domain of geriatric psychiatry. Cognitive impairment may take many forms, impairing memory, attention, as well as executive function. Empirical evidence indicates that with increasing age come neurobiological alterations, including reduced synaptic plasticity and changes to neurotransmitter systems, which are responsible for these impairments. It is interesting, however, that cognitive impairment does not occur with equal severity in all older persons; some are surprisingly resistant. This resilience is informed by a constellation of psychosocial and neurobiological processes that converge along the life course to establish individual vulnerability or resilience for cognitive decline. By understanding such dynamics, geriatric psychiatrists can recognize potential intervention targets that can potentially shield against cognitive health in older adults. Cognitive impairment in older adults calls for differential clinical management, particularly since it has been linked to various psychosocial and behavioral determinants. For instance, psychological constructs , such as self-efficacy and purpose in life can enhance cognitive resilience, suggesting that good mental health needs to be promoted to enable cognitive longevity. Furthermore, social support structures matter, in which people with intact social structures maintain better cognitive performance and lower rates of decline. The interactivity of cognitive function and psychosocial factors highlights the need for an integrated model of treatment that would incorporate the cognitive, emotional, and social dimensions. Cognitive and social interaction-based interventions could well be of actual benefit, thus the need to explore further in the context of geriatric psychiatry. Delirium, often occurring in the elderly with acute medical illness, is another age-related characteristic of significant relevance to cognitive function. It is associated with prolonged hospital stay and impaired cognitive outcomes, highlighting the importance of effective delirium management interventions in the elderly population. New evidence has explored new approaches like the incorporation of evening bright light therapy into delirium management units, yielding benefits on sleep and cognitive function in delirious patients. This multi-dimensional approach not only addresses the immediate cognitive deficits of delirium but also offers insight into how to improve overall cognitive function during and following hospitalization. Effectiveness in managing cognitive disturbance in the elderly can translate into functional improvement and, ultimately, improved quality of life, demonstrating the significant intersection of cognition and geriatric care (Ancoli-Israel et al., 2013; Laird et al., 2019).

12.1.3. The Role of Physical Health in Mental Well-Being

Physical well-being plays a crucial role in ensuring mental health, particularly in the case of the elderly, where the relationship between both is most apparent. Chronic physical illnesses , such as diabetes, cardiovascular illness, and neurodegenerative illness, exert a considerable impact on the psychological health of the elderly. This is a two-way interaction, as mental illnesses often lead to exacerbated physical conditions, thus creating a vicious cycle leading to poor quality of life. From the evidence of the neurochemical and endocrine responses to stress, physical disease treatment is not only necessary for physical well-being but also for the prevention of mental health disturbances. Physical health care can thus serve as a therapeutic process for enhancing mental health, putting stress on the coexistence of concurrent care measures , including medical and psychological care for the aged (Gautam et al., 2022). Among various interventions to support older individuals, promoting physical exercise offers itself as a significant process for enhancing mental health conditions. Regular exercise, even at moderate levels, has been found to assist in alleviating depression and anxiety symptoms as well as enhance cognitive function. Physical activities also provide social interaction, which is particularly vital for older adults who may be isolated. Social interaction also combats loneliness, a significant risk factor for depression among the elderly. Thus, physical health interventions not only optimize physical function but also foster an enabling environment to build mental resilience. Physical exercise must remain the first priority in treating clinicians because of its multi-dimensional advantages in optimizing both physical and mental health in older adults (Chan et al., 2020). Among geriatrics, the convergence of physical and mental health emphasizes the importance of taking up a holistic approach to healthcare delivery. Consultation-liaison psychiatry is central to this by ensuring the free flow of interaction between physical and mental health providers. The merged model supports early interaction with the psychological impact of physical illnesses, thereby improving overall health outcomes. Research has established that older adults with combined physical and mental illness exhibit worse adherence to treatment and higher healthcare costs. By developing tailored interventions that tackle both of these domains concurrently, health systems are in a position to achieve better clinical results and enhance the lives of older patients. Though the awareness of this link continues to increase, what is urgently required here is that practitioners and policymakers collaborate in an endeavor to bridge the gap between physical and mental health care among geriatric settings (Gautam et al., 2022) (Figure 12.5).

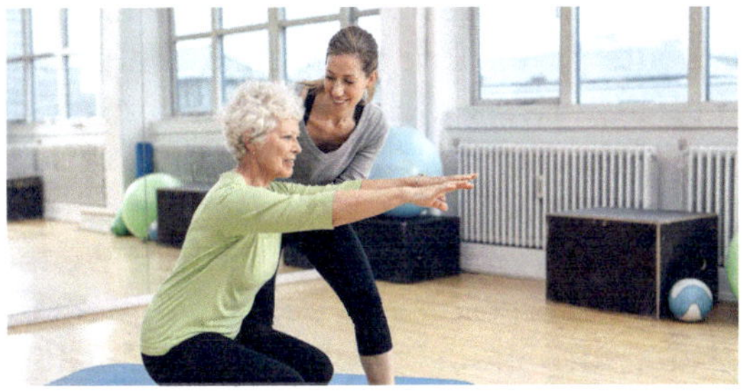

Figure 12.5. The role of physical health in mental well-being in the elderly.

Source: https://www.greatseniorliving.com/wp-content/uploads/2017/01/article-physical-health-@3X.jpg.

Test Your Knowledge

1. How does the aging process influence the prevalence and presentation of mental health conditions in older adults?
2. What are the most common mental health issues experienced by the elderly, such as depression, dementia, and anxiety?

12.2. Assessment and Diagnosis

Learning Outcome

1. Challenges in diagnosing mental illness in older adults.
2. Tools and techniques for assessment.
3. Importance of comprehensive evaluations.

The diagnosis and assessment process in geriatric psychiatry is necessarily complex due to the advanced age of the population treated and the multimodal character of the psychiatric disorders in older adults. Thorough assessments will commonly begin with a full clinical history, both acute psychiatric symptoms and previous medical histories. Variables , such as comorbidity, cognitive functioning, and psychosocial variables should be carefully explored so that an objective presentation of the subject's mental wellness is created. For example, Generalized Anxiety Disorder or Major Depressive Disorder is usually diagnosed by using subtle measurements through standardized tools , such as the Montreal Cognitive Assessment Test and the Geriatric Depression Scale, which measure cognitive and affective functioning, respectively (Kocakaya et al., 2023). An appreciation of the inter-relationships allows differential intervention that is responsive to the unique needs of older patients. In exploring geriatric syndromes, the assessment process can go beyond psychiatric symptomology to reflect overall geriatric health. Assessments , such as the Clinical Frailty Scale, the Katz Index of Independence in Activities of Daily Living, and the Informant Questionnaire on Cognitive Decline in the Elderly (IQCODE) are used in the measurement of frailty and disability (Guidet et al., 2019). These multi-dimensional assessments not only describe the probable interactions between these syndromes and psychiatric disorders but also allow for an integrated process of care. For example, a frail older patient with cognitive decline would elicit consideration of both their psychiatric interventions and their medical status, thereby encouraging a treatment plan that is holistic in its scope. This blended approach is particularly important in the geriatric age group, where comorbid disease states frequently complicate diagnosis and treatment. In addition, the assessment and diagnostic process in geriatric psychiatry also needs to consider the social environment in which older persons operate. Social health determinants, including socioeconomic status and social support networks, are fundamental to both the occurrence and treatment outcomes of psychiatric diseases. For instance, studies show a direct correlation between poverty and cognitive impairment, meaning that economic and social determinants are intricately associated with the identification of mental health within this group (Kocakaya et al., 2023). In addition, ongoing active engagement of patients in social activities can enhance psychological resilience to counteract depression and anxiety symptoms. Evaluating these social indicators, along with clinical symptoms, enables psychiatrists to formulate a comprehensive and effective treatment plan that ultimately enhances the quality of mental health care offered to elderly individuals (Figure 12.6).

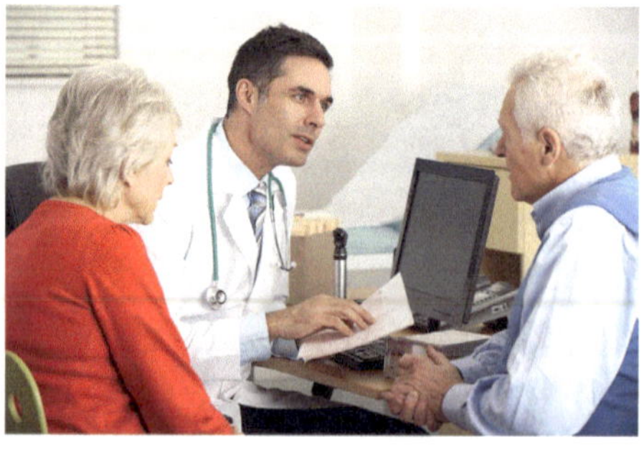

Figure 12.6. Assessment and diagnosis in the elderly.

Source: https://www.uhhospitals.org/-/media/images/blog/2015/07/screening-every-older-adult-should-get.jpg.

12.2.1. Challenges in Diagnosing Mental Illness in Older Adults

The complications of making a diagnosis of mental illness in older people are then compounded by other interconnected factors, one of which is the co-morbid overlap between psychiatric symptoms and illnesses. Geriatric patients, on the other hand, will often have concomitant chronic illnesses , such as heart disease, diabetes, or neurological illnesses, which mask, mimic, or confuse psychiatric symptoms. This diagnostic overshadowing thus represents an important challenge to healthcare practitioners as they navigate the intricate interplay between physical and psychological well-being. For instance, depression among the elderly may be confused with underlying physical illnesses, leading to misdiagnosis or delayed diagnosis. Further, older adults do not report psychological suffering because of stigma or the belief that it forms part of aging, making it challenging to establish diagnoses. There is also a barrier in the heterogeneity of symptom expression in older persons. Psychiatric conditions , such as depression, anxiety, and dementia, will manifest differently in the elderly than in younger individuals. Older persons, for example, may express less pronounced emotional presentations, which would be confused with cognitive impairment or normal aging processes. As mental illness is also a frequent symptom of dementia, clinicians must possess an advanced understanding of the ways these illnesses manifest differently among older patients. Additionally, cognitive impairment can also be an obstacle to the assessment process, as older people may not be able to verbalize their thoughts or feelings due to forgetfulness or confusion. All these pose greater challenges to the need for advanced training in geriatric psychiatry to achieve optimal diagnostic precision and, with it, corresponding treatment plans. The increasing prevalence of Alzheimer's disease among the elderly makes these diagnoses even more complicated. An estimated 6.7 million Americans aged 65 and older suffer from Alzheimer's, projected to increase exponentially over the next few decades and highlighting the desperate need for effective diagnostic and treatment techniques (Gautam et al, 2022). Given the intersecting symptomatologies of Alzheimer's and other psychiatric conditions, mental health clinicians must be competent to distinguish among these diseases, particularly in terms of the described relationship between somatic illness and suicidal thoughts among older adults (Mellqvist et al., 2015). It matters since incorrect or incomplete diagnoses lead to misplaced therapies, thereby worsening overall well-being and life quality. The convergence of these factors mandates that geriatric psychiatry must be a multidimensional, multidisciplinary specialty with a focus on holistic, individualized assessment to traverse the complexities involved in diagnosing mental illness in older people.

12.2.2. Tools and Techniques of Assessment

Assessment of the health condition of the elderly is of paramount importance in geriatric psychiatry, as it will enable care providerrs to provide interventions that are responsive to the unique needs of this population. Several instruments and methods have been created to support comprehensive assessments, with attention given to many areas , including physical health, mental health, and social functioning. Standardized assessments, including the Geriatric Depression Scale (GDS) and the Confusion Assessment Method (CAM), are powerful instruments that enable clinicians to screen for common psychiatric illnesses in geriatric patients. Utilizing these measures can lead to early identification of such conditions as depression and delirium, common among geriatric populations and with significant impacts on overall health outcomes. Early detection, coupled with adequate follow-up, can improve the quality of life for elderly patients, and therefore, effective assessment tools are a must in geriatric psychiatry practice (Gaikwad et al., 2025). In addition to formal screening instruments, careful examination always involves a multidisciplinary style, making use of the specialist expertise of various healthcare professionals. Multidisciplinary models with geriatricians, psychiatrists, nurses, and social workers can help in arriving at an integrated understanding of an older adult's health. A model, such as the Geriatric Recovery and Enhancement Alliance in Trauma (GREAT) demonstrates the benefit of an interprofessional process. With standardized processes, including screening tool use and specialty consultation, this program best addresses the combined needs of older trauma patients. Notably, through engagement of various stakeholders and ongoing monitoring of care processes, the GREAT initiative demonstrates how carefully designed assessment frameworks can maximize identification and treatment of geriatric psychiatric disorders and subsequently minimize complications and improve functional outcomes in elderly patients (Widder et al., 2021). The employment of tools and evaluation methods in geriatric psychiatry is not merely an issue of enhancing clinical outcomes, but also a form of quality assurance in health care systems. Regular assessment facilitates the identification of care deficiencies, which necessitate early intervention in accordance with the evolving needs of elderly patients. For instance, the creation of the geriatric trauma navigator role in the GREAT initiative indicates the necessity to constantly evaluate and update care practice. By monitoring relevant performance measures as well as through utilization of screening tools, healthcare providers can streamline their strategies to address patient needs more effectively, particularly in continually evolving areas like geriatric trauma and mental health treatment. Thus, application of rigorous evaluation methods ultimately fosters a culture of continuous improvement and all-around enhanced effectiveness in geriatric psychiatric treatment (Widder et al., 2021) (Figure 12.7).

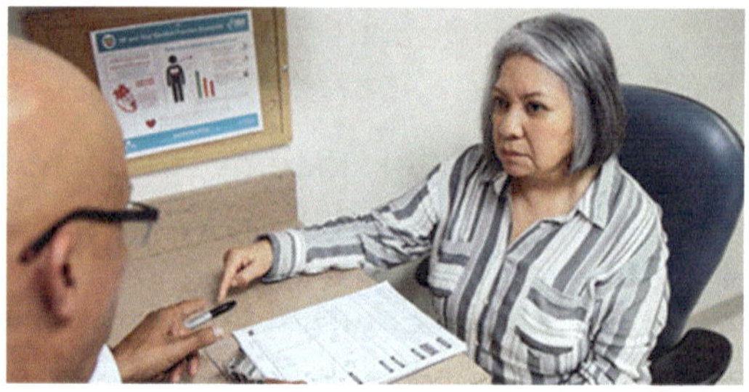

Figure 12.7. Cognitive assessment tools.

Source: https://www.alz.org/getmedia/b8afc199-0ad2-40ac-92fb-37b5d43ba20e/alzheimers-dementia-cognitive-tests-patient-assessment-teaserimage.jpg.

12.2.3. Importance of Comprehensive Evaluations

In the field of geriatric psychiatry, in-depth assessment is extremely significant to develop all-encompassing care for the patient. Comprehensive geriatric assessment (CGA) is a wide-ranging assessment of several areas of physical and cognitive and mental well-being, allowing clinicians to identify complicated health problems in older adults. By integrating various factors of evaluation, such as systemic disease conditions, cognitive functioning, and psychosocial issues, CGA encourages a highly evolved understanding of each patient's unique state of wellness. Through this multi-factor method, diagnosis of psychiatric conditions is not only essential, but treatment of co-morbid medical conditions that underlie mental health challenges is also imperative. With the aging population on the rise, applying CGA models is necessary in order to personalize treatment plans that align with individual patient needs, enhancing overall health outcomes and improving quality of life among this vulnerable group (Wongiam et al., 2025). In addition, detailed evaluations are of main importance in the management of malnutrition and other health-related hazards affecting the majority of older individuals. The overlooked malnutrition may lead to severe complications and negatively impact mental status and cognitive function. Through the implementation of CGA, healthcare providers can systematically assess nutrition status, comorbidities, and social determinants affecting diet.

For instance, as discussed in a case presentation, CGA recognized severe hypernatremia and malnutrition in an older hospitalized patient and thus enabled the development of a targeted nutrition intervention plan. Such a forward-looking approach not only addressed acute medical conditions but also caregiver training for continued nutritional care upon discharge. Effective early identification of conditions such as malnutrition, underscores the significance of CGA in the formulation of preventive strategies and enhancing the quality of life of complex, interrelated older patients with health issues (Park et al., 2025). Furthermore, coordination with multidisciplinary groups is key to the effectiveness of comprehensive geriatric psychiatry evaluations. Several healthcare providers, including physicians, nurses, dietitians, and social workers, contribute their skill sets to the evaluation process. This coordination enables the combination of all the parts of a patient's health in an attempt to provide individualized and comprehensive treatment plans. The recognition of mental health, physical health, and environmental considerations as interacting entities is the foundation for successful management of the multifaceted health profile of the elderly. Observations gained from team-oriented CGA sessions underlie treatment plans that are not only clinically appropriate but also address social and psychological concerns. Finally, this collaborative approach constructs a system of care that is adaptive to the complexities of geriatric psychiatry, consequently improving treatment outcomes and patient satisfaction (Wongiam et al., 2025).

Test Your Knowledge

1. How do clinicians differentiate between age-related cognitive decline and pathological conditions like dementia or delirium?
2. What assessment tools and screening tests are commonly used to evaluate mental health in older adults?

12.3. Treatment Approaches

Learning Outcome

1. Psychopharmacology in geriatric psychiatry.
2. Psychotherapy options for older adults.
3. Integrative and holistic treatment methods.

In geriatric psychiatry, treatment approaches must take into account the unique complexities of aged populations. Maybe the most pressing of these is the effective management of cognitive disorders, such as Alzheimer's disease (AD). The rapidly growing prevalence of AD requires that treatment models follow emerging research. Current interventions usually incorporate pharmacologic as well as non-pharmacologic interventions. Pharmacotherapeutic treatments try to modify the pathophysiological processes of AD, while psychosocial therapy, including cognitive behavioral therapy (CBT) and social interaction, is of maximal value in enhancing quality of life in affected patients. This integrated approach not only addresses the clinical manifestations of dementia but also lessens the psychosocial load, making treatment more acceptable for both caregivers and patients, eventually enhancing their overall well-being (N/A, 2023). Furthermore, older adults' treatment modalities during the COVID-19 pandemic present special challenges. Social isolation caused by this global crisis has affected the elderly disproportionately, with exacerbated psychiatric symptoms and declining cognitive health. Clinicians have grown to increasingly accept the need for adaptive care with flexibility, such as the implementation of telehealth services. Teletherapy not only increases access but also helps to reach patients who may struggle to manage traditional face-to-face visits. Innovative modalities, such as virtual support groups and online cognitive training, were found to relieve loneliness and social connectedness. Recognition of these shifts in the delivery of treatment is important in optimizing care response capabilities in geriatric psychiatry, specifically under the demanding conditions of the pandemic, which has deeply reordered the pattern of delivery of healthcare services (Ipsit, 2020). Incorporating family support in treatment plans also seems to be an essential concern for geriatric psychiatry. Engagement of families can provide a second line of care and emotional support to older patients with psychiatric illnesses. Family interventions not only enhance therapeutic intervention participation but also equip caregivers with the skills to support their relatives. Caregiver education programs have the goal of minimizing the emotional anguish for family members, ultimately creating better control of the patient's condition. This role consideration by the caregivers highlights the need for holistic strategies that go beyond the patient for enhancing the treatment environment in geriatric psychiatry. With ongoing research being conducted that further brings out the complex dynamics of family involvement in mental health care, an increasingly nuanced understanding can help in the development of tailored interventions that address the issues of patients and their families comprehensively (Gautam et al., 2022).

12.3.1. Psychopharmacology in Geriatric Psychiatry

The intricate realm of psychopharmacology holds significant significance in geriatric psychiatry, wherein physiological changes related to aging can influence the safety and efficacy of psychopharmacologic drugs. As the elderly patient typically has a comorbid medical condition, drug pharmacokinetics as well as pharmacodynamics may be vastly influenced. Elderly patients are prone to altered drug absorption, metabolism, and excretion, and thus, the process of prescribing must be rigorous and individualized. This is made more complex by the threat of polypharmacy, whereby patients are taking multiple drugs together that may cause adverse drug effects. Hence, geriatric psychiatrists need to carefully assess the benefit and risk parameters of psychopharmacological interventions in a manner that the drugs prescribed fall within the differential health factors and psychological needs of their patients. Understanding of these factors is essential to the facilitation of effective and safe treatment interventions for mental health conditions in older adults. The growing interest in new therapeutic strategies, particularly the application of psychedelics in geriatric psychiatry, has opened new doors to the treatment of treatment-resistant mental health conditions. Agents , such as psilocybin and MDMA have shown potential to treat such diseases as treatment-resistant depression and PTSD, particularly among the elderly who may be refractory to traditional antidepressants. Psychedelics , such as these bind to the serotonergic receptors, altering cognitive function and emotional behavior at their fundamental level, an action that may enhance neuroplasticity and overall mental health in older individuals. Interestingly, research indicates that the chemicals can lead to long-term changes in a matter of a few sessions for certain patients versus chronic medication with conventional therapies. However, the legal circumstances and potential risks in terms of increasing anxiety or cardiovascular issues imply that some serious deliberations must occur as to their application in clinics. (Shafique et al., 2025) Also, treatment engagement is a central aspect of geriatric psychiatry psychopharmacology because older adults typically face barriers that can discourage them from accessing care. The Raue and Sirey treatment engagement model highlights the importance of addressing individual and societal factors that influence patients' interactions with mental health care.

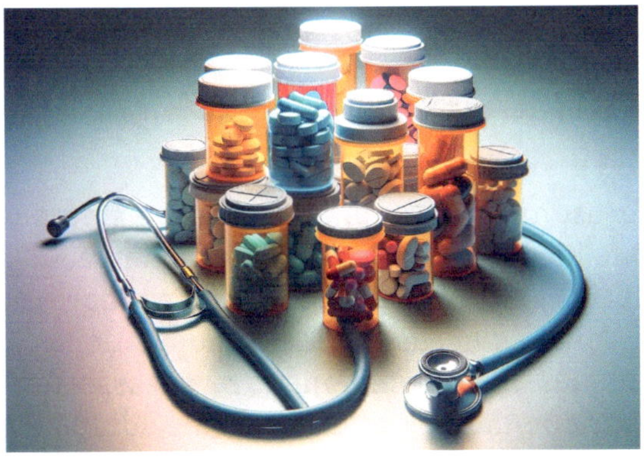

Figure 12.8. Psychopharmacology in geriatric psychiatry.

Source: https://external-content.duckduckgo.com/iu/?u=https%3A%2F%2Fpsychiatrynurses.com%2F_next%2Fimage%2F%3Furl%3Dhttps%3A%252F%252Fcdn.sanity.io%252Fimages%252Faire1hmi%252Fproduction% 252F3616c3ab85d562e70ae4b0e56fe27f427b3301cd-1792x1024.webp%253Fw%253D1792%2526q%253D100%2526auto %253Dformat %26w%3D3840%26q%3D100&f=1&nofb=1&ipt=069dcf469188cf0d1afdc5f60392ca6c2a3416a6cedf7 d6ed0f0be7cfb6a47b9.

Mental illness stigma and age bias can dissuade older patients from receiving treatment that they require, leading to passivity in terms of accepting their illnesses. Treatment expectation and decision-making themes displayed through interviews among older outpatients suggest that enhancing mental health literacy and psychoeducation has the potential to significantly increase patient involvement. By increasing knowledge and awareness of treatment approaches, medical professionals are better placed to support older adults in treating their mental health problems, ultimately leading to better outcomes in geriatric psychiatry. (Rosario et al., 2024) (Figure 12.8).

12.3.2. Psychotherapy Options for Older Adults

Psychotherapy is a core treatment strategy in geriatric psychiatry for the unique mental health issues of older adults. With this population of individuals increasingly struggling with loss, chronic illness, and isolation, evidence-based therapies are vital interventions in the toolkit of mental health professionals. Cognitive Behavioral Therapy (CBT) is an exceptionally powerful intervention, particularly for conditions like depression and anxiety. This goal-oriented, systematic treatment method assists older adults in reconditioning toxic thought patterns, enhancing their coping skills, and developing resilience against life's stresses. Additionally, techniques , such as supportive therapy and mindfulness have also been found to help promote emotional regulation and overall well-being among older adults, thereby maximizing their quality of life and a sense of self-efficacy in navigating their twilight years. In the presence of the pressing demand for effective therapeutic measures, coordination between medication management and psychotherapy is a novel avenue for elderly individuals with complex psychiatric disease. The highly developed pharmacological landscape demands wise scrutiny by virtue of the changes in drug metabolism relative to age, with relevance to efficacy as much as to safety. For instance, elderly individuals are possibly more susceptible to certain medications and therefore need individualized doses and stringent monitoring. Psychotherapy may be employed to enhance the effectiveness of pharmacotherapy by addressing underlying psychological causes of stress that, in turn, may potentially worsen symptoms. Evidence has indicated that the addition of psychotherapy with pharmacological interventions not only improves symptom remission but also leads to higher rates of treatment adherence, as individuals become more engaged in their recovery process. The combined modality underscores the value of the application of collaborative care models within geriatric psychiatry. As the field advances, studies continue to uncover creative psychotherapeutic techniques that may be particularly useful with older adults. For instance, technology-assisted interventions like teletherapy have expanded access to mental health treatment, enabling participants who may have mobility challenges or logistical concerns to be effectively reached by therapy.

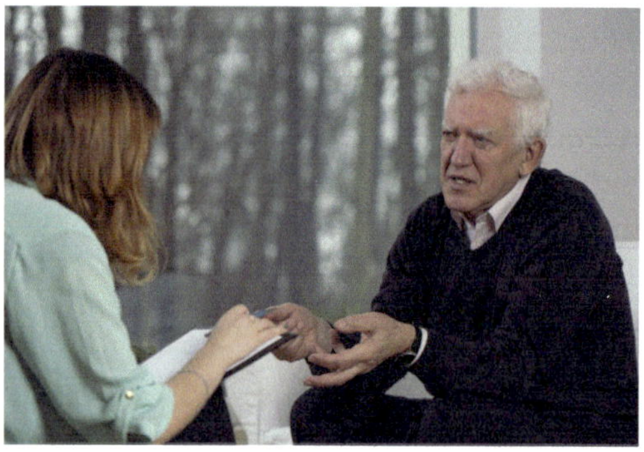

Figure 12.9. Psychotherapy options for older adults.

Source: https://external-content.duckduckgo.com/iu/?u=https%3A%2F%2Fmantracare.org%2Fwp-content%2Fuploads%2F2021%2F12%2FSupportive-Psychotherapy-Geriatric-Counseling.jpg&f=1&nofb=1&ipt=dc1e55d672fbc4230283aef4067a131c35addf48951622729a9aee2bd673192c.

Also, the recent emphasis on utilizing neuromodulation techniques, including Electroconvulsive Therapy (ECT) and Transcranial Magnetic Stimulation (TMS), underscores the potential to enhance standard psychotherapy in the management of extreme psychiatric illness, particularly in older adults who are not responsive to regular treatments (Gautam et al., 2022). Likewise, treatment protocols specifically aimed at addressing bipolar disorder in late life mirror the necessity for integrated approaches that encompass psychotherapeutic practices and psychopharmacologic therapies (Ljubic et al., 2023). Through amplification of interdisciplinary collaboration and incorporation of innovative modalities, geriatric psychiatry can make a real impact on the mental health of elderly persons (Figure 12.9).

12.3.3. Integrative and Holistic Treatment Methods

The use of holistic and alternative treatment modalities in geriatric psychiatry is increasingly valued today as an effective way of addressing the complex needs of elderly populations. The therapies most commonly are an assortment of various therapy modalities, including music therapy, art therapy, and pet therapy, all aimed at optimizing mental health and promoting emotional well-being. For instance, music therapy has been found to be effective for the reduction of depression and anxiety symptoms in older adults. Despite this, studies reveal a concerning deficit in intervention report quality, with less than 50% of the studies reporting on vital details , such as interventionist qualifications and treatment fidelity. This lack of standardization not only slows down the validity of outcomes but also presents obstacles in employing these treatments clinically (Allison et al., 2018). Establishment of better guidelines and uniform language is required for the advancement of employing music therapy in geriatric mental health treatment. Similarly, pet therapy has evolved as an adjuvant treatment for older patients suffering from mental health issues. The existing literature review indicates that interaction with therapy animals can lead to significant mood enhancement and symptom reduction of depression and anxiety symptoms (Pfeiffer et al., 2017). Promising as it is, pet therapy remains in short supply of robust evidence, with the majority of studies being methodologically poor. Anecdotal return and clinical observation prove its worth, but the lack of standardized studies restricts its widespread acceptance among psychiatrists. To support the utilization of pet therapy within treatment settings, there is a need to come up with additional research studies that employ robust methodologies and obtain qualitative findings to make more informed deductions about the impact on mental health among older adults. The integration of integrative and holistic treatment approaches into geriatric psychiatry offers varied therapeutic options and also honors a person-centered approach that respects the diverse experiences and personal preferences of older adults. This movement towards a more inclusive treatment approach recognizes the multi-dimensional basis of mental health and cares for not just the physiological aspects but also addresses the emotional, social, and spiritual needs. For instance, successful treatment with such therapies requires interdisciplinary coordination among caregivers to guarantee that the treatments are tailored to personal requirements. Ultimately, better reporting standards and research quality in holistic interventions will establish a more distinct understanding of their role in geriatric psychiatry and thus open the door to improved care and quality of life among the aging (Pfeiffer et al., 2017).

Test Your Knowledge

1. How do pharmacological treatments for older adults differ from those used in younger populations due to age-related physiological changes?
2. What roles do psychotherapy, cognitive stimulation, and lifestyle interventions play in managing mental health issues in the elderly?

12.4. The Role of Caregivers

Learning Outcome

1. Support systems for caregivers.
2. Training and resources for caregivers.
3. Impact of caregiving on mental health.

In geriatric psychiatry, caregivers are most important because they are essential support systems of the elderly individuals who suffer from mental illnesses. Caregivers provide necessary assistance not only in everyday activities but also in meeting the emotional and psychological needs of their loved ones. Their involvement can significantly contribute to the overall welfare of the aging, particularly those who are battling with diseases , such as dementia, depression, or anxiety. The stressors that caregivers undergo that influence their moods can hinder their performance in caring for their loved ones appropriately, a is why mental health interventions that address them are vital. Successful caregiver assistance can result in enhanced mental and physical health for both caregivers and the elderly, highlighting the mutual dependency of their well-being in this complex caregiving relationship. Thus, caregivers needs must be understood and addressed to promote enhanced psychiatric health for geriatric populations. Additionally, the COVID-19 pandemic has further magnified the issues faced by caregivers in the geriatric psychiatric context. As the hospitals were busy taking care of complex patients, informal home care has grown, and emphasis has been directed towards home-based caregiving assistance. Caregivers who have been mentioned to struggle with the burden of care delivery in their homes have been reported to have suffered more psychological distress and lack knowledge on health care requirements in this public health crisis. Informal caregivers who are not trained have also been required to master changing healthcare protocols under a short time frame, often without proper training or assistance. Understanding such dynamics is crucial since caregivers' health directly influences the quality of patient care. It is thus necessary to develop interventions and materials specifically for caregivers during crisis situations , such as COVID-19, to ensure the quality of geriatric psychiatric care (Gautam et al., 2022).

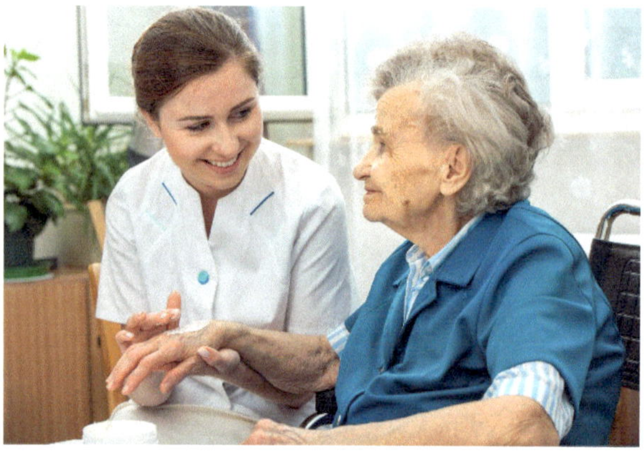

Figure 12.10. The role of caregivers for older adults.

Source: https://external-content.duckduckgo.com/iu/?u=https%3A%2F%2Fwww.optimumcareltd.co.uk%2Fwp-content%2Fuploads%2F2021%2F08%2Fpersonal-care.jpg&f=1&nofb=1&ipt=3a9202ba65c059f8024e9fe7df062276bf139794e54ed484fd26c386b08bc048.

The caregiving setting not only highlights the importance of caregiver support but also indicates the influence of the caregiver-patient relationship on treatment effectiveness. A quality caregiver relationship may facilitate easier compliance with treatment timing and patient compliance in general, leading to better control of psychiatric conditions prevalent in the elderly. The double burden on caregivers requires top-priority attention from the medical fraternity, as they lack proper support and recognition within the health care system. Health systems can, in turn, improve the quality of care for geriatric patients by integrating interventions that foster caregiver resilience through initiatives , such as training programs and mental health services. As geriatric psychiatry advances, addressing the complexities of caregiver roles will be crucial in working towards integrative mental health care for the aging (Chan et al., 2020) (Figure 12.10).

12.4.1. Support Systems for Caregivers

Among the areas of geriatric psychiatry, caregiver support systems' significance is more than ever before recognized as integral to enhancing the quality of care offered to older patients, and especially to those with mental illness. Caregiving can be stressful and continually imposes physical and emotional strain on relatives who are tasked with such activities. This can be further magnified when the caregivers themselves are elderly, as they may have their own health concerns to contend with. As research has demonstrated, caregiver stress is largely about undesirable psychological outcomes, including depression and anxiety. For that reason, formalizing systems—, such as respite care, educational programs, and counseling services, can mitigate these stressors and make for a more resilient caregiving arrangement. By identifying the necessity of such support systems, healthcare systems are themselves better equipped to prepare caregivers for responses to the needs of the elderly and thus achieve improved overall outcomes for care. Support systems are also essential not only for alleviating caregiver burden but for addressing the particular needs of particular populations within geriatric psychiatry. For instance, the caregivers who are caring for severely mentally ill patients, such as schizophrenics, have unique needs that need unique support approaches. An empirical study of older caregiver participants found significant levels of emotional distress, with 72% of the participants having moderate to severe burden and 46% having moderate to severe depression. This emphasizes the importance of inclusive support systems that not only take care of the patient's needs but also value caregiver mental health and well-being highly (Johnson et al., 2019).

These systems can include family therapy sessions and peer support groups where caregivers can share experiences and coping strategies, thereby increasing resilience in the caregiving process and enhancing the well-being of both the caregivers and the care recipients. Finally, the use of technology in care support systems presents a potential point of entry for expanding resources to caregivers. Computer-based systems can offer valuable assets , such as scheduling, medical reminders, and access to educational materials that equip caregivers with the knowledge and skills needed to handle complicated care demands. Also, online support forums and discussion groups can provide emotional support and friendship for the caregivers who might otherwise be lonely in their task. Telehealth access can also provide ready access to healthcare professionals so that caregivers are easily able to get timely advice without the inconvenience of traveling. With the utilization of technology, support systems can be made more accessible and personalized, allowing the caregivers to maintain their own well-being while still providing productive care to the elderly (Kotecha, 2022). Such innovations play a critical role in the development of a future where both the caregivers and their wards can thrive under the system of geriatric psychiatry.

12.4.2. Caregiver Training and Resources

The caregiver education landscape is critical to improving the quality of care for the elderly population, particularly in geriatric psychiatry. Caregivers frequently encounter new challenges as they work to address the complex conditions of aging patients, especially those with mental illness. As identified by research, ongoing education and assistance are the solution to enabling caregivers with the competencies and information needed to manage the shifting expectations of their jobs. Effective training programs with evidence-based practices can enhance care coordination and patient outcomes. It also assists in ensuring an environment where caregivers can have access to relevant resources to enable resilience and coping mechanisms necessary for their stressful work. According to evidence, effective training attention will optimize caregiver competency, which subsequently will optimize the overall health and well-being of older psychiatric patients. The need for specially tailored resources for caregivers has also increased due to the extensive demographic and socioeconomic representation of caregiving participants. Diversity in the caregiving participants' experiences makes extensive programs necessary. Customised resources aimed at various categories of caregivers—, such as those who are looking after people with cultural, ethnic, or age-related needs, can make caregiver education more inclusive. For example, interventions that focus on older caregivers' specific issues or hard-to-reach groups like BAME and LGBT communities are imperative. These customized programs not only enhance the capabilities of caregivers but also validate their practice, appreciating the complexity of the job. Furthermore, a targeted caregiver training program and allocation of resources can result in a higher competency and confidence level in caregivers, subsequently resulting in improved patient care in geriatric psychiatry (Henwood et al., 2017). Besides, the use of cooperative platforms among caregivers, healthcare professionals, and policymakers may promote the design of caregiver training programs and capacity. According to discussions in the literature, evidence-based policies can promote improvements in caregiver support systems. For instance, the incorporation of caregiver training modules into the study of health care can ensure that future practitioners will be qualified enough to recognize and address the issues faced by caregivers. Examination of the partnerships between research institutions and community-based organizations can make knowledge gaps easier to bridge and major resources more available. Such collaborative efforts are imperative in building a robust support system for caregivers, thereby strengthening the effectiveness of the healthcare workforce. Lastly, there is a need to advance the caregivers' training and support in ensuring high-quality, humane care for older persons, particularly their psychiatric needs (Morton et al., 2015) (Figure 12.11).

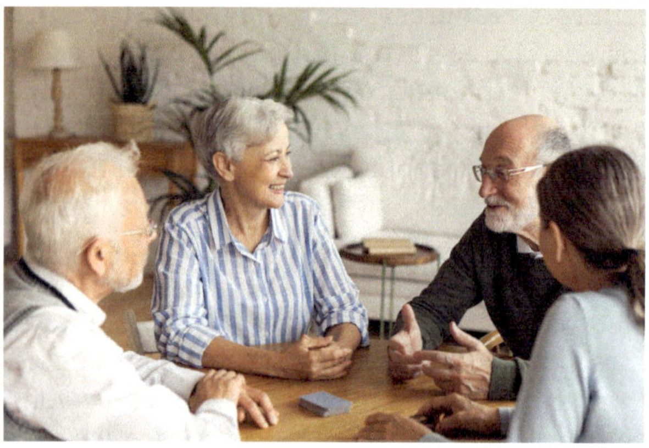

Figure 12.11. Training and resources for caregivers of older adults.

Source: https://external-content.duckduckgo.com/iu/?u=https%3A%2F%2Fallsaintsseniorliving.com%2Fwp-content%2Fuploads%2F2023%2F04%2FHow-Social-Connections-Keep-Seniors-Healthy-Hero.jpg&f=1&nofb=1&ipt=89e4049d5ebfba6e8d659841c673178b90a8f5d57e14195c8adbabe72c1a482a.

12.4.3. Impact of Caregiving on Mental Health

The caregiving function for the elderly can profoundly influence caregivers' mental health. Research suggests that individuals who assume the care of aging relatives are likely to exhibit high levels of stress, anxiety, and depression symptoms. Caregivers are often overwhelmed with demands, and that could lead to emotional exhaustion, social isolation, and neglect of health needs. With rising caregiving demands, particularly among informal caregivers, the psychological impact can become cumulative. This impact has taken center stage, especially during periods of crisis , such as the COVID-19 pandemic, that left many caregivers in prolonged and high levels of caregiving without adequate support. Caregiving's nature highlights the demand for interventions that are specific in lowering caregivers' mental health loads as well as boosting their own wellness in the area of geriatric psychiatry (Rahimi et al., 2025). Caregivers' support interventions are crucial in reducing the psychological impacts of caregiving. A recent online intervention study measured the outcomes of mental health among unpaid caregivers and found small but significant reductions in depression, anxiety, and stress scores over time. This reduction was not statistically significant but highlights the necessity of new support systems that cater to caregiver mental well-being. Having available structured educational resources and peer support forums can empower caregivers to manage their mental health effectively. These interventions, if specifically directed to address the specific needs of this group, can assist not only in decreasing psychological distress but also in increasing overall caregiving satisfaction and effectiveness. In integrating these strategies, geriatric psychiatry can play a key role in enhancing healthier caregiving settings (Rahimi et al., 2025). Secondarily, caregiving's mental health must be placed within the broader geriatric care context of balancing caregivers' and care recipients' psychological needs. The emotional challenges that are faced with aging, such as the existential pain of approaching end-of-life, also burden caregivers inordinately. Empowering caregivers emotionally through the engagement of religious and spiritual counseling can prove highly therapeutic and resilient. These interventions may enhance depressive and lonely mood and provide the individual with a sense of direction. These holistic initiatives address the interplay between mental health, spiritual well-being, and social connectivity. With the growing populations of elders, incorporating religious support in geriatric mental health models is increasingly significant towards promoting better overall outcomes for caregivers and their aging patients, pointing out the complex caregiving dynamics within the scope of geriatric psychiatry.

Test Your Knowledge

1. How do caregivers support daily functioning, emotional well-being, and treatment adherence in older adults with mental health conditions?
2. What challenges do caregivers face when managing behavioral or cognitive symptoms in elderly individuals?

12.5. Ethical Considerations

Learning Outcome

1. Informed consent and autonomy.
2. Confidentiality issues in geriatric care.
3. Addressing ageism in mental health treatment.

Ethical considerations in geriatric psychiatry are paramount in preserving the dignity and well-being of elderly patients, particularly neurocognitive disorder patients , such as dementia. Autonomy versus protective interventions is one of the core ethical challenges. Autonomy can be challenging for patients to communicate due to the fact that cognitive decline impedes decision-making abilities, and healthcare providers then have to take into account surrogate decision-makers. This reliance raises ethical issues about respecting the autonomy of patients while simultaneously ensuring their best interests are paramount in priority. Health care teams must embrace strategies in shared decision-making that involve the patients and their families and loved ones and establish an environment where individuals have room to make their decisions and informed decisions are made, hence enhancing the quality of geriatric mental health care. Furthermore, the integration of palliative care in the geriatric psychiatry specialty brings to the forefront significant ethical considerations involving end-of-life issues. Particularly in the scenario of chronic illness with neurocognitive disorder, the ethical principle of non-maleficence—avoiding causing harm—is the primary concern. The COVID-19 pandemic has emphasized these ethical concerns since patients with late-stage dementia were subjected to extensive hospitalizations that generally degraded their quality of life. An institution of a palliative care model within the geriatric care setting will serve to counteract this by making goal-of-care discussions and discussion of treatment preferences feasible among healthcare professionals, even when curative interventions are not appropriate (Cristina et al., 2021). The establishment of clear advance directives and quality communication about patients' desires regarding life-sustaining interventions comes into play in maintaining their dignity and avoiding incongruence with individualized values. Furthermore, health system problems within hospitals can further exacerbate ethical problems in geriatric psychiatry. Prompt diagnosis and effective treatment of individuals suffering from dementia are inadequate in most health systems, and treatment is delayed, which could alleviate suffering and improve quality of life (Gautam et al., 2022). The ethical implications of such system failures are profound, in that they can limit patients' ability to plan their futures and engage in decision-making about care. Resolution of these system issues requires not only a focus on enhancing diagnosis pathways but also stakeholder engagement in order to ensure ethical resource allocation. In recognizing the rich ethical landscape of geriatric psychiatry, healthcare providers are better able to negotiate the care complexities, ensuring that justice, beneficence, and respect for patient autonomy in practice are preserved.

12.5.1. Informed Consent and Autonomy

In geriatric psychiatry, principles of patient autonomy and informed consent have significant roles in treatment, particularly when addressing the complex problems of the elderly. Because of the cognitive impairments typical of this population, health care providers must tread a fine line between safeguarding patients' rights and well-being. In the past, medicine was more paternalistic, with the health care providers making decisions on behalf of patients while eroding their autonomy. But the modern focus on patient-centered care is an emphasis that patients ought to be informed of their treatment options and make well-informed decisions about their mental health care, particularly with regard to consent for treatment that has a very significant impact on their quality of life, such as medication management and psychosocial therapies. Good communication and education are therefore key to the informed consent process, making sure that the values and preferences of older patients are respected and become a part of their care plans. Informed consent in geriatric psychiatry also involves a nuanced understanding of the concept of capacity, and this can differ according to patients with different psychiatric illnesses. The assessment of decision-making capacity is of most importance since it directly influences the patients' ability to participate in their care and the validity of the informed consent that has been obtained. For instance, elderly patients with cognitive impairment will be unable to process information or express their will, thus making the process of consent challenging. Consequently, mental health professionals will be required to use methods of capacity assessment that take account not only of cognitive ability but also of social situation and overall welfare. Furthermore, the relationship between capacity and autonomy is emphasized by the necessity to foster caring cultures in which patients can contribute effectively to treatment discussions. By promoting an environment under which patients can be transparent with their wishes, clinicians can impose autonomy and respect for individuals as principles in geriatric mental healthcare. With enhanced medical innovations, such as cardiac implantable electronic devices, come additional pathways to informed consent through the imposition of new cybersecurity risks that older patients cannot fully comprehend. Since technology is now so embedded within health care, it is essential that patients are informed about potential risks—both medical and technological. Health professionals have a moral obligation to incorporate information on such risks into the process of informed consent so that patients can make fully informed decisions (Leanne et al., 2024). Since cyber-attacks pose a significant threat to the privacy and integrity of medical devices, no option should be weighed lightly in geriatrics, where the acceptance and faith in healthcare systems play an important role. Engaging patients in a dialogue that outlines these risks enhances patients' capabilities to take control of their health decisions, thereby supporting autonomy and being compatible with prevailing ethical standards in medical practice (Leanne et al., 2024). With advancing fields, it is essential to constantly re-examine and modify informed consent procedures to meet new challenges and maintain the autonomy of older patients effectively (Figure 12.12).

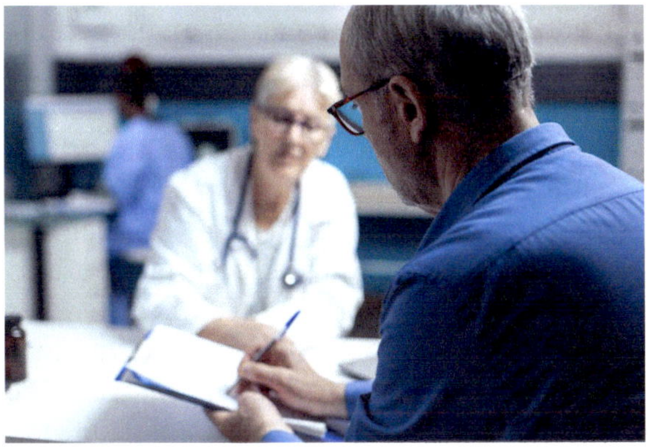

Figure 12.12. Informed consent and autonomy for older adults.

Source: https://external-content.duckduckgo.com/iu/?u=https%3A%2F%2Fwww.intelycare.com%2Fwp-content%2Fuploads%2F2024%2F11%2Fnurses-role-in-informed-consent.jpg&f=1&nofb=1&ipt=29c68bad4814a0f6844d79722bfd83d7c0ed24debac656250bef5142f640ea9f.

12.5.2. Confidentiality Issues in Geriatric Care

Confidentiality is also very difficult to maintain in gerontological care due to the multifaceted needs of older adults and the often multicomponent environments in which they are treated. Since older adults have multiple physical and mental illnesses, internal dynamics between families, caregivers, and health teams must be negotiated by care providers. This complexity is exacerbated when working with delicate matters , such as mental illnesses like depression, which are prevalent among older populations. Belief in thriving at advanced ages can be influenced by confidentiality being upheld during clinical sessions. Literature shows that practitioners working with older patients must be careful regarding their attitudes towards geriatric patients since these will influence patient disclosure and the effectiveness of treatment. By building a culture of understanding and trust, practitioners can maximize the practice of confidentiality and hence enhance the quality of care afforded to older patients. Legal and ethical obligations of confidentiality in geriatric psychiatry require meticulous adherence to guidelines that keep patient information secure without undermining the needs of holistic care. Health workers must be attuned to when breaching confidentiality might be required, such as where there is suspected abuse or threatened patient safety. This action, however, must be balanced thoughtfully against the potential impact on the patient-caretaker therapeutic relationship. Evidence shows that older adults may have privacy issues with their confidentiality, particularly when it comes to mental problems, which may restrict how far they are willing to receive treatment. It is thus crucial that there are learning activities aimed at increasing the extent of knowledge about confidentiality and its impacts among medical professionals. This may lead to better care and diagnostic capacities, particularly in recognizing and dealing with conditions like depression among such vulnerable individuals (Le et al., 2009). Furthermore, literature emphasizes the importance of integrating patient-centered practices in managing confidentiality in geriatric care. Patient agency can be established to facilitate older individuals to actively engage in health discussions, thus enhancing outcomes. Concerning the interplay between mental health, satisfaction with life, and social factors , such as loneliness and bereavement, it is evident that maintaining confidentiality is essential. Previous studies have cited correlations between higher depression risk and loneliness in older individuals, citing the need for openly available, confidential communication channels. Moreover, as health professionals attempt to create sensitive settings attuned to the unique challenges of aging patients, an emphasis on confidentiality can be used to enhance therapeutic partnership and good care practices. To manage these complexities effectively, training investments and policy reforms are required to deal with the issue of vulnerability not impinging upon the dignity and rights of geriatric patients (Mayhew et al., 1989) (Figure 12.13).

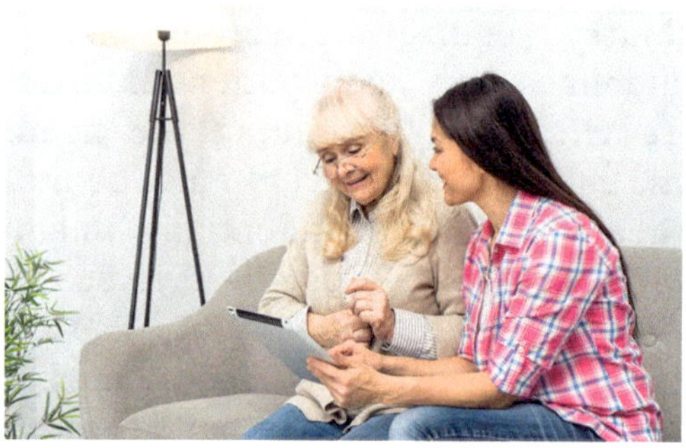

Figure 12.13. Confidentiality issues in geriatric care.

Source: https://external-content.duckduckgo.com/iu/?u=https%3A%2F%2Fcounselingchennai.com%2Fwp-content%2Fuploads%2F2023%2F04%2FGeriatric-Counselling-img.webp&f=1&nofb=1&ipt=15519469587ed959e37c81dd0485651e1e635c9849e2137dc8de3bf48bfcb198.

12.5.3. Addressing Ageism in Mental Health Treatment

Ageism remains one of the largest barriers to effective mental health treatment among older people. Such pervasive bias tends to lead to the denial of legitimate psychological problems, as mental health professionals are likely to immediately interpret aging patients in a stereotypical environment with a focus on incapacitation and decline. Older patients may then be deprived of an adequate array of quality mental health services, increasing isolation and powerlessness. For instance, alcohol use disorders among older people are under-diagnosed or ill-managed since ageist stereotypes lead to their underestimation (Prasad et al., 2024). Evading these prejudices requires intensive training and education of health professionals, with particular special focus being laid on the detection and overcoming of ageist biases to develop a more respectful mental health care environment. Moreover, the adverse effects of ageism not only include individual patients but also extend to system issues within healthcare. Mental health frameworks tend to overlook the distinct needs of older persons, particularly when adopting evidence-based interventions tailored to geriatric populations. As studies continue to highlight the importance of an integrated model of mental health, bridging the gap in care by age is more critical than ever. New research indicates that incorporating principles of positive psychiatry, where resilience and wisdom in old age are the main focus, can be used to combat stigma and enhance treatment outcomes (Reynolds et al., 2022). As clinicians promote a wider definition of geriatric psychiatry, including multidisciplinary teams and community resources, ageism needs to be actively confronted to promote the expectation that the mental health of older adults will be brought to the center rather than to the periphery. Finally, creating an empathy and awareness culture can significantly enhance the mental health care of older persons. Engaging family carers, the most common of whom bear the emotional and practical burden of managing mental illness in this population, is crucial towards creating a caring environment. By recognizing the significant role played by caregivers, healthcare systems can design interventions that address not only the psychological needs of older patients but also the health and well-being of those who care for them. Lastly, ongoing research on the cognitive wellness and mental health of older adults presents the potential for developing new strategies for eliminating ageism and promoting healthy conceptions of aging (Reynolds et al., 2022). Collectively, these may require effort to help bring a more inclusive and holistic mental health care approach where the dignity and humanness of older persons are respected for their needs.

Test Your Knowledge

1. How do issues related to autonomy, consent, and decision-making capacity impact mental health care for older adults?
2. What ethical dilemmas arise when balancing patient independence with safety, especially in cases of dementia?

12.6. Current Research and Trends

Learning Outcome

1. Advances in geriatric psychiatry.
2. The impact of technology on treatment.
3. Future directions in research.

The topic of geriatric psychiatry has seen a remarkable increase in research work during the past decade, bearing witness to the growing concerns regarding the unique mental health issues of elderly individuals. One bibliometric analysis of current research evidence evinced a 7.09% rate of annual increase, bearing witness to the accelerated interest in this critical area of inquiry among researchers. Of special note is the American Journal of Geriatric Psychiatry, the first-choice publication medium for groundbreaking work, with a range of topics from dementia to depression and psychiatric care targeted specifically to the older adult patient. This focus undoubtedly indicates the necessity of greater research concentration toward understanding and addressing the complex interaction of biological, psychological, and social determinants of mental illness in geriatric clients. Collaboration between institutions and countries is still a characteristic of these research endeavors, although in most cases, it is concentrated among a select group of powerful institutions, limiting worldwide participation in the discourse of geriatric mental health (Nwokedi, 2025). There is a particular area of worry that has taken center stage, such as the increased suicides among the elderly, a group seen to have several times the suicidal ideation compared to younger groups. Recent literature indicates that mental disorders, particularly depression, are the primary cause of heightened suicide risk in this population. A bibliometric analysis of suicide literature among the elderly showed an erratic increasing trend in published articles with a peak in 2021. The United States was a leading country in producing a substantial number of publications, with leading institutions playing a major role in spearheading massive research activity. Major journals, including the American Journal of Geriatric Psychiatry, are issuing critical research with emphasis on cultivating the utilization of certain interventions. In addition, repetitive keywords within this research indicate a growing emphasis on the identification of risk factors, diagnostic methods, and suicidal behavior prevention among older populations, thereby shaping current clinical interventions and public health initiatives (Kan et al., 2025). With the evolving practice of geriatric psychiatry, the emergence of interdisciplinary collaborations is increasingly necessary to address existing gaps in both clinical practice and research. Despite the multitude of information coming out of bibliometric studies, there are issues, such as the underrepresentation of non-English literature and the focus on quantitative indicators that can overlook qualitative dimensions of research impact. Subsequent studies need to engage a wider range of sources and methods in order to access a more comprehensive vision of the mental health environment of the older adult. In addition, guaranteeing international collaboration could widen the scope and the intensity of studies so that diverse perspectives inform the development of universal models of care. Through such limitations, the geriatric psychiatry field can move forward with the further creation of more efficient and universal treatments for mental health, eventually leading to better outcomes for an aging population faced with many psychological issues (Nwokedi, 2025).

12.6.1. Advances in Geriatric Psychiatry

New developments in the area of geriatric psychiatry have greatly enhanced our information and treatment of late-life mood and cognitive disorders. An example is the completion of the OPTIMUM study, which studied the efficacy of various augmentation strategies for treatment-resistant depression in elderly individuals. The study compared methods like switching to bupropion and augmenting with drugs , such as Lithium or nortriptyline. By evaluation of primary outcomes , such as remission rates and measures of well-being, the OPTIMUM study accentuates new interventions that are more effective and capable of reversing the unwanted effects of standard pharmacological treatment. The study accentuates the imperative of enhancing prevailing mechanisms of treatment to be in concordance with the sophistication of mental disease in old age, particularly when handling comorbidities and increasing complexity in reaction to treatment (Gautam et al., 2022). Besides mood disorders, geriatric psychiatry continues to struggle with significant problems in the field of neurocognitive disorders , such as Alzheimer's disease, where the management of apathy has become a significant concern. From existing studies on the prevalence and impact of apathy, it is evident that it significantly reduces quality of life in the affected individuals and poses an increased mortality risk. Accordingly, apathy has become a target amenable to treatment. New treatment approaches, particularly non-pharmacological interventions, are being developed to treat effectively anxiety and other behavioral symptoms of cognitive decline. For instance, research into customized cognitive-behavioral therapy and the use of virtual reality have promising avenues for treating anxiety in older adults with neurodegenerative diseases. These advancements point to a paradigm change in how the need of the older person for emotional and psychological care is addressed, going beyond traditional pharmacological intervention (Gautam et al., 2022).

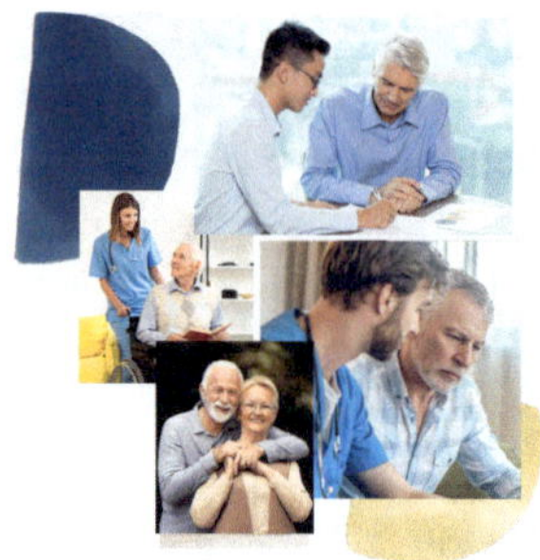

Figure 12.14. Psychiatric care in the elderly & old age.

Source: https://external-content.duckduckgo.com/iu/?u=https%3A%2F%2Fnairshospital.in%2Fwp-content%2Fuploads%2F2022%2F10%2FGeriatric-Psychiatry.jpg&f=1&nofb=1&ipt=fbcfea82f677a45f277872ce8564c5425f8fee4bdbbfa82e1b36d7b678db51f5.

The evolving landscape of geriatric psychiatry aims not only at the treatment of mental illnesses but also at the importance of successful aging and resilience in later years. Since the global population is aging, there has been a concomitant rise in mental illnesses that necessitates an integrated care system with both physical and mental health. Multidisciplinary teams offering comprehensive assessment and coordinated mental, physical, and social care have been advocated by more recent studies. The specific characteristics of older populations—overcoming ageism as well—are the reasons why it is with building a narrative that balances illness with health and resilience that support is given. Prospective research should work to enhance family caregivers' well-being while identifying moderators of treatment response heterogeneity, emphasizing the need for an integrative approach to geriatric psychiatric care that honors both the challenges and strengths inherent in aging (Figure 12.14).

12.6.2. The Impact of Technology on Treatment

The integration of technology into the treatment modalities of geriatric psychiatry has been transformative, enhancing the quality of care provided to older adults experiencing mental health issues. Telehealth services, for instance, have become increasingly vital, particularly in light of the COVID-19 pandemic, as they allow healthcare providers to reach patients in the safety of their homes. This accessibility is critical for seniors who may have mobility challenges or live in remote areas. Furthermore, technology-driven tools , such as mobile health applications facilitate ongoing monitoring of patients' mental states, enabling timely interventions. As individuals age, the prevalence of psychiatric conditions like Alzheimer's disease rises significantly, with an estimated 6.7 million seniors currently affected, a number projected to escalate to 13.8 million by 2060 without effective treatments or preventative strategies (Gautam et al., 2022). Thus, the role of innovative technologies in managing these conditions cannot be overstated. Emerging technologies in geriatric psychiatry also extend to predictive analytics, which harness machine learning and artificial intelligence to identify at-risk populations. For example, platforms that assess stress levels and emotional well-being can proactively highlight individuals who may be on the path to developing more serious mental health issues, such as depression or anxiety. Such predictive measures are essential in geriatric care, where early intervention significantly improves patient outcomes. By utilizing data-driven methods, healthcare providers can tailor their approaches to meet the unique psychological needs of older adults, ultimately fostering better recovery trajectories. The integration of these advanced technologies into practice not only streamlines care processes but also addresses the growing demand for psychiatric services, especially as the number of individuals requiring management of dementia-related conditions continues to rise (Chakraborty et al., 2023). Moreover, the financial implications of technology in geriatric psychiatry are significant, particularly in the context of the increased healthcare costs associated with mental illnesses. In 2023, estimates project that Medicare and Medicaid payments for individuals with dementia will be substantial, further underscoring the necessity for more efficient treatment methodologies (Gautam et al., 2022). The increase in healthcare spending necessitates the exploration of cost-effective technological solutions that can deliver quality care without overwhelming system resources.

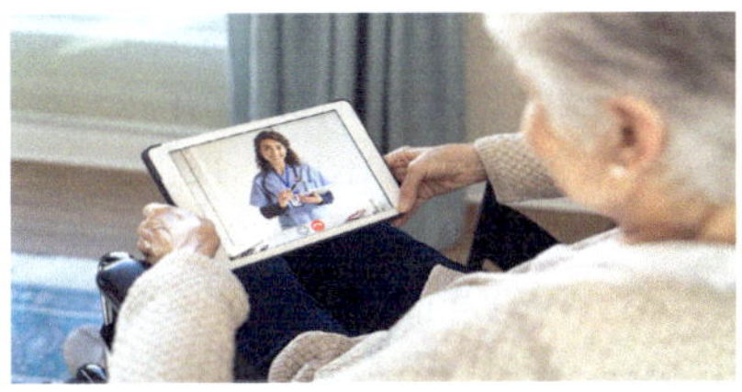

Figure 12.15. The impact of technology on treatment in geriatric psychiatry.

Source: https://external-content.duckduckgo.com/iu/?u=https%3A%2F%2Fwww.chenmed.com%2Fsites%2Fdefault%2Ffiles%2F2022-12%2F4%2520Benefits%2520of%2520Telemedicine%2520for%2520Seniors.jpg&f=1&nofb=1&ipt=09edcd17bb040738ce0d668362f6ba707dd19c1cc9b9bc83af3a65f449cb3073.

As technology continues to evolve, it holds the promise of improving not just the mental health outcomes for older adults but also the allocation of healthcare funds, ensuring that resources are utilized more effectively. This dual impact, enhancing patient care while addressing budgetary constraints, demonstrates that the embrace of technology in geriatric psychiatry could lead to a more sustainable healthcare model within this increasingly vulnerable demographic (Figure 12.15).

12.6.3. Future Directions in Research

Directions for the future of geriatric psychiatry require a concerted attention to the complex interplay between social isolation and mental illness in the elderly population. Evidence suggests that social isolation, defined by both objective, behavioral measures and subjective, self-reported experiences of loneliness, is profound in its impact on mental health, potently increasing the risk of depressive illness, anxiety disorders, and even suicidal attempts in this population. Despite the obvious connection, the mechanisms by which social isolation contributes to worsening mental illnesses are not well understood. Elucidating such relationships is important not only for the creation of specific therapeutic maneuvers but also for the optimization of currently available treatments. Future research will be needed to examine integrative methods that can tap into social connections to improve mental health outcomes, something that aligns with the National Institute of Mental Health's research agenda to transform the science of understanding and treating mental illness (Elizabeth et al., 2020). Furthermore, with aging populations increasing, particularly with an increase in those older than 65 outnumbering minors under age 18, interventions to combat Alzheimers disease provide glaring potential for research. A meta-analysis and systematic review of prevention of Alzheimers provided salient data, presenting 10 modifiable risk factors that have definitive evidence of their impact on the progression of the disease. These determinants highlight the need for future studies that assess these determinants and measure the effectiveness of comprehensive lifestyle interventions. By focusing on health behaviors like cognitive stimulation, exercise, and management of chronic diseases like hypertension and diabetes, investigators can offer evidence-based guidelines to practitioners and stakeholders in geriatric psychiatry. This direction emphasizes the necessity of bridging the gap between evidence-based research and practice, ultimately leading to the prevention of cognitive impairment, as well as enhancing quality of life in the elderly (Jin-Yu et al., 2020). In addition to bridging the gap for individual determinants, the future of geriatric psychiatric research will require a holistic examination of the biopsychosocial model. This model emphasizes the interplay between biological, psychological, and social determinants of mental health. The integration of social determinants of health into study designs could yield useful information regarding the effect of these determinants on the symptoms of mental illness as well as treatment outcomes in diverse populations. Notably, the National Institute of Mental Health's Research Domains Criteria framework emphasizes a multimensional approach that features social functioning as a vital component of mental health research. Investigating how environmental factors undermine or interact with genetic susceptibility can also illuminate the paths to mental disorder later in life, maximizing both etiology and therapeutic innovations. With advances in these avenues, it is crucial that results transfer to clinical practice to provide more effective, integrated mental health care to the elderly (Gautam et al., 2022).

Test Your Knowledge

1. How are advances in neuroimaging, genetics, and brain aging research improving understanding of late-life mental health disorders?
2. What current trends, such as digital mental health tools and community-based care models, are shaping the future of geriatric mental health?

SUMMARY

Geriatric psychiatry is increasingly becoming a field of importance to the treatment of the elderly as a whole. With the trend in demographics revealing greater numbers of older individuals susceptible to mental illnesses like depression and anxiety, it stands to reason that intervention must be developed. Research, like the inquiry into the rates and correlates of late-life depression, illuminates the complexity embedded in this elderly person's mental health picture. Despite numerous preventive measures during the last 10 years, the plateauing of depression rates underscores the necessity for innovative and comprehensive intervention approaches targeted at fostering mental well-being among the aging population (AshaRani et al., 2025). Such findings accentuate ongoing efforts at enhancing mental health care and making it both accessible and relevant to the specific situations of older people. Moreover, active engagement in treatment is an important determinant of success in geriatric psychiatric care. Raue and Sirey's theoretical model suggests the various steps involved in ensuring effective patient participation in their treatment of mental illness (Rosario et al., 2024). Higher mental health literacy, along with the reduction of stigma pertaining to mental illness among older adults, can significantly impact outcomes in treatment. It then becomes increasingly critical not only to identify mental illness but also to ensure that older adults are empowered through the treatment and referral process. Prioritizing individual and social determinants for treatment enrollment enables mental health professionals to better bridge gaps between patients and necessary services, ultimately improving overall mental health care for older adults. With these findings in mind, a comprehensive and community-based approach to geriatric psychiatry emerges as necessary in meeting the multifaceted needs of this demographic. Encouraging greater social interaction, reducing loneliness, and optimizing access to care are primary prescriptions for promoting psychological well-being in aging populations (AshaRani et al., 2025). By implementing these strategies within existing models of care, stakeholders can create an environment that supports the early detection and intervention, but also fosters resilience in older persons. Additional research must still explore the evolving needs of this population, delivering mental health care that will adapt to address the complexities of geriatric psychiatry. Lastly, collaboration between practitioners, families, and communities will be essential in realizing optimal mental health outcomes for the elderly.

In geriatric psychiatry, a particular issue of concern is elderly patients, particularly those battling multiple psychiatric disorders, and compliance with medications prescribed. Empirical findings report that patients' perceptions and attitudes towards treatment are key factors in compliance with prescribed medication regimes. For instance, a new study recently provided insightful viewpoints on how medication concerns can influence adherence behaviors in adolescents with psychiatric disorders, an experience that may parallel the same issues in the geriatric patient. Through understanding these dynamics, mental health clinicians can tailor interventions that not only address the effectiveness of medication but also enhance patient engagement and adherence. Emphasizing the necessity of considering these variables can lead to more effective treatment of the older adult with difficult medication regimens, ultimately leading to an enhanced holistic approach to the treatment of geriatric mental health. Another subject of paramount significance in geriatric psychiatry concerns the evolving dynamics of preventive interventions, particularly in vulnerable populations, for adverse mental health consequences. The recent meta-analysis and systematic review found that most active interventions, like cognitive behavioral therapy and drug therapies, lacked a robust evidence base behind them regarding their effectiveness in inhibiting progression to more serious psychiatric disorders among at-risk groups. This implies the need for newer treatment modalities specially tailored for the elderly age group. By recognizing the multiple determinants of geriatric treatment outcomes, researchers and clinicians are able to work towards creating evidence-based interventions that address the unique biological and social characteristics inherent in geriatric psychiatry. These improvements play a key role in reducing care protocols and offering better mental health outcomes for older adults. Finally, the integration of findings from both preventive intervention studies and medication adherence studies can guide future research and practice in geriatric psychiatry. As mental health professionals are treating the complicated problems of the elderly, they are also learning from thinking through what impact polypharmacy might have on making treatment more complicated. Imaging from pediatric patient populations regarding the primacy of side effects and attitudes in the compliance of medications just as readily carry over into geriatrics, so that just as much active intervention should be employed here. Knowing these factors' significance makes for improved care with a more holistic approach that promotes not only compliance but satisfaction with mental health care in general. Lastly, the learning from varied psychiatric populations reinforces the importance of adaptive models of treatment that incorporate the singular issues of older adults within mental health.

KEY TERMS FROM THIS CHAPTER

- Advance directives
- Capacity assessment
- Cognitive impairment
- Dementia
- Functional decline
- Geriatric psychiatry
- Mild cognitive impairment (MCI)
- Polypharmacy
- Reminiscence therapy
- Vascular dementia
- Alzheimer's disease
- Caregiver burden
- Delirium
- Elder abuse
- Geriatric assessment
- Late-onset depression
- Neurocognitive disorders
- Pseudodementia
- Sundowning

CRITICAL THINKING QUESTIONS

1. **The most common psychiatric disorder in the elderly is:**
   a. Schizophrenia
   b. Bipolar disorder
   c. Depression
   d. Personality disorder
2. **Which condition is characterized by an acute and fluctuating change in attention and cognition in elderly patients?**
   a. Dementia
   b. Delirium
   c. Generalized anxiety disorder
   d. Parkinson's disease
3. **Alzheimer's disease primarily affects which cognitive domain in its early stages?**
   a. Language comprehension
   b. Long-term memory
   c. Short-term memory
   d. Motor coordination
4. **Which of the following is a major risk factor for suicide in older adults?**
   a. Being married
   b. Financial wealth
   c. Chronic illness and social isolation
   d. High educational attainment
5. **The best initial approach to managing behavioral symptoms in dementia is:**
   a. Immediate use of antipsychotic medication
   b. Physical restraints
   c. Non-pharmacological interventions and environmental modifications
   d. Electroconvulsive therapy (ECT)

Short Answer Questions

1. What is geriatric psychiatry, and how does it differ from general psychiatry?
2. Name two common mental health disorders found in the elderly population.
3. What is the most common neurocognitive disorder seen in older adults?
4. How is depression in older adults different from depression in younger populations?
5. What role do physical illnesses and medications play in mental health issues among the elderly?

Answer to Critical Thinking Questions

1. (c); 2. (b); 3. (c); 4. (c); 5. (c)

REFERENCES

1. 2023 Alzheimer's disease facts and figures. (2023). *Alzheimer's & Dementia, 19*, 1598–1695. https://doi.org/10.1002/alz.13016 (accessed on 28th July 2025).
2. Addressing dementia. (2015). *OECD Health Policy Studies*. https://doi.org/10.1787/9789264231726-en (accessed on 28th July 2025).
3. Allison, M., Beloat, A., Daugherty, S., Hanson-Abromeit, D., et al. (2018). Reporting quality of music intervention research in healthcare: A systematic review. https://core.ac.uk/download/227054380.pdf (accessed on 28th July 2025).
4. Ancoli-Israel, S., Chong, M. S., Tan, K. T., Tay, L., et al. (2013). Bright light therapy as part of a multicomponent management program improves sleep and functional outcomes in delirious older hospitalized adults. https://core.ac.uk/download/323062309.pdf (accessed on 28th July 2025).
5. Appel, J. M. (2024). Capacity, informed consent and third-party decision-making. https://www.semanticscholar.org/paper/c1ab1ca3e64cd4261bee2be750330e91a77c8b69 (accessed on 28th July 2025).
6. AshaRani, P. V., Abdin, E., Roystonn, K., Devi, F., Wang, P., Shafie, S., Sagayadevan, V., et al. (2025). Tracking the prevalence of depression among older adults in Singapore: Results from the second wave of the Well-Being of Singapore Elderly Study. *Depression and Anxiety, 2025*. https://www.semanticscholar.org/paper/365f8988af93a4f55d7e2f9a009fb6e2b00b579b (accessed on 28th July 2025).
7. Bayraktar, I., Yalçın, N., Nalbant, K., Kültür, E., & Demirkan, K. (2025). Medication adherence and attitudes in adolescent psychiatry: Key influences. *Clinical Child Psychology and Psychiatry, 30*, 516–528. https://www.semanticscholar.org/paper/4a4381782fb6c25cf6c86bf0389ba80672254882 (accessed on 28th July 2025).
8. Caspersen, I. D., Fritzbøger, A. F. Ø., Petersen, J., Birkebæk, N., Christensen, A. M. R., Schou, A. J., Kristensen, K., et al. (2025). Effect of testosterone treatment during puberty in boys with Klinefelter syndrome (The TIPY Study): Protocol for a nationwide randomized, double-blinded, placebo-controlled study. *BMJ Open, 15*. https://www.semanticscholar.org/paper/0c7cc7092d375c5778d799b2e87960a757379447 (accessed on 28th July 2025).
9. Chakraborty, A., Banerjee, J. S., Bhadra, R., Dutta, A., Ganguly, S., Das, D., Kundu, S., et al. (2023). A framework of intelligent mental health monitoring in smart cities and societies. *IETE Journal of Research, 70*, 1328–1341. https://doi.org/10.1080/03772063.2023.2171918 (accessed on 28th July 2025).
10. Chan, E. Y. Y., Gobat, N., Kim, J. H., Newnham, E. A., Huang, Z., Hung, H., Dubois, C., et al. (2020). Informal home care providers: The forgotten health-care workers during the COVID-19 pandemic. *The Lancet, 395*, 1957–1959. https://doi.org/10.1016/s0140-6736(20)31254-x (accessed on 28th July 2025).
11. de Lasa, C., Brown, E. E., Colman, R. E., Rajji, T. K., & Colman, S. (2021). Invited letter: Integrated palliative care in a geriatric mental health setting during the COVID-19 pandemic. *International Journal of Geriatric Psychiatry, 37*. https://doi.org/10.1002/gps.5654 (accessed on 28th July 2025).

12. Del Rosario, N., Mackenzie, C. S., Koven, L. P., Reynolds, K. A., & Furer, P. (2024). 'Mental health is a mystery': Patient perspectives on treatment engagement in the referral process to specialty geriatric mental health services. *Aging & Mental Health, 29*, 478–487. https://www.semanticscholar.org/paper/647c4d46ced335e2b84fc288a4157e8a41fdabf3 (accessed on 28th July 2025).

13. Fässberg, M. M., Cheung, G., Canetto, S. S., Erlangsen, A., Lapierre, S., Lindner, R., Draper, B., et al. (2015). A systematic review of physical illness, functional disability, and suicidal behavior among older adults. *Aging & Mental Health, 20*, 166–194. https://doi.org/10.1080/13607863.2015.1083945 (accessed on 28th July 2025).

14. Laird, K. T., Krause, B., Funes, C., & Lavretsky, H. (2019). Psychobiological factors of resilience and depression in late life. *Translational psychiatry, 9*(1), 88. https://doi.org/10.1038/s41398-019-0424-7(accessed on 28th July 2025).

15. Gaikwad, R. A., & Durgawale, P. M. (2025). Comparative epidemiological assessment of quality of life (AQoL) among geriatric population in rural and urban Satara during the COVID-19 pandemic. *Journal of Neonatal Surgery*. https://www.semanticscholar.org/paper/0c40a426b96cb8c2ec46e87945ad6a27ee63ff87 (accessed on 28th July 2025).

16. Gautam, S., Gautam, M., Jain, A., & Yadav, A. N. (2022). Overview of practice of consultation-liaison psychiatry. *Indian Journal of Psychiatry, 64*(S), S201–S210. https://doi.org/10.4103/indianjpsychiatry.indianjpsychiatry_1019_21 (accessed on 28th July 2025).

17. Guidet, B., de Lange, D. D., Boumendil, A., Leaver, S., Watson, X., Boulanger, C., Szczeklik, W., et al. (2019). The contribution of frailty, cognition, activity of daily life and comorbidities on outcome in acutely admitted patients over 80 years in European ICUs: The VIP2 study. *Intensive Care Medicine, 46*, 57–69. https://www.semanticscholar.org/paper/d7cb5d0afb377ab15e2ec792c960fbce72cb4d7b (accessed on 28th July 2025).

18. Henwood, M., Larkin, M., & Milne, A. (2017). Seeing the wood for the trees. Carer related research and knowledge: A scoping review. https://core.ac.uk/download/145186527.pdf (accessed on 28th July 2025).

19. Johnson, S. L., Sebastian, T., Kuruvilla, A., & Manoranjitham, S. (2019). Burden and depression among the elderly care givers of patients with schizophrenia. *International Journal of Scientific Engineering and Research*. https://www.semanticscholar.org/paper/37eec59dfff65f20cd13d2a7c7f8d14a279d1d9f (accessed on 28th July 2025).

20. Kan, S. K., Zhang, Y. L., Bai, X. X., & Peng, B. (2025). Bibliometric and visual analysis of suicide in aged people over the past 20 years. *Frontiers in Psychiatry, 16*. https://www.semanticscholar.org/paper/35920247d5105de82b5bda844f2806e9762c6c04 (accessed on 28th July 2025).

21. Kocakaya, H., & Öztürk, H. M. (2023). Associates of cognitive functions in aged Turkish adults: Insights from a psychiatry outpatient clinic. *Turkish Journal of Geriatrics*. https://www.semanticscholar.org/paper/94f39f7cb835626f71e02fc808047a20cbd75d96 (accessed on 28th July 2025).

22. Kotecha, A. (2022). AKT question relating to abdominal pain. *InnovAiT, 15*, e77–e77. https://www.semanticscholar.org/paper/b99cb92850573cedd19a86da8057878a9a5da2b3 (accessed on 28th July 2025).

23. Lapid, M. I., Petrides, G., Hermida, A. P., & Forester, B. P. (2024). S2: Neuromodulation in geriatric psychiatry: Innovations and insights in ECT, TMS, tDCS, and cannabinoid therapies.

International Psychogeriatrics, 36, 9–9. https://www.semanticscholar.org/paper/1b6d154d1e0065731888183d67d5f08b0a687202 (accessed on 28th July 2025).

24. Le, G. (2009). Depression among the elderly: Screening practices and attitudes among nurse practitioners. https://core.ac.uk/download/223074313.pdf (accessed on 28th July 2025).
25. Ljubic, N., Ueberberg, B., Grunze, H., & Assion, H. J. (2023). Treatment of bipolar disorders in older adults: A review. *Focus, 21*(4), 434–443. https://www.semanticscholar.org/paper/365772f2e6aa9dcc73e0a633a2dcff2d4d9ff810 (accessed on 28th July 2025).
26. Maraqa, B., Nazzal, Z. A., Hamshari, S., Alutt, B., Rishmawi, E., & Qawasmeh, A. (2024). Prevalence of depression and anxiety among elderly primary care patients in Palestine. *Frontiers in Psychiatry, 14*. https://www.semanticscholar.org/paper/0ce45cf06db0cf5c7b627614e8bbfb220ed757bd (accessed on 28th July 2025).
27. Mayhew, K. M. (1989). An investigation of factors associated with depression in older adults. https://digitalscholarship.unlv.edu/cgi/viewcontent.cgi?article=1079&context=rtds (accessed on 28th July 2025).
28. Minichino, A., Davies, C., Karpenko, O., Christodoulou, N., Ramalho, R., Nandha, S., Damiani, S., et al. (2025). Preventing psychosis in people at clinical high risk: An updated meta-analysis by the World Psychiatric Association Preventive Psychiatry section. *Molecular Psychiatry, 30*, 2773–2782. https://www.semanticscholar.org/paper/bbd1eda59a59ead705a3efecd7301264ae0b9917 (accessed on 28th July 2025).
29. Morton, S., & Dunn, W. (2015). Addressing the health needs of an aging America: New opportunities for evidence-based policy solutions. https://core.ac.uk/download/75783019.pdf (accessed on 28th July 2025).
30. Mukherjee, S. (2020). 202–Psychosocial interventions for people with dementia as strategies to manage behavioral and psychological symptoms [Supported by European Association of Geriatric Psychiatry–EAGP]. *International Psychogeriatrics, 32*, 29–31. https://www.semanticscholar.org/paper/61787f0e19d52a7e62f6562ccdeacf6656ef55d8 (accessed on 28th July 2025).
31. Necka, E. A., Rowland, L. M., & Evans, J. D. (2020). Social disconnection in late life mental illness–Commentary from the National Institute of Mental Health. *American Journal of Geriatric Psychiatry, 29*, 727–730. https://doi.org/10.1016/j.jagp.2020.08.013 (accessed on 28th July 2025).
32. Nwokedi, V. U. (2025). Geriatric mental health research at a glance: A 10-year bibliometric mapping. *MOJ Gerontology & Geriatrics*. https://www.semanticscholar.org/paper/fdd2388d20b03038e802e2ef930d0520887c0f75 (accessed on 28th July 2025).
33. Park, D., Shin, A., & Park, Y. (2025). Nutrition intervention for older patients based on comprehensive geriatric assessment: A case report. *Clinical Nutrition Research, 14*, 91–99. https://www.semanticscholar.org/paper/75815418aa0b497e93771369eaf805f333172235 (accessed on 28th July 2025).
34. Pfeiffer, E. (2017). Grace Peterson Research Colloquium. https://core.ac.uk/download/232977413.pdf (accessed on 28th July 2025).
35. Pfister, T., Schröder, S., Heck, J., Bleich, S., Krüger, T. H. C., Wedegärtner, F., Groh, A., et al. (2024). Potentially inappropriate prescriptions of antibiotics in geriatric psychiatry—A

retrospective cohort study. *Frontiers in Psychiatry, 14*. https://www.semanticscholar.org/paper/70ad34d7c309073111bc794342d70d33c31089d6 (accessed on 28th July 2025).

36. Prasad, M. S. R., de Mendonça Lima, C. A., & Chong, D. (2024). S9: Addictions in later life an emerging crisis. *International Psychogeriatrics, 36*, 22–23. https://www.semanticscholar.org/paper/7fb0d48e1f8eeb513cccd76a7aa4f5a77c9cbbdc (accessed on 28th July 2025).

37. Rahimi, F., Shakibazadeh, E., Ashoorkhani, M., Hosseini, H., Foroughan, M., Aghayani, Z., & Farhandi, H. (2025). Effect of a web-based intervention on the mental health of informal caregivers of the elderly: A randomized controlled trial. *BMC Psychiatry, 25*. https://www.semanticscholar.org/paper/3eb8b491b68bad2b1f76855ca936487c33b88f88 (accessed on 28th July 2025).

38. Reynolds, C. F., Jeste, D., Sachdev, P., & Blazer, D. (2022). Mental health care for older adults: Recent advances and new directions in clinical practice and research. *World Psychiatry, 21*. https://www.semanticscholar.org/paper/9a3e77529b2edb85b4c4702606c0fda9524e73c5 (accessed on 28th July 2025).

39. S12: Recent advances in therapies for late-life neuropsychiatric disorder. (2023). *International Psychogeriatrics*. https://www.semanticscholar.org/paper/9999fbc5abd1c117351cf62ab6f2eb4fa5188e75 (accessed on 28th July 2025).

40. Scheffer, M., Bolhuis, J. E., Borsboom, D., Buchman, T. G., Gijzel, S. M. W., Goulson, D., Kammenga, J. E., et al. (2018). Quantifying resilience of humans and other animals. *Proceedings of the National Academy of Sciences, 115*, 11883–11890. https://doi.org/10.1073/pnas.1810630115 (accessed on 28th July 2025).

41. Shafique, H., Ahmad, M. W. A., ul Haq, U. (2025). Psychedelic pharmacology in psychiatry: The mechanisms and therapeutic potential of psilocybin, MDMA, and LSD in mental health disorders. *Journal of Medical & Health Sciences Review*. https://www.semanticscholar.org/paper/a690f3b608722bea66cd9c759de642a1a8fea928 (accessed on 28th July 2025).

42. Shiferaw, K. B., Yalew, E. S., Melese, A. Z., Chanie, S. T., Zeleke, G. A., Yitayal, M. M., & Fentanew, M. (2024). Depression and its associated factors among community dweller older adults in Gondar town, Northwest Ethiopia: A cross-sectional study. *Journal of Psychiatry Research*. https://www.semanticscholar.org/paper/e2ac6c00864df1587bc6bf1900a85bd7a8c40480 (accessed on 28th July 2025).

43. Torgersen, L. N. S., Schulz, S. M., Lugo, R., & Sütterlin, S. (2024). Patient informed consent, ethical and legal considerations in the context of digital vulnerability with smart, cardiac implantable electronic devices. *PLOS Digital Health, 3*. https://www.semanticscholar.org/paper/e14abcce9cdb166d45b3640462351ec830d915b2 (accessed on 28th July 2025).

44. Ukpo, S. D., Imohiosen, C. E., Owot, J. A., & Ajuluchukwu, P. (2024). The impact of religious and spiritual counseling on mental health outcomes in geriatric care. *International Journal of Multidisciplinary Research and Growth Evaluation*. https://www.semanticscholar.org/paper/bb242e4de5010e7dbce622ad7dab627a03c54900 (accessed on 28th July 2025).

45. Vahia, I. V. (2020). COVID-19, aging, and mental health: Lessons from the first six months. *American Journal of Geriatric Psychiatry, 28*, 691–694. https://doi.org/10.1016/j.jagp.2020.05.029 (accessed on 28th July 2025).

46. Widder, S., Mørch, K., Bradley, N., Ternan, L., & Lam, N. (2021). Geriatric Recovery and Enhancement Alliance in Trauma (GREAT) multidisciplinary quality improvement initiative:

Improving rates of successful resuscitation, rehabilitation and reintegration of geriatric trauma patients across the trauma spectrum of care. *Canadian Journal of Emergency Nursing*. https://www.semanticscholar.org/paper/957ec90a11747a812c2481e9c198b55d4cb2e962 (accessed on 28th July 2025).

47. Wongiam, N., Praditpornsilpa, K., & Vacharaksa, A. (2025). Comprehensive geriatric assessment for oral care in older adults: A focus group study. *BMC Geriatrics, 25*. https://www.semanticscholar.org/paper/46333a6e8ab489e234c6de91a394a2e44608dbc0 (accessed on 28th July 2025).

48. Yu, J. T., Xu, W., Tan, C. C., Andrieu, S., Suckling, J., Evangelou, E., Pan, A., et al. (2020). Evidence-based prevention of Alzheimer's disease: Systematic review and meta-analysis of 243 observational prospective studies and 153 randomized controlled trials. *Journal of Neurology Neurosurgery & Psychiatry, 91*, 1201–1209. https://doi.org/10.1136/jnnp-2019-321913 (accessed on 28th July 2025).

SOMATIC SYMPTOM AND RELATED DISORDERS

13

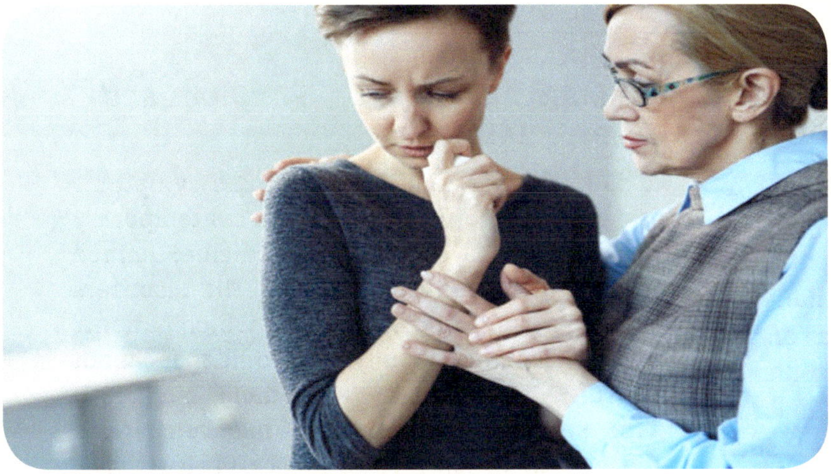

LEARNING OBJECTIVES

After studying this chapter, you will be able to:

1. Give historical context of somatic symptom and related disorders;
2. Explain the types of somatic symptom disorders;
3. Identify the symptoms and diagnosis;
4. List the causes and risk factors;
5. Discuss the treatment approaches;
6. Focus on the impact on quality of life.

Introduction

The research on somatic symptom and related disorders is a critical field of investigation in the fields of psychology and psychiatry. The disorders, which are a manifestation of bodily complaints not fully explainable by medical diseases, involve an interplay of psychological and physiologic processes that is complex. It disrupts the lives of patients and provokes extreme distress and impairment. As the Diagnostic and Statistical Manual of Mental Disorders (DSM) has evolved, so too has our understanding of such disorders. Interestingly, even the diagnostic criteria themselves have shifted, in reflection of a longstanding debate about the interaction between mind and body. Understanding the history of the definitions is important for clinicians who want to provide effective intervention, as appropriate interventions have a huge impact on improving patients' health by addressing both psychological and somatic processes of their condition. Historically, studies of somatic symptoms led to dichotomies between psychological and physiological explanations, which inclined towards concealing the causal processes operating. As past classifications within psychiatric textbooks illustrate, such as those evident in descriptions in the instance of paranoia and associated disorders, symptoms presented by patients are often described in rigid terms that fail to encompass the full nuance of their experience. Recent critiques of classical psychiatric literature have identified that numerous symptoms now falling under the umbrella of somatic disorders continue to be poorly concordant with modern diagnostic classification, leaving the possibility for disconnection between historical and contemporary clinical knowledge (Kendler, 2017).

Clarification of this discrepancy can serve to draw forth more nuanced modes of diagnostics that are attuned to the nuances of patients' subjective experience, thereby enhancing integrative treatment. Moreover, research on the biological and psychological markers of resilience opens up doors to what allows individuals to cope with somatic symptoms. Resilience is such a plastic, adaptive process from one person to the next that it varies significantly from person to person, particularly in response to life stresses that can exacerbate somatic symptoms. Standard self-ratings of resilience are helpful but not ideal, since they can be non-objective (Carnevali et al., 2018). New studies investigate the relationship between physiological markers, such as heart rate variability, and individual resilience profiles, and suggest a neurobiological component in how people deal with somatic events. By merging biological, psychological, and social accounts, a more comprehensive model can be constructed to support treatment for those with somatic symptoms and related disorders, thereby providing improved therapeutic results and an integrative understanding of health (Figure 13.1).

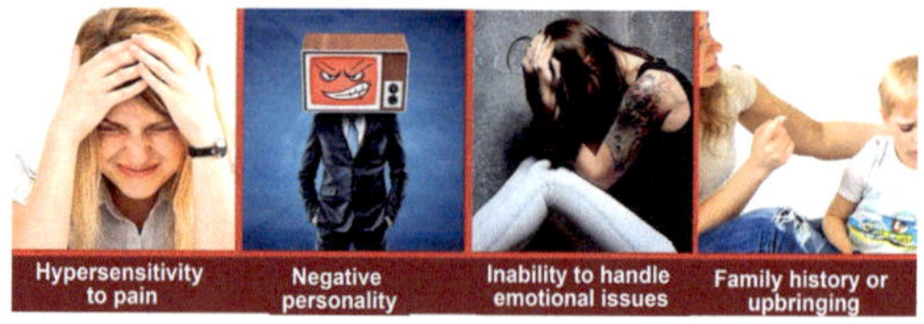
Hypersensitivity to pain
Negative personality
Inability to handle emotional issues
Family history or upbringing

Figure 13.1. Somatic symptom and related disorders.

Source: https://images.medindia.net/patientinfo/950_400/causes-of-somatoform-disorders.jpg.

Definition of Somatic Symptom and Related Disorders

A sound understanding of somatic symptoms and related disorders is critical in contemporary paradigms of psychology and medicine. Defined mainly in the context of DSM-5, the disorders refer to a range of conditions in which patients display prominent bodily symptoms that cannot be fully explained by a medical diagnosis. This shift in categorization has reassigned the way in which mental health professionals work with these illnesses, from the stigmating term of somatoform disorders to the more descriptive term of somatic symptom disorders. This shift illustrates a vital recognition that psychological and emotional concerns can have a tremendous influence over physical wellness, and as such, treatment needs to extend past the body's physical symptoms to also target the underlying psychological concerns (Testal et al., 2014). Somatic symptom disorders are not only distinguished by the presence of physical complaints but also by preoccupation with them, and most often by significant distress and impairment in daily functioning. This can be manifested in a number of ways, such as heightened concern about health, amplified reactions to symptoms, and overutilization of medical services. Besides, these conditions express the intricate interdependence between the body and mind, reaffirming the need for health practitioners to adopt the biopsychosocial perspective in diagnosing and treating such diseases. Research has established that factors , such as anxiety, stress, and even cultural nuances tend to exacerbate such symptoms (Akiki et al., 2018). Understanding the multi-dimensional features of somatic symptom disorders is important in order to adopt effective intervention strategies. Somatic symptom misinterpretation often leads to ineffective therapies or misdirected interventions. As the DSM-5 categorizes, effective treatment must thus encompass both psychological and medical care for health, taking a holistic approach to cope with the complexities surrounding these disorders. The clinicians are encouraged to make open communication with the patients possible and help the patients understand how they can explain their experiences and help them develop coping mechanisms that will resist stress and anxiety. Lastly, an empathetic comprehension of the definition and character of somatic symptoms and related disorders serves as the foundation for improved therapeutic outcomes and quality of life in patients (Testal et al., 2014).

Importance of Understanding These Disorders

The complexity of somatic symptoms and related disorders calls for a subtle understanding of the disorders. A thorough understanding of these disorders is important not only for correct diagnosis but also for correct treatment and management of the patients. Overlapping symptoms with the physical illnesses in the majority of the patients with these disorders result in improper diagnoses and inappropriate interventions. For instance, defining the distinctive presentations of depression and anxiety, that is, the integration of repetitive negative thinking with symptom clusters, highlights clinical heterogeneity that can complicate patient treatment. Toward this end, the understanding of these relationships is crucial in the development of individualized treatment plans addressing the particular experiences of each patient, with the possible improvement in overall prognosis and quality of life. Furthermore, making clear the specific symptoms that accompany somatic symptom and related disorders can strengthen the patient-provider therapeutic relationship. As an example, recent studies have indicated that muscle tension is highly linked to pathological worry but not with concentration difficulty, which is more akin to depressive symptoms. By pointing out such differences, providers can engage in more fruitful discussions with patients about their symptoms and foster collaborative treatment decisions.

This collaborative approach not only helps demystify the illnesses but also establishes a trusting, sympathetic environment necessary for treatment adherence. In essence, an understanding of the complexity of these illnesses enhances the therapeutic relationship, ultimately leading to healthier outcomes. Additionally, knowledge of somatic symptoms and related disorders is integral to advancing the research and public policy. As studies further reveal intricate associations between symptoms and underlying psychological processes, findings can guide next-generation diagnostic criteria and treatments. For example, studies have shown that repetitive negative thinking contributes centrally to intercorrelating depression and anxiety symptoms, which has implications for prevention programs. This report establishes the necessity for increased integration of mental health treatment into primary medical care so that detection may occur earlier and with reduced stigma of these disorders. In this manner, both society and the health care system can facilitate more compassionate-mindedness toward mental health and, in turn, enhance well-being in assorted populations as well as enhance overall public health efforts (Figure 13.2).

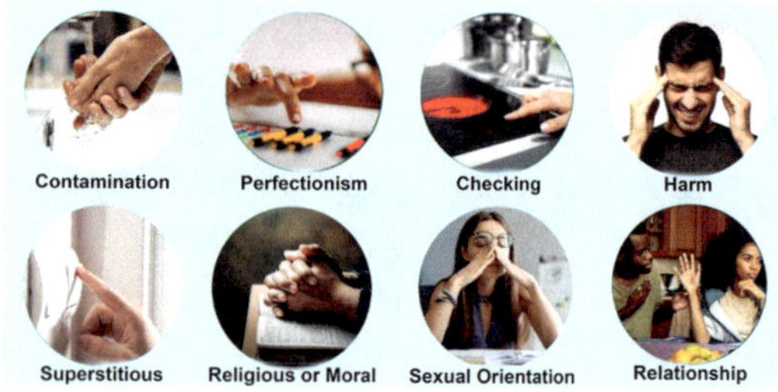

Figure 13.2. Importance of understanding these disorders.

Source: https://www.simplypsychology.org/wp-content/uploads/types-of-OCD-1.jpg.

13.1. Historical Context

Learning Outcome

1. Evolution of the concept of somatic symptoms.
2. Key figures in the development of somatic symptom theory.
3. Changes in diagnostic criteria over time.

History of somatic symptom and related disorders is a complex one of changing diagnostic criteria and understanding in psychiatric literature. Ever since the somatoform disorders were coded in early diagnostic manuals , such as the DSM-III, there has been ongoing debate about how the disorders should be diagnosed and categorized. Publication of the fifth edition of the DSM has ignited controversies initiated by the earlier versions about the nature of such conditions. More significantly, the change from classical somatoform disorders to somatic symptom disorders is a significant step towards accepting interaction among psychological and physiological forces, as reflected in proposed revisions of diagnostic criteria by the APA. Secondarily, the movement towards identifying an expanded array of signs is a critical evolution in psychiatric epistemology, aiming to refine diagnosis while handling contemporary clinical practices in genetics and neurology (Testal et al., 2014). Lastly, the trajectory of somatic symptom disorders is characterized by the continuous battle between psychosocial and biomedical paradigms. Early psychiatric comprehension was to view somatic symptoms as secondary to mental distress, but this reductionist view has more and more been altered. The inclusion of a dimensional approach allows for the capture of the experience of the person more closely, which appreciates the complexity of the somatic symptoms beyond mere psychogenic etiology. This paradigm change is an evolving appreciation that physical symptoms may have psychological as well as biological causation. The thorough investigation of somatic symptom disorders is a sustained attempt to improve on the shortcomings of earlier classifications, as indicated by criticism directed toward earlier versions that were confusing and invalid (Kendler, 2017).

The change in definitions and criteria attests to a continued striving for a better definition of our knowledge of psychological phenomena. The development of somatic symptoms and related disorders in psychiatric nomenclature also illustrates the strength of historical discourses in mental health sciences. Just as the knowledge of mental disorders has grown, so too has the categorization of somatic symptoms, as the history of paranoid disorders and how they have been represented in DSM volumes shows. This reference leads to the broader thematic problem in psychiatry regarding the stability and predictability of diagnostic criteria. Historical analyses of paranoia, for example, reveal spectacular changes in the emphasized clinical features in different DSM revisions, representing a significant inconsistency over the past century (Kendler, 2016). These shifts underscore the necessity of putting current conceptualizations of somatic symptom disorders into the broader context of psychiatric history, which underscores the dynamic tension between developing clinical understanding and historical context.

Such a conversation continues to shape current clinical practicc and research to understand the complexity of somatic experiences.

13.1.1. Evolution of the Concept of Somatic Symptoms

The knowledge about somatic symptoms has evolved over time, as has associated scientific information and clinician techniques. Somatic symptoms in the past have often been dismissed as having a sole psychological origin, and thus, proper medical attention was not provided and diagnoses were inappropriate. With time, the realization that there is an intricate relationship between body and mind increased, and clinicians realized how distressful experiences of the mind appear physically. This paradigm change has led to the trend towards a departure from an exclusively psychosomatic model, with demands for a more integrated concept that accounts for biological, psychological, and social variables. As the topic evolved, so did the implication that somatic symptoms are capable of having a dramatic impact on the quality of life of an individual, demanding holistic assessment and management practices. In recent work, the intersection of inflammatory processes with somatic symptomatology has emerged as a topic of interest for clinicians and researchers. Of particular interest is the finding that there is a significant phenomenological convergence between sickness behavior caused by biological stressors and clinical depression. This overlap implies that inflammatory pathways may both underlie these two conditions, pointing to a common neurobiologic substrate. For instance, as noted recently in the literature, the pro-inflammatory cytokines associated with sickness behavior can mimic depressive symptoms , including fatigue and anhedonia. Moreover, if not treated, chronic inflammation can exacerbate depressive episodes with irreparable harm and functional damage. Thus, the dialogue of somatic symptoms has evolved to encompass not only somatic complaints but also their biological underpinnings and cognitive consequences, presaging an increasingly complex appreciation for these multifaceted illnesses. Contemporary understanding of somatic symptoms is clearly reflected in diagnostic standards, including the DSM-5, which reconceptualizes and reconfigures the diagnosis and treatment of these disorders.

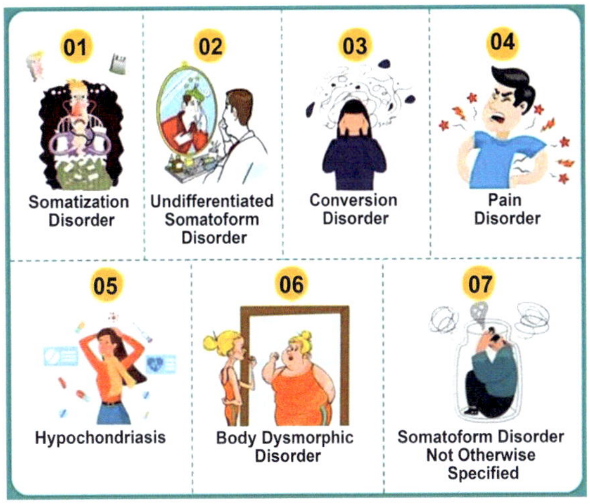

Figure 13.3. Evolution of the concept of somatic symptoms.

Source: https://naxlex.com/nursing/assets/images/study_guides/somatic-symptom-illnesses-and-sleepwakefulness-disorders-types_1695643767.jpg.

The guidebooks change from the use of somatoform disorders to somatic symptom and related disorders, illustrating this progressive direction, asserting that somatic symptoms are real experiences regardless of there not being an evident medical cause. This change provides a more integrated strategy that takes into account patients' subjective experience and their significant influence on health-related quality of life, emphasized in evidence of a general practice prevalence of 16% for psychosomatic disorders. Hence, an enhanced sensitivity to somatic symptoms in clinical practice calls for enhanced training of psychiatric and non-psychiatric clinicians alike to deal with such disorders skillfully and compassionately, ultimately leading to patient outcomes and care quality improvement (Bosutti et al., 2012; Guerrero et al., 2015) (Figure 13.3).

13.1.2. Key Figures in the Development Of Somatic Symptom Theory

The development of somatic symptom theory has been largely influenced by profound minds that articulated the dynamics of the interaction between psychological phenomena and somatic symptomatology. Freud is best described as a pioneer in this regard, considering that his work emphasized the complex interaction between emotional trauma and somatic symptoms, a concept that was the precursor to modern-day somatic symptom theory. His psychoanalytic research demonstrated how unconscious conflict might appear in the form of physical disease, thus reversing the mind and body duality. This exploration into the unconscious mind provided the platform for later researchers to expand further on the mechanisms by which psychological issues could cause somatic disturbances, illustrating Freud's long-lasting impact within the discipline. With the foundation for a biopsychosocial theory established, Freud's work set the stage for future theorists, who expanded on his theories to create a more multifaceted explanation for somatic symptoms as deeply interwoven with emotional and cognitive processes. Assisting with Freud's early ideas, people like George Engel went on to advance the theory in the form of the biopsychosocial model. According to Engel, health and illness do not solely result from biological determinants; they are of utmost importance and, in fact, influenced by psychological and social aspects to a huge extent. Such an integrated model provides a very comprehensive view of somatic symptom disorders, especially looking into how these factors work together to produce and experience the symptoms. The work of Engels emphasizes that personal experiences, culture, and social support have a lot to do with health. Moreover, his findings regarding patient-centered care encourage clinicians to be more empathetic in care, encouraging consciousness that somatic symptoms have to be assessed in the overall context of a patient's existence. Engel's work remains at the forefront of controversy surrounding somatic symptoms and related disorders today, bridging gaps between different disciplines. More recent theory in somatic symptoms has been influenced by research on disorders like generalized anxiety disorder (GAD) and obsessive-compulsive disorder (OCD), where somatic symptoms are often the focal symptom. The Intolerance of Uncertainty Model (IUM) of Generalized Anxiety Disorder (GAD), for instance, describes how cognitive mechanisms, such as Negative Problem Orientation (NPO) and Cognitive Avoidance (CA), interact with uncertainty to manifest as worry and somatic anxiety (Bottesi et al., 2016). This modern model reflects the prominence of cognitive-behavioral theories in the formulation and treatment of somatic symptoms, showing the theory's alignment with new paradigms of mental health. Similarly, studies of disorders like SO-OCD illustrate how somatic presentation can complicate diagnoses, for example, sexual orientation fears, where expert assessment tools are required for intervention (Ching et al., 2018). All of these works join an ongoing conversation in the field, illustrating the complexity and diversity of experience of somatic symptoms from historical and contemporary authorities in psychology.

13.1.3. Changes in Diagnostic Criteria Over Time

The development of diagnostic criteria highlights a paradigm shift in mental health understanding and its convergence with physical symptoms. That changing paradigm is amply demonstrated in the shift from somatoform disorders to somatic symptom disorder (SSD), where a more subtle assessment strategy will be required to capture complexity in patient experience. The DSM-5 revision aims to reduce stigma surrounding such diagnoses by embracing the legitimacy of somatic symptoms without prima facie labeling them as being purely psychological. This reconsideration recognizes that somatic symptoms can be concurrent with or independent of traceant medical conditions, thereby allowing for increased understanding of patient presentations and enhancing general clinical practice. In addition, the increased dimensionality in DSM-5 diagnostic criteria allows for a more dynamic conceptualization of somatic symptom disorders. This shift not only harmonizes with current neurological and genetic insight but also transcends the limitations of previous categorical models, which typically did not account for the variety of symptoms. The examination of the relationship between excessive thoughts, feelings, and actions associated with these symptoms has been instrumental in defining SSD. As noted, symptoms can be demonstrated by patients disproportionate to other patients with similar medical conditions, leading to excessive distress and impairment in daily living. The use of such presentations as standard within the DSM framework facilitates clinicians to treat numerous cases without risking the likelihood of misdiagnosis or misinterpretation, thus facilitating a more compassionate treatment of patients (Levenson et al., 2017). Implications of such conceptual shifts pose serious basic challenges to questions regarding the validity and usefulness of newer categories of diagnoses. While the DSM-5 has difficulty imposing concision to the classification of somatic symptoms, it also invites attention to whether or not its architecture is successful in everyday practice, particularly within primary care, where these disorders most frequently occur. Merging the erstwhile somatoform disorders into a category of somatic symptom disorder requires strict scrutiny of clinical outcome and long-term efficacy. Most importantly, as understanding of mental health and overall medical health evolves, recurring scrutiny and debate have to be undertaken to further refine criteria for diagnosis to continue to keep in mind prevailing clinical realities and patients' lives on a basis that is simultaneously scientifically sound and empathetic (Testal et al., 2014).

Test Your Knowledge

1. How did early concepts such as hysteria and conversion disorders influence modern understanding of somatic symptom and related disorders?
2. What major shifts occurred in diagnostic classification from earlier editions of DSM to the current DSM-5-TR for these disorders?

13.2. Types of Somatic Symptom Disorders

Learning Outcome

1. Somatic symptom disorder.
2. Illness anxiety disorder.
3. Conversion disorder.

Somatic symptom disorders encompass a range of diseases that present with somatic symptoms that are not explicable by medical illness, typically resulting in high distress and functional impairment. Somatic Symptom Disorder is one type in which one or more somatic symptoms occur together with excessive thoughts, feelings, or behaviors regarding the symptoms that result in significant interference with daily functioning. Patients may become stuck in a persistent preoccupation with their health, leading them to desire extensive medical testing despite assurances from clinicians. The disorder highlights the intricate dynamic between psychological distress and physical findings, as patients identify a variety of symptoms that may involve multiple bodily systems, leading to excessive healthcare use and provider frustration. Another significant type of somatic symptom disorder is Illness Anxiety Disorder (IAD), previously known as hypochondriasis. Individuals with IAD experience an extreme fear of developing or having a serious illness, even if they do not have any somatic symptoms or only minor ones. Their excessive, inappropriate health concern usually leads to habitual compulsive health checking or avoiding medical care. Kroenke (2003) theorizes that over 33% of somatic complaints remain medically unexplained and that fears have a tendency to exacerbate body sensation perception, thus promoting increased levels of anxiety and distress. Subsequently, the vicious cycle of worry persists, which tends to complicate both psychiatric and medical management. Cognitive-behavioral therapy that targets altering maladaptive beliefs associated with health and behaviors has been theorized as a likely advantage for individuals with IAD. Last but not least, Conversion Disorder (CD) is a special expression of the somatic symptom disorders in which patients present with neurological symptoms , such as weakness or movement abnormality, with no neurological basis. Symptoms may be tremors, paralysis, or seizures that are very distressing and interfering, typically following psychological stressors or trauma. Patients tend to struggle with the authenticity of their symptoms, as they can be overwhelmingly real but lack any clear medical basis. Research indicates that conversion symptoms are often found to co-occur with other psychiatric illnesses, particularly anxiety and depressive disorders, with the psychological explanations behind the development of these symptoms being emphasized (Bekhuis et al., 2015). Treatment is typically multidisciplinary, combining physical rehabilitation and psychotherapy directed at physical and psychological factors to facilitate recovery and improve functioning (Figure 13.4).

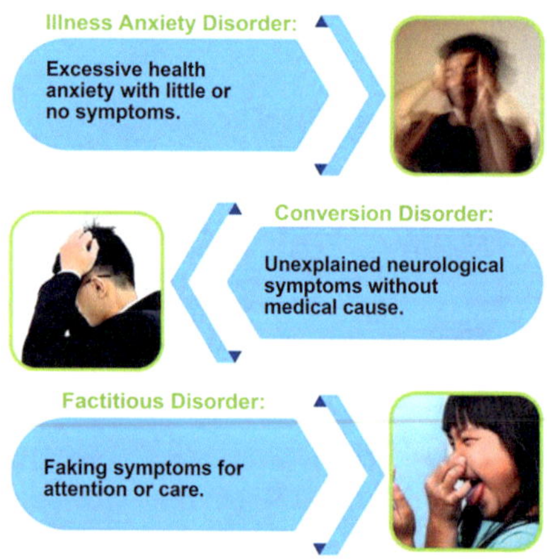
Illness Anxiety Disorder:
Excessive health anxiety with little or no symptoms.
Conversion Disorder:
Unexplained neurological symptoms without medical cause.
Factitious Disorder:
Faking symptoms for attention or care.

Figure 13.4. Types of somatic symptom disorders.

Source: https://www.brightpathbh.com/wp-content/uploads/Types-819x1024.jpg.

13.2.1. Somatic Symptom Disorder

Identification of Somatic Symptom Disorder (SSD) is vital to the identification of the way physical symptoms manifest underlying psychological issues. SSD is characterized by excessive distress and impairment resulting from somatic symptoms, which might be further accompanied by irrational attitudes, feelings, and behaviors towards the symptoms. Individuals suffering from SSD will become overly concerned with their health when there is no or little physical illness. This can lead to redundant physician visits and unnecessary diagnostic testing, therefore stressing not only health care resources but also the emotional system of the patient. Visibility of these signs is not merely the reflection of comorbid medical disease but is indicative of more insidious interplay between physical and psychological health. The challenge is in distinguishing SSD from other psychiatric conditions, requiring professional evaluation by medical practitioners (Levenson et al., 2017). The reclassification of somatoform disorders to SSD in the fifth edition of the Diagnostic and Statistical Manual of Mental Disorders (DSM-5) has generated significant controversy among doctors. This reclassification underscores the necessity of developing a better concept of mental and physical health interaction. By the inclusion of a dimensional model of diagnosis, the DSM-5 invites clinicians to examine the severity and implications of somatic symptoms rather than holding out for categorical definitions. This is an acknowledgment that the fact of the matter is that many individuals present with clusters of symptoms that do not readily fit into previous traditional diagnostic categories. Moreover, reorganization of the disorders anticipates going toward the integration of neurology and genetics developments into psychiatric practice. It highlights the need for considering biological, psychological, and social determinants while diagnosing and treating SSD (Testal et al., 2014). Effective treatment of SSD often requires a multidisciplinary approach with psychological as well as medical therapies in mind. Cognitive-behavioral therapy (CBT) has been shown to be an effective treatment as it informs patients about and modifies maladaptive cognitive patterns related to their symptoms. In addition, an interdisciplinary group of healthcare providers can assist with enhancing treatment outcomes. Promotion of a therapeutic relationship between the healthcare provider and patient can also improve treatment outcomes. Treatment of the psychological components of SSD can assist with managing somatic symptoms in patients, which will further reduce their overall level of distress and improve their quality of life. Treatment strategies should be tailored based on case complexity. As research into the processes of SSD continues, it is to be expected that more targeted treatment interventions will emerge, further bridging the gap between somatic and psychotherapy treatments (Levenson et al., 2017) (Figure 13.5).

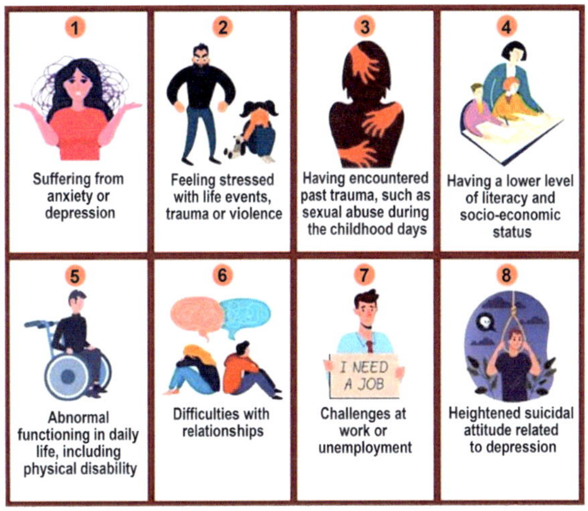
1
Suffering from anxiety or depression
2
Feeling stressed with life events, trauma or violence
3
Having encountered past trauma, such as sexual abuse during the childhood days
4
Having a lower level of literacy and socio-economic status
5
Abnormal functioning in daily life, including physical disability
6
Difficulties with relationships
7
I NEED A JOB
Challenges at work or unemployment
8
Heightened suicidal attitude related to depression

Figure 13.5. Somatic symptom disorder.

Source: https://mind.help/wp-content/uploads/2022/03/Risks-Complications-Of-Somatic-Symptom-Disorder-768x786.jpg.

13.2.2. Illness Anxiety Disorder

Illness anxiety disorder (IAD), previously referred to as hypochondriasis, is a condition involving excessive concern about serious illness with little medical evidence to justify such concerns. Individuals with IAD misinterpret bodily sensations as indicators of serious illness and, in most instances, exhibit excess health behavior or maladaptive avoidance. This health concern can lead to severe impairment in social, occupational, or other significant areas of functioning. Current diagnostic criteria emphasized the point that, for individuals afflicted by IAD, there is a protracted concern of at least six months regarding their health status, pointing towards the chronic nature of this disorder. Moreover, unlike patients with genuine medical illnesses, IAD-diagnosed individuals do not have a large number of somatic symptoms, which further highlights the psychological nature of their suffering and the requirement for an approach more focused on subtlety while making treatment decisions. The publication of the DSM-5 readjusted the category of somatic symptoms and related disorders and led to the redistribution of IAD in this system. By focusing on the anxiety experienced about health issues, the DSM-5 allows one to better comprehend how such disorders manifest themselves in patients. This classification goes along with the expanding recognition of psychological factors' role in explaining somatic symptoms. Furthermore, by placing IAD within the broader category of somatic symptom disorders, clinicians are better positioned to identify comorbid conditions, such as depression and generalized anxiety disorder, which tend to coincide with IAD. Identification of these co-occurring conditions is essential in order to administer targeted treatment regimens that address both the psychological and somatic components of affected individuals (Levenson et al., 2017). In exploring the treatment modalities for illness anxiety disorder, optimal practice dictates that cognitive-behavioral therapy (CBT) is particularly helpful. CBT targets the distortion of thought patterns responsible for undue concern for health, encouraging a more realistic interpretation of sensations in the body. Patients are taught to confront their fears gradually, thereby abandoning avoidance behaviors for health anxiety. Moreover, psychoeducation on the nature of the IAD and its underlying psychological foundations can enable individuals to overcome their irrational beliefs about illness. As the understanding of somatic symptom disorders develops, the need for an integrated model addressing both psychological and physiological perspectives remains fundamental. Treating the complex nature of conditions like IAD can enhance the outcomes of treatment and the quality of care for patients with such disabling diseases (Testal et al., 2014).

13.2.3. Conversion Disorder

Conversion disorder, which is among the somatic symptoms and related disorders, is an illness that presents in the form of neurological symptoms that have no identified medical cause. It is most commonly defined by symptoms , such as paralysis, tremor, or non-epileptic seizures that can dramatically affect an individual's functioning. These symptoms can be triggered by psychological precipitants and produce distress to an extent comparable to that associated with recognized physical diseases. Since the patients cannot reconcile the physical symptoms with the absence of a medical diagnosis, the psychological component is irrevocably interconnected with their experience, causing further psychological distress. In the absence of physical explanations, conversion disorder tests the boundaries of usual medical understanding, and treatment calls for an integrated methodology that includes both psychological evaluation and somatic assessment. The new standards under the DSM-5 have also questioned the classification and definition of conversion disorder, which was put under somatic symptom disorders. The dimensional diagnosis now considers the severity and impact of an individual's symptoms, emphasizing the significance of the contribution of psychological aspects that may exacerbate physical manifestations. Such a categorization acknowledges that even though certain patients may present overt physical symptoms, others may have more covert forms that nonetheless produce a lot of distress and disability in their everyday lives. By placing conversion disorder in this broader context, clinicians are in the best position to explore the intricate interconnection between emotional and physical wellness. Moreover, the reclassification of somatoform disorders as somatic symptom disorders reinforces a multi-dimensional consideration of patient experiences, affirming the value of a broad, multi-disciplinary treatment strategy, addressing both symptom and mental health (Testal et al., 2014). Conversion disorder treatment necessitates a needs-adjusted therapy balancing both physical and psychological interventions. Cognitive Behavior Therapy (CBT) has also become an anchor treatment, helping patients to unlearn adaptive cognition and behavior linked to symptoms. Supportive therapies , such as physical rehabilitation are also important in restoring functionality and exercising self-efficacy. Moreover, engagement in psychoeducation can acclimatize the patient to more insight into their state, which can minimize anxiety concerning their symptoms. Given the profound impact of trauma and stress on conversion disorder symptomatology, an interdisciplinary treatment solution that addresses these psychological origins is imperative. The interfacing among healthcare professionals of different specialties ultimately aims to empower patients and facilitate their way forward in recovery despite the disabling nature of conversion disorder (Levenson et al., 2017) (Figure 13.6).

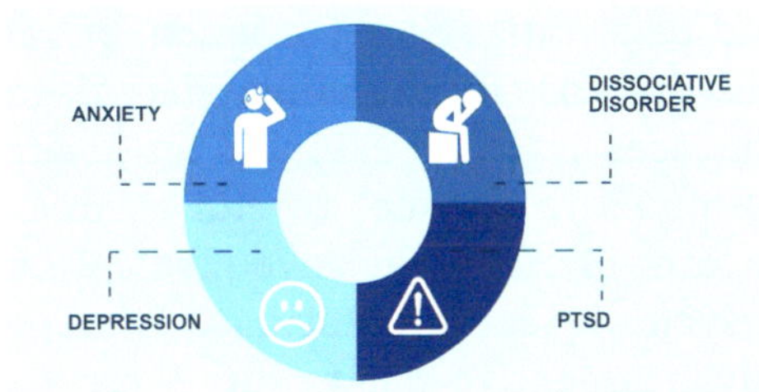

Figure 13.6. Conversion disorder.

Source: https://www.therecoveryvillage.com/wp-content/uploads/2022/01/Conversion-Disorder-co-occuring-disorders.webp.

Test Your Knowledge

1. What distinguishes somatic symptom disorder, illness anxiety disorder, and conversion disorder from each other?
2. How do psychological factors affecting other medical conditions differ from factitious disorder and malingering?

13.3. Symptoms and Diagnosis

Learning Outcome

1. Common symptoms associated with somatic symptom disorders.
2. Diagnostic criteria according to DSM-5.
3. Challenges in diagnosing these disorders.

Symptoms of somatic symptoms and related disorders (SSRD) need to be understood for proper management and diagnosis. SSRD has a complicated combination of unexplained medical and physical complaints that cause the patient tremendous distress. Symptoms may be pain, fatigue, and gastrointestinal symptoms, and this makes clinicians look for psychosomatic linkages that connect physiological symptoms to psychological distress. The classification of these disorders has evolved with time, particularly with the release of the DSM-5, which reduced the traditional somatoform disorders to a model based on the dimensionality of symptom presentation. This is believed to enable easy understanding of the emotional and physical dimensions of these disorders, thus allowing clinicians to make an accurate diagnosis, which is important for developing a proper treatment plan (Testal et al., 2014). The diagnostic evaluation of somatic symptom disorders requires careful inspection to distinguish medically explained illnesses from those of psychological cause. Chronic pain, fatigue, or sensation in various systems can obscure the underlying diagnosis. In such cases, it is very essential for healthcare professionals to conduct careful assessments in the form of comprehensive medical history and psychological evaluations. Fortunately, the advancement in diagnostic criteria leads clinicians to diagnose SSRD with great emphasis laid on interdisciplinary collaboration. Additionally, the overlap of SSRD symptoms with other neurological or psychological illnesses complicates the diagnosis even further. For instance, symptoms of multiple sclerosis , such as vertigo, sleep disorder, and dysphagia, can bring about a challenge in terms of the appropriate underlying disease, leading to heightened clinical suspicion (Balla et al., 2018). In addition to enhancing diagnostic precision, an understanding of the temporal and functional aspects of symptoms plays a pivotal role in the treatment of SSRD. The presentation of symptoms will vary from one phase of the disorder to another, while they will persist or abruptly exacerbate in response to psychological stressors or major life events. Understanding this dynamic allows clinicians to assess symptom exacerbation and psychological deterioration, thereby guiding therapeutic interventions. Moreover, incorporating a patient-centered strategy that reinforces communication and empathic listening is vital in creating a therapeutic climate. This type of approach not only lowers the stigma of somatic symptoms but also helps patients assume an active role in diagnosis and treatment. This comprehensive understanding emphasizes the need for individualized approaches to improve the patient outcomes and the quality of life in patients with somatic symptoms and related disorders (Figure 13.7).

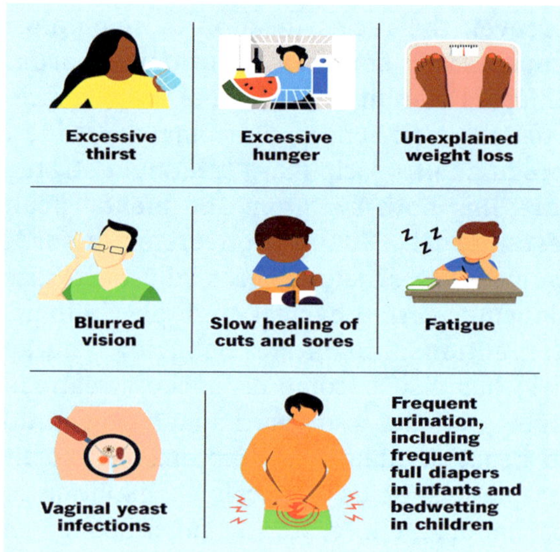

Excessive thirst
Excessive hunger
Unexplained weight loss
Blurred vision
Slow healing of cuts and sores
Fatigue
Vaginal yeast infections
Frequent urination, including frequent full diapers in infants and bedwetting in children

Figure 13.7. Symptoms and diagnosis.

Source: https://my.clevelandclinic.org/-/scassets/images/org/health/articles/21500-type-1-diabetes.

13.3.1. Common Symptoms Associated With Somatic Symptom Disorders

Somatic symptom disorders are characterized by the presence of physical symptoms that cannot be explained by a medical illness. Common symptoms of such disorders tend to manifest themselves in the form of persistent complaints, for example, pain, fatigue, and nausea, which have a significant effect on the individual's functioning. Patients tend to report vague or unexplainable body symptoms, leading to an abnormal frequency of medical visits and potential conflicts with healthcare providers. Distress generated by these symptoms may build on illness perception, further raising the levels of anxiety and somatic preoccupations. These symptoms need to be appreciated because they represent an entry point for so many individuals presenting for help without any recognizable medical basis, so making the diagnosis of somatic symptom disorders particularly challenging. Of the enormous quantity of presentations in somatic symptom disorders, the incidence of insomnia and other somatic symptoms is particularly significant. Existing literature indicates that insomnia and somatic symptom items reliably rank among the highest in affected populations, validating the interconnectedness of body and mental distress. For instance, individuals with such disorders often present with complaints of not only bodily symptoms, but also helplessness and vulnerability, which further exacerbate their sleep issues. The co-prevalence of somatic and insomnia symptoms may be a marker of atypical presentations of mood disorders, and one should carefully assess sleep behavior while diagnosing and treating somatic symptom disorders. This relationship underscores the complex interplay among psychiatric disorders and bodily symptomatology, thus necessitating a multi-dimensional assessment and treatment strategy. Repeated somatic symptoms impose significant morbidity on patients' quality of life and overall health status. Approximately a third of medically unexplained somatic symptoms presented in primary care are followed by a significant portion of these patients with co-morbid depressive and anxiety disorders (Kroenke, 2003). Such psychiatric co-morbidities can be anticipated based on recent life stressors and a higher severity of somatic symptoms, showing the need for comprehensive assessments taking into account medical, psychological, and social parameters. Efficacious treatments usually consist of a combination of antidepressants and cognitive behavior therapy, both for the mental health syndromes as well as for somatic symptoms (Kroenke et al., 2003). By utilizing stepped care, health practitioners may channel interventions into symptom duration and severity, approaching patients with better results in dealing with the complexities of somatic symptom disorders. By these strategies, not only are symptoms individually reduced but also the holistic approach to understanding patient care in this subtle domain, improved outcomes are facilitated (Figure 13.8).

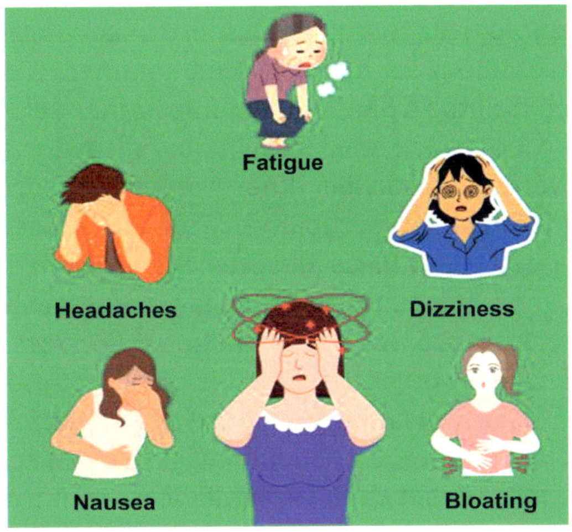

Figure 13.8. Common symptoms associated with somatic symptom disorders.

Source: https://lh7-rt.googleusercontent.com/docsz/AD_4nXcORAznDzlwuQGKnhvIrqTaVp480wq_75PiQeAc5uS5lTm2-CXVt-Mpg8rHL01ioE3f8yO8n_pEKn34Q7kQHXL-GErQnkdDGFf0HzQl98AHF9KfYLPMpG4h579WFv-KPAw4jSFAmUizpuQSdvexEp_dBTi3?key=fv6YbaasIB8yy1Dhnz5n_Q.

13.3.2. Diagnostic Criteria According to DSM-5

The Diagnostic and Statistical Manual of Mental Disorders, Fifth Edition (DSM-5), also contains precise criteria for the diagnosis of somatic symptoms and related disorders, which acknowledge the important intersection between psychological and medical health. According to the manual, somatic symptom disorder (SSD) is defined as comprising one or more distressing or disruptive somatic symptoms that interfere with daily life. Probingly, the DSM-5 mandates that excess and disproportion in the person's thoughts, feelings, or behaviors concerning such symptoms be present, highlighting a point of focus on psychological facets in evaluating somatic experience. Such a system allows clinicians to detect patients who not only complain of physical distress but also exhibit inner emotional suffering, thus both medical and psychological interventions are incorporated in treatment in an advanced manner. Apart from SSD, the DSM-5 also defines other related disorders , such as illness anxiety disorder and conversion disorder. Illness anxiety disorder delineates a preoccupation with the presence of a serious illness despite the presence of little or no somatic symptoms, suggesting a persistence in health anxiety. Conversion disorder, on the other hand, involves symptoms of a neurological kind that are not explainable through medical conditions, suggesting an acute relationship between psychological tension and bodily expression. The diagnostic definition for such disorders is crucial in the differentiation between primary psychological pathology and medically reversible disorders, thereby enabling optimized intervention that addresses both the physical and mental dimensions of the patient's experience. Such diagnostic precision is imperative in minimizing misdiagnosis and ensuring proper management. Comprehension of these diagnostic definitions not only facilitates effective identification but also facilitates the structuring of the treatment approaches that such disorders necessitate. The emphasis on SSD's abnormal feelings, thoughts, and behavior, particularly in contrast to patients who have the same signs and symptoms, underscores the importance of mental health practitioners inquiring into the internal lives of their patients (Levenson et al., 2017). Further, research indicates that disorders , such as generalized anxiety disorder, with somatic symptoms of muscle tension, could be helped by more differentiated diagnostic criteria that prioritize specific stress-related symptoms (Joormann et al., 1999). Overall, the DSM-5 is a valuable resource in guiding clinicians to a proper conceptualization of somatic symptoms and related disorders, hence enhancing diagnosis, treatment, and patient outcomes.

13.3.3. Difficulties in Diagnosing These Disorders

Diagnosis of Somatic Symptom and Related Disorders is complicated with an array of challenges, primarily caused by the complicated co-mingling of physical and psychological symptoms. Clinicians would typically be challenged by the subjective nature of the symptoms characterized by patients, thus causing dismissive attitudes or misdiagnosis. For instance, symptoms , such as pain or fatigue are used in association with a multitude of medical conditions, thereby compounding the diagnosis. The Diagnostic and Statistical Manual of Mental Disorders emphasizes cautious diagnosis, but the blurring of lines between psychological disease and somatic complaint so often produces a diagnostic morass. Mental illness also may be underreported by patients due to stigma, adding to the difficulty of the diagnostic process. This complex interaction necessitates a delicate approach that integrates psychosocial and medical perspectives, ultimately presenting challenges to healthcare professionals in making accurate diagnoses. Another monumental challenge in the diagnosis of Somatic Symptom and Related Disorders is that there are no consistent diagnostic criteria among various healthcare professionals. While some criteria are outlined in the DSM, variations in interpretation and application may lead to incongruent diagnoses. As a result, patients may receive conflicting diagnoses or treatment strategies, particularly in settings that have fluctuating medical norms. Moreover, patient self-report, particularly with young children or those who cannot articulate their symptoms clearly, aggravates these challenges. This challenge is particularly emphasized in the childhood symptoms of anxiety, where the delineation of distinct anxiety disorders from normative developmental behavior is slippery. The use of advanced analytical techniques, such as confirmatory and exploratory factor analyses, has been a potential way of enhancing diagnostic accuracy, but these techniques have not been widely used in clinical environments, leading to an absence of valid diagnosis (Briggs-Gowan et al., 2012). Lastly, the co-morbid conditions generally conceal the Somatic Symptom and Related Disorders diagnosis. Patients present with a combination of psychiatric and somatic complaints that may be indicative of many underlying pathologies. In multiple sclerosis, for instance, otolaryngologic symptoms are unfairly attributed solely to neurological dysfunction although they have a direct impact on quality of life. They often occur at various stages of illness and could be to blame for a delay in appropriate diagnosis and treatment (Balla et al., 2018). Besides, such co-morbidity will lead to overemphasis on the physical interventions that could overlook the need for psychological interventions. The practitioners must thus create a deep understanding of both physical and emotional dimensions of each patient's experience. Such holistic practice is critical in boosting diagnostic accuracy and treatment outcomes in Somatic Symptom and Related Disorders (Figure 13.9).

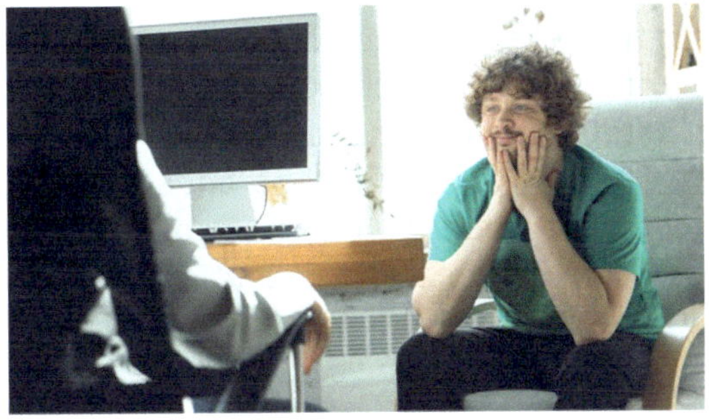

Figure 13.9. Challenges in diagnosing these disorders.

Source: https://www.seniorfitness.org/wp-content/uploads/2024/08/Challenges-in-Diagnosing-Anxiety-Disorders-768x432.jpg.

Test Your Knowledge

1. What key symptoms—such as excessive thoughts, anxiety, or behaviors related to physical complaints—characterize somatic symptom disorders?
2. How do clinicians use clinical interviews, medical evaluations, and DSM-5-TR criteria to diagnose these disorders?

13.4. Causes and Risk Factors

Learning Outcome

1. Biological factors contributing to somatic symptoms.
2. Psychological influences and stressors.
3. Sociocultural factors affecting prevalence and perception.

The etiology of somatic symptoms and related disorders is closely associated with an assortment of causes and risk factors encompassing biological, psychological, as well as social factors. Among them is the existence of chronic illness, which could stimulate heightened awareness of the body and focus on somatic symptoms. These clinical facts are typically accompanied by psychological factors , such as depression and anxiety, further complicating the somatic symptoms phenomenon. The entwining of the relationship is brought out by findings that show patients presenting for medical care with somatic symptoms also have co-morbid mental health disorders like anxiety and depressive disorders. Hence, chronic disease patients can be particularly vulnerable to the development of somatic symptom disorders, and thus careful evaluation and combined treatment modalities that respect physical and mental health considerations are necessary (Kroenke, 2003). Stress plays a key role in the development of somatic symptom disorders since recent life stressors can significantly impact an individual's vulnerability towards these disorders. Research suggests that stressful events of life could be the precipitants, and one ends up having an over-preoccupation with bodily feelings, which can culminate in somatic complaints. Low self-rated health members might have more prevalent somatic complaints, suggesting that how individuals rate themselves on their health status can influence their mental status. Chronic stressor exposure can also result in maladaptive coping mechanisms that express themselves in the form of somatic complaints. Therefore, it is crucial to comprehend how stress interacts with sick role behavior and self-concept to discern which groups are at risk and implement preventative interventions with the aim of offsetting the impact of stress on health outcomes (Mayston et al., 2012). Healthcare utilization patterns are also a significant risk factor for somatic symptom and related disorders. Increased exposure to medical attention can sometimes reinforce the cycle of somatic complaints as patients will begin relying on medical attention in order to verify what they are going through rather than face underlying psychological grievances. Excessive healthcare utilization is frequently associated with the complexity of care required, difficulties of patient-provider interaction, and feelings of lack of achievement in outcome from intervention. These interactions risk escalating an individual's sense of illness and exaggerating somatic complaints. Further, poor communication between the patients and the healthcare professionals can exacerbate frustration and confusion, thus exacerbating the vicious cycle of somatic symptom presentation. Treatment of somatic symptom disorders becomes paramount by interrupting these loops through enhanced provider training and improving patient support services (Kroenke, 2003).

13.4.1. Biological Factors Contributing to Somatic Symptoms

The relationship between somatic and biological symptoms becomes increasingly recognized in psychological research, particularly in the treatment of somatic symptoms and related disorders. One of the critical biological mechanisms is the function of cytokines, which are proteins used in cell signaling within the immune response. Higher levels of some cytokines, such as interleukin-1 receptor antagonist (IL-1ra), have been positively correlated with somatic symptoms among depressed cancer patients, suggesting that biological mechanisms contribute to the occurrence of somatic symptoms. Interestingly enough, somatic symptom scores among cancer patients are typically rather high relative to those of their caregivers, implying that the magnitude of such symptoms may be established both by biological stressors and psychological demands of coping with chronic illness. Clarification of these relationships bears critical relevance for the creation of individualized interventions that integrate both biological and psychological dimensions of care (Li et al., 2017). A second important biological factor relates to the neurobiological mechanism of aging and its effect on mental health, specifically geriatric depression. Research indicates that with increasing age, biological changes, such as altered neuroendocrine function and inflammatory responses, can induce psychological distress and somatic symptoms. Psychological experience of health, life satisfaction, and loneliness in older adults further complicate this cycle. As with geriatric populations that have been studied, depression not only impacts emotional health but can also be evidenced by physical complaints, making diagnosis more difficult

(Mayhew et al., 1989). The linking of these physical complaints with biological aging serves to reinforce the proposition that psychological and physiological processes are interrelated, ultimately serving to underscore the necessity of knowing these biological factors in responding to somatic symptoms. The scope of biological factors has since been expanded into more comprehensive contexts, such as stress response systems and their impact on somatic symptoms among diverse populations. Chronic stress induces a chain of neurobiological processes that, in the end, cause the malfunctioning of the hypothalamic-pituitary-adrenal (HPA) axis, which finally triggers the emergence of somatic symptoms. This dysregulation is generally manifested in the form of alterations in immune response, manifesting as increased inflammation, which has been related to somatic presentation in patients suffering from stress-related disorders. Furthermore, environmental as well as genetic tendencies may promote these biological alterations, and hence it is essential to discuss each patient's own biological background. Understanding of these intricate biological determinants is able to assist clinicians in accurate diagnosis and therapy of somatic symptoms so as to enhance patient outcomes and care in somatic symptom and other similar disorders (Mayhew, 1989; Li et al., 2017) (Figure 13.10).

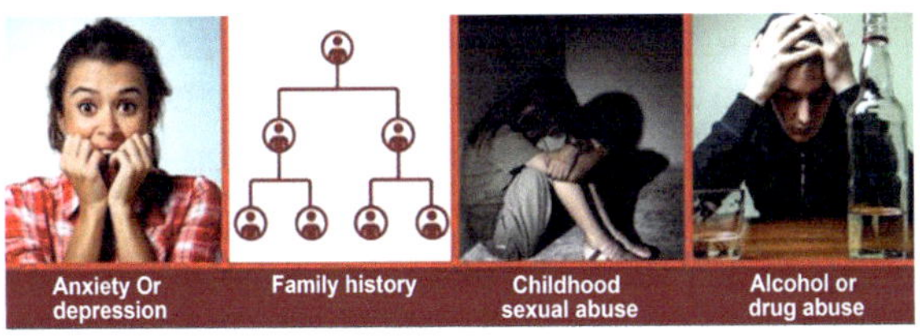
Anxiety Or depression
Family history
Childhood sexual abuse
Alcohol or drug abuse

Figure 13.10. Biological factors contributing to somatic symptoms.

Source: https://mantracare.org/wp-content/uploads/2021/12/Risk-Factors-Of-Somatic-Symptom-Disorder-e1639202313686-768x310.jpg.

13.4.2. Psychological Influences and Stressors

The dynamic between psychological issues and somatic symptoms and related disorders is key to understanding how mental states can be translated into physical expression. Psychological and emotional pain through depression and anxiety has been found to exert a profound effect on the intensity and the experience of somatic symptoms. Anxious children, for instance, may express their internal agonies through physical complaints. This approach makes evident the importance of psychological health in treatment settings. The prevalence of somatic, anxiety, and depressive disorders in children demonstrates the complex interdependence of emotional wellness and somatic expressions. Research shows that certain psychological interventions, particularly in early childhood, are effective in reversing the onset and severity of these disorders and resulting in global health and functioning (Storey & Smith, 2008). Thus, psychological considerations must take priority in treatment to achieve maximum recovery and quality of life. Stressors, either psychological or physical, are the main causal factors for the generation and perception of somatic symptoms. Research has shown that many various types of stressors, from traumatic life experiences to chronic stress, are causally involved in developing conditions , such as irritable bowel syndrome and define the interaction between emotional tension and biological reactions. These stressors may enhance visceral sensitivity, with augmented pain response or discomfort and no organic disease. This relation is optimally characterized in experimental models of stress in which the impact of acute and chronic stress on physiological processes is assessed, that order to confirm the significant influence of stress on visceral responses. Awareness of these interactions promotes the identification of potential therapeutic targets to decrease stress-related somatic symptoms. Therefore, the incorporation of stress management therapies in treatment becomes essential for improvement in therapeutic outcomes and the management of the multidimensional nature of somatic symptom disorders (Larauche et al., 2011). Furthermore, the psychological nature of stressors necessitates the incorporation of an integrative approach in treatment procedures for somatic symptoms and related disorders. A majority of individuals undergo a combination of psychological stressors that could exacerbate their somatic symptoms, thus leading them into a distress cycle. The more anxious or depressed the patients become, the more they focus on body sensations and utilize them as evidence for severe illness. Therefore, it is critical to develop effective psychological therapies to break the pattern. Cognitive-behavioral intervention-based evidence-based therapies can provide the patients with the necessary tools for reinterpretation of the symptoms and management of their emotions. This interdisciplinary strategy not only addresses the psychological stressors at hand but also enables patients to regain mastery over their health narratives. Further interfacing of psychological insight with medical management forms an integral framework for addressing somatic symptom-related disorders effectively (Smith et al., 2008).

13.4.3. Sociocultural Determinants That Affect Prevalence and Perception

Sociocultural influences have significant effects on somatic symptoms and related disorders because they shape people's experiences and expressions of distress. Various cultures' conceptualization and definition of mental health disorders differ, hence affecting symptom expression and interpretation. For instance, in certain societies where stigmas of mental illnesses are prevalent, individuals react with somatic symptoms as a socially acceptable way of expressing emotional distress. This behavior pattern can lead to increased reporting of somatic symptoms since the individual is concerned about the social impact associated with a mental illness diagnosis. In this manner, sociocultural milieux do not allow for proper diagnosis and treatment, hence further increasing the cycle of mislabeling and misinterpreting mental health issues among groups. Moreover, some sociocultural aspects , such as urbanization, drug abuse, and population variables, equally correlate with the incidence of depression and anxiety, directly attributed to somatic symptom disorders.

Evidence has revealed that individuals in urban areas tend to have increased levels of anxiety compared to rural residents, as proven in various studies conducted across various populations from Nepal (Holen et al., 2016). Furthermore, culturally determined behaviors like the use of psychoactive drugs like marijuana have also been associated with increased depressive symptoms, further complicating the picture of somatic symptom disorder. The dynamic interplay among these extremely variable sociocultural determinants emphasizes the necessity of applied mechanisms in mental health care that account for the particular context of given populations, thus maximizing understanding as well as outcome. Finally, an externalist perspective offers useful ideas in accounting for somatic symptoms within the broader sociocultural setting. It suggests that psychiatric disorders cannot be fully accounted for based on strictly biological characteristics, as they are inescapably bound up with social and cultural ones (Glackin et al., 2019). For instance, cultural norms and societal expectations may determine how distress is communicated, which might make somatic symptoms valid health issues or simply expressions of hidden emotional distress. Once the complex interrelation of sociocultural factors affecting mental health is understood, practitioners can construct more comprehensive treatments that target not only the client's symptoms but also their lived realities. Such harmonization is likely to enhance the detection of somatic symptom disorders, with higher awareness and less stigma surrounding mental health in general (Figure 13.11).

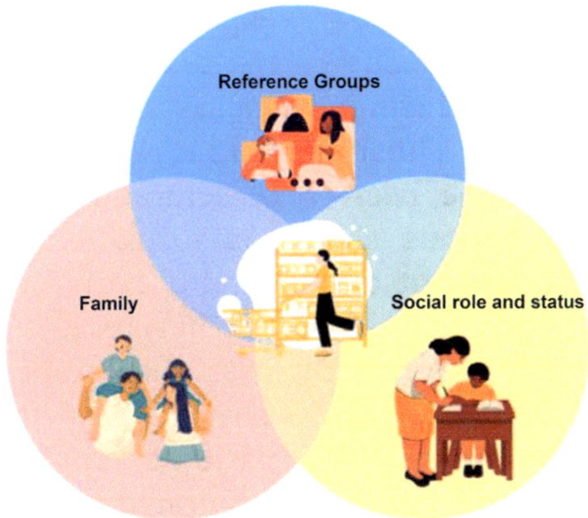

Figure 13.11. Sociocultural factors affecting prevalence and perception.

Source: https://www.superheuristics.com/wp-content/uploads/2023/02/Sage-Green-Abstract-Floral-Social-Networking-Venn-Diagram-Graph-1-768x576.png.

Test Your Knowledge

1. How do biological, psychological, and social factors contribute to the development of somatic symptom and related disorders?
2. What role do trauma, stress, and maladaptive cognitive patterns play as risk factors?

13.5. Treatment Approaches

Learning Outcome

1. Psychotherapy options for somatic symptom disorders.
2. Role of medication in treatment.
3. Importance of a multidisciplinary approach.

Treatment interventions of somatic symptoms and related disorders need multi-modal intervention that embodies psychological, physical, and social dimensions of care. The presumption underlying successful treatment is that these disorders are often the product of interaction among biological, psychological, and social determinants. The most commonly used technique is cognitive-behavioral therapy (CBT), which enables patients to recognize and restructure negative thought patterns that cause their somatic symptoms. This model of treatment not only alleviates symptoms but also educates for coping, strengthening itself against future assault. In addition, the addition of psychoeducation to the process empowers patients by providing them with the knowledge and information to better understand their illnesses and become more actively involved in the healing process. In clinical practice, new models , such as The BodyMind Approach (TBMA)®, particularly in the treatment of medically unexplained symptoms (MUS), have emerged. This approach combines elements of dance movement psychotherapy within a biopsychosocial framework to treat the complex interplay of somatic symptoms and emotional well-being. The TBMA-based treatment programs are designed to treat patients who tend to traverse healthcare networks without ever coming to a resolution, thereby reducing unwanted medical interventions. These structured group interventions not only offer peer support in groups but also augment traditional therapy techniques through reinforcement of the body movement-emotional expression link. Practitioners are able to more effectively treat the chronic nature of such disorders as well as increase patient satisfaction with their care by utilizing such integrative models. (Payne, 2015) Additionally, measures of prevention cannot be overstated, especially about the high prevalence rate of somatic symptoms among adolescents and children. Evidence provides that the treatment of psychological early detection and intervention of anxiety and depression disorders has been able to reduce the prevalence of somatic symptoms among younger populations. Cognitive-behavioral skills and techniques training programs hold particular promise because they support adaptive coping skills that can prevent the risk of future somatic difficulties. Programs work more effectively with this population when they are developmentally sensitive and culturally responsive, so that they respond to the distinctive needs of ethnically different children. Thus, effective prevention and treatment interventions require a combined program incorporating both psychological therapy and strong family and social support systems. (Smith et al., 2008)

13.5.1. Psychotherapy for Somatic Symptom Disorders

Psychotherapy is the cornerstone in the treatment of somatic symptom disorders, allowing individuals an avenue to become more informed and cope more effectively with the psychological issues associated with their body symptoms. Cognitive Behavior Therapy (CBT) is particularly useful as it allows patients an opportunity to challenge and rework irrational thought processes involved in their somatic experiences. Through the focus on maladaptive patterns, the patients are able to reattribute their symptoms and reduce anxiety, eventually leading to improved coping abilities. The structured nature of CBT also enables realistic goal formation, which enhances the motivation of the individuals towards the treatment. Furthermore, evidence suggests that, along with the medical treatment, psychotherapy can actually improve the outcomes of the patients, supporting the necessity for an integrated approach towards the treatment of somatic symptom disorders. The second viable option of psychotherapy is mindfulness-based interventions that are aimed at enhancing the patient's awareness and acceptance of his/her somatic experience in a nonjudgmental manner. These therapies encourage the development of skills that enhance psychological resilience and emotional regulation, which are central to managing chronic physical symptoms. Perhaps patients may reduce the symptom-distressing impact by developing awareness that is non-reactive to bodily sensations. Research has indicated that mindfulness interventions can decrease the severity of symptoms and enhance psychological functioning. Additionally, pairing mindfulness with conventional medical care not only gets patients more in touch with their own abilities to manage their health but also encourages a more integrative understanding of the mind-body relationship, a central focus in the narrative of somatic symptom disorders. Group therapy may also assume an important role in the psychotherapeutic management of somatic symptom disorders. A part of being in group sessions provides patients with a unique space to communicate, a chance for patients to be part of a shared experience, and to foster mutual empathy. This feeling of peer community and belonging may even replace feelings of loneliness that patients can feel and foster a sense of healing and camaraderie. Group therapy encourages the articulation of coping behaviors and adaptive skills among the group members. It also supports their reciprocal experience validation to enhance self-acceptance and decrease additional stigma for having symptoms. As research attests to the efficacy of group therapy in improving emotional functioning, its inclusion within models of treatment for somatic symptom disorders would be a significant step towards optimizing patient care and outcomes, echoing demands for multi-modal therapeutic strategies in this field (Soyka & Horak, 2004; Van Damme et al., 2018) (Figure 13.12).

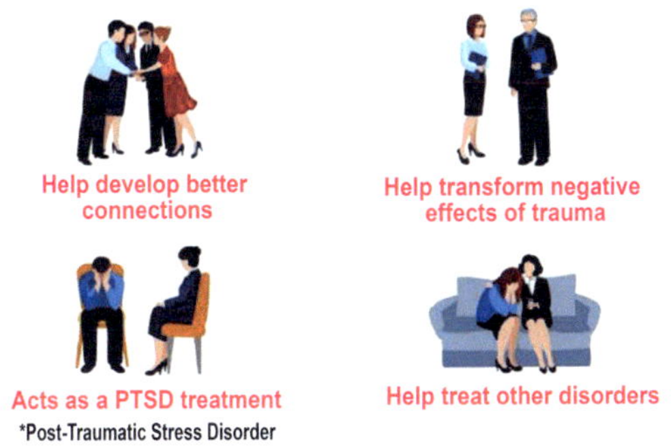

Figure 13.12. Psychotherapy options for somatic symptom disorders.

Source: https://thepleasantmind.com/wp-content/uploads/2019/10/The-Benefits-of-Somatic-Therapy-for-Treating-Trauma-Patients-1024x1024.jpg.

13.5.2. Role of Medication in Treatment

The role of medicine in managing somatic symptoms and related disorders cannot be downplayed because it offers a means of intervening in both the physical and psychological aspects of such disorders. Medications , such as antidepressants and anxiolytics can minimize symptoms of depression and anxiety that usually accompany somatic disorders, making it easier to introduce psychotherapeutic intervention. Studies have shown that the co-treatment of pharmacotherapy and psychological therapy is superior to psychotherapy alone. For instance, in the treatment of a particular symptom, titrating doses based on each patient's requirements can make treatment far more likely to adhere to and more successful overall, ultimately resulting in more integrated functioning. A multimodal treatment approach that incorporates medication can therefore successfully treat the complex interaction between somatic experience and affective disturbance in these disorders. Psychotropic medications have been shown to enhance motivation and participation in treatment programs, particularly in substance use disorders, which comorbidly occur with somatic symptom disorders. As a study on an outpatient model of detoxification shows, psychotropic medication was common practice, and a high percentage of patients benefited from the combination of pharmacotherapy and motivational psychotherapy. The results of this treatment approach show that medication not only serves to address withdrawal or coping symptoms but also operates to encourage patients to pursue further therapeutic services. It is apparent that effective medication management in these instances can become an important gateway to broader treatment, enhancing the prospects of long-term recovery and symptom diminishment in individuals with complex needs. Also, one has to consider how the drug can be tailored to accommodate the special characteristics of every patient's condition. Current studies indicate that there are several drivers of treatment decisions, including symptom reports, comorbidities, and lifestyle. These drivers are significant in determining the appropriate medication pathway to pursue, thus the impetus for a personalized approach. In the management of somatic symptoms and related disorders, identification of these influences can help clinicians optimize treatment options, including medications in combination with other modes of treatment as needed. By treating not only the biological but also the psychological components of these illnesses, clinicians can facilitate more effective management strategies, with the end result being improved patient outcomes and quality of life for those patients who are experiencing these challenging disorders.

13.5.3. Importance of a Multidisciplinary Process

For somatic symptoms and related disorders, a multidisciplinary framework is more than a necessity. It enables an in-depth understanding of the complex interaction between psychological and physiological causes of these conditions. By incorporating a range of healthcare professionals , such as psychologists, physical therapists, and primary care doctors, patients are best able to obtain a comprehensive evaluation and customized treatment regimen. Such collaboration can reveal some underlying issues not apparent when care is delivered in a siloed way. For example, treating musculoskeletal disorders might remove symptoms , such as pain or discomfort and thus improve overall patient well-being. Secondly, this balanced perspective also encourages teamwork among specialists that can ultimately lead to innovative treatment methods, where intricate solutions to the multidimensional issues presented by somatic symptom disorders can be better attained, leading to improved patient outcomes. Also, there is mounting evidence in favor of the efficacy of multidisciplinary treatment for conditions like somatic tinnitus, wherein psychological factors are responsible for a great deal of the physical symptoms. Where tinnitus is linked with somatic disease, accurate evaluation by professionals in audiology and musculoskeletal medicine is crucial in the provision of a correct diagnosis and care. Intervention that respects the co-relationship between auditory and somatosensory systems can be very rewarding, as outlined in many research works. For example, in tinnitus: the typical modulation by specific physical activity highlights the requirement for understanding the complex interaction between somatic disorders and sensory input. Accordingly, collaboration among audiology experts with specialization in somatic disorders can not only give a more elaborate diagnosis but can, with therapy, also enhance efficiency, empowering the patient by addressing both their sensory and somatic aspects with a combined approach (Cialente et al., 2017). In pediatric populations as well, the need for multidisciplinary treatment is no less pressing, especially in the management of Functional Neurological Symptom Disorder (FNSD). When symptoms are triggered by atypical nervous system stimulation, a unitary treatment model in most instances proves insufficient.

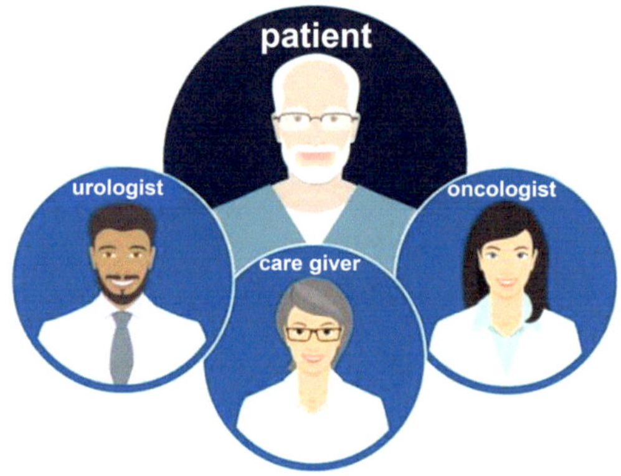

Figure 13.13. Importance of a multidisciplinary approach.

Source: https://slideplayer.com/slide/14978226/91/images/13/Importance+of+Multidisciplinary+Approach.jpg.

The integration of modalities , such as Dance Movement Therapy (DMT) with more traditional medical approaches encourages an environment of care that compromises between psychological and somatic concerns for the patient. DMTs emphasize body awareness and communication without words, also play an important role in mind-body integration, an indispensable factor for children with FNSD. The study has proven that the integration of psychotherapeutic techniques with physical therapy and family involvement can enhance the healing process by making a support system available to buffer against symptom-focused attention that tends to hinder recovery. Hence, the interdisciplinary model is of greatest utility in creating integrated treatment plans that acknowledge the complex factors influencing a child's health (Powers, 2024) (Figure 13.13).

Test Your Knowledge

1. How do cognitive-behavioral therapy (CBT) and psychoeducation help individuals manage somatic symptom disorders?
2. What role do medication, regular follow-up, and a collaborative care approach play in treatment?

13.6. Impact on Quality of Life

Learning Outcome

1. Effects on daily functioning and relationships.
2. Economic implications of somatic symptom disorders.
3. Stigma and its influence on treatment seeking.

The impact of somatic symptoms and related disorders on the quality of life can be extensive and far-reaching. Individuals with such disorders would complain of chronic, inexplicable physical symptoms that elicit significant emotional and psychological distress. This crossover between physical and mental illness can be a debilitating cycle, where the symptoms reinforce the feelings of depression and anxiety. As observed from recent studies, overuse of the internet has been associated with increasing somatic symptoms among adolescents, illustrating the manner in which lifestyle variables of today might be to blame for declining mental well-being. This interaction shows that the quality of life is not only determined by the presence of physical symptoms but has strong associations with broader psychosocial factors , such as social interaction and the ability to perform daily activities effectively (Cerutti et al., 2017). Also, the prevalence of conditions , such as premenstrual syndrome (PMS) among female university students is another instance of somatic symptoms' detrimental impact on quality of life. It is estimated that nearly 63% of Lebanese female university students have PMS, which causes both physical distress and psychological issues, such as irritable behavior and heightened emotional reactivity. This cross-interaction of somatic and affective symptoms not only disrupts academic functioning but also affects interpersonal relationships and general well-being. The high association between lifestyle variables, such as caffeine consumption and drug use, and PMS severity supports the use of comprehensive health interventions to improve the quality of life among patients (Akiki et al., 2018). These findings emphasize the need for interventions that are specifically crafted and address both somatic symptoms and psychological dimensions to enhance satisfaction with life and to reduce the burden of somatic disorders. Finally, the effects of somatic symptoms and related disorders extend to long-term outcomes for health. Long-term difficulties resulting from these disorders can lead to social retreat and decreased coping ability, further fixating individuals in a cycle of poor quality of life. Because research indicates that the impact of lifestyle on somatic symptoms yields valuable insights into the mechanisms for these disorders. For instance, excessive users of the internet are found to have greater depression and more somatic complaints, which indicate that interventions aimed at encouraging healthier digital habits are advisable. With these findings, promoting environments that activate physical activity and mental health awareness is crucial because these interventions can be very helpful in improving quality of life for patients with somatic symptoms and related disorders (Cerutti et al., 2017).

13.6.1. Effect on Daily Living and Interpersonal Relationships

Somatic symptoms and related disorders exert a significant impact on everyday functioning and interpersonal relationships, often falling into the trap of distressing themselves by exaggerating psychological and somatic symptoms. The patients who have these disorders usually fall into the trap of constant somatic complaints that lead to disturbance in their routine activities, for example, their job or school. This disturbance in daily activity further increases the sense of frustration and hopelessness. Adolescents, actually, have shown a measurable relationship between heavy internet use and more somatic symptoms, which also makes it challenging for them to engage constructively in academic and social settings. Cited in research, heightened use of the internet among adolescents has been linked not only to somatic complaints but also to emotional and behavioral problems, emphasizing the significance of understanding such connections in depth to mitigate further deterioration in functioning (Cerutti et al., 2017). Somatic symptoms and associated disorders have effects that spread beyond personal experience, having significant effects on interpersonal relationships. Collateral peers and members may struggle with understanding the nonvisible nature of these symptoms, leading to miscommunication and frustration. Individuals will stay away from social interactions due to a fear of experiencing a somatic symptom when in public or being labeled as attention-seeking. Solitude breeds through avoidance, diminishing supportive social networks necessary for well-being. In teenagers and kids, the impact is particularly severe; such a population might be at greater risk of developing depressive symptoms along with somatic complaints, thus creating a vicious cycle feedback that sustains stress in parent, peer, and teacher relationships (Smith et al., 2008). Addressing the pervasive impact of somatic symptoms and related disorders in daily functioning and relationships calls for integrated interventions that extend beyond symptom control. Interventions that enhance emotional regulation and adaptive coping are necessary to counteract the psychological impact of these disorders. Importantly, including psychological therapies as opposed to the use of pharmacological interventions alone has been demonstrated to improve outcomes for affected children (Smith et al., 2008). Moreover, education programs to de-mystify somatic symptoms can also foster peer and family understanding, further supporting systems. As the evidence shows, enhancing everyday functioning and healthy interpersonal relationships entails a strategy that addresses both the individual's symptoms and the broader implications for his or her social environment (Figure 13.14).

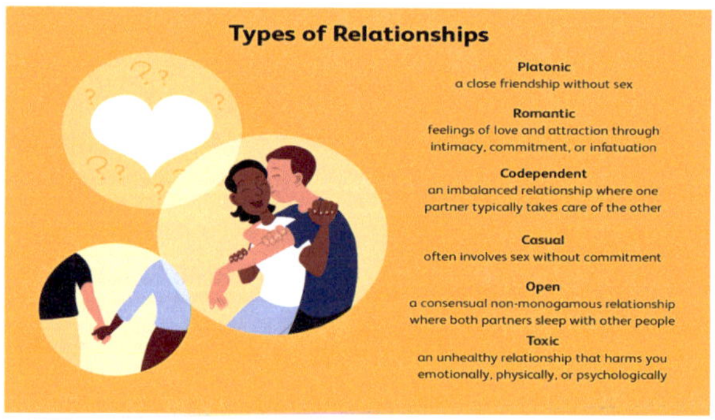

Figure 13.14. Effects on daily functioning and relationships.

Source: https://www.verywellmind.com/thmb/GAI6XG8GTBAfFNYixX-cemjEinc=/1500x0/filters:no_upscale():max_bytes(150000):strip_icc()/6-types-of-relationships-and-their-effect-on-your-life-5209431_V1-a0f57cea6a114b9cbfa1553c0142ec92.png.

13.6.2. Economic Implications of Somatic Symptom Disorders

The economic implications of somatic symptom disorders are far-reaching and impose a significant burden on health systems, workplace functioning, and overall quality of life in society. The disorders are multifaceted in nature, and this complicates their diagnosis and treatment, thus leading to increased healthcare costs. The patients will report a plethora of physical symptoms that lack an obvious medical etiology, which translates to expensive medical evaluations and visits. This diagnostic odyssey can take up significant healthcare resources, distracting from simpler problems and piling up medical costs. As seen in numerous studies, the chronic aspects of these disorders weigh heavily on finances, demanding continuous treatment that can overburden both public and private health systems. Further, the entwinement of symptoms of both the mind and the body complicates treatment as, in most instances, mental health issues are not adequately addressed, creating a circle of economic strain on healthcare resources (Mayston et al., 2012). Finally, somatic symptom disorders severely disrupt a patient's ability to function within the workplace, leading to lost productivity as well as increased absenteeism. Such people are often disadvantaged in stable jobs due to their unstable physical and mental conditions. The resultant work loss not only affects the financial condition of the person but can extend its effects to employers, too, where frequent replacement and high turnover inflate operational costs. Moreover, mental illness stigma will dissuade individuals from seeking treatment, thus sustaining suffering as well as additional economic loss. Failure to address serious somatic symptom disorders will see businesses pay increased healthcare premiums as well as decreased employee morale, hence a less competitive business environment (Etkin et al., 2020). Lastly, societal influence from somatic symptom disorders also points towards their economic impact. The populations with the highest burden of these disorders ultimately have increased healthcare expenditures, which can put pressure on public health budgets. The effects are most pronounced in low- and middle-income settings, where the availability of mental health care remains suboptimal. The economic burden extends to the productivity lost on a macroeconomic scale, since populations with these disorders contribute less to the workforce. Treatment of somatic symptom disorders using integrated treatment approaches may potentially offset some of these economic burdens, and investments in mental health infrastructure have the potential for huge long-term returns for the healthcare system and society at large. It is therefore necessary to appreciate the links between physical and mental health as core to developing effective interventions that diminish the economic impact of such under-researched disorders (Mayston et al., 2012) (Figure 13.15).

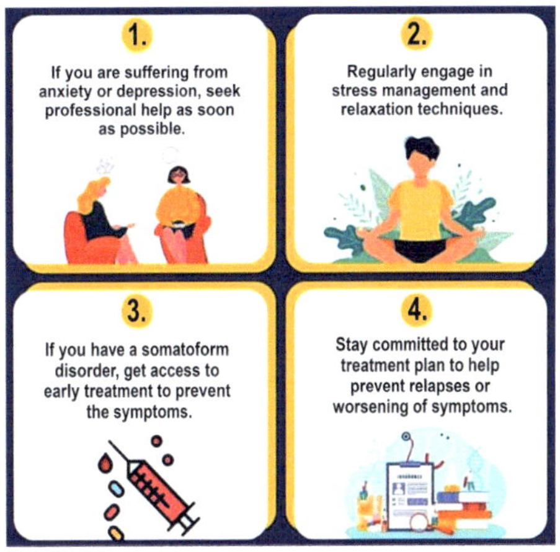

Figure 13.15. Economic implications of somatic symptom disorders.

Source: https://mind.help/wp-content/uploads/2022/03/Self-help-Strategies-For-Somatic-Symptom-Disorder.jpg.

13.6.3. Stigma and Its Influence on Treatment Seeking

Stigma is of considerable importance in shaping individuals' experiences with somatic symptoms and related disorders, particularly in determining whether they will ever approach treatment or not. Stigma takes the form of public views that equate mental illness with personal weakness, and thus shame and internalization of stigmatizing stereotypes. Consequently, individuals avoid seeking help out of fear of labeling and judgment, and hence exacerbate their conditions. This aversion to treatment not only hinders recovery but also creates a cycle of suffering wherein people silently suffer from symptoms rather than meeting their needs. It is important to understand the psychological effect of stigma in devising effective interventions to facilitate open discussions about mental health and in formulating culturally responsive strategies towards seeking treatment among different groups, which not only reverses existing obstacles that prevent people from seeking care but also narrows down necessary care. Cultural differences also complicate the stigmatization of somatic symptoms by affecting the way people convey and understand psychological distress. In some cultures, like those of the Chinese, emotional distress can be conveyed through physical complaints, a process referred to as somatization. Such adaptation by culture can amplify stigma when the detection of psychological conditions is perceived negatively. Instead of seeking psychological treatment, they may seek physical therapy, hoping that the outward manifestation of their distress will be more acceptable and understandable in a social context. The tension between cultural expectations and stigma creates increased challenges for seeking treatment among individuals with somatic symptom disorders and emphasizes the need for culturally sensitive practice in clinical work. By integrating cultural knowledge into treatment models, clinicians can better tailor their services to address the unique demands of individuals from different cultures, reducing stigma and promoting greater acceptance of psych treatment (Heine et al., 2002). Stigma has also been shown to influence the quality of care that is delivered following presentation to the health care system. Stigmatized groups are usually discriminated against by medical practitioners, which can lead to misdiagnosis and poor treatment plans. Institutional bias can also deter people from seeking care, creating the cycle of oppression started by stigma. In combating these consequences, healthcare systems must ensure that they offer training that will help reduce implicit biases and enhance patient empathy in those afflicted with somatic symptoms. A deep understanding of how stigma operates on both the personal and the systemic levels is needed so that help-seeking is viewed as a strength rather than a weakness. In our discussion as we walk through the various treatment methods, an integral component will be ensuring that techniques targeting stigma are infused in order to improve health outcomes for individuals suffering from somatic symptoms and related disorders (Bee et al., 2016) (Figure 13.16).

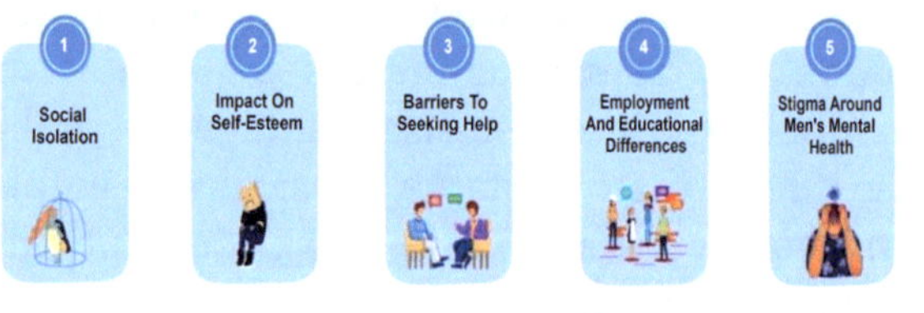
1
Social Isolation
2
Impact On Self-Esteem
3
Barriers To Seeking Help
4
Employment And Educational Differences
5
Stigma Around Men's Mental Health

Figure 13.16. Stigma and its influence on treatment-seeking equate mental health.

Source: https://www.psychologs.com/wp-content/uploads/2024/03/addressing-mental-health-stigma-and-its-impact-on-society-2-1024x553.jpg.

Test Your Knowledge

1. How do somatic symptom disorders interfere with daily functioning, emotional well-being, and social relationships?
2. What challenges do individuals face regarding work, physical activity, and healthcare utilization due to persistent physical symptoms?

SUMMARY

In explaining the complexities involved in somatic symptom and related disorders, it is imperative that one highlights the interaction between psychological and physiological issues which make these conditions complex. Research has indicated that the onset of somatic symptoms can be an indication of underlying psychological distress, which makes diagnosis and treatment complicated. The findings indicate that the cancer patients' somatic symptom scores are higher than those of the caregivers, and this indicates the unique challenge of individuals undergoing bodily illness as well as mental illness. This finding of the link between somatic complaints and psychological health not only has significant implications for clinicians to understand but highlights the importance of designing targeted interventions to treat biological and behavioral aspects of such illnesses. Thus, the recognition and treatment of somatic symptoms in the realm of mental illness can lead to improved treatment outcomes as well as increased patient quality of life (Li et al., 2017). In addition, the two-way interaction between psychological disorders and somatic symptoms, such as anxiety and depression, suggests that patients who come in with illnesses like irritable bowel syndrome can have a variety of disturbances in emotion. This overlap between physical and mental illness is a significant field of study, as it sets up the necessity for an integration of treatment approaches. For instance, patients with irritable bowel syndrome have shown intermediate levels of depressive and anxiety symptoms compared to non-clinical populations. These findings emphasize the necessity for clinicians to treat both the physical and affective aspects of patient care in cases of somatic symptom disorders. Increased advanced learning in this field would lead to more integrative treatment protocols that include medical and psychological care networks to address patients' complicated needs (Hendry et al., 2008). In conclusion, the overlap between somatic symptoms and related psychological disorders is a significant field for continued research and clinical practice. Understanding of the mechanisms of these disorders will be required to develop successful treatments and to reduce stigma associated with mental illness in somatic disorders. The evidence pointing toward major cytokine correlations in particular patient groups suggests potential pathways for targeted therapeutic interventions, which can decrease both somatic and psychiatric symptoms. With the significant influence that these disorders can have on one's life, ongoing research is necessary to continue to improve our knowledge and methods so that patients can receive comprehensive and helpful care that is suited to their individual experiences. From the confluence of knowledge between both biological and psychological fields, healthcare professionals can establish a more empathic and therapeutic environment for patients with somatic symptoms and related disorders ((Hendry et al., 2008; Li et al., 2017).

The discovery of somatic symptoms and related disorders shows strong links between psychological well-being and physical health. All through the discussion, it is a recurring theme that mental health has an overarching effect on experiencing somatic symptoms. Patients frequently discover that their physical conditions are intrinsically connected to emotional experiences, making it a cycle that becomes hard to diagnose and treat. Integrated care approaches are emphasized as being needed, as mental health issues have the potential to lead to somatic symptoms, leading to higher healthcare utilization and poorer outcomes. The combination of these two factors is what displays the need for healthcare providers to recognize the psychological foundations of somatic complaints, thereby ensuring treatments that target the body and mind equally. Moreover, evidence demonstrates that systematic assessment of mental health is most likely to enhance somatic symptom disorder treatment. Proper screening tools are a crucial part of the detection of those patients at risk of debilitating somatic symptoms that are induced by underlying psychiatric illness. As an example, a recent meta-review depicted varied depression screening measures with specific reference to their application in oncology. As documented within the review, the Hospital Anxiety Depression Scale (HADS) is very effective for screening purposes, but its limitations suggest that a tailored approach might be necessary for different patient groups. This indicates a clear line of future work in identifying the optimal tools to evaluate mental health symptoms within patients who present with somatic disorders (Andersen et al., 2015). Finally, the relationship between treatment outcome and mental health is particularly poignant in low-income and middle-income environments, where somatic symptom disorders are likely to be underdiagnosed. Inherent disadvantageous conditions are also typically interwoven with limited access to healthcare resources, generating a vicious feedback loop that influences patient adherence to treatment protocols. Systematic review has identified mental illness disorders that clearly impair uptake of care and adherence, especially to chronic conditions , such as HIV/AIDS. From this research, it is clearly evident that psychosocial elements like depression can affect clinical outcomes significantly, thereby reaffirming the need to treat mental health as part of integral care approaches. This evidence supports the case for incorporating mental health interventions into care plans to improve the overall effectiveness of treatment (Mayston et al., 2012).

KEY TERMS FROM THIS CHAPTER

- Alexithymia
- Conversion disorder
- Factitious disorder
- Health anxiety
- Illness anxiety disorder
- Medically unexplained symptoms
- Primary gain
- Psychogenic pain
- Secondary gain
- Somatization
- Body preoccupation
- Doctor shopping
- Functional neurological symptom disorder
- Hypochondriasis
- Malingering
- Mind-body connection
- Pseudo seizures
- Reassurance seeking
- Somatic symptom disorder
- Symptom amplification

CRITICAL THINKING QUESTIONS

1. **Somatic Symptom Disorder is characterized by:**
   a. Intentional faking of symptoms for personal gain
   b. Physical symptoms that are explained by a medical condition
   c. Excessive focus, anxiety, or behavior related to physical symptoms
   d. Absence of any physical complaints
2. **In Illness Anxiety Disorder, the primary concern is:**
   a. Actual physical symptoms
   b. Preoccupation with having or acquiring a serious illness
   c. Substance abuse
   d. Impulsivity and risk-taking behaviors
3. **Conversion Disorder typically presents with:**
   a. Neurological symptoms incompatible with medical findings
   b. A strong desire to receive medication
   c. Recurrent abdominal pain
   d. Chronic fatigue and fibromyalgia
4. **Factitious Disorder involves:**
   a. Malingering for financial gain
   b. Producing or faking symptoms to assume a sick role
   c. Denial of all medical treatment
   d. Unconscious creation of symptoms
5. **Which of the following best distinguishes malingering from Factitious Disorder?**
   a. The severity of symptoms
   b. The absence of physical complaints
   c. The presence of an external incentive in malingering
   d. The involvement of multiple body systems

Short Answer Questions

1. What are somatic symptom and related disorders primarily characterized by?
2. How does Somatic Symptom Disorder differ from Illness Anxiety Disorder?
3. What is the main psychological factor that contributes to Conversion Disorder (Functional Neurological Symptom Disorder)?
4. Name two common physical symptoms that might be reported in Somatic Symptom Disorder.
5. Define Factitious Disorder and explain how it differs from malingering.

Answer to Critical Thinking Questions

1. (c); 2. (b); 3. (a); 4. (b); 5. (c)

REFERENCES

1. Mayston, R., Kinyanda, E., Chishinga, N., Prince, M., & Patel, V. (2012). Mental disorder and the outcome of HIV/AIDS in low-income and middle-income countries: a systematic review. *AIDS (London, England), 26 Suppl 2*, S117–S135. https://doi.org/10.1097/QAD.0b013e32835bde0f
2. Rodríguez Testal, Juan Francisco; Senín Calderón, Cristina; Perona Garcelán, Salvador Del DSM-IV-TR al DSM-5: análisis de algunos cambios International Journal of Clinical and Health Psychology, vol. 14, núm. 3, septiembre-diciembre, 2014, pp. 221-231 Asociación Española de Psicología Conductual Granada, España (accessed on 28th July 2025).
3. Akiki, Z., Assaad, S., Costanian, C., Daou, D., et al. (2018). Factors associated with premenstrual syndrome and its different symptom domains among university students in Lebanon. https://core.ac.uk/download/287659543.pdf (accessed on 28th July 2025).
4. Andersen, B. L., Becker, G., Carey, M., Carlson, L. E., Cella, D., et al. (2015). Patient-reported depression measures in cancer: A meta-review. https://core.ac.uk/download/42138163.pdf (accessed on 28th July 2025).
5. Balla, M. P., De Vincentiis, M., Di Stadio, A., Greco, A., et al. (2018). Otolaryngologic symptoms in multiple sclerosis: A review. https://core.ac.uk/download/188830242.pdf (accessed on 28th July 2025).
6. Bottesi, G., Ghisi, M., Carraro, E., Barclay, N., Payne, R., & Freeston, M. H. (2016). Revising the Intolerance of Uncertainty Model of Generalized Anxiety Disorder: Evidence from UK and Italian Undergraduate Samples. *Frontiers in psychology*, *7*, 1723. https://doi.org/10.3389/fpsyg.2016.01723 (accessed on 28th July 2025).
7. Bee, P., Lovell, K., MacFarlane, G. J., McBeth, J., et al. (2016). Managing chronic widespread pain in primary care: A qualitative study of patient perspectives and implications for treatment delivery. https://core.ac.uk/download/77614574.pdf (accessed on 28th July 2025).
8. Bekhuis, E., Boschloo, L., Rosmalen, J. G. M., Schoevers, R. A., et al. (2015). Differential associations of specific depressive and anxiety disorders with somatic symptoms. https://core.ac.uk/download/518960486.pdf (accessed on 28th July 2025).
9. Bosutti, A., Jellema, A., Laugeray, A., Peters, A., Rossi-George, A., Schaffner, A., Wadee, A. A., et al. (2012). Depression and sickness behavior are Janus-faced responses to shared inflammatory pathways. https://core.ac.uk/download/9652296.pdf (accessed on 28th July 2025).
10. Li, M., Kouzmina, E., McCusker, M., Rodin, D., Boutros, P. C., Paige, C. J., & Rodin, G. (2017). Cytokines and depression in cancer patients and caregivers. *Neuropsychiatric disease and treatment*, *13*, 2903–2911. https://doi.org/10.2147/NDT.S144774 (accessed on 28th July 2025).
11. Briggs-Gowan, M. J., Carter, A. S., Godoy, L., Mian, N. D., et al. (2012). Patterns of anxiety symptoms in toddlers and preschool-age children: Evidence of early differentiation. https://core.ac.uk/download/215508112.pdf (accessed on 28th July 2025).
12. Carnevali, L., Koenig, J., Ottaviani, C., Sgoifo, A., et al. (2018). Autonomic and brain morphological predictors of stress resilience. https://core.ac.uk/download/157570373.pdf (accessed on 28th July 2025).
13. Cerruti, R., Spensieri, V., Presaghi, F., Valastro, C., Fontana, A., & Guidetti, V. (2017). An exploratory study on Internet addiction, somatic symptoms and emotional and behavioral

functioning in school-aged adolescents. Clinical Neuropsychiatry: Journal of Treatment Evaluation, 14(6), 374–383.(accessed on 28th July 2025).

14. Ching, T. H. W., Dowell, J., Schauldt, V., Siev, J., et al. (2018). Assessing sexual orientation symptoms in obsessive-compulsive disorder: Development and validation of the Sexual Orientation Obsessions and Reactions Test (SORT). https://core.ac.uk/download/153166511.pdf (accessed on 28th July 2025).
15. Cialente, F., Cianfrone, G., Ciofalo, A., De Vincentiis, M., et al. (2017). Somatic tinnitus. https://core.ac.uk/download/98350252.pdf (accessed on 28th July 2025).
16. Cubała, W. J., Landowski, J., Michalak, L., Wiglusz, M. S., et al. (2015). Symptom frequency characteristics of the Hamilton Depression Rating Scale of major depressive disorder in epilepsy. https://core.ac.uk/download/512496548.pdf (accessed on 28th July 2025).
17. Van Damme, A., Declercq, T., Lemey, L., Tandt, H., & Petrovic, M. (2018). Late-life depression: issues for the general practitioner. *International journal of general medicine*, *11*, 113–120. https://doi.org/10.2147/IJGM.S154876(accessed on 28th July 2025).
18. Etkin, P., Ibáñez, M. I., López-Fernández, F., Mezquita, L., et al. (2020). Five Factor Model of personality and structure of psychopathological symptoms in adolescents. https://core.ac.uk/download/323287852.pdf (accessed on 28th July 2025).
19. Everaert, J., & Joormann, J. (2019). Emotion regulation difficulties related to depression and anxiety: A network approach to model relations among symptoms, positive reappraisal, and repetitive negative thinking. https://core.ac.uk/download/237010850.pdf (accessed on 28th July 2025).
20. Garza Guerrero, C., Ibarra Patrón, D., & Medina Vidales, G. (2015). Case report: Diagnostic reconceptualization in the DSM-V on somatoform disorders. https://core.ac.uk/download/76602724.pdf (accessed on 28th July 2025).
21. Glackin, S., Krueger, J., & Roberts, T. (2019). Psychiatry beyond the brain: Externalism, mental health, and autistic spectrum disorder. https://core.ac.uk/download/186331930.pdf (accessed on 28th July 2025).
22. Heine, S. J., Ryder, A. G., & Yang, J. (2002). Somatization vs. psychologization of emotional distress: A paradigmatic example for cultural psychopathology. https://core.ac.uk/download/10687096.pdf (accessed on 28th July 2025).
23. Hendry, J., Hince, D. A., Hood, S. D., Potokar, J., et al. (2008). Irritable bowel syndrome patients exhibit depressive and anxiety scores in the subsyndromal range. https://core.ac.uk/download/61299561.pdf (accessed on 28th July 2025).
24. Hirani, S., Hyam, J. A., Newman, S. P., Shaefi, S., et al. (2006). An examination of factors influencing the choice of therapy for patients with coronary artery disease. https://core.ac.uk/download/1737093.pdf (accessed on 28th July 2025).
25. Holen, A., Linde, M., Manandhar, K., Risal, A., et al. (2016). Anxiety and depression in Nepal: Prevalence, comorbidity and associations. https://core.ac.uk/download/77011297.pdf (accessed on 28th July 2025).
26. Soyka, M., & Horak, M. (2004). Outpatient alcohol detoxification: implementation efficacy and outcome effectiveness of a model project. *European addiction research*, *10*(4), 180–187. https://doi.org/10.1159/000079840 (accessed on 28th July 2025).

27. Joormann, J., & Stoeber, J. (1999). Somatic symptoms of generalized anxiety disorder from the DSM-IV: Associations with pathological worry and depression symptoms in a nonclinical sample. https://core.ac.uk/download/63727.pdf (accessed on 28th July 2025).

28. Kendler K. S. (2017). The Clinical Features of Paranoia in the 20th Century and Their Representation in Diagnostic Criteria From DSM-III Through DSM-5. *Schizophrenia bulletin*, *43*(2), 332–343. https://doi.org/10.1093/schbul/sbw161(accessed on 28th July 2025).

29. Kroenke, K. (2003). Patients presenting with somatic complaints: Epidemiology, psychiatric comorbidity and management. https://core.ac.uk/download/288845950.pdf (accessed on 28th July 2025).

30. Larauche, M., Mulak, A., & Taché, Y. (2011). Stress-related alterations of visceral sensation: Animal models for irritable bowel syndrome study. https://core.ac.uk/download/323080393.pdf (accessed on 28th July 2025).

31. Levenson, J. L., Sharma, A. A., & Ortega-Loayza, A. G. (2017). Somatic symptom disorder in dermatology. *Clinics in dermatology*, *35*(3), 246–251. https://doi.org/10.1016/j.clindermatol.2017.01.010(accessed on 28th July 2025).

32. Mayhew, K. M. (1989). An investigation of factors associated with depression in older adults. https://digitalscholarship.unlv.edu/cgi/viewcontent.cgi?article=1079&context=rtds (accessed on 28th July 2025).

33. Payne, H. (2015). The body speaks its mind: The BodyMind Approach® for patients with medically unexplained symptoms in primary care in England. https://core.ac.uk/download/29850393.pdf (accessed on 28th July 2025).

34. Powers, E. (2024). Utilizing dance movement therapy in the treatment of functional neurological symptom disorder. https://core.ac.uk/download/604141236.pdf (accessed on 28th July 2025).

35. Pamela Storey and Marjorie Smith Thomas Coram Research Unit, Institute of Education, University of London (2008). Methods and approaches to improving the emotional health and well-being of children: A briefing paper concerning interventions to prevent internalizing disorders. A briefing paper concerning interventions to prevent internalising disorders https://core.ac.uk/download/pdf/82102.pdf (accessed on 28th July 2025).

PSYCHIATRIC EMERGENCIES

14

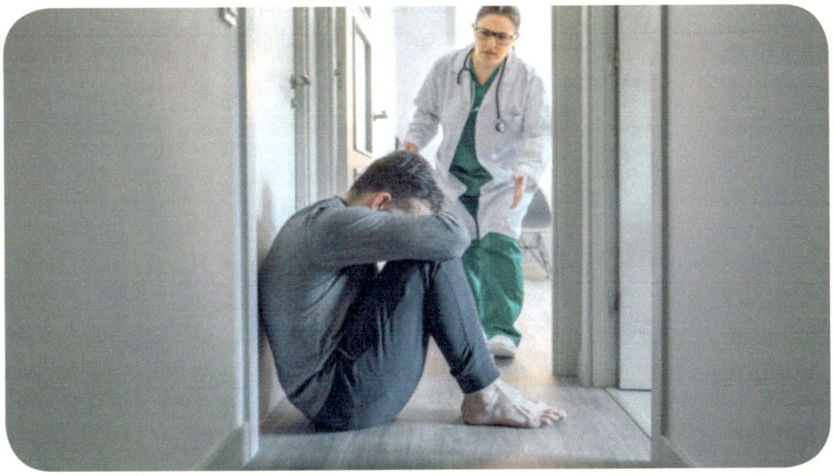

Introduction

In the mental health care environment, psychiatric emergencies pose distinctive challenges requiring instant and urgent response with knowledge. These emergencies may occur due to various conditions , such as severe psychotic breaks, suicidal thoughts, and extreme cases of anxiety attacks, usually compounded by other forms of mental illness , such as depression or schizophrenia. The seriousness of these situations is compounded by the vulnerable condition of mental health services in most areas, where resources are already strained. As established in the literature, five individuals out of every one hundred living in conflict environments suffer from mental disorders, illustrating an intrinsic concurrence between environmental stressors and psychiatric presentation (Weissbecker et al., 2023). The development of new frameworks and modalities, such as the Mental Health and Psychosocial Support Minimum Service Package (MHPSS MSP), is intended to promote coordination and effectiveness in the management of these emergencies and thereby optimize outcomes for affected

LEARNING OBJECTIVES

After studying this chapter, you will be able to:

1. List the types of psychiatric emergencies;
2. Identify the signs and symptoms;
3. Illustrate the risk factors;
4. Explain assessment and diagnosis;
5. Focus on the immediate interventions;
6. Define long-term management.

populations. Effective intervention in psychiatric emergencies requires a multidisciplinary approach whereby multiple health care services are coordinated and existing resources are optimized. The role of consultation-liaison psychiatry (CLP) is pivotal since it acts as a broker between mental and physical health care systems, rendering in-depth assessments and tailor-made interventions for comorbid patients. Historically, the evolution of psychiatry, which has been interrupted by significant advances , such as the discovery of psychotropic drugs and therapy treatments, has transformed how emergencies are managed (Gautam et al., 2022). Such historical advancements are important in understanding the current practice of psychiatric care and the need for professionals knowledgeable in both physical and mental health disciplines. The close interconnection between psychological determinants and bodily health outcomes serves to emphasize the value of an interdisciplinary approach to responding suitably to psychiatric emergencies.

The continued advancement in knowledge about mental health and its integration with general health systems reflects increasing recognition of the value of responding to psychiatric emergencies. As health care professionals recognize the interrelationship between physical and mental health, they are more likely to formulate effective response strategies. Investment in training and utilization of resources for CLP services can enhance the ability to manage psychological crises in diverse medical settings, enhancing patient outcomes and reducing the load on the overall health system. Lastly, emphasis on an integrated and coordinated strategy in psychiatric emergencies is not only a clinical necessity but also a moral necessity, as it is directly connected with the well-being of vulnerable populations who must be dealt with timely, humane care (Gautam et al., 2022; Weissbecker et al., 2023).

Explanation of Psychiatric Emergencies

Psychiatric emergencies are a range of acute mental health crises that require immediate action. They manifest in the form of suicidal ideation, severe depression, psychotic disintegration, or unexpected attacks of anxiety, severely endangering individuals safety and well-being. The seriousness of such attacks normally calls for immediate assessment and intervention from mental health professionals to stabilize the individual and prevent further deterioration.

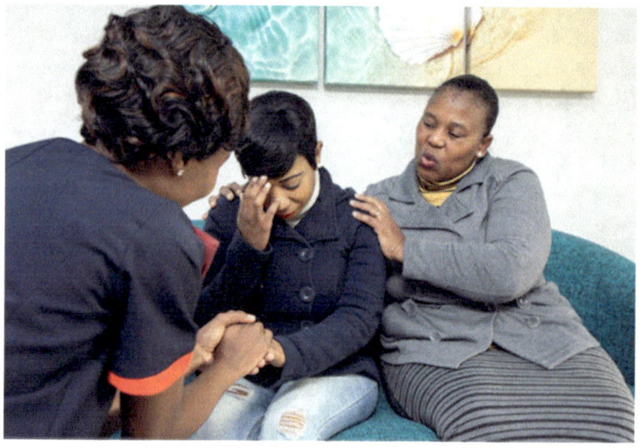

Figure 14.1. Psychiatric emergencies.

Source: https://external-content.duckduckgo.com/iu/?u=https%3A%2F%2Fwww.lifehealthcare.co.za%2Fmedia%2F3430%2Fpsychiatriclife-article-730x488.jpg&f=1&nofb=1&ipt=f1d1afbb9d2c499dc560435ce5928fdaa9c27ae33525efacd41712b237e7c36b.

Most importantly, psychiatric emergencies are not only destructive to the people experiencing them but also affect their families and communities because their ripple effects become overwhelming to social services and health systems. The interaction between mental illness disorders, socio-economic factors, and environmental stressors drives the occurrence of these emergencies, and the need to establish well-functioning community support systems and empathetic healthcare platforms to deal with the increasing number of people overwhelmed by these emergencies. In psychiatric emergencies, socio-economic considerations are prominent, as has been shown in some studies examining concomitant health problems. For instance, it was revealed in a systematic analysis that alcohol abuse-related disorders could result in substantial economic costs through concomitant healthcare costs and lost productivity (Lima & Esquerdo, 2003) (Figure 14.1).

This is one example of how mental illness can extend beyond single crises and become a general public health concerns that necessitate prompt systemic intervention. In psychiatric crises, the need for rapid intervention is further complicated by the potential co-morbid substance abuse disorders and medical illness that may require multi-modal interventions. Therefore, resolution of psychiatric emergencies is not only a question of acute clinical intervention but one of fulfilling the socio-economic determinants that led to the individual's mental health emergency. Being aware of how psychiatric emergencies are presented and dealt with is also an inquiry into society's attitude and the role of the criminal justice system. The policy of deinstitutionalization, which sought to integrate the mentally ill into society, has instead led to additional stigmatization and "transinstitutionalisation," in which such individuals end up in prison or other facilities rather than receiving proper mental health care (Cummins et al., 2013). This diversion makes it harder to address psychiatric emergencies since it is a sign of overall social failure to address the mental health crisis. Therefore, police officers and emergency workers are often at the frontlines of such interactions, highlighting the need for better training and equipment to manage such emergencies with compassion and effectiveness. With the changing face of mental health, it is essential to understand these dynamics to create effective policies and interventions that focus on the welfare of such individuals and facilitate their reintegration into society.

Significance of Early Intervention

In psychiatric emergencies, the importance of prompt intervention cannot be overstressed. Mental crises generally require prompt treatment, as delayed intervention will worsen the symptoms and introduce additional complications. Prompt intervention, particularly through the implementation of de-escalation strategies by experts, greatly influences patient outcomes. Forensic nursing, for instance, uses strategies , such as empathetic listening and active listening in minimizing potentially volatile interactions and agitating patients. This active management not only facilitates the management of the crisis in the short run but also supports a therapeutic environment to enhance future treatment engagement. Focusing on timely and suitable intervention in psychiatric emergencies enables healthcare professionals to enhance patient safety and support more positive recovery processes, highlighting the important influence of timely interventions in mental health cases (Ruth et al., 2025). Additionally, early recognition of psychiatric emergencies is typically associated with reduced morbidity and mortality. Conditions , such as acute depression, psychosis, or suicide ideation need to be evaluated and treated immediately to prevent disastrous consequences. If the warning signs of a crisis are recognized early by medical professionals, they can implement evidence-based interventions that stabilize the patient and prevent worsening. For instance, the implementation of proper pharmacological intervention or the development of therapeutic communication can be critical first interventions in crisis management. Research reveals how early psychiatric evaluation not only reduces the risk of self-harm but also supports overall patterns of mental health recovery. Without immediate intervention, the risk of escalating crises increases, requiring the application of early intervention as a central element of effective psychiatric intervention (Borie et al., 2024). Apart from immediate patient care, response in psychiatric emergencies also involves coordination among interdisciplinary teams to offer complete crisis management. When mental health professionals, emergency responders, and forensic nurses are coordinated in a team framework, they create an integrated system of dealing with complex issues arising from emergencies. A collaborative model fosters shared decision-making as well as access to the right resources and interventions. Early intervention by multidisciplinary teams has evidenced reductions in hospital stays and enhanced effective outpatient follow-ups. As the character of psychiatric emergencies continues to evolve, the need for timely interventions and collaborative measures will be crucial in enhancing quality care, safeguarding patient rights, and ultimately increasing health outcomes among the vulnerable population (Ruth et al., 2025).

14.1. Types of Psychiatric Emergencies

Learning Outcome

1. Suicidal ideation and attempts.
2. Acute psychosis.
3. Severe substance abuse crises.

In psychiatry, psychiatric emergencies present in various forms with certain responses and interventions. Suicidal crises are one of the frequent presentations where individuals arrive with acute self-injurious thoughts or intent. The urgency of such situations is evident because of the risk of suicide completion, hence the need for immediate intervention. Underlying mental illness, critical life stressors, or substance abuse are frequent underlying causes for suicidal crises. Identification of warning signs, for example, threatening words or acute changes in behavior, can be lifesaving for professionals and caregivers. Research has revealed that an integrated approach that includes psychological support along with crisis stabilization can significantly reduce short-term threats, thus redirecting individuals into long-term therapeutic possibilities and support structures, thus enhancing the prognosis for recovery (Oving et al., 2019). A second critical category of psychiatric emergencies is acute psychotic crises, which commonly present with a break from reality, hallucinations, or delusions. These episodes can occur as a consequence of many conditions, including schizophrenia or severe mood disorders, but may also be secondary to substance intoxication or withdrawal. These types of presentations are unpredictable, so emergent evaluation and treatment are required to avoid harm to the patient and others. Recommended interventions would include de-escalation of the crisis and, if necessary, antipsychotic drug therapy to sedate the patient. Further, adequate follow-up treatment is essential to manage any underlying disease and avert subsequent attacks (Oving et al., 2019). Awareness of the nuances of such emergencies can be a great difference in the efficacy of treatment administered during the crisis situation. Lastly, substance-induced psychiatric emergencies are a growing concern as the opioid crisis and other substance use issues continue to plague society. Acutely intoxicated or withdrawing patients may present with a variety of behaviors ranging from agitation to extreme mood syndromes or cognitive impairment. The nature of the psychiatric emergency is determined to some extent by the substance used, leading to a myriad of presenting clinical scenarios that confound diagnosis and treatment. Responders must differentiate between primary psychiatric disorders and drug-use-triggered or drug-use-influenced disorders so that they can provide appropriate care. Effective management can involve immediate medical treatment, possibly with supportive therapy and antidote administration as needed, along with psychiatric evaluation (Chan et al., 2017). The relationship between psychiatric well-being and drug use requires comprehensive treatment frameworks that accommodate the psychological and medical demands in emergency rooms.

14.1.1. Suicidal Behavior and Attempts

The suicidal ideation and attempt process has received tremendous attention when considered in the context of psychiatric emergencies, particularly in children and adolescents. Based on research, a significant number of youths have been found to struggle with non-suicidal self-injury behaviors, with a specific survey reporting that 10% of children aged between 4 and 17 had reported engaging in non-suicidal self-injury (NSSI). Alarmingly, within the 12 to 17-year-old demographic, one in 13 contemplated suicide within the past year, while one in 40 made an attempt (O\u27Gorman et al., 2019).

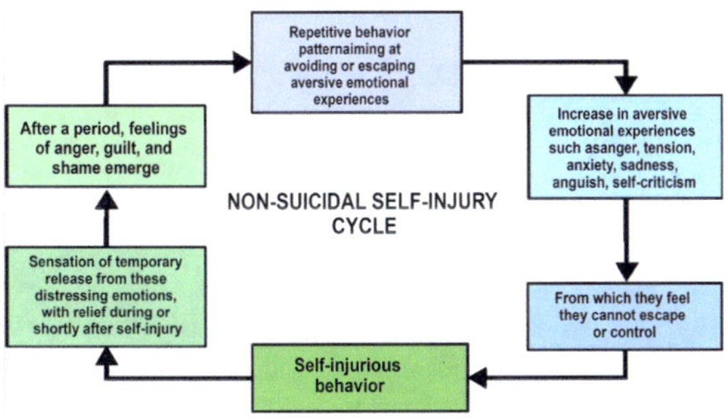

Figure 14.2. Non-suicidal self-injury cycle. (NSSI).

Source: https://www.jped.com.br/en-profile-non-suicidal-self-injury-in-adolescents-articulo-S0021755719303250#imagen.

These statistics underscore the urgent need for educational institutions to adopt proactive measures in addressing these critical mental health issues. As schools are generally the point of entry for adolescents, it is important that they establish an open environment for the cause of mental health and train staff with the ability to identify risk behavior and intervene appropriately. Suicidal ideation should be subjected to close scrutiny and an understanding of the underlying mental illnesses. Psychiatric emergencies encompass a variety of acute disturbances , including suicide attempts, severe depression, and psychosis (Colombo et al., 2022) (Figure 14.2).

Effective initial assessments should include comprehensive histories, physical examinations, and lab screens to preclude possible medical etiologies. This full protocol is important in the safeguarding of patient safety and directs healthcare professionals towards appropriate interventions. A case in point would be adolescent sites where adolescents express ideation of self-harm; psychiatric evaluation and crisis stabilization, if required, become integral parts of treatment immediately. By the recognition of suicidal ideation as a legitimate psychiatric emergency, mental health professionals will be in a position to cope with the complexity of the treatment, and as such, minimize the risk of subsequent suicide attempts. Prevention and postvention practices are crucial components of the mitigation of the impact of suicidal ideation and attempts in schools. Schools are in a strategic position to take a leading role in suicide prevention by establishing supportive environments in which students can safely talk about their mental health issues and experiences (Gorman et al., 2019). Putting structured programs based on the principles of the Queensland Suicide Action Prevention Plan, prevention, intervention, and postvention, can provide structures that build student resilience and enhance mental well-being. Secondly, collaboration with mental health professionals ensures staff members receive the proper training to effectively intervene when a crisis is presented. By tackling the topic of a holistic approach to mental health, schools can focus on developing a community culture mindful of signs of distress and providing support services to those in need in a timely fashion.

14.1.2. Acute Psychosis

The development of acute psychosis presents severe challenges to psychiatric emergencies in that it tends to produce a wide array of disturbing symptoms. Acute psychotic patients are in the habit of presenting symptoms ranging from violence and hallucinations to delusions and, in very severe cases, violent reactions. For this reason, emergency room psychiatrists need to take an immediate and systematic approach to dealing with these patients. Acute psychosis identification is essential not just to facilitate timely intervention but also to create safety for both patient and staff. Diagnostic ambiguity implies that clinicians need to try to determine emergent conditions , such as suicidal ideation or other life-endangering behavior, during the process of assessment, underlining the importance of effective triage efforts under these conditions (Adams et al., 2002). Pharmacological intervention is a significant component of the management of acute psychosis, particularly in the emergency room. One of the most common approaches is the use of antipsychotic drugs, often supplemented with sedatives, to rapidly stabilize the patient. For instance, in Rio de Janeiro, a major study found that the combination of haloperidol and promethazine was used extensively for rapid tranquilization due to clinicians' perception of safety and efficacy in psychiatric emergency rooms (Adams et al., 2002). But although the application of this treatment is common, the truth is that there is a lack of further scientific evaluation of other pharmacological interventions to prove their efficacy. This lack of empirical evidence means re-examining existing treatments carefully so as to guarantee the administration of the best and evidence-based interventions to patients so that they might cope better with the disorganized process of acute psychosis. Other than pharmacotherapy, the management of acute psychosis in emergency settings is otherwise supported by non-pharmacological interventions aimed at providing a supportive and protective environment. These may include de-escalation techniques, patient reassurance, and therapeutic interaction to reduce agitation and facilitate trust. Emergency physicians must also consider the general context of each patient's presentation, including potential organic etiologies or concurrent medical illnesses that may exacerbate psychiatric illness (Diner et al., 2011). Interpersonal communication and team care in interprofessional team environments are also paramount, providing an integrated management of both mental health emergencies and underlying medical conditions. With increasing knowledge of mental health in the world, maximization of acute psychosis management remains a critical objective in psychiatric emergencies, leading to improved outcomes and safety of the patient (Figure 14.3).

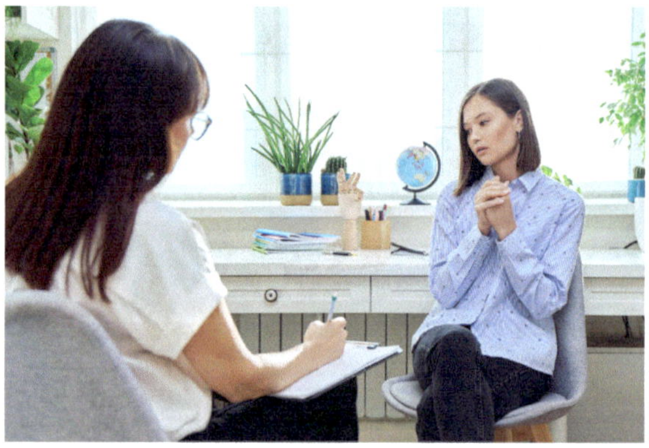

Figure 14.3. Acute psychosis.

Source: https://external-content.duckduckgo.com/iu/?u=https%3A%2F%2Fassets.betterhelp.com%2Fadvice%2Fimages%2F9c2664008f1dd72e952fd752aca39654-borderline-personality-disorder-awareness-month-spotlight-on-a-misunderstood-condition_7_l.jpg&f=1&nofb=1&ipt=b18cb4db5188dc7ca70b6d0258725cce5bc2387e2f857d874c6b9e7205194042.

14.1.3. Severe Substance Abuse Crises

The state of severe substance abuse crises is one that has become a pressing concern within the broader category of psychiatric crises. The complex nature of the crises is further augmented by the convergence of psychological disorders and the pharmacologic management of aggression and violent behavior. For instance, patients with severe substance abuse often present with numerous forms of psychosis, which manifest as immediate behavioral disturbances necessitating prompt intervention. In a majority of emergency settings, the generic application of pharmacological treatments, such as the haloperidol-promethazine combination, has been shown to effectively control acute agitation and psychosis, though comprehensive evaluation of such interventions remains the exception (Adams et al., 2002). Practitioners are thus obligated to possess expertise in the complexities presented by both the dynamics of substance-induced disorders and the modalities of treatment in effect to effectively handle such psychiatric emergencies. Also, crisis intervention is reliant on trained staff to perform the interventions needed. Physical restraints, even though a debated crisis intervention technique for dealing with highly agitated patients, prove to assist in preserving patient safety during severe emergencies. Legal regulations mandate trained medical staff to closely monitor patients restrained at all times, but the quality and intensity of the monitoring efforts can have a life-altering impact on the patient (Allen, 2018). Application of more intense surveillance procedures, including more intense registered nurse assessment, has been shown to decrease the duration of restraint episodes. This evidence recommends immediate action by healthcare systems in adopting best practices in the care of patients experiencing severe substance abuse crisis episodes, focusing on continuous psychiatric monitoring to minimize the harms of such interventions. Lastly, a need exists to comprehend the overall societal effect of extreme substance abuse emergencies in the context of psychiatric emergencies. In addition to overwhelming the healthcare system, the increasing prevalence of substance use disorders also adds to increased homelessness, violence, and incarceration among the psychiatrically ill. This social cost calls for intervention that is not only multifaceted in scope, including emergency psychiatric care, but prevention and community support mechanisms as well. Resolution of the root causes of drug abuse, that is, socioeconomic disadvantage, and availability of mental health services, is necessary to avert extreme crises. By encouraging a more holistic model that combines immediate clinical treatment with ongoing preventative measures, the mental health industry can begin confronting the severe issues of serious substance abuse for the ultimate benefit of public health and safety (Figure 14.4).

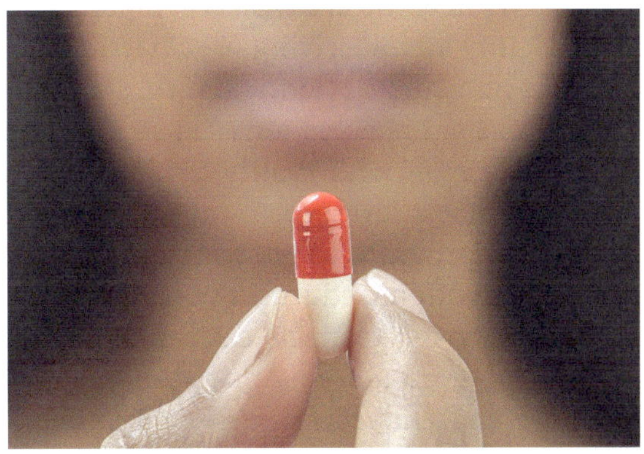

Figure 14.4. Substance abuse.

Source: https://www.verywellmind.com/thmb/CFoJkG5bKG97uaYfLzGzKeZhcIY=/1500x0/filters:no_upscale():max_bytes(150000):strip_icc()/close-up-of-mixed-race-woman-holding-medication-capsule-543195329-594ac4ae5f9b58f0fc9ea72f.jpg.

Test Your Knowledge

1. How do suicidal behavior, acute psychosis, and severe agitation differ as forms of psychiatric emergencies?
2. What distinguishes substance-induced emergencies from mood-related or anxiety-related crises?

14.2. Signs and Symptoms

Learning Outcome

1. Behavioral indicators.
2. Emotional and psychological signs.
3. Physical manifestations.

For psychiatric emergencies, recognition of signs and symptoms is key to effective intervention and management. Familiarity with the fundamentals of these signs can make a huge difference in deciding the fate of victims of mental health emergencies. Excessive anxiety, mood alterations, and social withdrawal are typical symptoms that usually signify an underlying psychiatric illness that needs immediate attention. Also, symptoms like delusions or hallucinations can be indicators of a deeper break with reality that spirals out of control if not addressed in time. As the staff development program, as described in (Smith et al., 2016), mentions, educating teachers about warning signs for teenage depression makes the environment more supportive and also maximizes the chance for early intervention, which is crucial for reducing psychiatric emergencies. In adolescents, the presentation of psychiatric disorders is unique, with symptoms often manifesting as changes in behavior rather than readily apparent emotional distress. Symptoms , such as increased irritability, extreme variability of sleep or appetite patterns, and concentration impairment can readily be attributed to typical developmental changes. Caregivers and educators must be aware of differentiating normal adolescent behavior from potential indicators of mental illness. The program in Smith et al. (2016) showed that teachers can indeed detect these more subtle signs with proper training, ultimately leading to increased referral rates and a drastic reduction in psychiatric emergencies. These preventative measures not only enhance the well-being of the students but also create a culture of sensitivity towards mental health within institutions. The implications of observing signs and symptoms extend beyond immediate responses to psychiatric crisis; they also influence long-term mental health strategies.

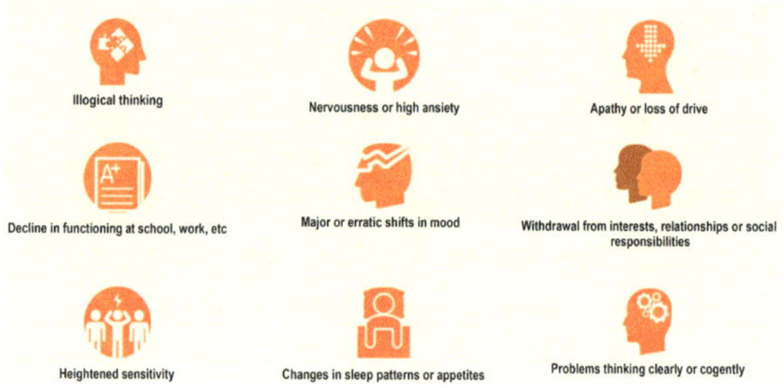

Figure 14.5. Symptoms of psychiatric disorders.

Source: https://www.facebook.com/photo/?fbid=10156359212318367&set=a.10151153608848367.

A systematic review indicated that inadequate knowledge by mental health professionals of emergency situations would frequently hinder appropriate responses and interventions for patients in crisis who are deteriorating. This gap emphasizes the need for integrated training of teachers as well as mental health professionals to make them more attuned to symptomatology in times of high pressure. If mental health professionals are trained to pick up cues of psychological distress early on, then they can implement appropriate interventions that defuse a crisis to ease the perceived burden on emergency services and overall patient management (Figure 14.5).

14.2.1. Behavioral Indicators

Behavioral cues play a strong role in identifying psychiatric emergencies, particularly in teenagers. Emotionally reactive (ER) teenagers are more likely to engage in self-injurious behavior, which makes their interpersonal interactions and emotional presentation important to track. Studies have documented that higher emotional reactivity presents as the major symptom underlying self-injury, with it further showing the bidirectionality of the relationship; individuals exhibiting self-injurious acts (NSSI) tend to show increased emotional reactivity that can enhance the risk status. Keeping track of these behavioral markers can thus serve as key determinants to understand an adolescent's mental status, with timely interventions possible. Following proper assessments, identifying emotional reactivity patterns may aid clinicians in guiding certain interventions aimed at reducing such behavior, minimizing psychiatric emergencies (Kandsperger et al., 2022). Participation of bystanding individuals cannot be overlooked when developing behavioral indicators in psychiatric emergencies. Far too frequently, those surrounding potential victims or individuals in crisis possess critical information about suspicious activity before any act of violence or self-harm ever being done. Research indicates that peers themselves frequently recognize warning signs, such as disruptive patterns of emotion or threatening communication, that lead up to an attack or self-mutilation. Through engaging with bystander observations and rewarding reporting of such behavioral indicators, groups are able to develop preventive measures for psychiatric emergencies. The approach highlights the importance of integrating bystander observations into threat assessment systems, thereby enhancing the likelihood of earlier intervention and support for at-risk individuals (Borum et al., 2021). Apart from the importance of social and affective markers, other behavioral markers may also point to a looming psychiatric crisis. Changes in daily routines , such as withdrawing from friends and family, sudden academic decline, or increased agitation, are most often precursors to a more severe mental health crisis. Clinicians must be attentive to these patterns because they might indicate a need for immediate psychological assessment and intervention. For example, studies have found that adolescents who engage in self-injurious thoughts or behaviors most often have high variability in their psychological functioning over time. Through the use of a broad evaluation approach that includes measures of behavior, mental health clinicians can make targeted interventions, addressing the problems early before they become full-blown crises (Kandsperger et al., 2022).

14.2.2. Emotional and Psychological Signs

In emergencies of a psychiatric nature, psychological and emotional cues are the most important signs of a person's mental state, typically pointing towards causatives underneath. Patients may express increased anxiety, depression dominating everyday life, or alternate mood swings episodically, suggesting an alteration from the normal emotional function. Such an emotional crisis can be triggered by many reasons, including subjective experiences of trauma, environmental stress, or significant life changes. For instance, psychological distress resulting from relegation from a professional league has been documented, with evidence showing that affected fans display clinically significant scores of psychological distress on standardized measures (Banyard & Shevlin, 2001). Recognition of these symptoms together with other behavioral symptoms, such as withdrawal from others or changes in appetite and sleep, is central to early intervention, underscoring emotional alertness within personal and clinical settings. Emotional symptoms that become evident within psychiatric emergencies generally contribute to the worsening of psychological disturbance and endanger people's safety and health. Despair and hopelessness can lead to suicidal ideation or self-injurious behavior, with immediate danger needing to be treated. Disturbance of cognition, along with mood disturbance, can become apparent; patients become distractible, unable to make decisions, and forgetful, thus increasing feelings of inadequacy and frustration. For example, the long-duration astronauts in space suffer from psychological stressors that worsen with time, necessitating proper coping mechanisms and psychological support for maintaining mental health (Leveton et al., 2025) (Figure 14.6).

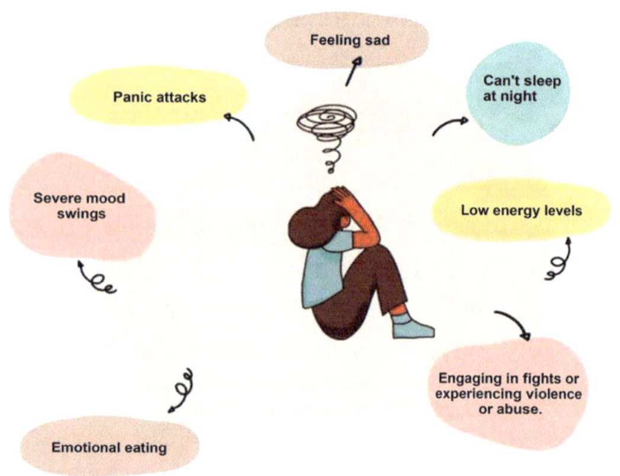

Figure 14.6. Emotional and psychological signs.

Source: https://www.unicef.org/jordan/sites/unicef.org.jordan/files/styles/media_large_image/public/6_7.png.webp?itok=-lzKJD2K.

Successful monitoring and early detection of these signs of cognition and emotion are essential in averting the threat of psychiatric emergencies, facilitating return to stability, and enhancing resilience. Therapeutic intervention-wise, detection and reaction to emotional and psychological signs are essential in formulating effective intervention strategies. Mental health professionals tend to use interventions , such as cognitive-behavioral therapy (CBT) and mindfulness training, which can improve an individual's capacity for responding to emotional cues in crisis situations. These interventions focus on reconditioning negative thought patterns and enhancing coping skills to provide a more adaptive emotional response to stressors. The applicability of one-on-one psychological treatment is especially apparent in cases of extreme stress, such as space missions, where psychological factors can hinder operational effectiveness as well as individual well-being (Leveton et al., 2025). Overall, acknowledgment and intervention of emotional and psychological symptoms not only prevent psychiatric crises but also enable individuals with the tools to endure elaborate emotional places, ultimately leading to recovery and toughness.

14.2.3. Physical Manifestations

The physical presentation process in psychiatric emergencies tends to complicate the diagnosis and treatment of mental illnesses. Patients presenting at the emergency department with psychiatric symptoms may present with a range of physical symptoms, such as agitation, tachycardia, and hyperventilation. The presentations can be linked with an underlying psychiatric illness or the impact of acute stressors. For instance, severe anxiety can trigger physiological responses that are equivalent to medical emergencies, including panic attacks. Management of these physical symptoms is critical, as they overshadow the central psychiatric issue and result in misdiagnosis. Thorough evaluation of physical and mental condition is therefore essential, especially since physical symptoms tend to fuel heightened distress and complicate treatment. Knowledge of the association between physical symptoms and psychiatric disorders allows clinicians to provide more effective and multidisciplinary care within the emergency setting. Psychiatric emergencies in some cases are caused by some conditions, such as tinnitus, and result in severe distress, which leads individuals to seek emergency treatment. Tinnitus patients report varying physical and emotional symptoms that may escalate into a psychiatric emergency. (Altissimi et al., 2016) identifies that chronic cases of tinnitus are frequently associated with psychiatric comorbidities like depression and anxiety. Acute or worsening patients suffering from tinnitus may exhibit physical symptoms ranging from irritability to suicidal ideation, which further supports the need for medical treatment. Moreover, the gravity of tinnitus treatment as a part of a psychiatric condition necessitates familiarity with both auditory and psychological features. Because patients with such complaints present to emergency departments, clinicians must address not only the physiological aspects of tinnitus but also remain mindful of psychiatrists' eyes to circumvent associated psychiatric distress (Figure 14.7).

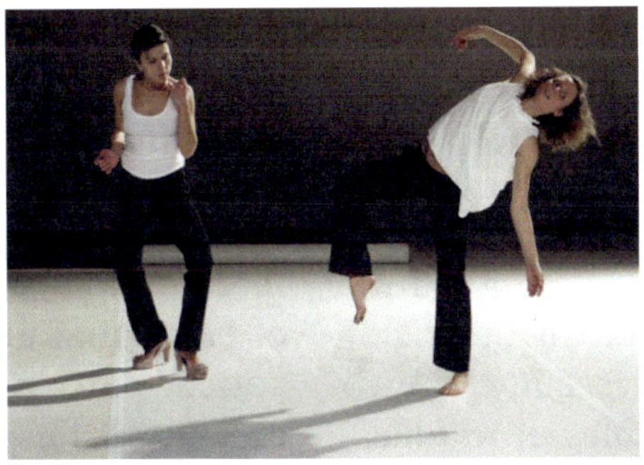

Figure 14.7. Physical manifestations.

Source: https://gibanica.info/wp-content/uploads/2020/04/MAD_Fizic%C2%A6%C3%AEne-manifestacije1.jpg.

Along with this, an understanding of physical symptom management in psychiatric emergencies must include a critical assessment of pharmacotherapy. Adams (2002) indicates the following common application of intramuscular medications for acute tranquilization in emergency departments, particularly in cases involving intimidating or assaultive behavior. Haloperidol and promethazine have proved helpful in acute agitation management, which is normally the situation in psychiatric emergencies. However, the lack of extensive scientific scrutiny of most pharmacological interventions generates gaps in knowledge about their long-term impact. Clinicians are thus forced to precisely weigh the benefits and risks of these interventions, particularly when they treat patients who have extremely prominent physical signs. Lastly, the treatment of both the psychological and physical dimensions of psychiatric emergencies is required to achieve maximum patient outcomes, underscoring the importance of an integrated treatment approach incorporating medical and psychiatric evaluation.

Test Your Knowledge

1. What warning signs indicate imminent risk of self-harm, violence, or loss of behavioral control in psychiatric emergencies?
2. How can symptoms such as hallucinations, extreme confusion, or sudden mood instability signal an acute psychiatric crisis?

14.3. Risk Factors

Learning Outcome

1. Pre-existing mental health conditions.
2. Environmental and social influences.
3. Biological and genetic predispositions.

Recognition of the multifaceted and multidimensional causative sources of risk factors in psychiatric emergencies is crucial for effective intervention and management. Triggers of psychiatric crises can be occasioned by an assortment of factors, spanning from biological, psychological, to social. Biological precipitates , such as genetic vulnerabilities, neural disorganization, and comorbid medical illnesses may be pivotal in the risk of development of a psychiatric emergency. Further, the psychological variables of trauma history, drug and alcohol abuse, and psychiatric disorders raise the risk, most typically resulting in heightened agitation or behavioral storms. Social determinants , including socioeconomic status, family relationships, and social support networks also affect patients' vulnerability to psychiatric emergencies. Recognizing this synergy of factors allows for increased consideration of patient needs and flexibility of intervention strategies. The COVID-19 pandemic has substantially magnified already existing risk factors for psychiatric emergencies and posed specialized challenges to health systems. Unrivaled stress, anxiety, and social isolation during the pandemic further overwhelmed those at risk for mental health emergencies. The majority of patients have experienced increased symptoms due to fear of being exposed to the virus and disruption of routine care, leading to increased agitation and behavior disturbances. In addition, even the healthcare workers have experienced burnout and emotional exhaustion when managing these increased demands, further complicating emergency delivery of care. The impact of COVID-19 only underscores the importance of early identification and intervention strategies to combat the risks inherent in extreme behavioral symptoms in emergency settings. The coordination of these risk factors is addressed through collaboration among healthcare providers and commitment towards creating support environments for patients and staff, particularly during crises. Nursing interventions in psychiatric emergencies cannot be ignored, particularly in the context of high-risk procedures , such as mechanical restraint. The application of frequent monitoring and evaluation of restrained patients has been found to minimize the duration of restraint episodes, according to existing research studies. Increasing the frequency of evaluation by registered nurses offers timely intervention that can prevent the escalation of crises and ultimately translate to improved patient outcomes. In recognizing the complex risk factors for psychiatric emergencies, such as those exacerbated by the pandemic, healthcare providers are in a stronger position to promote policies that support continued psychiatric care. Enhanced observation practices not only reduce the risks of restraint but establish a therapeutic environment conducive to healing, thereby both effectively meeting immediate safety concerns and continuous psychiatric well-being.

14.3.1. Pre-Existing Mental Health Conditions

The presence of prior mental illness can most often be a significant factor in the situation of psychiatric emergencies, particularly due to stressful situations , such as the COVID-19 pandemic. Individuals with a diagnosed condition of mental illness might experience worsening symptoms in periods of heightened tension or anxiety, and this can complicate things for them as well as lead to psychiatric emergencies. For example, research has established that pandemic-induced fears and anxieties have sharply increased levels of stress in the population, particularly among individuals who were already disadvantaged as far as their mental well-being was concerned. Such high levels of anxiety have been demonstrated to trigger severe symptoms in individuals with conditions , such as anxiety disorders, depression, and bipolar disorder, where extreme psychiatric intervention is necessitated to prevent further degeneration (Nava et al., 2024). A review of mental health trends during the pandemic focuses on the varied ways pre-existing conditions affect service use and treatment outcomes. The post-COVID-19 period was associated with a sharp decline in psychiatric hospitalizations, partly due to realignment of healthcare systems and more extensive use of outpatient services. Yet, people with existing conditions were much hindered from accessing early care, and this often led to increased crises and involuntary hospitalizations (Figure 14.8).

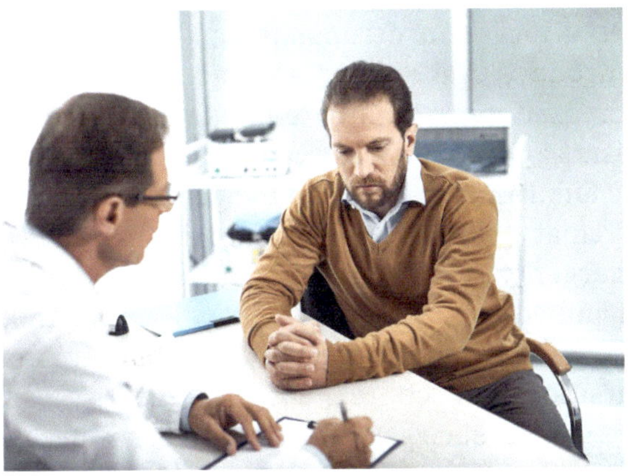

Figure 14.8. Pre-existing medical condition.

Source: https://external-content.duckduckgo.com/iu/?u=https%3A%2F%2Fstatic.wixstatic.com%2Fmedia%2Fc04786_87e20bcb13ea457e9ee022bcc7272a99~mv2.jpeg%2Fv1%2Ffill%2Fw_980%2Ch_653%2Cal_c%2Cq_85%2Cusm_0.66_1.00_0.01%2Cenc_auto%2Fc04786_87e20bcb13ea457e9ee022bcc7272a99~mv2.jpeg&f=1&nofb=1&ipt=fff7b6d65762854385e1aa720ef97137ae6a9b58839787034996633e037f9f03.

Demographic and clinical presentation studies of patients admitted in the challenging period indicate a shift in diagnosed conditions, with schizophrenia becoming more frequent, as compared to earlier trends where mood disorders dominated (Freitas et al., 2024). The shift is indicative of how outside pressures can significantly alter the presentation of psychiatric emergencies and the nature of illnesses presented to healthcare providers. The consequences of a history of mental illness in psychiatric crises are not merely applicable to crisis clinical management but also extend to the long-term course of people's mental health. Individuals with a history of psychiatric disorders may be at increased risk of building lasting sequelae from emergencies, including possibly developing new or worsening symptoms to stressors in society. Such a vicious cycle may be potentially created by the interaction of fear with existing mental health issues, as shown by the evidence accrued during the COVID-19 pandemic. These complications underscore the importance for mental health treatment providers to adopt a model of care that includes respect for patients' histories, the potential for symptom provocation, and the development of tailored interventions to prevent the threat of psychiatric emergencies (Nava et al., 2024).

14.3.2. Environmental and Social Influences

Interconnectedness between environmental and social variables is most significant in the aetiology of mental health and therefore impacts the development of psychiatric crises. Environmental determinants , such as pollution, urbanization, and housing conditions have been revealed to initiate the deterioration in mental health. For instance, kids living in extremely polluted areas are vulnerable to developing anxiety and depressive disorders, highlighting the importance of healthy environments for mental health. In addition, the social environment, from family to community support, also influences one's resilience to mental illnesses. Residents of well-strong, supportive social networks do better in crisis situations because social networks can reverse mental health stressors. Environmental and social measurements are the key to knowledge on how to apply overall strategies for the proper management of psychiatric emergencies. The healthcare systems also need to recognize the importance of environmental and social determinants in managing psychiatric emergencies. Socioeconomic status has a direct bearing on access to mental health treatment; individuals from lower socioeconomic status often face numerous obstacles, such as economic restrictions, lack of access to transportation, and stigmatization. The interconnection between environmental stressors and psychiatric disorders calls for an interdisciplinary approach in healthcare paradigms. Initiatives focused on the improvement of social conditions, for example, housing stability, education, financial assistance, and social participation, can significantly reduce the emergence of psychiatric emergencies. Moreover, policymakers need to make the integration of mental health care into public health measures, to diminish environmental obstacles, a top priority to enhance overall mental health outcomes (Wasserman et al., 2023). Without policymakers attempting to tackle such underlying social factors, actions taken to manage psychiatric emergencies may be short-sighted and unsustainable. Education and mental health advocacy also play important roles in mitigating the risk of environmental and social forces in psychiatric emergencies. Educational campaigns for the public must aim at drawing attention to the integration of mental health, social support systems, and community health. Through generating learning settings concerning mental well-being, communities can positively cultivate supportive settings in which individuals are well-educated on healthy living choices and have adequate channels for support. Strengthening public mental health programs in accordance with the Sustainable Development Goals aims at expanding access to mental health care and healthy lifestyles (Wasserman et al., 2023). In addition, equipping community leaders and healthcare workers with skills to identify signs of psychological distress can enable them to respond quickly when there is a crisis. Lastly, encouraging the debate on environmental and social determinants offers a ground for an increased responsive and good quality mental health care system capable of managing psychiatric emergencies.

14.3.3. Biological and Genetic Predispositions

Understanding psychiatric emergencies demands the investigation of intrinsic genetic and biological propensities that significantly influence mental well-being. Genetics has been studied to strongly contribute to susceptibility to various psychiatric conditions like mood disorders, anxiety disorders, and psychotic disorders. For instance, variations in genetics can affect neurotransmitter functions and neurodevelopmental mechanisms, leading to increased vulnerability to mental health crises. Besides, a subject's history of mental illness in the family may also reveal the genetic aspects of psychiatric disorders, meaning that psychiatric emergencies may be predisposed towards in an individual by biological factors, and those emergent conditions may be caused by stressors outside their coping abilities. Lastly, early detection of such genetic risk factors may become an important step towards tailoring prevention strategies since personalized interventions could temper the adverse effects of psychiatric emergencies among susceptible individuals. Apart from genetics, biological mechanisms , such as neurochemical imbalance and hormonal fluctuation are capable of inducing psychiatric emergencies. Neurotransmitter processes , such as dopamine and serotonin pathways, directly correlate with the regulation of emotions and stability of mood. Impairment of these processes could lead to the generation of acute psychiatric emergencies. For example, patients whose serotonin levels have altered would develop heightened anxiety or depressive states, which then would instigate emergencies that must be attended to urgently (Figure 14.9).

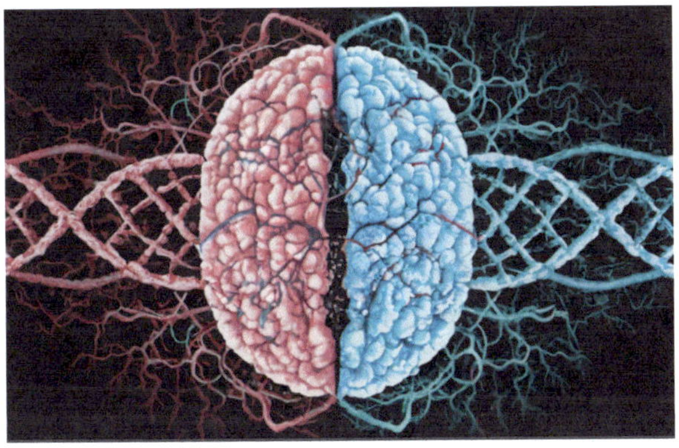

Figure 14.9. The connection between genetics and mental health disorders.

Source: https://mapmygenome.in/cdn/shop/articles/The_Connection_Between_Genetics_and_Mental_Health_Disorders.webp?v=1725084413.

Moreover, endocrine fluctuations, as might be indicated in stress reactions, can compound these issues, since elevated levels of cortisol have been shown to exacerbate underlying mental fragilities. By learning about the interrelated complexity of bodily systems, therefore, information about the sources of psychiatric emergencies and optimal methods for intervention is refined to respond to the differential requirements of those concerned. Enhanced recognition of the interplay between biological and genetic weaknesses with environmental factors points to the complexity of psychiatric crises. Researchers promote a model that considers not just genetic vulnerabilities but also the effect of environmental stressors on mental status, as illustrated by research into diseases like Myalgic Encephalomyelitis/Chronic Fatigue Syndrome (ME/CFS). The etiology of ME/CFS illustrates the power of genetic susceptibility interacting with environmental exposures to enhance the risk of developing disabling psychiatric symptoms later in life (Nacul et al., 2020). Psychopathy, with its potent association with extreme violence in some individuals, similarly illustrates the power of genetic underpinnings to guide public health prevention programs aimed at avoiding psychiatric catastrophes (N/A). By acknowledging such multilevel influences, mental health practitioners are better able to design prevention and intervention measures, adequately addressing the immediate needs of individuals at risk for crisis episodes while not losing sight of long-term management and recovery alternatives.

Test Your Knowledge

1. What biological, psychological, and social risk factors increase the likelihood of a psychiatric emergency?
2. How do substance misuse, trauma history, or poor treatment adherence contribute to emergency presentations?

14.4. Assessment and Diagnosis

Learning Outcome

1. Initial evaluation techniques.
2. Use of standardized assessment tools.
3. Importance of differential diagnosis.

For psychiatric evaluation and diagnosis, mental health is essential, especially during psychiatric emergencies. A judicious assessment would typically begin with a comprehensive history-taking process of the patient's presenting symptoms, past psychiatric history, and relevant social circumstances. This multifaceted approach is necessary to realize the multifaceted nature of psychiatric disorders, which are never singular in occurrence. For instance, in child psychiatric emergencies, research indicates that depressive disorders are among the most frequently diagnosed conditions, and they account for a large proportion of psychiatric emergency service admissions (Ocako et al., 2024). This prioritizing of thorough assessment not only informs the patient's initial management but also determines long-term treatment planning, enabling healthcare workers to tailor interventions according to specific needs effectively. The diagnostic process is done by deciphering different clinical signs and symptoms using standardized diagnostic criteria, for example, the DSM-5. The subjectivity in psychiatric diagnosis, however, creates issues that have to be carefully navigated by mental health professionals. In spite of the development of technology, including the use of artificial intelligence tools, the clinician's expertise cannot be replaced if disorders are to be diagnosed correctly. Actually, one recent study proved the potential of AI to contribute to this process using diagnostic options derived from first assessments, with moderate agreement with clinical diagnoses (Laherrán et al., 2024). Technology like this has the potential to make diagnoses more precise, but emotional complexity and human behavior nuances usually require the human element in the assessment process, which reinforces the importance of clinician-patient interaction in psychiatric emergencies. Besides, the rapidly transforming climate of psychiatric assessment also reflects the criticality of interventions in the situation of crisis on schedule. The immediacy of psychiatric emergencies calls for prompt and effective diagnostic procedures, resorting to screening tools and formal interviews. In children, for example, the rapid increase in psychiatric admissions due to depressive disorders shows the need for efficient, timely diagnosis in pediatric psychiatric emergency departments (Ocako et al., 2024). Use of evidence-based assessment protocols is crucial to allow for the identification of at-risk persons as speedily as possible and consequently provide proper treatment and forestall further worsening. Ultimately, effective evaluation and diagnosis not only eliminate acute symptoms but also serve as a foundation for intensive, long-term psychiatric care in the treatment of psychiatric emergencies.

14.4.1. Early Evaluation Methods

Initial assessment techniques in psychiatric emergencies are critical to enable timely and effective diagnosis and interventions. They involve thorough evaluations that apply clinical interviews as well as standardized assessment tools to quantify the severity of psychiatric symptoms. A full history-taking is one of the initial steps, such as recent behavioral change, medical history, and psychosocial stressors. Establishing rapport is crucial during this initial meeting because crisis patients may be reticent to share sensitive information. By employing standardized tools , such as the Mental Status Examination (MSE), clinicians can systematically assess such factors as appearance, behavior, mood, cognition, and thought content. Prioritizing these factors, healthcare practitioners can develop vital considerations in arriving at rapid decisions about care, such as whether or not to hospitalize or intervene pharmacologically. In psychiatric emergencies, it is also crucial to screen for any underlying medical conditions that may be leading to a patient's presenting symptoms. Techniques , such as collateral history taking from family and/or friends or previous providers can be very informative and shed further light on the situation. Also, laboratory investigations and neuroimaging may be requested in order to exclude non-psychiatric causes of the symptoms, for example, infections, metabolic disorders, or intracranial lesions. The observation of an order on the diagnostic process allows significant improvements in the patient outcome (Gul et al., 2024) (Figure 14.10).

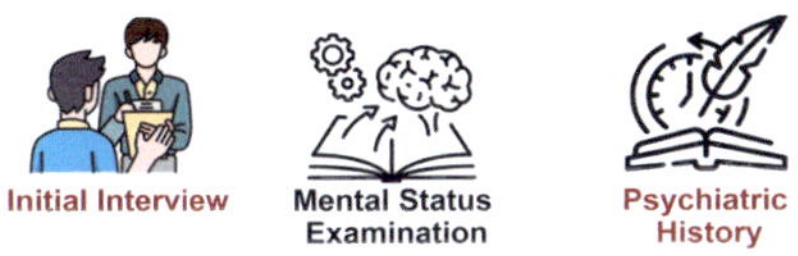

Figure 14.10. Initial evaluation techniques in psychiatric emergencies.

Source: https://cherryhillrecoverycenter.com/wp-content/uploads/2023/07/Step-by-Step-Process-of-a-Psychiatric-Evaluation.png.

Interdisciplinary collaboration into the assessment process, where psychiatric professionals can collaborate with medical teams, enhances the validity of the diagnosis and establishes an integrated care plan addressing psychiatric and medical requirements. Also, initial assessment procedures must include risk assessment for harm to self or others, which is imperative during emergencies. Healthcare professionals are taught to use evidence-based best practices to screen for suicide risk, considering previous attempts, acute ideation, and psychosocial stressors impacting the patient's mental status. Closely reviewing environmental factors, for example, drug use or social isolation, can also help to establish the context of the emergency. According to a recent audit, only 60% of cases adhered to recommended protocol procedures for initial evaluation in psychiatric emergencies (Gul N et al., 2024). It becomes essential to keep conducting training for staff on risk assessment and intervention methods. Having an integrated, well-documented process for evaluation not only adds to patient safety but also supports a more efficient management of psychiatric emergencies.

14.4.2. Use of Standard Assessment Tools

The use of standardized evaluation tools is essential in psychiatric emergency management since they provide a methodical process of evaluating the conditions of patients. Standardized questionnaires and assessment scales are some of the instruments that aid practitioners in gathering and analyzing information from patients in an organized way, which is essential during times of high pressure. Use of the same provides not only speed in diagnosis but also enhances the standardization and authenticity of services delivered. For emergency conditions, where speed counts, standardized measures make sure none of the key factors are omitted, thereby improving patient outcomes. Through the application of evidence-based assessment instruments, mental health professionals can more effectively determine a patient's condition severity and interventions best suited, eventually resulting in the quality of psychiatric emergency care overall. Furthermore, standardized assessment tools can promote communication and coordination between multidisciplinary teams in emergent conditions. When caregivers from various specialties apply common assessment templates, they can better share important findings and observations. These collaborative efforts add to a more comprehensive understanding of patients' needs and facilitate integrated care, as indicated in research that addresses the use of standard screening procedures in emergency departments. For instance, collaborative efforts, as pointed out by Berlin et al. (2015), can facilitate greater patient engagement and participation in assessments, as clinicians get an opportunity to ask pertinent questions guided by the standardized format (Figure 14.11).

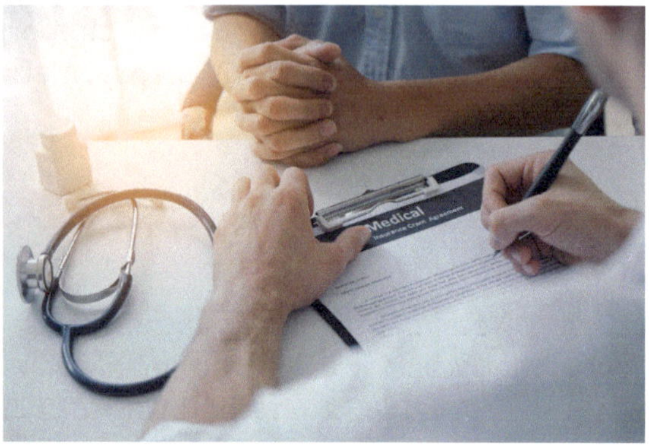

Figure 14.11. Standardized assessment tools is vital in managing psychiatric emergencies.

Source: https://external-content.duckduckgo.com/iu/?u=https%3A%2F%2Fblog.proemhealth.com%2Fhubfs%2FStandardized%2520Mental%2520Health%2520Assessment%2520Tools.jpeg&f=1&nofb=1&ipt=dcca32ba6e4263e29b66edd394cd1ac49ecbf05bfa9d28185c21d1eea16aaf61.

Thus, facilitating cooperation via standardized evaluation not only enhances the assessment process but also provides a better supportive environment for the patient in cases of acute psychological distress. Additional evidence suggests that the optimization of , such assessment mechanisms can have a direct influence on the duration and resolution of psychiatric crises. For example, implementation of increased frequent checks by trained health practitioners in cases of restraint has led to drastic reductions in the time span of the same, presented as outcomes for Allen (2018). Monitoring and frequent check-ups enable health practitioners to modify care plans in a timely fashion, diminishing opportunities for prolonged psychiatric crises. The consistent use of standardized tools in these facilities not only makes it easier to make quick decisions but also clearly demonstrates clear lines for intervention, leading to patient safety and well-being. As mental health care evolved, the employment of standardized assessment tools remains a pillar for ensuring successful treatment of psychiatric emergencies, leading to improved results and preservation of patient dignity.

14.4.3. Importance of Differential Diagnosis

In the case of psychiatric emergencies, the importance of differential diagnosis cannot be overstated. Correct diagnosis of mental illnesses on time is essential, particularly when patients present with acute symptoms that resemble other diseases. Differential diagnosis serves to assist clinicians in excluding overlapping psychiatric conditions, such as distinguishing between bipolar disorder and schizophrenia, and this will profoundly affect outcomes in treatment. Specifically, diagnostic stability of illnesses like schizophrenia and bipolar disorder has been shown to be convincingly established by emergency evaluation, and even more transient illnesses like brief psychotic disorder can involve unbridled confusion (Azevedo-Marques et al., 2010). This highlights the necessity for clinicians to adopt a formal approach based on standardized criteria and observation guidelines in order to obtain the maximum diagnostic accuracy. A proper differential diagnosis not only enables one to determine the underlying condition of the psychology but also to treat any comorbid conditions that could be aggravating the original psychiatric disorder. For instance, psychotic states have been reported to develop as a result of substance abuse, which complicates the diagnosis further (Azevedo-Marques et al., 2010). Therefore, a proper investigation into the history of substance abuse and the patient's current health conditions is important. Moreover, psychiatric emergencies are often compounded by co-existing medical problems, which make an in-depth understanding of the patient's general health profile very important. Through examination of relevant medical histories and utilization of proper diagnostic instruments, clinicians can ascertain that both psychiatric and general medical conditions are properly taken into consideration, hence avoiding misdiagnosis and the consequent effects on patient treatment. Moreover, the consequences of incompetent differential diagnosis during psychiatric emergencies may not only be severe for the course of treatment in the patient but, worst of all, can lead to a higher morbidity and mortality. Literature indicates that undiagnosed psychiatric disease tends to worsen distress and, in certain patients, predispose them to suicide. This demonstrates the critical role played by mental health professionals in reducing such risks by conducting early and accurate assessments. By practicing differential diagnosis actively, clinicians are in a better position to design appropriate therapeutic interventions that respond to both immediate treatment and long-term care of crisis patients. For this reason, the application of evidence-based practices remains essential in the psychiatric emergency setting in an effort to optimize patient outcomes and prevent the incidence of adverse events.

Test Your Knowledge

1. What steps are involved in conducting a rapid mental status examination during a psychiatric emergency?
2. How do clinicians evaluate risk levels for suicide, aggression, or medical complications during emergency assessments?

14.5. Immediate Interventions

Learning Outcome

1. Crisis intervention strategies.
2. Role of emergency services.
3. Importance of safety planning.

Psychiatric emergencies require immediate interventions aimed at stabilizing and safeguarding the individuals at risk. Onset of acute mental conditions, such as severe anxiety, psychosis, or suicidal intent, requires urgent intervention by mental health professionals and care systems. Crisis counseling, medication management, and establishing a favorable environment are crucial interventions for the prevention of harm to the individual or others. Above all, these early interventions lay the foundation for the balance of therapeutic work to be done, offering a more comprehensive plan for the mental health treatment of the individual. The interventions are also capable of alleviating distress, opening the way to further mental health treatment and services. By expediently responding to these crises, professionals can limit the long-term impact of acute psychiatric incidents on the individual and the community. The issue of immediate interventions calls for an understanding of the uniqueness of each psychiatric emergency. Practitioners have to balance responding in a manner that caters to the unique nature of the crisis, including the individual's history, mental state at presentation, and social context. Equally important is the recognition of response capacity variations across various healthcare environments, which necessitates having structured, well-coordinated emergency processes in place. For instance, following a disaster, immediate mental health intervention must not only be administered to the victims but also to emergency responders who experience secondary traumatic stress. A sensitive approach that considers the full spectrum of psychological responses, such as major depressive disorder and bereavement, must be ensured to provide proper and effective immediate interventions to meet diverse needs (McFarlane & Williams, 2012). The evolving landscape of psychiatric emergencies, particularly substance-related emergencies, highlights the importance of harm reduction principles to be embedded in acute interventions. In response to the rising opioid overdoses, acute responses must incorporate evidence-based interventions on overdose prevention and response. It is necessary to conduct a risk and protective factor assessment since it enables practitioners to tailor interventions based on individuals' and communities' needs. For instance, identifying the different levels of risk presented by diverse populations can greatly increase the effectiveness of interventions on a short-term basis. This initiative not only provides an immediate solution to acute crises but can also form the basis for longer-term rehabilitation and support. In the end, the inclusion of intervention strategies targeting the complex character of such emergencies has the potential to lead to positive results and promote resilience among impacted groups (Baldacchino et al., 2012).

14.5.1. Crisis Intervention Strategies

Crisis intervention skills are required for managing psychiatric emergencies, as they facilitate immediate relief and restoration in cases of intense distress. Crisis intervention strategies typically involve a formal psychological and emotional assessment of the individual to allow professionals to determine the most appropriate course of action. Effective crisis intervention typically involves coordinating the efforts of different actors, including health professionals, social organizations, and the state. These coordinated efforts, as studied by research, demonstrate that the regulatory approach of a government is capable of driving positive behavioral practices among healthcare facilities and the population overall, therefore enhancing the general efficacy of crisis interventions (Chen et al., 2023). Through incorporating these several facets of care in a strategic manner, experts can formulate a comprehensive intervention plan that considers the needs of the affected individuals and optimally utilizes the available resources. Moreover, sound crisis intervention techniques must address establishing rapport and trust between the responding team and crisis persons. The initial contact sets the tone for the intervention, and it should be ensured that the professionals exercise empathy and compassion. Active listening and emotional validation are a few of the major techniques applied in this case, enabling people to be heard and valued. In addition, the use of evidence-informed practices, such as those identified by professionals in crisis intervention, underscores the merit of a coordinated response to such crises. Through the use of measures that professionals have already agreed upon, the interventions are not only effective but also sensitive to the unique circumstances of each individual (Xi et al., 2019) (Figure 14.12).

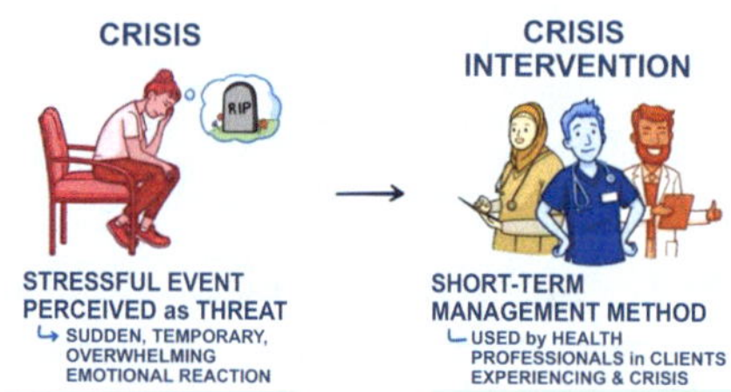

Figure 14.12. Crisis intervention.

Source: https://external-content.duckduckgo.com/iu/?u=https%3A%2F%2Fosmose-it.s3.amazonaws.com%2FRnjkfJheT3OMkp-H_h8-TJaKT2W0zbLt%2F_.jpg&f=1&nofb=1&ipt=98b26e96be27389837753fb970b7ea33bee1acb4022a2d357825ccd22596f445.

Such systematic systems can finally allow individuals to reclaim control and navigate their emotional disturbances more effectively. In addition, establishing the success of crisis intervention approaches is also important to maximize future practice. Regular assessment allows for the determination of success and aspects of improvement, which can promote a cycle of learning and adaptation. Scholarship has proved that intervention decisions made strategically have a robust impact on the behavior and psychological reaction of people affected during crises (Chen et al., 2023). The procedure enhances the effect of interventions while providing an avenue for developing resilience in the community as individuals learn how to handle crises more constructively. By building a culture of support and recovery, such interventions can contribute to long-term mental health within communities, ultimately warding off future psychiatric crises.

14.5.2. Role of Emergency Services

Emergency services play a central role in addressing psychiatric emergencies as the front line workers in addressing acute mental health crises. Emergency services are usually the first point of contact for crisis patients, highlighting the importance of having specially trained staff who can efficiently screen and address mental illnesses. The installation of mental health crisis stabilization units , such as the Transitional Care Area (TCA) at Central Vermont Medical Center, is a clear instance of innovative emergency service practices. Through having a dedicated space for psychiatric care within emergency departments, the TCA not only reduces the length of stay for psychiatric patients in hospitals but also prevents inappropriate inpatient admissions through greater access to timely treatment (Burzynski et al., 2017). This model illustrates the evolving nature of emergency services to address the complexity of mental health crises. The incorporation of some guidelines and practices in emergency services is very critical in impacting patient outcomes throughout psychiatric emergencies. For instance, the requirement for constant observation and assessment of patients under mechanical restraint has emerged as fundamental in diminishing the duration of restraint episodes and general safety. A project that resulted in more frequent registered nurse checks showed a 44% decrease in restraint use duration, highlighting the way better oversight is central to crisis management in psychiatric care (Allen, 2018) (Figure 14.13).

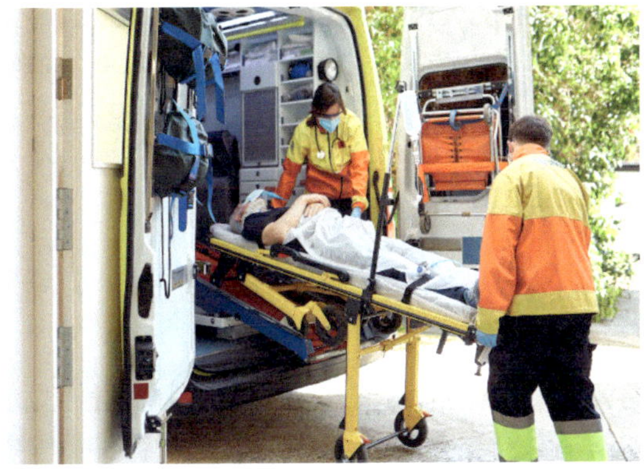

Figure 14.13. Emergency services in psychiatric emergencies.

Source: https://external-content.duckduckgo.com/iu/?u=https%3A%2F%2Fwww.columbiasouthern.edu%2Fmedia%2Fvl1jnvdz%2Fems-administrator.jpg&f=1&nofb=1&ipt=ee78e0f97737e52df974c331751b4a6480520bcb384d0be2f80e4b98bb159d99.

Emergency departments can benefit from integrating such evidence-based practice to provide patients with comprehensive, continuous care when managing acute psychiatric challenges. Such reforms not only improve patient safety but also align with the greater purpose of recovery-oriented care in emergency departments. Besides, emergency services have a role beyond an immediate crisis intervention function, such as prevention and post-crisis intervention. Through cooperative partnerships with community mental health agencies, emergency services ensure that patients receive ongoing support and services following an emergency. Continuity of care is essential in effectively treating mental health issues and preventing future emergencies. Experience that has been obtained from models like the TCA is essential in inspiring such programs for other emergency services, advocating for adequate staffing and a particular setting conducive to therapeutic interventions (Burzynski et al., 2017). Breaking the barriers to emergency services for psychiatric emergencies requires an integrated approach that prioritizes both acute care and long-term mental health outcomes, ultimately optimizing the effectiveness of the mental health crisis response system.

14.5.3. Significance of Safety Planning

Safety planning is an essential component of active psychiatric care in psychiatric emergencies. Effective safety planning comes from collaboration with patients to define personal triggers, coping strategies, and support pathways that increase resilience and empower the patient. With set plans for navigating the crisis, safety plans are helpful resources that guide patients and caregivers through intense periods of distress. Today's studies emphasize the reality that patients who are made to feel invested in their safety planning have greater ownership of their mental health process, encouraging a sense of agency that is key to thwarting undesirable outcomes of psychiatric crisis. Further, the incorporation of community resources into safety plans would render them more potent, providing patients with a broader support base for crises. Such general strategies not only alleviate transient distress but also are a plus for long-term mental health. The necessity for safety planning is also brought out by the complexity of mental health crises, particularly in the wake of disasters or traumatic events that occur suddenly. Disasters pose unique challenges to individuals and to medical systems, as the diverse mental health requirements that they create can testify. Research has established that such an incident can cause a variety of psychiatric illnesses, ranging from depression and anxiety to post-traumatic stress disorder (PTSD), not only for the primary victims but also for responding personnel. Safety planning is crucial in such a situation, as it enables the individual to navigate the psychological impact of trauma successfully. Implementing formalized safety plans not only facilitates immediate psychiatric crisis management but also has potential application in the long-term recovery process by ensuring that individuals are receiving required mental health interventions tailored to their personal circumstances, as evidenced in (McFarlane & Williams, 2012). The applicability of developing safety plans is not limited to adolescents but also extends to school communities where self-injurious behavior and suicidal ideation risks are of specific frequency. Schools are responsible for addressing such challenges, as highlighted in recent studies with high incidence rates of non-suicidal self-injury among adolescents. With a population of adolescents at risk of suicide, schools have to implement effective suicide safety planning models that prioritize the welfare of students. Schools need to be capable of identifying warning signs, delivering supportive interventions, and fostering a setting that welcomes open discussion of mental health. Furthermore, working with mental health professionals and integrating individualized safety plans can be used to strengthen intervention methods. Such proactive approaches not only mitigate risks associated with psychiatric emergencies but also foster resilience among students, fundamentally promoting a culture of openness and support within educational settings as articulated in (Gorman et al., 2019).

Test Your Knowledge

1. What are the key principles of de-escalation, safety measures, and crisis stabilization in psychiatric emergencies?
2. How do medications, such as sedatives or antipsychotics, help manage acute agitation or psychosis in emergency settings?

14.6. Long-Term Management

Learning Outcome

1. Follow-up care and treatment options.
2. Role of therapy and counseling.
3. Support systems and community resources.

In psychiatric crises, long-term plans of management have a critical role to play in the establishment of long-term patient stability and recovery. These include a comprehensive system of treatment that transcends stabilization during the crisis. For patients experiencing psychiatric crises, there is a significant benefit to good long-term management planning in enhancing their quality of life and frequency of crises. Treatment of causative factors of mental health-related conditions has to be a multidimensional approach in conjunction with therapeutic treatments and regular medication. Studies suggest that more emphasis on long-term interventions probably tends to produce better outcomes, allowing healthcare professionals to address not only symptoms but also causative factors of psychiatric conditions, thus providing real support for treatment and recovery and resilience in the patient (Haryanto, 2024). Also supporting the value of long-term management is the potential for multiple psychiatric crises. Good management requires frequent contact with patients, supporting the importance of a regular follow-up regime. This should include regular appointments, crisis planning, and family involvement to enable patients to feel understood and reassured. Evidence indicates that patients receiving regular care are less likely to be hospitalized and have improved global functioning. By investing in long-term management, mental health professionals are able to minimize future crises and provide patients with skills in coping that strengthen their symptom management skillset (Nguyen et al., 2024). This model of prevention not only addresses immediate risk but also prepares patients for a healthy and independent life. Finally, incorporating community resources and support systems in long-term care plans can also enhance the success of treatment. Multilevel collaborative care models that involve the collaboration of community mental health services, support groups, and rehabilitation programs go a long way in enhancing patient resilience.

These resources provide patients with outlets for social support, education, and skill acquisition that are pivotal in targeting the complexities of mental health disorders. Application of such resources assists in developing a sense of belonging and being, which are critical in the process of healing. Like in effective models, an equilibrium approach to long-term management can significantly mitigate the impacts of psychiatric emergencies, thus ensuring sustainability within mental health recovery processes (Haryanto, 2024). Placing emphasis on long-term measures, the field of psychiatry can assure better outcomes among patients, eventually making society healthier.

14.6.1. Treatment and Follow-Up Options

In cases of psychiatric emergencies, the urgency of follow-up care and treatment cannot be overstated. Following a sudden exacerbation, patients are likely to face an array of issues from their symptom control to resumption of normal life. Effective follow-up care is important to ensure that the long-term needs of the patient are met, ultimately determining the path of their recovery. It is crucial to have a solid support system, in the manner of regular therapeutic visits, medicine and life modifications, when dealing with disorders , such as depression, anxiety, and PTSD. Regular monitoring and therapeutic intervention by health care professionals are critical in helping strengthen resilience and adaptive coping strategies, consequently reducing the chance of relapse and enhancing overall patient outcomes. A new treatment in the continuum of follow-up care is Ketamine-assisted psychotherapy (KAP). This approach has much potential for decreasing treatment-resistant mood disorders and can be very beneficial after a psychiatric crisis. Research suggests that KAP can induce lasting symptom decreases for depression, anxiety, and PTSD, even after the treatment session has finished. Since many patients show clinically significant improvement, KAP is a useful choice for those who have already failed to respond to traditional treatments. However, there are some concerns, including the significant attrition rates that exist in treatment studies. As KAP gains popularity, further exploration of its long-term effects and integration into present-day psychiatric care models will be required in an attempt to make the most of its application for patients (Yermus et al., 2024). Research on digital interventions in mental health is another focus for the advancement of follow-up care in psychiatric settings, especially in low and middle-income countries (LMICs) with high rates of mental health problems. Programs , such as Step-by-Step (SbS) have been successful in the management of depression and anxiety in at-risk populations, including humanitarian emergency-affected populations. With the application of technology to provide scalable mental health interventions, SbS addresses accessibility hurdles and creates low-cost treatment options. Evidence from systematic reviews shows that such technology-mediated guided interventions not only deliver positive health effects but also economic gains for patients, as increased productivity generally offsets healthcare costs. As decision-makers begin to turn to sustainable alternatives for mental health crises, the incorporation of digital interventions in the grand design of follow-up care may be a turning point (Hana et al., 2023).

14.6.2. Role of Therapy and Counseling

Of specific significance in psychiatric emergencies is counseling and therapy in stabilizing individuals with acute crises of their mental health. These interventions are direct means of emotional support and skill development, aiming at diminishing distress and facilitating recovery. Community-based interventions underscore the importance of organized mental health interventions by emphasizing resilience-building and stability. For instance, lessons learnt from Project Liberty indicate the manner in which the integration of mental health care within support systems in the community constructs integrated systems for psychiatric emergencies. This not only addresses the immediate psychological needs but also yields a supportive environment that enhances access to assistance, thus improving mental health in emergencies (Henley et al., 2018). Counselors and therapists working in psychiatric emergency settings must be able to effectively maneuver the complexities of mental illnesses while rendering appropriate interventions. Such health professionals make use of an eclectic approach consisting of assessing the severity of an individual's condition, establishing rapport, and offering specific therapeutic interventions intended for crises. The evidence indicates that formal guidelines for the provision of psychiatric emergency services make services of higher quality (Hersrud et al., 1977) (Figure 14.14).

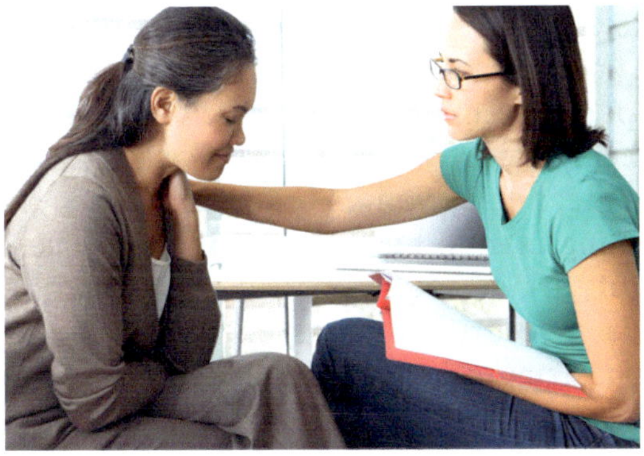

Figure 14.14. Counseling in psychiatric emergencies.

Source: https://external-content.duckduckgo.com/iu/?u=https%3A%2F%2Fwww.one-eighty.org%2Fwp-content%2Fuploads%2F2021%2F08%2FAdobeStock_52601999.jpg&f=1&nofb=1&ipt=7d149592c15513725871b1ef7d50a2642c00b349b8c5826cd23236fb3e996bb4.

Such responsiveness is of critical significance as timely interventions can significantly lower the incidence of long-term psychological consequences. Further, effective communication between multidisciplinary teams ensures comprehensive care for clients and therefore addresses psychological as well as social determinants leading to crises. Last but not least, integrating therapy and counseling with more comprehensive mental health services enables continuous support following the acute phase of a psychiatric emergency. Long-term therapeutic relationships facilitate coping mechanisms, resilience, and personal development, which are instrumental for people who are recovering from crises. Once initial interventions have taken place, subsequent counseling can be directed toward the discovery of underlying issues of, say, trauma or unresolved conflicts that precipitated the emergency. Such long-term engagement supports self-responsibility and empowerment, allowing individuals to regain control over their own mental health. Moreover, the teamwork-driven recommendation under efficient emergency service structures points toward the incorporation of therapy with community services in order to ensure complete care, thereby enhancing the general competence of psychiatric emergency interventions (Henley et al., 2018).

14.6.3. Support Systems and Community Resources

While addressing psychiatric emergencies, it is of the utmost importance to recognize the significance of robust support systems and community resources in a bid to intervene and bring about recovery. In acute mental health crisis conditions, individuals also require emergency access to professional as well as social support systems. These can include mental healthcare programs, crisis intervention units, and neighborhood community groups that provide critical resources. The utility of these support systems can directly influence the resolution of psychiatric emergencies. Not only do these systems offer relief on an immediate basis, but they also place a lot of value on long-term recovery interventions, and these help create individual and community resilience. Proper coordination of current networks of community support ensures that emergency responses are not only timely but also lasting, and this brings an integrated response to mental health care. In a crisis, specifically following disasters, civil administrations and health authorities are tested for their capacity to respond and coordinate effectively. Each disaster poses specific conditions, and responses must be tailored to respect the specific psychological needs of the populations involved. As emphasized, most of the focus has gone to posttraumatic stress disorder while other mental health conditions, such as major depressive disorder and complicated grief, are overlooked. This inequality indicates the necessity for community services to be flexible and adaptive to the varying psychological impacts endured by victims and emergency service workers. Not only is the creation of support groups a must short-term after a disaster, but it is also necessary to address long-term mental health effects, which are commonly underestimated. Well-being organized services can extend their usefulness beyond the immediate emergency to serve general community health in ways that resonate long after the crisis has passed (McFarlane & Williams, 2012). The recent COVID-19 pandemic provides an example of how psychiatric emergencies are confounded by more general sociocultural tensions. The increased segregation and worry because of the pandemic have had a germane bearing on patients and healthcare providers both, highlighting the need for accessible community resources. In ERs, the delivery of care for behavioral emergencies, such as agitation, has been transformed with the double effect of the virus. Timely intervention and identification, coupled with appropriate support systems, can guarantee the diminution of the mental strain on patients and healthcare providers as well. Community resources enabling mental health assistance in times so full of turmoil are important in establishing a sense of security for everyone involved. Lastly, emphasizing cooperation between community services and health responses can enhance the overall management of psychiatric emergencies, yielding improved results for everyone involved (Wiseman & O'Gorman, 2019).

Test Your Knowledge

1. How do follow-up care, therapy, and medication management contribute to preventing future psychiatric emergencies?
2. What roles do support systems, community resources, and relapse-prevention strategies play in long-term stabilization?

SUMMARY

In the psychiatric emergency literature, it is essential to recognize the central role of systematic interventions in optimizing patient safety and care. Mechanical restraint use is one such high-risk emergency intervention that necessitates emergent but calculated evaluation. Recent research indicated that increasing the frequency of registered nurse assessments during restraint periods can dramatically enhance patient outcomes by curtailing the duration of interventions. The findings reveal that the transition from intermittent to continuous monitoring not only safeguards the patient but also offers a more responsive care environment. These shifts, grounded in empirical data, highlight the necessity of the integration of advances in evidence-based practice within psychiatric settings to solidify the appeal for modifying clinical standards to meet the evolving needs of crisis patients (Allen, 2018). Also, the broader implications of improved psychiatric care extend well past crisis intervention to longer-term mental illness. As has been demonstrated in various disaster scenarios, healthcare systems are faced with very different challenges that need flexible and integrated responses. Incorporation of mental health services into emergency planning is not only beneficial but mandatory. Disasters expose the shortcomings of existing healthcare infrastructures in handling the psychological impact experienced by not only the direct victims but also by emergency responders. With an appreciation of the existing psychiatric morbidity in the affected population, health services become better equipped to transform and, therefore, improve their overall effectiveness and resilience to both acute and chronic forms of psychological trauma (McFarlane & Williams, 2012). Lastly, the results of such observations validate the need for ongoing training and policy initiatives to enhance the quality of psychiatric emergency care. More support for nursing staff and other front-line health care workers, particularly under high-pressure situations, is crucial to achieving optimum care standards. The evidence of decreased durations of restraint also demonstrates that improved practice adjustments with relevant information can lead to significant improvements in patient outcomes. By becoming committed to a culture of continuous assessment, education, and enhancement, the mental health field can embark on a path that not only effectively resolves crises but can also assist in informing the broader trajectory of mental health treatment paradigms (Allen, 2018).

As one reads through the major characteristics of psychiatric emergencies, one can observe that early assessment and intervention are crucial for best management. The significance of early recognition of signs associated with mental health emergencies cannot be overstated. Psychiatric emergencies manifest in various forms , such as suicidal ideas, acute psychosis, or severe anxiety. Identification of prevailing signs and associated risk factors is at the core of developing appropriately tailored care trajectories. The literature emphasizes the need to prepare healthcare professionals to recognize such indicators early enough so that the patients can be given the immediate help they require. As noted by recent studies, the implementation of integrative response procedures by local authorities can enhance the capacity of healthcare systems to manage such crises efficiently, hence the overall better outcomes for crisis individuals (DeVries, 2021). Moreover, the multidisciplinary model of psychiatric emergency treatment is vital in ensuring holistic care. Through bringing together various healthcare providers, including psychiatrists, psychologists, social workers, and emergency services, teams can implement specialized interventions to address the complex needs of patients presenting with psychiatric emergencies. The collaborative model of treatment enhances the quality of treatment and facilitates an environment in which patients feel nurtured and comprehended.

Engaging different disciplines not only improves the efficiency of treatment plans but also offers better communication and coordination among service providers during emergencies. The integrated method is required in the wake of contemporary challenges , such as the COVID-19 pandemic, which has necessitated responsive interventions in our healthcare systems to respond effectively to ongoing psychological distress (Akori et al., 2024). Overall, the key elements in managing psychiatric emergencies rely on rapid response, multidisciplinary collaboration, and anticipatory education for healthcare professionals. The integration of these factors provides a firm basis for coping with the intricacies involved in managing mental health emergencies, thereby benefiting patients and the overall healthcare system collectively. While continuing to assess and enhance emergency response measures, it is important to draw on past experiences and research, as shown in municipal case studies of emergency preparedness. By the application of lessons learned from past crises and evidence-based practice, healthcare systems can much better equip themselves to respond to psychiatric emergencies. The research conclusions regarding the effectiveness of community-based methods underscore the value of resilience and being prepared to confront future issues in mental health treatment (DeVries, 2021).

KEY TERMS FROM THIS CHAPTER

- Acute psychosis
- Agitation
- Catatonia
- Crisis intervention
- Decompensation
- Delirium
- Emergency medication
- Homicidal ideation
- Involuntary commitment
- Mania
- Mental status examination
- Panic attack
- Psychiatric hold
- Restraint
- Seclusion
- Substance intoxication
- Substance withdrawal
- Suicidal ideation
- Suicide attempt
- Violence risk assessment

CRITICAL THINKING QUESTIONS

1. **A patient presenting with suicidal thoughts and a detailed plan should be:**
   a. Discharged with a follow-up appointment
   b. Referred for outpatient therapy
   c. Monitored by family at home
   d. Admitted immediately for psychiatric evaluation and safety
2. **Which of the following is a key feature of a manic episode that may require emergency intervention?**
   a. Mild sadness
   b. Decreased need for sleep, increased risk-taking behavior, and aggression
   c. Excessive daydreaming
   d. Stable mood with occasional irritability
3. **A psychiatric emergency involving violent behavior should be initially managed with:**
   a. Verbal de-escalation and safety precautions
   b. Immediate restraints without communication
   c. Ignoring the patient until they calm down
   d. Forcing medication without consent
4. **Neuroleptic Malignant Syndrome (NMS) is a life-threatening condition associated with:**
   a. Antidepressants
   b. Benzodiazepines
   c. Antipsychotic medications
   d. Mood stabilizers
5. **Which of the following symptoms is most concerning in a potential case of serotonin syndrome?**
   a. Dry mouth
   b. Mild fatigue
   c. Hyperreflexia and agitation with high fever
   d. Constipation

Short Answer Questions

1. What constitutes a psychiatric emergency? Provide two examples.
2. Which mental health condition is most commonly associated with suicidal ideation in emergencies?
3. What are the warning signs of an imminent suicide attempt?
4. Define acute psychosis and name two potential causes.
5. How does a mental health professional assess a patient's risk for violence during an emergency?

Answer to Critical Thinking Questions

1. (d); 2. (b); 3. (a); 4. (c); 5. (c)

REFERENCES

1. Abi Hana, R., Abi Ramia, J., Burchert, S., Carswell, K., Cuijpers, P., Heim, E., Knaevelsrud, C., et al. (2023). Cost-effectiveness of digital mental health versus usual care during humanitarian crises in Lebanon: Pragmatic randomized trial. *JMIR Mental Health, 11*. https://www.semanticscholar.org/paper/57cb14a94cce7905be2b707151c6d25e1ea85975 (accessed on 28th July 2025).
2. Adams, C. E., Carvalho, A., Coutinho, E., et al. (2002). Current practices in managing acutely disturbed patients at three hospitals in Rio de Janeiro–Brazil: A prevalence study. https://core.ac.uk/download/60238.pdf (accessed on 28th July 2025).
3. Akori, S., Ali, S., Barageine, J., et al. (2024). Development and pilot test of a multi-component intervention to support women's recovery from female genital fistula. https://core.ac.uk/download/617035268.pdf (accessed on 28th July 2025).
4. Allen, Diane, "Decreasing Duration of Mechanical Restraint Episodes by Increasing Registered Nurse Assessment and Surveillance in an Acute Psychiatric Hospital" (2018). *DNP Scholarly Projects*. 5. https://scholars.unh.edu/scholarly_projects/5(accessed on 28th July 2025).
5. Altissimi, G., Cianfrone, G., Ciofalo, A., et al. (2016). When alarm bells ring: Emergency tinnitus. https://core.ac.uk/download/54538689.pdf (accessed on 28th July 2025).
6. Alzheimer's Association. (2023). 2023 Alzheimer's disease facts and figures. *Alzheimer's & Dementia, 19*, 1598–1695. https://doi.org/10.1002/alz.13016 (accessed on 28th July 2025).
7. Azevedo-Marques, J. M. de, Del-Ben, C. M., Menezes, P. R., et al. (2010). Differential diagnosis of first episode psychosis: Importance of optimal approach in psychiatric emergencies. https://core.ac.uk/download/pdf/37451890.pdf (accessed on 28th July 2025).
8. Baldacchino, A., Bloor, R., Crome, I., et al. (2012). Preventing opioid overdoses in Europe: A critical assessment of known risk factors and preventative measures. https://core.ac.uk/download/20457694.pdf (accessed on 28th July 2025).
9. Banyard, P., & Shevlin, M. (2001). Responses of football fans to relegation of their team from the English Premier League: PTS?. *Irish journal of psychological medicine, 18*(2), 66–67. https://doi.org/10.1017/S0790966700006352 (accessed on 28th July 2025).
10. Barlow, E. M., Dickens, G. L., Endrawes, G., et al. (2019). Effectiveness and experiences of mental health nurses in cases of medical emergency and severe physiological deterioration. https://core.ac.uk/download/322475718.pdf (accessed on 28th July 2025).
11. Berlin, J. S., Gutierrez, P. M., Petrik, M. L., et al. (2015). Barriers and facilitators of suicide risk assessment in emergency departments: A qualitative study of provider perspectives. https://core.ac.uk/download/213077361.pdf (accessed on 28th July 2025).
12. Binay Kayan Ocakoğlu, G. E., Alkaş Karaca, M. C., Erata, F. T., Ocakoğlu, E. Y., Oral, G., & Karacetin, G. (2024). Assessment of children and adolescents' admissions to pediatric psychiatric emergency department. *Psychiatry, 88*, 41–54. https://www.semanticscholar.org/paper/8b5b0e1ed7620f32b25bdbc85d6bfe4fd0ed55a0 (accessed on 28th July 2025).
13. Borie, M. H., Alsharif, K. A., Alzahrani, M. S., & Aljohani, A. (2024). Critical assessment and intervention in young patients with neurological emergencies. *International Journal of Community Medicine and Public Health*. https://www.semanticscholar.org/paper/5d3b00bec44b69487f893da7ecaf493aa20bb076 (accessed on 28th July 2025).

14. Borum, R., & Rowe, M. (2021). The importance of bystanders in threat assessment and management. https://www.semanticscholar.org/paper/71e283a9c3063fd021c593fdeee1ee43e696749e (accessed on 28th July 2025).

15. Burzynski, A. E. (2017). Emergency crisis services for psychiatric boarder patients at Central Vermont Hospital ED. https://core.ac.uk/download/215152687.pdf (accessed on 28th July 2025).

16. Chan, M., Leung, P., Ho, T., Hung, S., Lee, C., Tang, C., Cheung, K., et al. (2017). Are psychiatric comorbidities and associated cognitive functions related to treatment response to methylphenidate in boys with attention-deficit/hyperactivity disorder? *Neuropsychiatric Disease and Treatment, 13*, 1071–1080. https://www.semanticscholar.org/paper/35a91061c4453c2ef75c988158c53c9db9790eb4 (accessed on 28th July 2025).

17. Chang, B. P., Powsner, S., Roppolo, L. P., et al. (2020). Management of agitation during the COVID-19 pandemic. https://core.ac.uk/download/323311338.pdf (accessed on 28th July 2025).

18. Chen, L., Li, H., Tian, F., Xie, C., & Zhao, L. (2023). Research on psychological crisis intervention strategies under emergencies: An analysis based on the four-party evolutionary game. *Sustainability*. https://www.semanticscholar.org/paper/d29712c7ec5e75ceef5e07e0e1dc7b61506e1ce4 (accessed on 28th July 2025).

19. Nacul, L., O'Boyle, S., Palla, L., Nacul, F. E., Mudie, K., Kingdon, C. C., Cliff, J. M., Clark, T. G., Dockrell, H. M., & Lacerda, E. M. (2020). How Myalgic Encephalomyelitis/Chronic Fatigue Syndrome (ME/CFS) Progresses: The Natural History of ME/CFS. *Frontiers in neurology, 11*, 826. https://doi.org/10.3389/fneur.2020.00826(accessed on 28th July 2025).

20. Colombo, C., Fregna, L., Locatelli, M., Manfredi, E., Martini, F., Perrozzi, G., & Pratesi, D. (2022). Psychiatric emergencies. https://core.ac.uk/download/559263449.pdf (accessed on 28th July 2025).

21. Cummins, I. D. (2013). Policing and mental illness in the era of deinstitutionalization and mass incarceration: A UK perspective. https://core.ac.uk/download/19331353.pdf (accessed on 28th July 2025).

22. DeVries, Joe, "The Impact of Emergency Preparedness on Improving Recovery, Trust in Government and Employee Morale" (2021). *EMPA Capstones*. 67. https://digitalcommons.law.ggu.edu/capstones/67(accessed on 28th July 2025).

23. Diner, B. C., Kyser, J. G., et al. (2011). A practical approach to the assessment and management of psychiatric emergencies. https://core.ac.uk/download/46967190.pdf (accessed on 28th July 2025).

24. Freitas, J. R., Desport, C., Martins, D. O., Santos, M., & Fonseca, C. (2024). The impact of the COVID-19 pandemic on psychiatric hospitalizations in a Portuguese department: A retrospective observational study. *European Psychiatry, 67*, S512–S512. https://www.semanticscholar.org/paper/6b570bfc4b77e490125e0d287cc3f9555c6bb385 (accessed on 28th July 2025).

25. Gautam, S., Gautam, M., Jain, A., & Yadav, A. N. (2022). Overview of practice of consultation-liaison psychiatry. *Indian Journal of Psychiatry, 64*, S201–S210. https://doi.org/10.4103/indianjpsychiatry.indianjpsychiatry_1019_21 (accessed on 28th July 2025).

26. Gul, N., & Nizami, A. T. (2024). Evaluating adherence to rapid tranquilization protocols in

psychiatric emergencies: An audit of a tertiary care facility in Pakistan. *BJPsych Open, 10*, S233–S234. https://www.semanticscholar.org/paper/4813f3fe4d5330c19a99e260de9ffa724c31411e (accessed on 28th July 2025).

27. Gul, N., & Nizami, A. T. (2024). Service evaluation of diagnostic evolution in psychiatric patients at Benazir Bhutto Hospital: Comparing OPD and ER admissions. *BJPsych Open, 10*, S189–S189. https://www.semanticscholar.org/paper/44204dfc4de9b7b63df8dab95216e1edaea9f6fc (accessed on 28th July 2025).

28. Haryanto, J. (2024). Short-term versus long-term portfolio management strategies and the selection of securities. *Advances in Management & Financial Reporting*. https://www.semanticscholar.org/paper/d42aef922574daaf06dda243312abc611945ada7 (accessed on 28th July 2025).

29. Henley, R., Marshall, R., & Vetter, S. (2018). Integrating mental health services into humanitarian relief responses to social emergencies, disasters, and conflicts: A case study. https://core.ac.uk/download/159149249.pdf (accessed on 28th July 2025).

30. Hersrud, Maren L.; Kiser, Karalee; and Knox, Catherine M., "Psychiatric Emergency Services in Oregon" (1977). Dissertations and Theses. Paper 2597. https://doi.org/10.15760/etd.2594(accessed on 28th July 2025).

31. Kandsperger, S., Schleicher, D., Ecker, A., Keck, F., Bentheimer, S., Brunner, R., & Jarvers, I. (2022). Emotional reactivity in adolescents with non-suicidal self-injury and its predictors: A longitudinal study. *Frontiers in Psychiatry, 13*. https://www.semanticscholar.org/paper/cc004fc2d8220d4d4a527e14e9e296c6813da51b (accessed on 28th July 2025).

32. Laherrán, N., Palacios, R., & Vázquez, A. (2024). Assessment of the capability of artificial intelligence for psychiatric diagnosis. *European Psychiatry, 67*, S825–S825. https://www.semanticscholar.org/paper/805e0f04e92b0d5f9d86d11cacb204ceb6b97afc (accessed on 28th July 2025).

33. Leveton, L. B., Picano, J. J., Schneiderman, J. S., et al. (2025). Risk of adverse cognitive or behavioral conditions and psychiatric disorders. https://core.ac.uk/download/pdf/42706622.pdf (accessed on 28th July 2025).

34. Lima, E., & Esquerdo, T. J. (2003). The economic costs of alcohol misuse in Portugal. No 24, NIMA Working Papers from Núcleo de Investigação em Microeconomia Aplicada (NIMA), Universidade do Minho(accessed on 28th July 2025).

35. McFarlane, A. C., & Williams, R. (2012). Mental health services required after disasters: learning from the lasting effects of disasters. *Depression research and treatment, 2012*, 970194. https://doi.org/10.1155/2012/970194(accessed on 28th July 2025).

36. Nava, R., Benatti, B., Girone, N., Macellaro, M., Pellicioli, C., Maggioni, L., Marcatili, M., et al. (2024). Assessing the fear of COVID-19 in psychiatric patients: Results from an Italian multicentric study. *Clinical Neuropsychiatry, 21*, 529–537. https://www.semanticscholar.org/paper/630c5dd724a1d0b2f9eb744ce49a90ea59d117b0 (accessed on 28th July 2025).

37. Nguyen, T. N. H., Khuu, T. P. D., Nguyen, Q. H., & Nguyen, M. C. (2024). Can sustainable supply chain strategies of company enhance for mitigation of risk damages and long-term resilience? An empirical analysis for the context of COVID-19 pandemic. *WPOM – Working Papers on Operations Management*. https://www.semanticscholar.org/paper/d349c070da15bc8935c2fbc43cb5030c8325ba24 (accessed on 28th July 2025).

38. Wiseman, Martin and O'Gorman, Shannon (2019) "School Based Responses to Non-Suicidal Self Injury and Suicide: Literature Considerations When Framing a Policy Response," eJournal of Catholic Education in Australasia: Vol. 3 : Iss. 1 , Article 12. Available at: https://researchonline.nd.edu.au/ecea/vol3/iss1/12 (accessed on 28th July 2025).

39. Oving, I., Masterson, S., Tjelmeland, I., Jonsson, M., Semeraro, F., Ringh, M., Truhlář, A., et al. (2019). First-response treatment after out-of-hospital cardiac arrest: A survey of current practices across 29 countries in Europe. *Scandinavian Journal of Trauma, Resuscitation and Emergency Medicine, 27.* https://www.semanticscholar.org/paper/74058bfadf55dfcd84914048573fdabba21b7adc (accessed on 28th July 2025).

40. Ruth, K., Ahlawat, P., & Kaur, R. (2025). Forensic nursing approaches to de-escalation and crisis management in psychiatric emergencies: A systematic review. *D Y Patil Journal of Health Sciences.* https://www.semanticscholar.org/paper/ba34f04e44e76cefaaaf4fa2112a9de0ccfa5d5c (accessed on 28th July 2025).

41. Smith, Y. (2016). School mental health guide for educators. https://core.ac.uk/download/84457996.pdf (accessed on 28th July 2025).

42. Wasserman, D., Arango, C., Fiorillo, A., Levin, S., Peters, A. C., Rao, G. P., Sylla, A., et al. (2023). Pushing forward public mental health agenda and promotion of mental health. *World Psychiatry, 22*, 170, 171. https://doi.org/10.1002/wps.21052 (accessed on 28th July 2025).

43. Weissbecker, I., Nic A. Bhaird, C., Alves, V., Ventevogel, P., Willhoite, A., Hijazi, Z., Hanna, F., et al. (2023). A minimum service package (MSP) to improve response to mental health and psychosocial needs in emergency situations. *World Psychiatry, 22*, 161, 162. https://doi.org/10.1002/wps.21048 (accessed on 28th July 2025).

44. Xi, Y., Shi, K., Yao, Y., Chen, R., He, Y., Jia, C., Qi, S., et al. (2019). A preliminary study on psychological crisis intervention strategies used in public emergencies. *13*, 133–138. https://www.semanticscholar.org/paper/500db8b2cab4abc357350d43c3d0179e82122deb (accessed on 28th July 2025).

45. Yermus, R., Bottos, J., Bryson, N., De Leo, J. A., Earleywine, M., Hackenburg, E., Kennedy, S., et al. (2024). Ketamine-assisted psychotherapy provides lasting and effective results in the treatment of depression, anxiety, and post-traumatic stress disorder at 3 and 6 months: Findings from a large retrospective effectiveness study. *Psychedelic Medicine, 2(2)*, 87–95. https://www.semanticscholar.org/paper/c84c515f051df7d5bc9305e7367a8497745429af (accessed on 28th July 2025).

TREATMENT MODALITIES IN PSYCHIATRY

15

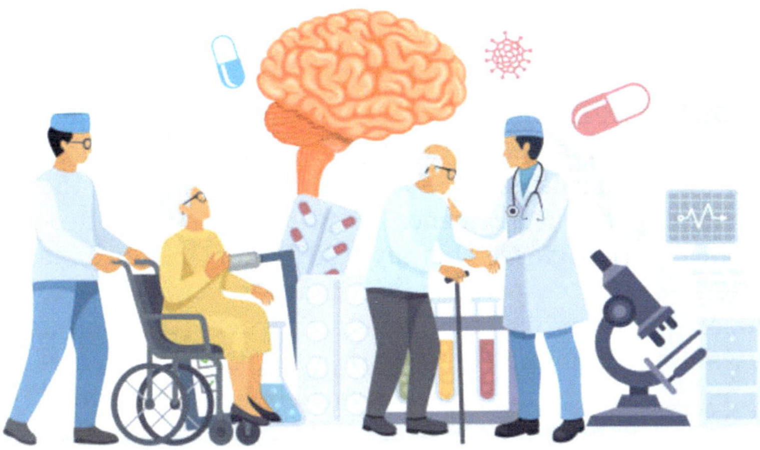

LEARNING OBJECTIVES

After studying this chapter, you will be able to:

1. Discuss psychopharmacology;
2. Define psychotherapy;
3. Explain about electroconvulsive therapy (ECT);
4. Explore transcranial magnetic stimulation (TMS);
5. Describe lifestyle and holistic approaches;
6. List the emerging treatment modalities.

Introduction

Psychiatric treatment modalities constitute a wide range of interventions employed to manage mental health disorders and improve the quality of life of patients. The global increase in mental health disorders necessitates an exhaustive familiarity with the treatment modalities present, which can be categorized into pharmacological and non-pharmacological modalities. They have their own advantages and disadvantages, and each contributes significantly towards determining treatment outcomes. Emerging evidence indicates that a multidimensional model is essential to effective intervention, integrating biological, psychological, and sociocultural dimensions. This essay aims to critically analyze various modalities of treatment in psychiatry, detailing their effectiveness, usefulness, and theoretical underpinnings, which guide them, in the hope of lending support to more evidence-based practice. The shift to integrative treatment models is reflected in greater acceptance of newer methods , such as sensory modulation therapy. This form of therapeutic treatment can address the varied sensory processing dysfunction in patients with mental disorders, as delineated by Dr. Ayres' Sensory Integration Theory (Hoque, 2016). Sensorimotor function may be used as evidence to show that sensory modulation can serve as an effective alternative to coercive routine practices and facilitate safer environments for upset or angry patients. The use of these modalities has shown promising results in the promotion of patient outcomes through the emphasis on the importance of personalized care plans that meet the specific needs of each individual. With the development of the field of psychiatry, the inclusion of sensory-based approaches to mainstream treatment can have the potential to enhance the efficacy and acceptability of psychiatric treatment. Further, exploring the nuances of specific populations under psychiatric treatment brings to light the complexities of managing illnesses like personality disorders with self-injurious behavior. Findings indicate that clinical symptoms are more severe among patients with personality disorders with deliberate self-injury and are less amenable to treatment modalities overall (Chiesa et al., 2011). This emphasizes the necessity of tailor-made treatment approaches that react to the unique presentations of such patients, leading to better therapy outcomes. As mental health professionals continue to strive to understand the meaning of self-injury and contain it, the discovery of effective treatment models continues to be essential. This essay aims to provide an overview of these treatment modalities so that there is an improved understanding of psychiatric care as it develops to meet the diverse needs of patients.

Definition of Psychiatry

The meaning of psychiatry comprises a branch of medicine that is dedicated to detecting, comprehending, and healing mental diseases. The field blends biological and psychological principles to address the complexity of the human mind and behavior. Psychiatry aims not only to heal symptoms of mental illnesses but to enhance overall psychological well-being. With the surge of mental illness disorders in contemporary society, the role of a psychiatrist is currently central to how comprehensive care is delivered to an individual patient, including how many various treatment models are required, such as drug management, psychotherapy, and other types of techniques, with an emphasis on holistic healing of a patient. The interaction of the evolving landscape of mental health with the evolving definitions that enshroud psychiatry elucidates the growing understanding of mental health's impact on physical health, eventually leading to a more refined respect for patient treatment modalities in the field. Over the past few decades, the sophistication of treatment modalities in psychiatry has emphasized the need for evidence-based practices. Cognitive-behavioral therapy (CBT), for instance, is today a premier treatment for conditions like obsessive-compulsive disorder (OCD). But significant barriers prevent access to these life-saving therapies. Stigma surrounding mental illness and the pain of coming forward to seek treatment deter patients from undergoing necessary care. Additionally, external factors, which comprise a shortage of trained therapists and the cost of psychotherapy, would in most cases result in suboptimal treatment for worthy individuals. New methods, such as the utilization of neuroimaging techniques, have the promise of initiating change by being able to predict patients' long-term treatment outcomes and hence improving treatment access and treatment modality efficacy in psychiatry (O'Neill & Feusner, 2015). Understanding the attachment styles casts yet another insight into the definition of psychiatry as well as its treatment modalities. Research has provided some insight into how adult attachment styles influence caregiving behavior and subsequently treatment outcome. For instance, an individual's attachment style could be what makes an individual receptive to various treatments with an impact on his/her treatment engagement level. There is evidence to suggest that there is a correspondence between an individual's attachment style and caregiving behavior preference. As a result, such knowledge can guide the therapeutic engagement of patients and psychiatrists so that interventions become tailored to activate patients' respective emotional constellations. Drawing inferences from attachment research and caregiving research into psychiatry can guide its treatment strategy to optimize patient response, towards an integrative model of knowledge encompassing psychological, emotional, and relational dimensions of mental health (Carli et al., 2016).

Importance of Treatment Modalities

The importance of the treatment modalities in psychiatry can hardly be overemphasized, as they constitute the frameworks in which mental health professionals work with a wide variety of psychiatric disorders. Various modalities, ranging from psychotherapy and pharmacotherapy to novel sensory modulation techniques, provide essential tools for the tailoring of treatments. For instance, Dr. Ayres' Sensory Integration Theory outlines the significance of processing sensors in mental health and demonstrates the impact that interruptions in sensory integration can have on resulting in adverse emotional effects, including anxiety and depression (Hoque, 2016). Thus, incorporating sensory-focused techniques may act as a prevention strategy, providing both patients and practitioners with the ability to control behavior in a productive way and reduce reliance on more coercive interventions like seclusion or restraint. This demonstrates not only the adaptability of treatment modalities but also the critical importance of their contribution to the enhancement of patient care. Furthermore, the presence of a broad range of treatment modalities facilitates the holistic treatment of mental illness conditions. Clinical social workers, who constitute a significant percentage of the mental health professional workforce, are likely to apply multiple modalities learned from their extensive training to treat clients with mental illness disorders (Masiriri, 2008). This multi-dimensional care offers the diversity to plan interventions that are not only aimed at treating the psychiatric symptoms but also sociocultural variables influencing an individual's mental illness. By recognizing how differently people respond to treatment, practitioners are best able to optimize therapeutic gain and achieve recovery. With the increasing recognition of the places of different therapeutic approaches, there is a need for ongoing research and pedagogical enhancements, as well as to prepare professionals with the abilities required to maneuver through the complex nature of mental health care. Moreover, the integration of evidence-based processes into treatment modalities enhances their effectiveness and usability in psychiatric settings. Continuous monitoring of treatment outcomes, as represented by the success of sensory modulated approaches as reported in current educational in-services, reflects how evidence-based practice leads to long-term changes in patient outcomes and staff attitudes (Hoque, 2016). The necessity to evaluate these modalities is underscored by the need to maintain quality care in relation to the ethical issues likely to arise from managed behavioral healthcare, such as reimbursement levels and availability of services (Masiriri, 2008). The support of evidence-based practices asserts the commitment to the welfare of patients and ensures that practitioners use techniques not just effective but ethically sound, providing a more compassionate approach to the treatment of mental illness.

15.1. Psychopharmacology

Learning Outcome

1. Types of psychiatric medications.
2. Mechanisms of action.
3. Benefits and risks of medication.

Psychopharmacology is a dynamic field of treatment for the majority of psychiatric disorders, and it offers a biochemical underpinning of the mechanism of mental illness. With the application of drugs to alter the neurochemical mechanisms of mood, cognition, and behavior, psychopharmacology enhances the therapeutic armamentarium in psychiatry. Antidepressants, antipsychotics, mood stabilizers, and anxiolytics are some of the main classes of psychotropic medications that have effects on specific neurotransmitter systems. As a case in point, selective serotonin reuptake inhibitors (SSRIs) influence serotonin concentrations to a significant extent, and this has been observed to reduce symptoms of depression and anxiety. Clinical psychopharmacology practice, however, might exceed the pharmacological focus because it is possible to pair it with psychotherapy and obtain synergistic effects that can amount to more holistic treatment outcomes. The journey of attaining optimal mental health requires careful balancing of medication regimens appropriate to the unique needs of individual patients. The active field of psychopharmacology is increasingly shaped by neuroscientific advances that illuminate the core biological underpinnings of psychiatric illness. As researchers reveal the complexity of neural circuits as well as the balance of various neurotransmitters, psychopharmacology reacts in equal measure to more effectively address the multi-factorial nature of mental illness. Different patients show remarkable heterogeneity in their response to psychiatric medications, highlighting the importance of personalized medicine in psychopharmacologic approaches. One such idea is that of creative psychopharmacotherapy, where treatments need to be considered as a whole. This will involve finding medication options to complement the person's individual history and individual symptomology, as psychological and biological determinants have a powerful impact upon each other. By synthesizing psychopharmacotherapy with psychotherapy, clinicians achieve a greater comprehension of the patient and therefore, enhance outcomes within all clinical settings (Avdibegović et al., 2021). Furthermore, the confluence of psychopharmacology and addiction treatment accentuates the need for individualized approaches based on endophenotypic heterogeneity among patients. Addiction is a complex interplay of biological and environmental factors with meaningful variability in symptom expression and treatment response. Studies suggest that integration of goal-directed (model-based) and habitual (model-free) systems is a significant consideration in addiction behavior. Different endophenotypes may have identical addiction characteristics but respond to treatments in different ways, indicating a move towards the development of pharmacologic treatments targeted at these inherited characteristics. This subtle insight is well-suited for the optimization of recovery through the ability of clinicians to tailor treatment in a manner that speaks to the unique pathophysiological set of each patient (Adinoff et al., 2018). Consequently, the acceptance of the complexities of psychopharmacology and individualized treatment models has the ability to change the effectiveness of psychiatric treatment.

15.1.1. Types of Psychiatric Medications

The field of psychiatric medications is extensive, with several classes dealing with many disorders of mental illness. The main categorizations of the pharmacological medications include antidepressants, antipsychotics, anxiolytics, mood stabilizers, and stimulants. Depressing drugs, primarily selective serotonin reuptake inhibitors (SSRIs) like fluoxetine and fluvoxamine, are commonly prescribed to treat depression and anxiety disorders. Their activity is usually the augmentation of brain levels of neurotransmitters like serotonin, thereby increasing mood and emotional well-being.

Recent findings suggest that there is a large utilization of SSRIs in treating conditions like obsessive-compulsive disorder (OCD), where fluoxetine and fluvoxamine were the most frequently used medications in an international population of patients receiving treatment for this disorder. Understanding these medications' mechanisms is crucial to effective psychiatric care. In addition to antidepressants, antipsychotic medications play a critical role in the control of major mental illness, including schizophrenia and bipolar disorder. Antipsychotics are first-generation (typical) or second-generation (atypical) (Figure 15.1).

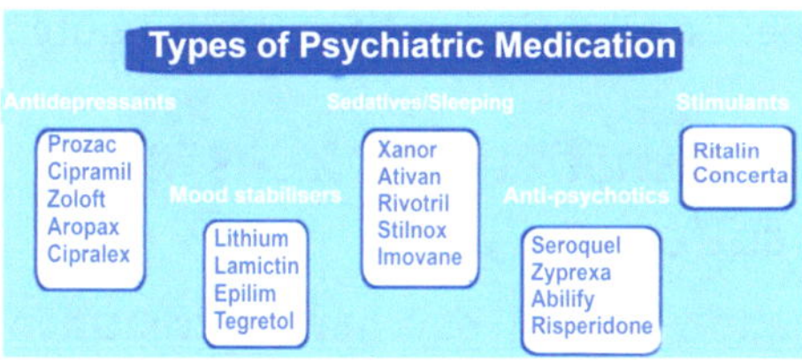

Figure 15.1. Common categories of psychiatric medications.

Source: https://external-content.duckduckgo.com/iu/?u=https%3A%2F%2Fwww.dramiric.co.za%2Fwp-content%2Fuploads%2F2016%2F02%2Ftypesofpsychdrugs450px.jpg&f=1&nofb=1&ipt=260a5b074a7de3c8cad2966a1f569d0811ae5074a1d9bad4c123b61d52e3e1f7.

The older generation, including drugs like haloperidol, has its main action on dopamine receptors to produce serious side effects, for example, extrapyramidal symptoms. Atypical antipsychotics, for example, risperidone and aripiprazole, possess a different kind of action by influencing more than one neurotransmitter system, thereby reducing side effects while exerting therapeutic effects. Recent research indicates a new trend in the use of atypical antipsychotics, with proof submitted on their increased prescription to patients undergoing treatment for disorders like OCD (Micallef-Trigona, 2014). This change reflects increased awareness of the complex and dynamic nature of psychiatric disease and the need for tailored treatment plans. The development of neurostimulation techniques is a recent advance in psychiatric modalities of treatment, particularly for treatment-resistant patients who can no longer be treated with drug therapy. Therapies , such as electroconvulsive therapy (ECT) have been shown to be effective in the management of severe depression but are normally accompanied by side effects, for example, memory loss. Alternatively, repetitive transcranial magnetic stimulation (rTMS) is gaining popularity considering its promising results and minimal side effects, providing a potential alternative to ECT treatment for refractory depression (Micallef-Trigona, 2014). This action reflects an important re-examination of traditional modes of treatment while highlighting the need for reconciliation of drug and non-drug modalities to treat mental disorders. This diversification in treatment modalities supports the utility of personalized interventions that address unique patient needs and facilitate recovery.

15.1.2. Mechanisms of Action

The mechanism-of-action idea is the foundation for understanding how treatments in psychiatry bring about change in patients. Every treatment modality brings about change through distinct psychological, biological, or sociocultural mechanisms that ultimately determine success. Cognitive therapy, for example, is aimed at altering inappropriately distorted thought patterns, while cognitive-behavioral therapy uses behavioral techniques to alter behavior along with cognition. This multi-layered paradigm presents clinicians with a model to select the optimal treatments for specific patient conditions and the mechanisms involved in psychiatric illness. Efficacy usually depends on a well-developed comprehension of these mechanisms so that practitioners can organize interventions that are consistent with each treatment's distinct features and patient group, maximizing therapeutic efficiency (Carbajal, 2018). Various trauma treatment modalities emphasize the role of mechanisms of action to treat particular disorders, most notably post-traumatic stress disorder (PTSD). The research suggests various evidence-based therapies with diverse mechanisms for symptom reduction, such as cognitive processing therapy (CPT) and eye movement desensitization and reprocessing (EMDR). CPT, for instance, entails cognitive restructuring by way of asking patients to clarify distorted beliefs regarding trauma so they can re-interpret their experiences. EMDR, on the other hand, applies bilateral sensory stimulation to help patients integrate traumatic memories. Both treatments are based on distinct mechanisms to promote recovery, but their combined efficacy in the treatment of PTSD highlights the need to identify how these modalities interact at the psychological level to ensure optimal outcomes (Carbajal, 2018) (Figure 15.2).

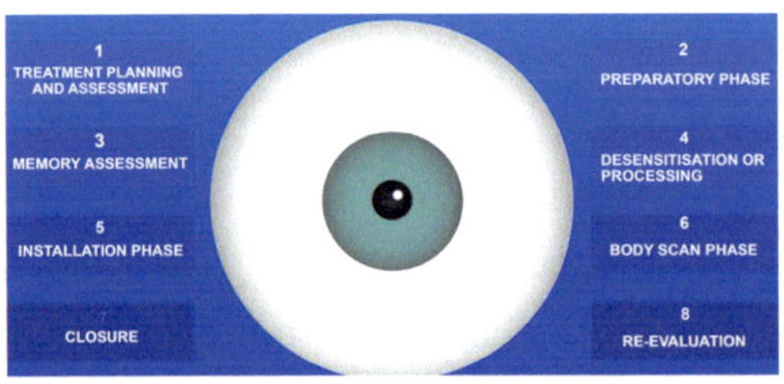

Figure 15.2. The eight phases of EMDR therapy.

Source: https://external-content.duckduckgo.com/iu/?u=https%3A%2F%2Fcdn-wordpress-info.futurelearn.com%2Finfo%2Fwp-content%2Fuploads%2F0cf5638e-f7f6-4c4c-9707-605a85c87295-768x432.png&f=1&nofb=1&ipt=a071c8034b6f37f4bb2aebf4322dc169e4381488428cf671048ab35f40dae725.

In addition to traditional psychotherapeutic methods, the impact of recovery tales is a promising approach to intervention in treating mental illness. Recovery tales allow individuals to relate to others' experiences and, therefore, empathize and form ties important to healing. A study of the acceptance of these tales revealed that the respondents would reflect on their own problems as they compared themselves to the storytellers' experiences. This reflection is significant because it increases emotional engagement and enables personal comprehension. The identified mechanisms for connection, self-comparison, experiential learning, and empathy, are central to how stories can be employed as a treatment mechanism that not only reaffirms personal identities but also triggers recovery. An appreciation of these connections further illustrates why narrative-based approaches can be integrated into current treatments to optimize therapeutic outcomes.

15.1.3. Benefits and Risks of Medication

Medication use in psychiatric treatment has numerous benefits, and therefore, it is a very important modality for the majority of patients. Drugs , such as antidepressants, antipsychotics, and mood stabilizers can significantly decrease symptoms of diseases , such as depression, schizophrenia, and bipolar disorder, thereby improving the lives of patients. For instance, research indicates that medication can make a patient's mood better, increase functionality, and even allow the patient to engage more actively in therapeutic interventions like cognitive-behavioral therapy (CBT) (O'Neill & Feusner, 2015). Moreover, drugs are often the central component of the treatment of chronic psychiatric conditions, allowing patients to lead normal lives. However, as with all medical treatments, the efficacy of these drugs can vary from person to person, depending on biochemistry and adherence to regimens prescribed, and must be closely monitored on the part of healthcare providers. While the advantages exist, the risk is not in psychiatric medications. Side effects, minor to severe, can occur, potentially deterring patients from continued treatment. Side effects like weight gain, sexual dysfunction, and increased anxiety will undermine the effectiveness of medication and lead to discontinuation (Noel et al., 2017). Additionally, potential interactions between drugs can render treatment regimens cumbersome, particularly for comorbid patients who require multiple drugs. The risk of dependence or withdrawal also must be accounted for, especially with benzodiazepines and other anxiolytics, because they can lead to patients seeking alternative treatment modalities. These risks highlight the need for patient education and informed consent so that patients are informed about both the therapeutic effects and limitations of the drugs they are prescribed as part of a total treatment program. With the evolution of the specialty of psychiatry, increasing demands are made for an integrative model where drugs are complemented by psychotherapeutic techniques for better results. Not only does this integration facilitate symptom care but also addresses the deeper cognitive and emotional problems suffered by patients. Technologies , such as neuroimaging forecasting therapeutic outcomes to therapies like CBT are under investigation (O'Neill & Feusner, 2015). Such advances can refine treatment programs by standardizing medication consumption in line with individual patient needs and feedback. At the same time, incorporating medications into integrative care will always be accompanied by constant evaluation of benefits and risks to ensure evidence-based treatment, always patient-centered. The overall strategy aims at empowering the patient to be in control of their mental health, thus being in cooperative efforts with clinicians for good therapeutic outcomes.

Test Your Knowledge

1. How do different classes of psychotropic medications (e.g., antidepressants, antipsychotics, anxiolytics) work to alter brain chemistry?
2. What factors influence medication selection, dosage, and monitoring in psychiatric treatment?

15.2. Psychotherapy

Learning Outcome

1. Types of psychotherapy (e.g., CBT, DBT).
2. Effectiveness of psychotherapy.
3. Role of the therapist.

Psychotherapy is at the center of treatment approaches in psychiatry when it comes to the therapeutic relationship between the clinician and the patient. Through this process, there can be the intentional examination of various facets of mental health: emotional, cognitive, and behavioral. Specific psychotherapeutic methods, for example, psychodynamic therapy and cognitive-behavioral therapy, present different perspectives on mental illness and its resolution. Both modalities emphasize the importance of understanding the patients personal history and subjective experience in guiding treatment interventions. In addition, whether psychotherapy is a success depends heavily on the therapists ability to create a working environment that is non-judgmental and supportive in which clients can freely discuss their feelings and thoughts. Such an environment facilitates self-examination and personal growth, both of which are essential factors of successful therapeutic interventions. Among the trauma-focused interventions, psychotherapy has been found to be effective in treating disorders , such as post-traumatic stress disorder (PTSD). Evidence recognizes five principal interventions:

cognitive therapy (CT), cognitive-behavioral therapy (CBT), cognitive processing therapy (CPT), prolonged exposure (PE) therapy, and eye movement desensitization and reprocessing (EMDR) therapy. Both modalities have gentle techniques for engaging with and processing trauma, but their effectiveness can vary greatly depending on the client's individual situation and circumstances. An evidence-based application of these therapies necessitates an unambiguous evaluation of histories and treatment histories to guide practitioners in selecting the most suitable intervention. Through attention to shaping treatment approaches to the population's unique characteristics, therapists can optimize clients' outcomes and enhance the overall efficacy of psychotherapeutic interventions (Carbajal, 2018) (Figure 15.3).

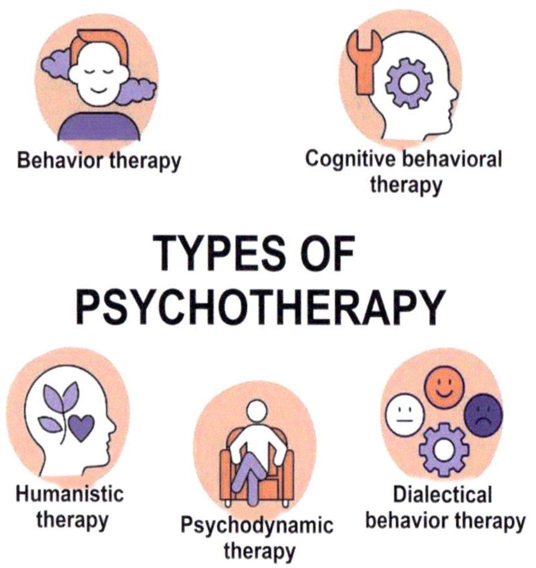

Figure 15.3. Types of psychotherapy.

Source: https://external-content.duckduckgo.com/iu/?u=https%3A%2F%2Fwww.simplypsychology.org%2Fwp-content%2Fuploads%2FTypes-of-psychotherapy.jpg&f=1&nofb=1&ipt=c06b4016d7dbcf8e113a7423ab24dea8b9d4af8495ad054c6b4bc8b8d14cebb7.

Additionally, the assessment of psychotherapy effectiveness contributes significantly to measuring the impact of psychotherapy as a critical dimension of determining treatment effectiveness and guiding future practice. Developing a framework of outcomes in psychotherapy not only supports clinicians in sharpening their skills but also contributes toward developing an understanding about the subtle interplay operating in the process of therapy. These areas of measurement comprise therapy outcome, therapy process, client predictors, and training outcome, which address the need for multidimensional methods of evaluation. Practitioners can learn what works and for whom with a systematic data-gathering process, which optimizes the flexibility of psychotherapy in a variety of settings. This is consistent with the overall objective to more effectively assess therapy modalities in research, ultimately creating a robust evidence base to inform training regimens and clinical practice (Elliott et al., 2006).

15.2.1. Types of Psychotherapy (e.g., CBT, DBT)

Psychotherapy is a broad field with numerous modalities that are suited to specific psychological disorders and patient needs. Of the most commonly known forms, Cognitive Behavioral Therapy (CBT) and Dialectical Behavior Therapy (DBT) are two of them. CBT is about recognizing and altering negative thought patterns so an individual can replace unhealthy behavior with healthier ones. Emotional and behavioral control through cognitive processes is the fundamental assumption of CBT, which has proven to be exceptionally effective for the treatment of conditions , such as depression, anxiety disorders, and eating disorders. As a systematic modality, CBT allows patients to learn problem-solving skills for coping with distress, resulting in improved overall psychosocial adaptation and functioning, which is also the basis for its extensive use in contemporary therapeutic practice. In the past few years, Dialectical Behavior Therapy (DBT) has been established as a concentrated form of cognitive-behavioral treatment designed initially for borderline personality disorder. DBT synthesizes mindfulness, emotional regulation, distress tolerance, and interpersonal effectiveness principles in order to offer effective treatment to individuals who are experiencing severe emotional dysregulation. The group and interactive character of DBT, typically in the form of a combination of individual and group therapy sessions, fosters an alliance capable of producing dramatic gains in self-esteem and interpersonal functioning. Findings suggest that DBT has proven effective in reducing suicidal behavior and increasing emotional regulation, emphasizing the life-transforming potential of DBT and offering a viable intervention for patients whose symptoms have been unresponsive to more traditional forms of therapy (Figure 15.4).

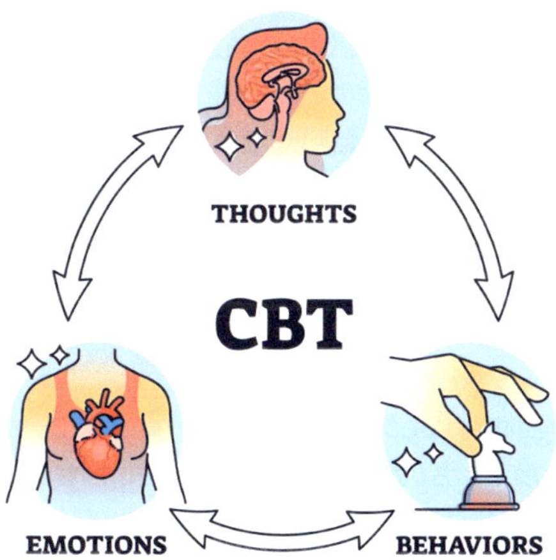

Figure 15.4. Cognitive behavioral therapy (CBT).

Source: https://www.simplypsychology.org/wp-content/uploads/CBT.jpg.

Exploring the landscape of psychotherapy also comes with the investigation of the effectiveness of treatment for a range of conditions. Findings suggest that psychosocial treatments, namely those designed for eating disorders like Binge Eating Disorder (BED), have essential significance for recovery and the quality of life. As highlighted in recent literature, CBT is especially effective against bulimia nervosa and BED, while family therapy approaches have been promising for anorexia nervosa. An integrative intervention with interpersonal psychotherapy and supportive therapies can also enhance treatment outcomes, especially when handling complex psychosocial dynamics. The multisectoral orientation of these interventions emphasizes the importance of tailoring therapeutic modalities to individual differences, as it is through tailoring that one manages to develop resilience, prevent relapse, and achieve sustained change (Costa & Melnik, 2016; Marzilli et al., 2018) (Figure 15.5).

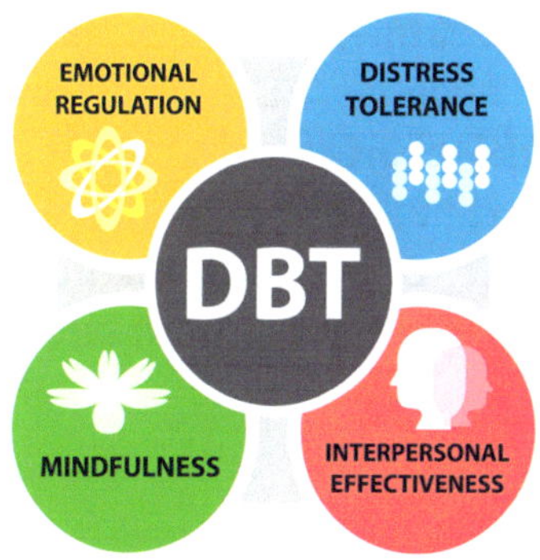

Figure 15.5. Dialectical behavior therapy (DBT).

Source: https://www.simplypsychology.org/wp-content/uploads/Dialectical-Behavior-Therapy.jpeg.

15.2.2. Effectiveness of Psychotherapy

The effectiveness of psychotherapy has become a prime focus of psychiatric treatment modalities that include heterogeneous theoretical orientations and specific therapeutic modalities. While psychotherapy is composed of many techniques, its ultimate purpose is the enhancement of emotional functioning through relief of psychological distress. It has been proven through research that different forms of psychotherapy, such as cognitive-behavioral therapy, psychosocial interventions, and trauma-focused therapies, have different results based on the patient population and the complexity of their psychopathology. Specifically, results have been improved in conditions such as depression and anxiety through ordered psychotherapeutic interventions.

Through thé capacity to modify therapy to suit the individual's requirements, psychotherapy can achieve enduring and profound alteration, highlighting the merit of psychotherapy as an area of psychiatric treatment. Furthermore, the effectiveness of these modalities is constantly enhanced by research, and thus, psychotherapy is a good choice for many individuals requiring psychiatric treatment. Analysis of particular conditions, such as PD, accounts for more regarding the character of psychotherapy in accurate treatment. For instance, PD patients who also use DSI exhibit higher levels of severity of symptoms, which require specialized treatment.

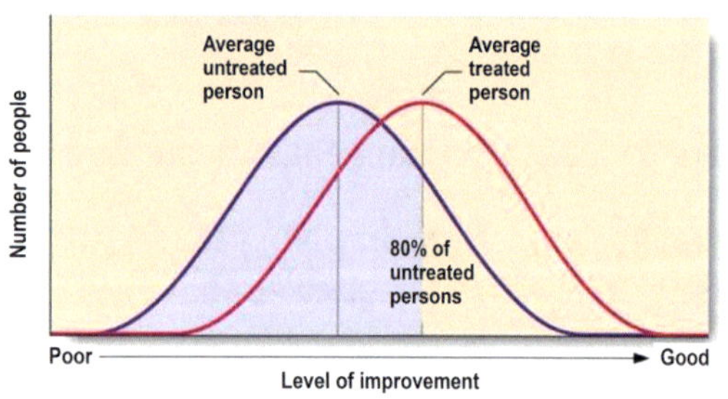

Figure 15.6. Effectiveness of psychotherapy.

Source: https://external-content.duckduckgo.com/iu/?u=https%3A%2F%2Fimage.slideserve.com%2F484990%2Feffectiveness-of-psychotherapy-l.jpg&f=1&nofb=1&ipt=a042ca8dde15a2291607de8be08c9e82b907311c0219917a2572e17fafda1306.

A recent research offers data regarding the various outcomes of strategies applied to the treatment of PD patients, differentiating between those with and without DSI. DSI participants in outpatient treatment programs demonstrated considerably enhanced symptom control and decreased recidivism of self-injurious behavior compared to their inpatient counterparts. This finding illuminates the requirement for treatment protocols tailored to account for the subtleties of DSI, that is, that effective psychotherapy must vary with patient severity and specific attributes. Greater awareness of such distinctions is required for the maximization of treatment methods in psychiatry (Figure 15.6).

Furthermore, the meta-analysis of trauma-focused treatments puts the spotlight on evidence-based psychotherapy for the treatment of disorders like Post-Traumatic Stress Disorder (PTSD). Literature points to several modalities as being highly efficacious, including cognitive therapy, cognitive-behavioral therapy, and eye movement desensitization and reprocessing (EMDR) therapy. All modalities are shown to be effective, but there are subtleties regarding the treatment modality that are important to practitioners to consider when determining the best fit for certain populations. For example, cognitive-processing therapy may yield improved outcomes among other trauma victims, whereas others may be helped by prolonged exposure therapy. With continued evolution in psychotherapy, having practitioners with the knowledge to make the optimal choice of interventions on empirical grounds can lead treatments forward to work across various patient populations and thereby lead to better mental health outcomes in psychiatry.

15.2.3. Therapist's Role

The role of the therapist in psychiatric treatment modalities is crucial in that it serves as a guide and support for the patient during the mental health process. The therapeutic process is rooted at its core in the establishment of an effective therapeutic relationship between the client and therapist, which is conceptualized as trust, empathy, and cooperation. This is important to effective treatment outcomes, as therapists help clients verbalize feelings and thoughts and, therefore, gain a more extensive understanding of conditions. Through the literature, the effectiveness of treatment modalities , such as cognitive-behavioral therapy (CBT) relies heavily on this bond. A healthy alliance not only enhances client engagement but also diminishes barriers to accessibility, such as stigma and the lack of motivation to attend therapy (O'Neill & Feusner, 2015). Hence, therapists play a key role in creating a safe and therapeutic environment that allows for personal development and exploration. Therapists are also responsible for modifying treatment techniques to accommodate individual clients' needs. In CBT, for example, therapists will have to modify interventions through responses and scenarios provided by the client so that interventions are effective and relevant. Adaptation is particularly important for client groups with particular mental health conditions, such as OCD and chronic tic disorders. Literature indicates significant barriers to effective treatments like CBT, including shortages of trained practitioners and logistics difficulties clients may encounter (O'Neill & Feusner, 2015). The therapists, therefore, must not only possess intimate knowledge of various treatment techniques but also devise innovative solutions—like teletherapy options—to expand their reach and help clients overcome such barriers. Aside from direct client contact, therapists' work involves ongoing self-reflection and professional development. To be effective, therapists must keep up with recent studies, treatment strategies, and psychiatric treatment advancements. Staying updated on this education enables them to be prepared to continue building on the therapeutic relationship and adapting their practices based on new evidence-based therapies. The efficacy of treatments like Comprehensive Behavioral Intervention for Tics (CBIT), for instance, relies on therapists receiving proper training regarding the latest methodologies and technologies facilitating remote delivery of care. By committing to lifelong learning, therapists are able to advance their practice and influence the entire field of mental health treatment, finally making a difference in clients' lives and the effectiveness of treatment modalities in psychiatry.

Test Your Knowledge

1. How do major psychotherapy approaches—such as CBT, psychodynamic therapy, and humanistic therapy—differ in their goals and techniques?
2. In what ways does psychotherapy complement psychopharmacological treatment in managing mental health disorders?

15.3. Electroconvulsive Therapy (ECT)

Learning Outcome

1. Indications for ECT.
2. Procedure and administration.
3. Side effects and controversies.

Electroconvulsive Therapy (ECT) is a standard of care in psychiatry for patients with severe mood disorders , such as major depressive disorder (MDD). All the advances in pharmacotherapy and psychotherapy notwithstanding, there remain a considerable number of patients—around one-third—who are resistant to conventional treatment modalities despite repeated trials, showing that other interventions are needed (Borrione et al., 2020). ECT operates by inducing controlled seizures through electrically stimulating the brain, and it is believed to normalize chemical balance and improve neuronal function. The therapy is typically reserved if other treatments fail, testifying to its usefulness in the treatment of treatment-resistant depression cases and other severe psychiatric disorders. Although ECT is effective, it is not without its challenges, predominantly cognitive side effects due to its convulsive nature. Usage is typically accompanied by short-term memory loss and some patients have chronic cognitive impairment that deters individuals from undergoing this therapy (Abedinzadeh et al., 2013). Recent research on fine-tuning of ECT protocols is seeking to reduce these side effects, for example, by adjusting seizure duration and employing adjunctive drugs , such as lidocaine to maximize therapeutic outcome. Research indicates that these techniques are capable of maximizing overall tolerability of ECT without diminishing its effectiveness in the treatment of serious psychiatric illnesses. Establishing an accurate and tailored medical approach for ECT may thus have significant repercussions for its uptake and utilization within the clinic. In addition, the clinical applications and technical applications of ECT evolve, with ongoing research aimed at the potential contribution of implementing neuroscience and technology into treatment modalities. New treatments , such as non-invasive neuromodulation therapies, such as transcranial magnetic stimulation and magnetic seizure therapy, are under investigation in combination with ECT, providing new possibilities for innovative psychiatric treatment (Borrione et al., 2020). As psychiatry advances toward individualized treatment, the potential for optimizing ECT through the use of customized interventions , such as closed-loop systems and computer-modeling of electrical fields, could further optimize its efficacy as well as curtail associated risks. Thus, the future of ECT is not only behind but also in its flexibility and integration into a total system of modalities of treatment tailored to the individual needs of each patient (Figure 15.7).

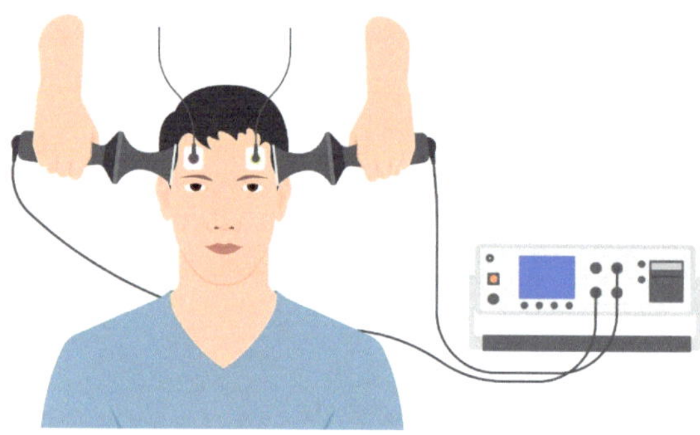

Figure 15.7. Electroconvulsive therapy (ECT).

Source: https://external-content.duckduckgo.com/iu/?u=https%3A%2F%2Fmood-disorders.co.uk%2FASSETS%2FIMG%2Fresources%2FECT-AdobeStock_433757000.jpg&f=1&nofb=1&ipt=8310c8eaf6e47eadb65b627dca013f488f42a623e3f8d3a3fa1341a8fb02adbd.

15.3.1. Indications for ECT

Electroconvulsive therapy (ECT) remains an institution of care in psychiatry, particularly for those with severe psychiatric illnesses who are not adequately responsive to routine pharmacologic interventions. ECT's primary indications are major depressive disorder, bipolar disorder, and treatment-resistant schizophrenia. Major depressive disorder, especially when it is the psychotic or suicidal ideation type, exhibits strong sensitivity to ECT, with research indicating patients to respond rapidly to their symptoms compared to other standard treatments. In the case of bipolar disorders, ECT is used for manic and depressive states in cases where the condition is dangerous or threatening to life, again emphasizing that it is a critical intervention in psychiatry (Certa et al., 2012). The clinical utility of ECT is established, particularly where equivalent pharmacotherapy trials have been unsuccessful or are contraindicated. Additionally, ECT is invaluable in acute illnesses in which rapid alleviation of symptoms is required, such as severe catatonia or suicidal depression. As borne out by the practice of medicine, the prescription for ECT often follows failure of therapy; it also involves those situations in which patients experience inordinate psychological distress that necessitates expedient action. Significantly, the effective integration of ECTs into treatment plans also reflects broader shifts in psychiatric practice, demonstrating its effectiveness and relevance, particularly with patients having complex or refractory disorders (Gazdag et al., 2014) (Figure 15.8).

ECT indications

Psychiatric	Medical
Mood disorders	NMS
Psychotic disorders	Status epilepticus
Catatonia	Parkinson's
	Catatonia

Figure 15.8. ECT indicators.

Source: https://external-content.duckduckgo.com/iu/?u=https%3A%2F%2Fwww.the-hospitalist.org%2Fwp-content%2Fuploads%2Flegacy%2Ffiles%2F139329a_graphic_web.png&f=1&nofb=1&ipt=2df333dd23c4dc2707b07dbd706a5438aae6fae0085cacb1ab7b8fe6434f32f9.

Although effective, the availability and uptake of ECT can vary widely according to geographical and clinical settings and influence outcomes for patients. In countries like Serbia, for instance, there is evidence of a very low usage rate of ECT despite the recognized necessity for treatment of severe exacerbations of recurrent depressive disorder. With 66.7% of ECT treatments applied for this condition being recorded in clinical evaluations, the lack of treatment consequently reaffirms substantial psychiatric care infrastructure shortages (Gazdag et al., 2014). The necessity for more services and recent trends to offer a continued alternative for individuals with an urgent need for ECT is increased by this shortage. Hence, offering alternatives to these constraints in the mental health system is crucial to provide comprehensive care to individuals with severe psychiatric disturbances.

15.3.2. Procedure and Administration

In the context of psychiatric counseling, treatment processes and intervention delivery are essential to ensuring effective outcomes. The formalized nature of such processes allows for customization of treatment protocols based on the specific needs of individual patients, which enhances the prospects of therapeutic success. This is particularly crucial in working with personality disorders (PDs), which are notoriously hard to treat due to the complexity of their psychopathology. An intense understanding of such complexities enables therapists to be more focused on the inherent characteristics of personality pathology, potentially enhancing engagement and retention in treatment. The incorporation of strategies that address metacognition—essentially the understanding and consciousness of one's mental states, can help to influence the trajectory of treatment and results. Thus, strengthening metacognitive abilities is key to optimizing general function and symptom diminution associated with PDs, indicating the importance of prudent process in psychiatric treatment. Coupled with understanding patient profiles, psychiatric management occasionally relies on a variety of modalities, including psychotherapy, pharmacotherapy, or blended approaches. One critical aspect of the success of such modalities is the systematic screening of patient histories and symptoms before the implementation of interventions. This first step is crucial as it guides the clinician's choice of treatment modality, thereby influencing the overall effectiveness of treatment provided. For instance, extensive research work on the cost-effectiveness of treatment of major depressive episodes identified a decline in costs between 1991 and 1996. This kind of evidence is critical for the necessity for both administrative and procedural psychiatric treatment to be viewed from a monetary viewpoint, potentially with long-term consequences on resources and availability of treatment (Bir et al., 2025). Moreover, effective administration of psychiatric care extends beyond direct patient contact to encompass an organizational framework for supportive, comprehensive care. Coordination of care among care providers, adherence to recommendations from best practice guidelines, and routine monitoring of therapeutic activity, for instance, are essential elements of effective administration. In this context, incorporating metacognitive training as part of treatment interventions may prove beneficial to the improvement of patient outcomes in personality disorder therapies. Studies have indicated that enhancement of metacognitive performance has been able to predict general symptomatic, interpersonal, and general well-being improvement, as evident in studies conducted on a large population of outpatients receiving formal psychotherapy. Thus, effective procedures and administration, if adjusted as per patient profile, not only improve the therapeutic alliance but also achieve optimal resource utilization and patient satisfaction (Carcione et al., 2019).

15.3.3. Side Effects and Controversies

The area of psychiatric treatment modalities is typically shrouded in problems involving side effects and controversy. Among these modalities, drugs , such as antidepressants and antipsychotics are more scrutinized by virtue of their side effects. Patients usually report difficulties , such as weight gain, sexual dysfunction, and cognitive impairment, leading to non-compliance and treatment discontinuation.

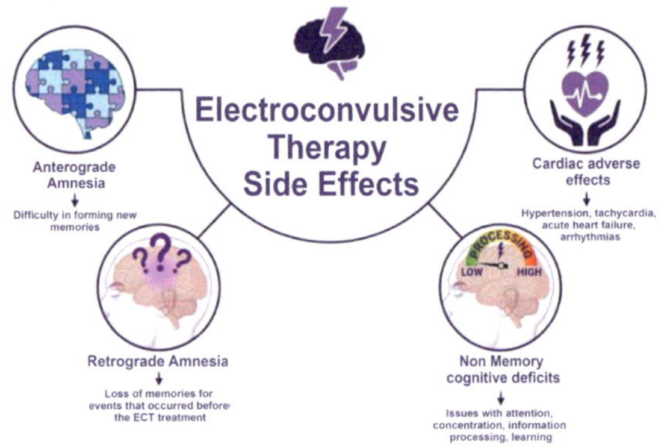

Figure 15.9. Side effects of ECT.

Source: https://www.researchgate.net/publication/383898454/figure/fig1/AS:11431281277123594@1725956164379/Possible-adverse-effects-of-Electroconvulsive-Therapy-ECT.png.

The intricacy of managing such side effects makes it difficult to make clinical decisions, as one has to weigh the potential good against the danger of patient harm. Moreover, discussion of psychiatric drugs is often polarized in that some are convinced of their indispensable role in the treatment of severe mental illness, whereas others advocate more naturalistic approaches with the focus on lifestyle modifications and psychotherapeutic interventions. The debate draws to the fore the thin line that practitioners have to draw when weighing the appropriateness of drug interventions in patient populations of variable backgrounds. Electroconvulsive therapy, although considered an effective treatment for severe depression and selected psychotic disorders, is a treatment frequently called into question by its possible side effects: loss of memory and impairment of cognitive function. The stigma attached to ECT, fueled by sensationalized media representation, has resulted in strong resistance by patients and families. However, the evidence does suggest that when applied cautiously, as seen in geriatric patient studies, ECT does produce excellent response rates, at times as high as 80% in specific groups (Snyder et al., 2017) (Figure 15.9).

This is to highlight a profound controversy in the practice of psychiatry: the superimposition of tangible advantages over the horizon of perceived danger. As doctors insist on wise treatment choices, there exists a categorical necessity for open conversations regarding both the effectiveness and side effects of ECT to design a greater degree of patient awareness and increase compliance. Recent advancements in behavioral treatments also reveal unwanted controversies and side effects. For instance, Comprehensive Behavioral Intervention for Tics (CBIT) holds promise, but problems with availability, such as a shortage of trained providers and challenges with logistics, can slow its implementation (Bauer et al., 2016). This is a significant equity concern in mental health care because not all families can locate this evidence-based practice. Furthermore, while the pilot studies indicate favorable outcomes in tic severity reduction, inconsistent response among the children indicates that not all patients experience significant benefit, which may lead to frustration and disappointment. As behavior therapy assumes its center stage role, it is more important than ever that mental health clinicians properly inform patients about the anticipated benefit and limitations so that families are adequately informed and well-supported throughout treatment.

Test Your Knowledge

1. What clinical conditions are most commonly treated with ECT, and why is it considered effective in severe cases?
2. What are the typical steps involved in administering ECT, and what safety precautions are taken during the procedure?

15.4. Transcranial Magnetic Stimulation (TMS)

Learning Outcome

1. Mechanism of TMS.
2. Clinical Applications.
3. Comparison with ECT.

Transcranial Magnetic Stimulation (TMS) has emerged as a leading non-invasive treatment approach in psychiatry, particularly in patients with major depressive disorder (MDD) who have been unresponsive to standard therapy. The technique utilizes pulses of alternating magnetic fields to induce small electrical currents in specific sites within the brain associated with mood regulation. Unlike pharmacological therapies, TMS avoids systemic side effects that are traditionally associated with drugs. Apart from this, the increasing application of precision medicine principles to TMS interventions optimizes treatment outcomes by tailoring interventions to the patient's neurobiological profile, for instance. Such innovation underlines why TMS holds the potential not only to alleviate depressive symptoms but also to provide a more tailored strategy for therapy, eventually addressing the untreated needs of treatment-resistant MDD patients, who represent a considerable proportion of those accessing psychiatric services (Verdejo-Garcia et al., 2019). Despite the potential of TMS, attention should be given to its limitations and existing problems in routine clinical practice. While findings from ongoing studies support the efficacy of TMS, overall response rates are narrow, and problems with optimal treatment parameters, such as treatment duration and frequency of sessions, exist. The value of the methods can also be contextually enhanced by simultaneous coupling to neuroimaging and cognitive testing, allowing for the determination of specific brain regions and cognitive functions most affected by depressive illness. As suggested in the initial activity of the Neuroscience Interest Group, the development of harmonized protocols and open channels of clinical relevance will be key to maximizing TMS benefit. Addressing these concerns through large-scale, multi-site research studies will cement the body of evidence needed to guide clinicians on best TMS practice, in the end, bridging the gap between neuroscientific research and clinical care (Verdejo-Garcia et al., 2019). Research into brain stimulation techniques like TMS aligns with a larger trend toward individualized psychiatric care. As therapeutic models evolve, clinicians and researchers are challenged to give top priority to the identification of biomarkers capable of predicting treatment response to TMS. This aligns with suggestions that precision-based models can maximize the overall effectiveness of neuromodulatory procedures. The inclusion of customized cognitive interventions and the integration of machine learning algorithms may offer monumental improvements in the precision of applying TMS. Notwithstanding this, the environment continues to be limited, with small sample sizes in studies and a lack of cost-effectiveness analyses. Filling these lacunae through instituting strong clinical trials and incorporating a precision medicine framework has the potential to lead to optimized treatment regimens and improved patient outcomes, reflecting improved understanding of mental illness and its neurobiology (Borrione et al., 2020) (Figure 15.10).

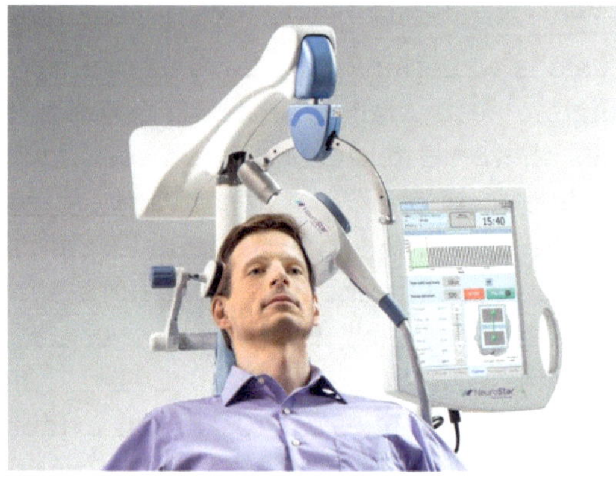

Figure 15.10. Transcranial magnetic stimulation (TMS)

Source: https://sa1s3optim.patientpop.com/assets/images/provider/photos/2627674.jpg.

15.4.1. Mechanism of TMS

Transcranial Magnetic Stimulation (TMS) is an invasive neuromodulation that is better realized to be effective in the treatment of major depressive disorder (MDD) and several psychiatric illnesses. The technology involves the delivery of brief magnetic pulses to the scalp that induce electrical currents in the brain that have the ability to affect neuronal excitability. TMS targets specifically the prefrontal cortex, an area involved in mood regulation. The mechanism is via the creation of an electromagnetic field that can modulate cortical neurons' excitability, increase synaptic plasticity, and even enable higher levels of connectivity in depressed neural networks. The result is that TMS not only enables mood improvement but can even rewire depression's neurobiological substrates, thus providing a bountiful addition to the treatment arsenal of psychiatry (Borrione et al., 2020). Despite its promising advantages, TMS is not free from limitations, particularly its relative inconstancy of effect among different patients. The success of therapy is contingent on factors like stimulation frequency, duration, and the patient's own brain pathology or anatomy. Recent research promotes more accuracy by adapting TMS protocols to individual characteristics, which could boost its efficacy. This would involve adding cognitive therapies to enhance the neurological effects of TMS, as well as employing multimodal biomarkers to improve the detection of the right patient profiles for treatment. With the application of high-technology techniques like computer electric field modeling and machine learning algorithms, clinicians can individualize TMS applications for optimum clinical outcomes. Such advances have the potential to individualize TMS treatment, aiming at minute differences in patient response (Ahmed et al., 2014).

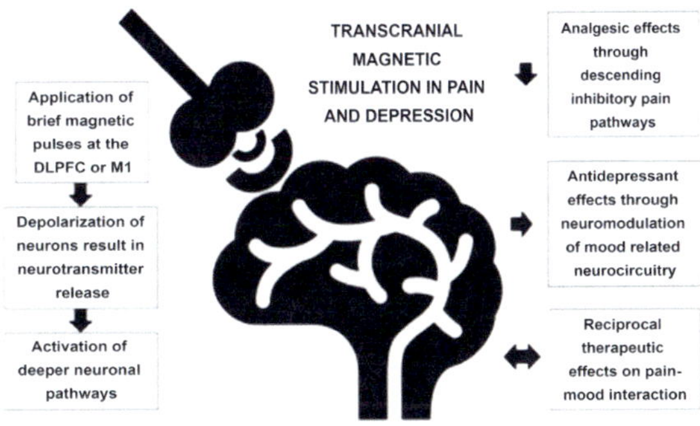

Figure 15.11. Possible mechanisms of action of repetitive transcranial magnetic stimulation in pain and depression.

Source: https://www.researchgate.net/figure/Possible-mechanisms-of-action-of-repetitive-transcranial-magnetic-stimulation-in-pain-and_fig1_325765273.

Moreover, while TMS has great promise, particularly for MDD, there is a need for ongoing research to help explain the full array of its benefits and limitations. Among the major challenges is incomplete knowledge regarding the physiological processes governing TMS response and the cognitive side effects that may emerge. Although TMS is tolerable, the interaction between this therapy and distinct neurobiological variables may induce differential effects that warrant further study of the pathophysiologic response. The growing literature suggests the necessity of full clinical trials that not only indicate TMS efficacy but also evaluate safety and cost-containment measures. This focus on a precision-targeted approach may ultimately make TMS a cornerstone of effective intervention strategies in psychiatry, thereby making sure that it is able to utilize its potential in transforming patient treatment in mental health (Borrione et al., 2020) (Figure 15.11).

15.4.2. Clinical Applications

The application of functional near-infrared spectroscopy (fNIRS) in clinical psychiatry represents a groundbreaking advancement in the diagnostic and monitoring functions of mental health professionals. For over two decades, fNIRS has emerged as a highly promising neuroimaging technology due to its unique advantages, such as portability, relative low cost, and capacity for assessing brain function in real time with no need for burdensome patient preparation. fNIRS measurement can complement the traditional clinical interview and mental state assessment and enhance the validity of psychiatric diagnoses. Furthermore, this modality facilitates the use of continuous measurements of treatment outcome by allowing clinicians to observe physiological changes in patients' brain function under therapeutic intervention. Increased studies on fNIRS show its potential for transforming clinical practice in psychiatry to provide a more educated treatment approach towards patients based on empirical evidence and neurobiological understanding (Charmaine et al., 2017). Multimodal neuroimaging approaches are another critical component of psychiatric intervention in clinical applications. By integrating a variety of neuroimaging techniques, such as structural and functional magnetic resonance imaging (MRI), healthcare professionals can design more accurate diagnostic classifiers for psychiatric conditions. For instance, studies have shown that a multimodal classification model used to classify alcohol dependence not only yields an accuracy of 79.3% in diagnosis but also surpasses individual imaging modalities, including grey-matter density measures (Guggenmos et al., 2020) (Figure 15.12).

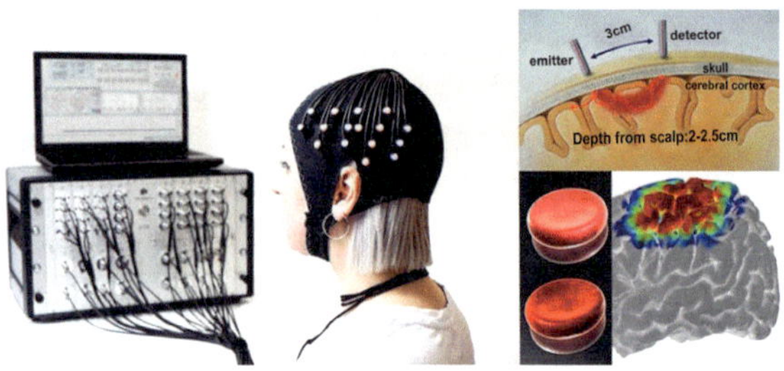

Figure 15.12. Functional near infrared spectroscopy.

Source: https://external-content.duckduckgo.com/iu/?u=https%3A%2F%2Fwww.cookchildrens.org%2Fsiteassets%2Fimages%2Fspecialties%2Fneurology%2Fneuro-research%2Ffnirs-figure-1---left.jpg&f=1&nofb=1&ipt=c77c87b239fcda0b576d40b1e899be39e4870000d579836220af3473b453278c.

This evolution signals the need to capitalize on multispectral neuroimaging data to build long-lasting, data-based models with the ability to differentiate healthy controls from ailing psychiatric patients. Leveraging the capabilities of various imaging modalities, clinicians and researchers are able to better understand the intrinsic neurobiological underpinnings of disorders, thus individualizing treatment programs more effectively for each patient. Having these technological advances meet the practice of psychiatry has several ramifications for the practice in the future. The ongoing development of cutting-edge neuroimaging technology, such as fNIRS and multimodal classifiers, heralds a revolution in mental health care that heralds the transition towards precision psychiatry. With the application of these groundbreaking approaches, clinicians can enhance their rate of diagnosis and make treatment plans for patients more optimal based on individualized neurobiological data. With continuous research asking further questions into new techniques and extension of the presently known methods, the future of neuroimaging in psychiatry promises even greater scope, perhaps resulting in the identification of new interventions and better outcomes. The integration of neuroscience with clinical practice promises not only improved treatment modalities but also emphasizes the need for further research into understanding mental health disorders in a more holistic approach (Charmaine et al., 2017; Guggenmos et al., 2020).

15.4.3. Comparison with ECT

The creation of Repetitive Transcranial Magnetic Stimulation (rTMS) is a fascinating alternative to Electroconvulsive Therapy (ECT) in the treatment of severe depression. While ECT has been used as a treatment gold standard for decades, it is often accompanied by substantial side effects, notably memory impairment, which acts as a deterrent for patients undertaking this option. In contrast, rTMS has become an intriguing treatment with a favorable safety profile, having the potential to deliver therapeutic effects without significant cognitive liabilities. Researchers are now eager to compare rTMS and ECT to see if rTMS can replace ECT in clinical practice safely. This study has important issues of whether rTMS can produce similar or superior outcomes with fewer side effects, and it will affect the treatment decision in psychiatrists and also patients (Micallef-Trigona, 2014). Moreover, the instantaneous effect of ECT in alleviating depressive symptoms also varies with the longer duration needed for rTMS to have significant effects. Despite the shorter duration of treatment using ECT, the challenge is identifying predictive biomarkers for individualized patient responses to the treatment. Studies , such as those applying connectome-based predictive modeling (CPM) in ECT-treated patients will attempt to establish correlations between pre-treatment patterns of functional brain connectivity and outcomes following the treatment. Such findings have shown that particular networks in the brain in the prefrontal cortex and subcortical areas may be potentially utilized as significant predictors of the efficacy of ECT. Identifying these biomarkers could make personalized treatment methods for ECT more effective, potentially making it a more targeted method without compromising on its established rapid benefits (Sun et al., 2020). When comparing rTMS with ECT, it should be considered not just their efficacy but also the tangible patient experience and preference. While some might appreciate the non-invasive nature of rTMS and a lower rate of side effects, others with extremely severe and treatment-resistant depression might prefer ECT due to its proven immediate effect. However, the currently dominant empirical studies emphasize the necessity of close comparative examination, and in particular randomized clinical trials, to clarify the advantages and disadvantages of both modalities. Through systematic comparison of parameters , such as remission duration, treatment response rates, and quality of life outcomes, clinicians can navigate these protocols more effectively. Overall, sustained investigation of the efficacy and safety of rTMS versus ECT not only aims to define the best therapeutic alternatives but also contributes to broader psychiatric treatment strategies (Micallef-Trigona, 2014).

Test Your Knowledge

1. How does TMS work to modulate brain activity, and what disorders is it commonly used to treat?
2. What advantages and limitations does TMS have compared to other neurostimulation therapies like ECT?

15.5. Lifestyle and Holistic Approaches

Learning Outcome

1. Importance of nutrition and exercise.
2. Mindfulness and stress reduction techniques.
3. Role of support systems.

The increased popularity of lifestyle and holistic approaches among psychiatrists indicates a radical shift in the perception and management of mental illness. Traditional psychiatric modalities specialize in pharmacological interventions, yet awareness is increasing on the importance of lifestyle components to overall mental health. Elements of diet, exercise, sleep patterns, and stress management are increasingly prominent as core treatment components. This integrated approach recognizes that mental and physical health cannot be separated and validates the value of addressing the person as a whole through a whole-person approach. With consideration for the interrelated nature of body, mind, and external influences, practitioners are able to advance more long-lasting health outcomes, ultimately enhancing patients' overall well-being in the face of mental health complications. Holistic models, such as Ayurveda, are templates for making lifestyle changes part of psychiatric therapy. Drawing from ancient practices, Ayurveda is focused on keeping the body's unique types of energies, or doshas, in a state of equilibrium so that optimal health is maintained. Ayurveda emphasizes treating each person according to their constitution, so it is suited for more tailored and effective interventions. Noted, as is initial genomic research suggesting doshic constitutional associations with particular genetic profiles, and a suggestion of insight at a deeper level of how individualized care can increase mental health treatment effectiveness. Moreover, as practices like Ayurveda are increasingly being researched in Western settings, their emphasis on prevention and health can potentially redescribe classical psychiatric practice, inducing a broader vision from which to view mental illness and health (Rhoda, 2014). Technological advances also intersect with lifestyle and holistic practices in fresh ways. The advent of brain-computer interfaces (BCIs) is an exemplary illustration of how modern neuroscience can shape treatment approaches that are in alignment with holistic ideals. These neurotechnologies are particularly relevant for patients who have extensive communication and mobility impairment, as they provide enhanced interaction with the environment. BCIs offer solutions that aim not only to improve the quality of life but also remain consistent with overarching holistic principles by considering several factors , including behavioral patterns, environmental contexts, and capabilities. By the integration of technology and holistic methods, there is potential for the development of dynamic and adaptive treatment modalities that capture the multi-dimensional nature of human experience, and hence contribute towards a broader knowledge of mental health (Kerick et al., 2012).

15.5.1. Importance of Exercise and Nutrition

Over the past few years, there has been extensive recognition of the worth of nutrition and exercise as adjunctive treatments in psychiatry. A proper diet can do a lot to improve mental health, and it is responsible for influencing mood stability and symptom improvement in many psychiatric conditions. For instance, studies have shown that specific dietary patterns, with lots of fruit, vegetables, whole grains, and healthy fats, correlate with less depression and anxiety. The inclusion of formal exercise provides an additional advantage since exercise has been demonstrated to release endorphins and create a sense of well-being. It encourages not just physical but also mental well-being and thus these lifestyle modifications are part of overall psychiatric treatment. Therefore, nutrition and exercise serve not just as prevention but as adjunct therapy that enhances the effectiveness of more conventional treatment modalities. Furthermore, evidence indicates that lifestyle intervention in the areas of diet and exercise can significantly improve the quality of life of severe mental illness patients. As an example, a large lifestyle intervention trial among survivors of breast cancer reported improvement in psychological health with weight management through dietary change and regular physical activity (Campbell et al., 2006) (Figure 15.13).

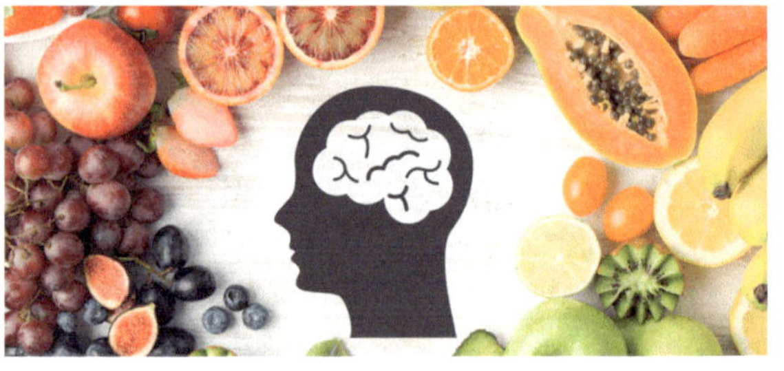

Figure 15.13. The role of nutrition and exercise in psychiatric disorders.

Source: https://external-content.duckduckgo.com/iu/?u=https%3A%2F%2Fcareme.health%2F_next%2Fimage%3Furl%3Dhttps%3A%252F%252Fvideo.curegrid.co%252Fdj%252Fmedia%252Fpost_banners%252FScreenshot_2024-10-11_at_9.47.40AM.png%26w%3D3840%26q%3D75&f=1&nofb=1&ipt=64a790d8b9660757d31d8261260b77242cae22ad25536a779980e8d5626862c4.

This implies that the same methods can prove useful for mental health patients, further attesting to the fact that physical and mental health are interconnected. Such treatments can prove beneficial in treating not only psychological symptoms of disorders but also physical health issues that accompany them, thus creating better treatment results. Establishment of a routine with regular diet and exercise can enhance compliance and treatment outcome and pave the way to long-term recovery in psychiatric patients. Exercise counseling as part of psychiatric practice is also necessary for the optimal outcome of depressive disorders. A current study demonstrated the manner in which comprehensive training in education for healthcare workers led to a significant rise in exercise counseling for depressed patients, representing an immense loophole within the conventional treatment approach (Pace & Roscoe, 2023). Through the emphasis on the therapeutic ability of physical exercise as an easily accessible intervention tactic, healthcare workers can act as facilitators for patients to get actively involved in their therapy. This not only reduces shame around seeking assistance but also instills a sense of agency and autonomy regarding one's own health. Lastly, the incorporation of exercise and nutrition into psychiatric care not only addresses physical as well as mental illness but also represents a paradigm shift to a more coordinated, patient-focused system of mental healthcare.

15.5.2. Mindfulness and Stress-Reduction Techniques

Mindfulness has become a hot tool in psychiatric treatment modalities over recent years. This intervention is founded in Buddhist practices, where mindfulness is defined as developing awareness of the present moment and further maintaining control over thoughts and emotions. This activity provides the individual with the possibility of stepping back from their mental struggle and creating an enhanced level of control over their internal experiences. The spike in scientific research over the past decade attests to the efficacy of mindfulness interventions for curing many mental health disorders, including depression and anxiety. Notably, the focus on empirical evidence has revealed that even though the promise of mindfulness interventions has been extremely high, there is a significant imperative for continued research to validate long-term findings and potential negative effects obtained from these interventions, as reflected in the new literature on mindfulness across mental health contexts (Griffiths et al., 2015). Mindfulness-based stress reduction techniques have also been identified as being most effective in eliminating the symptoms of anxiety disorders. A systematic review of various psychological interventions indicated that embodiment practices, which generally overlap with mindfulness strategies, consistently yield moderate to large state anxiety reductions (Beck et al., 2024) (Figure 15.14).

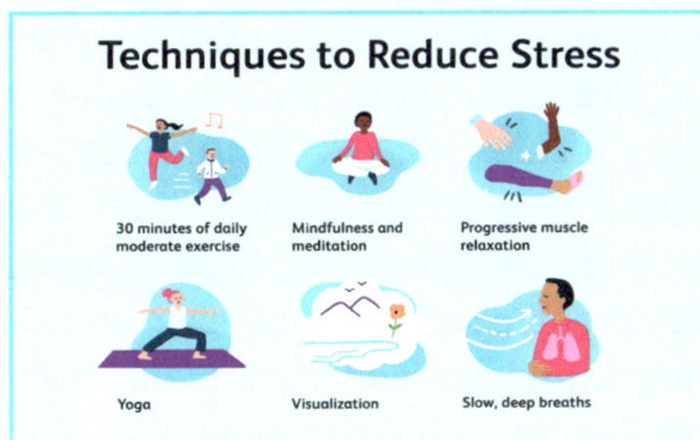
Techniques to Reduce Stress
30 minutes of daily moderate exercise
Mindfulness and meditation
Progressive muscle relaxation
Yoga
Visualization
Slow, deep breaths

Figure 15.14. Techniques to reduce stress.

Source: https://www.verywellhealth.com/thmb/_zdHPRT3b9Y92Yim-OdtH7ly_dU=/1500x0/filters:no_upscale():max_bytes(150000):strip_icc()/how-to-reduce-stress-5207327_FINAL-907db114a640431ba1e8ecbb9e81b77f.jpg.

These techniques, grounded in heightened body awareness and breathing regulation, meet the underlying disconnection that can occur between intellectual assessment and somatic responses to stress. Because stress is often experienced somatically, consistent practice in mindfulness allows people to better align their reactions, establishing a healthier connection with stressors. This exchange involves the importance of a sense of how the body is responding to emotional states and serves to further reinforce the integrated connection between mind and body in stress management intervention. In addition, including mindfulness as an intervention strategy serves to incorporate mainstream traditions of psychotherapy and to cultivate an integrated system for therapeutic intervention. The combined application of mindfulness, cognitive strategies, and breathing exercises permits a balanced approach that confronts both cognitive distortion and emotional dysregulation. This multidimensional strategy encourages the integration of mindfulness skills within daily existence and establishes a foundation for sustained mental health enhancement. Nevertheless, care must be exercised to remain responsive to the varied effectiveness of individual breathing practices and individual responsiveness among these exercises. This places mindfulness-based therapies alongside the changing nature of the treatment of mental health, hence broadening the treatment experience of each patient by ensuring individualized care plans that take into consideration the personal experiences of different patients (Beck et al., 2024).

15.5.3. Role of Support Systems

Support systems play an important role as part of the treatment interventions implemented in psychiatry and significantly impact the outcome of patients and their recovery paths. Family, friends, peer support groups, and mental health workers all contribute to environments that encourage healing and development. A strong support system can potentially reinforce a patient's participation and compliance with treatment interventions, whether they be pharmacological or psychotherapeutic. Studies indicate that individuals who feel supported are more likely to cope with the adversity associated with mental illness and ultimately offer better compliance with treatment and overall mental health outcomes. Within this context, support systems work as vehicles of change; they engage communication, encourage participation, and provoke callings, all of which are critical with regard to managing psychiatric illnesses. Recovery stories in therapy are the best way to show how the support system can be integrated into the protocol of the treatment. It has been investigated by many modalities, text, audio, and video, that recovery stories can create a sense of shared experience, thus reaffirming the concept of community and mutual comprehension among people going through similar experiences. These narratives tend to make the patients reflect on their experiences, then comfort them in acknowledging the struggles. The identification with narrators makes the sense of belonging and empathy crucial for recovery. The processes by which the patients identify with these stories could result in life-changing effects, like increased sensitivity and desire to seek recovery, as discussed in the studies of recovery stories' influence (Ng et al., 2019). Newer forms of therapy have also been included within support networks, such as sensory modulation. It draws on the best use of potential through sensory processing in order to reduce suffering among patients. Research works indicate that sensory integration methods present real-world alternatives to traditional treatments, such as in the stressful environments of psychiatric programs, and it reduces the likelihood of coercive strategies like seclusion and restraint (Hoque, 2016). Staff training in sensory modulation practices allows mental health centers to build better support networks for patients, encouraging environments where people feel empowered and supported. This would not only strengthen the therapeutic relationship between the staff and patients but also contribute toward a community-based model of mental health care, which places high emphasis on collective support, fueling the improvement in patient care and outcomes.

Test Your Knowledge

1. How do factors such as nutrition, exercise, sleep, and stress management contribute to mental health improvement?
2. What roles do mindfulness, yoga, meditation, and complementary therapies play in holistic mental health care?

15.6. Emerging Treatment Modalities

Learning Outcome

1. Use of psychedelics in therapy.
2. Advances in neurotechnology.
3. Future directions in psychiatric treatment.

New psychosocial modalities in psychiatry are a reflection of the vibrant developments in mental health interventions, driven by scientific breakthroughs and changing needs of society. Among the notable trends is the integration of technology in treatment practice. Teletherapy, for instance, has become increasingly widespread, allowing patients to receive mental health treatment from the comfort and safety of their own homes. This modality not only expands access to care but also bypasses barriers , such as transportation issues and in-person visit stigma. Also, mental health treatments on the internet are becoming more sophisticated, enabling users to track symptoms and apply evidence-based approaches to self-management. These therapies are evidence of a shift from traditional, in-person forms of therapy to more adaptive, accessible therapies that can be provided to diverse populations and their related needs, optimizing the overall breadth and reach of psychiatric therapy in today's world. Another increasingly prominent area of emerging treatment modalities involves the use of psychobiotics and neurostimulation therapies. Psychobiotics, which are supposed to enhance mental health using live bacteria, are on the list as potential candidates for influencing the gut-brain axis in order to regulate mood and behavior. Research indicates that these microbial treatments have promise as an adjunctive psychiatric treatment by minimizing symptoms of depression and anxiety. Concurrently, neurostimulation techniques , such as transcranial magnetic stimulation (TMS) and electroconvulsive therapy (ECT) are evolving, increasingly being applied to treatment-resistant depression. These modalities are increasingly popular, spurred by continuing advances in efficacy and safety, and have the potential to revolutionize treatment paradigms in psychiatric care. Thus, these novel modalities not only provide an extension of therapy options but also pose a challenge to further research into interdisciplinarity, potentially enhancing patient care outcomes. In addition, awareness of the socio-emotional impact of events like harassment on mental health mandates interventions directed at at-risk groups. Harassment's trend, particularly against figures who are public in nature like politicians, offers a timely intersection of mental health care and public safety. Recent studies have shown that harassers are likely to exhibit evidence of untreated mental illness, thereby leaving room for proactive mental health intervention. Mental health professionals can not only assist the victim but also prevent the occurrence of risks of un-treated mental illness in harassers by designing targeted programs related to the psychological dynamics of harassment. Such a dual-focus model prioritizes the need for innovation in treatment approaches, including understanding mental health's socio-political context and actively fostering public education and supports, hence building community resilience and mental health literacy in society.

15.6.1. Therapeutic Use of Psychedelics

As the stigma regarding psychedelic drugs dissolves gradually, their therapeutic potential in psychiatry is gaining a lot of interest. It has been observed that psychedelics like psilocybin and MDMA have good reports for treating numerous mental illnesses like depression, anxiety, and post-traumatic stress disorder (PTSD). This new interest, also referred to as the psychedelic renaissance, is a testament to a fundamental change in perceiving these drugs as anything more than recreational use; they are being recognized for their ability to facilitate profound psychological healing. Even with this possibility, the clinical promise of these psychedelics is stunted by legal barriers. Several countries, including the United States, are gradually researching protocols that could potentially offer increased access to psychedelic therapy, with a foreseen change in policies that will significantly alter modalities of treatment for mental health (Kusumaningrum et al., 2024). Optimism regarding psychedelic therapy must be tempered, however, with caution in considering findings. Although previous studies have advocated for the effectiveness of psychedelics in treatment, scientists advise that the results may not be as definite as suggested. The presentation context within the media may also be a contributory element towards overestimating the risks and benefits of such drugs, creating inflated public expectations. The preliminary nature of current findings warrants taking the empirical research on psychedelics very seriously. Over time, there has been a trend wherein the effect sizes of certain therapies, like cognitive behavioral therapy and other conventional therapies, have decreased. This trend raises concerns about whether psychedelics are losing their potency with an increase in studies being conducted (Meling et al., 2024). Lastly, integration of psychedelics in therapeutics requires an open discussion of their potential and limitations. In a backdrop drawn in sensationalized reports and occasionally, misleading data, it is imperative that stakeholders like policymakers, practitioners, and patients have their information grounded in sound research. Good communication is imperative in setting realistic expectations and making informed policies on psychedelic interventions. Examination of legal models, in addition to an evidence-based approach to assessing risk and benefit, can foster a culture in which therapeutic psychedelics use is a viable option for the treatment of severe psychiatric disease (Kusumaningrum et al., 2024; Meling et al., 2024).

15.6.2. Advances in Neurotechnology

Application of neurotechnology for psychiatric treatment methodologies has been a significant landmark in addressing and treating mental illness disorders. Advances in neuroimaging technologies have enabled a better understanding of brain-behavior correlations, particularly where disorders , such as depression and schizophrenia are concerned. Efforts , such as the Enhancing Neuroimaging Genetics through Meta-Analysis (ENIGMA) Stroke Recovery working group represent this trajectory, as they bring massive data sets from diverse populations together with rigorous methodologies to analyze brain function and structure. ENIGMA's capacity to draw on the data of over 2,100 stroke patients across a number of studies is a testament to the capacity of large-scale collaborations to uncover patterns and correlations masked by local small-scale studies in the past. This approach not only facilitates our comprehension of neurobiological underpinnings but also directs the development of more focused and efficient treatment regimens in psychiatry (Assogna et al., 2020). In addition, the area of neuromodulation has seen groundbreaking developments that have the possibility of treating a vast array of psychiatric illnesses. DBS is one important example, providing a strong alternative for refractory patients. Recent discussion among experts at the DBS Think Tank annual meeting marks the necessity for challenging the boundaries of neurophysiological approaches and new stimulation modalities. These advances affirm the promise of adaptive DBS systems, capable of responding in real time to neural activity, and pave the way toward individually customized treatment regimens. Greater emphasis on brain network mapping through connectomics provides increasing significance to a shift towards network-centered interventions, suggesting psychiatric disorders are tractable at a systems level as opposed to specific brain regions. Such advances promise more efficient and advanced therapeutic interventions for patients suffering from complex mental health complexities (Ramirez-Zamora et al., 2019) (Figure 15.15).

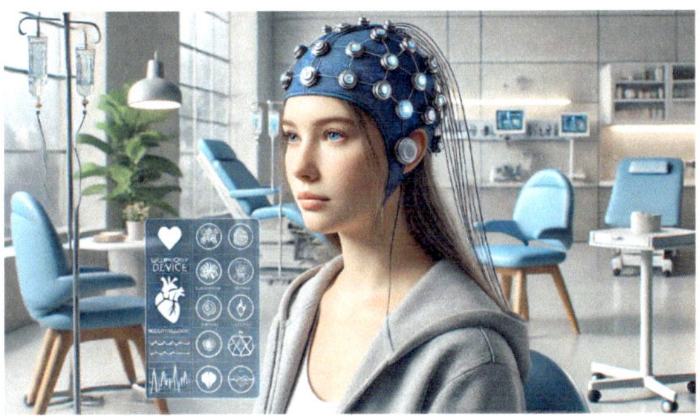

Figure 15.15. Neurotechnology in psychiatric treatment.

Source: https://external-content.duckduckgo.com/iu/?u=https%3A%2F%2Fmiro.medium.com%2Fv2%2Fresize%3Afit%3A1358%2F1*ehRkTjK6bqPrK9qI0zW_JA.jpeg&f=1&nofb=1&ipt=8226c395524576631a43fa89779a6cb004033090b9a14ac01039d278d9b26548.

As neurotechnology advances and expands, ethics need to be incorporated in the development of therapeutic modalities in psychiatry. The use of technologies , such as DBS and its adaptive forms raises serious ethical questions, primarily concerning patient autonomy, informed consent, and implications of changing neural circuits. Furthermore, the integration of neuroimaging in clinical practice needs the creation of formal ethics guidelines to maintain patient confidentiality and address concerns regarding neuroenhancement. Resolving these ethical issues is most important to ensure that advances in neurotechnology are not only available but also distributive, avoiding disparities in mental health care. Thus, as innovations in neurotechnology promise to revolutionize psychiatric therapies, an equitable discussion of their effects on society should accompany their evolution, ultimately fostering a comprehensive approach to psychiatric care that is both effective and morally responsible.

15.6.3. Future Directions in Psychiatric Treatment

The field of psychiatric treatment is forever evolving because of the developments in research and improved understanding of mental illnesses. One such promising field of work is the integration of couples therapy into the treatment of disorders like posttraumatic stress disorder (PTSD). Research in recent years has indicated that interpersonal issues have a central role to play in the treatment of veterans with PTSD, making it essential to involve partners in the treatment. Cognitive-behavioral conjoint therapy for posttraumatic stress disorder (CBCT) is one of the structured interventions applied to enhance relationship function alongside the treatment of PTSD. Surprisingly, research suggests that briefer versions of CBCT, when combined with innovative models of delivery , such as clinical video teleconferencing (CVT), may promote greater ease and efficacy of treatment, suggesting a possible trend toward increased flexibility and patient responsiveness to treatment within psychiatric contexts (Morland et al., 2019). Future directions of the treatment of schizophrenia also require attention, in particular with respect to treating negative symptoms, which have historically been under-treated in psychiatry. While current psychosocial treatments tend to prioritize relief of positive symptoms, there is an unmet priority need for suitable approaches to the management of negative symptoms due to their association with reduced quality of life. There is new evidence to suggest that cognitive behavior therapy (CBT) and social skills training (SST) may offer significant benefits to patients with negative symptoms. Researchers recommend a change in current treatment strategies and stress that combined treatment modalities comprising positive and negative symptom treatment should be developed in parallel. Such methods would facilitate inclusive patient treatment and promote improved long-term results, stretching the psychiatric community to broaden its treatment model (Caponigro et al., 2013). Also, integration of technology into psychiatric treatment represents an essential frontier that holds much promise for the future. Telehealth options like CVT not only expand access but also help individuals who may have difficulty with in-person face-to-face treatment. This method has become popular, particularly among veterans, who have expressed a preference for virtual sessions. With the growth of the field, ongoing research remains crucial in determining the effectiveness of these emerging delivery channels. With the exploitation of technology, mental health providers can provide an increasingly flexible method, increasing patient satisfaction and treatment adherence. The integration of innovative technology solutions with established treatment protocols can ultimately redefine the boundaries of psychiatric care, resulting in a more embracing and receptive health atmosphere (Caponigro et al., 2013; Morland et al., 2019).

Test Your Knowledge

1. How are innovations such as digital therapeutics, VR therapy, and AI-based mental health tools shaping future treatment approaches?
2. What new developments in neurostimulation, psychedelic-assisted therapy, and precision psychiatry are currently being explored?

SUMMARY

The psychiatric treatment modalities horizon is wide and constantly opening up. Different therapies , such as medication, psychotherapy, and other novel treatment methodologies , such as Electroconvulsive Therapy (ECT) and repetitive Transcranial Magnetic Stimulation (rTMS), have significantly entered into the treatment of mental illness disorders. The established efficacy of ECT in the treatment of severe depression is weighed against its side effect possibility, most importantly memory impairment. Conversely, rTMS offers a promising option with fewer reported side effects and mounting support for its effectiveness, ranking high among the search for optimal treatment modalities for psychiatry. Thus, weighing the pros and cons of both modalities in determining the optimum treatment approach for each patient is the need for individualized treatment plans for psychiatric practice (Micallef-Trigona, 2014). In addition, integrating sensory processing methods into psychiatric therapy is a progressive step away from traditional methods. Research has demonstrated sensory-modulated approaches as potentially effective in alleviating anxiety and distress symptoms, providing productive alternatives to coercive practices , such as seclusion and restraint. These promising findings reflect the importance of adopting broad, multi-component approaches addressing the sensory issues of patients. Through training mental health staff on these modalities, as has been documented by recent programs, medical personnel can considerably enhance their ability to design therapeutic environments. The favorable response of sensory integration interventions by caregivers and learners signifies a shift towards more empathetic and effective treatment modalities, an essential step in psychiatric treatment (Hoque, 2016). The last conclusion drawn from previous research and clinical practices in psychiatric treatment emphasizes the necessity for more innovation in treatment modalities. The comparison between old interventions like ECT and novel options like rTMS and sensory processing methods highlights the dynamic nature of mental health treatment. Mental health professionals need to keep pace with ongoing research and training to render their practice progressively refined. As understanding of various treatment modalities improves, the potential for improved patient outcomes will improve, leading to a move towards new paradigms of mental health treatment. Future directions should not only be towards innovation but also towards evidence-based assessments that call new therapies to account for efficacy and ensure that psychiatric treatment remains patient-centered as well as efficient in the face of the fast-changing context (Micallef-Trigona, 2014; Hoque, 2016).

Understanding the effectiveness of various treatment modalities in psychiatry entails a critical review of traditional and emergent methods. One such prevailing topic that emerges with the reading of the literature is the increased application of technology in mental illness management. Patients with bipolar disorder, for instance, have reported significant benefits provided by self-monitoring practices facilitated by the use of electronic avenues. These technologies enable individuals to track moods and activities, leading to self-reflection and better communication with health care providers. The findings suggest that engaged technology use can be an empowered approach to self-management, yet problems related to usability and interpretation remain fairly prevalent. This highlights the pressing need to user-design technologies that are responsive to the particular needs of users who work with psychiatric diseases, as noted in a study examining the conduct of people with bipolar disorder (Chang et al., 2016). Apart from technology, sensory processing approaches are being understood as excellent therapy interventions in psychiatric rehabilitation. Sensory processing abnormalities can have numerous negative consequences, including depression and anxiety. Dr. Ayres' Theory of Sensory Integration illustrates the efficacy of sensory modulation techniques in enhancing patients' emotional balance and feeling of well-being. Research indicates that these interventions can abate distress and agitation in patients with a variety of psychiatric diagnoses, including anxiety and post-traumatic stress disorder. When sensory modulated treatments are added to treatment protocols, mental health professionals can provide viable alternatives to more coercive interventions , such as seclusion and restraint. These modalities empower staff and patients equally to build supportive therapeutic relationships, showing the more holistic face of psychiatric treatment beyond conventional medications (Hoque, 2016). The terminology of treatment modalities in psychiatry also speaks to the necessity of ongoing staff training and education. Initiatives for heightening awareness regarding sensory integration techniques among psychiatric staff have also produced promising results. Educational interventions can significantly improve staff competency in utilizing sensory resources in an effective manner. Positive feedback from training exercises indicates that sensory approaches are beneficial to clinical practice for both experienced therapists and students. Thus, staff knowledge affects both the therapeutic environment and patients' outcomes. There exists an important need for continuous research to evaluate the real impact of these education programs in practice, so that fresh, evidence-based solutions are implemented effectively in psychiatric treatment facilities. This step enhances the general quality of care, showing commitment to empowering patients and improving staff in mental health treatment.

KEY TERMS FROM THIS CHAPTER

- Antidepressants
- Antipsychotics
- Anxiolytics
- Behavioral activation
- Cognitive Behavioral Therapy (CBT)
- Deep Brain Stimulation (DBS)
- Dialectical Behavior Therapy (DBT)
- Electroconvulsive therapy (ECT)
- Exposure therapy
- Family therapy
- Group therapy
- Mindfulness-based therapy
- Mood stabilizers
- Motivational interviewing
- Pharmacotherapy
- Psychodynamic therapy
- Psychoeducation
- Psychotherapy
- Supportive therapy
- Transcranial Magnetic Stimulation (TMS)

CRITICAL THINKING QUESTIONS

1. **Which of the following is considered a first-line treatment for major depressive disorder?**
   a. Electroconvulsive therapy (ECT)
   b. Psychodynamic therapy
   c. Selective serotonin reuptake inhibitors (SSRIs)
   d. Antipsychotic medications
2. **Cognitive Behavioral Therapy (CBT) is especially effective for:**
   a. Schizophrenia
   b. Bipolar disorder
   c. Obsessive-compulsive and anxiety disorders
   d. Dementia
3. **Electroconvulsive Therapy (ECT) is primarily used when:**
   a. Patients refuse to take any medication
   b. Depression is mild and short-term
   c. Rapid improvement is needed in severe depression or treatment-resistant cases
   d. For treating insomnia
4. **Which class of drugs is most commonly used for acute anxiety relief?**
   a. Antipsychotics
   b. Beta-blockers
   c. Benzodiazepines
   d. Mood stabilizers
5. **Psychoeducation is an important treatment component that:**
   a. Focuses on providing information and coping strategies to patients and families
   b. Involves only group therapy
   c. Uses hypnosis for trauma recovery
   d. Encourages complete medication avoidance

Short Answer Questions

1. What is the difference between pharmacotherapy and psychotherapy in psychiatric treatment?
2. Name two commonly used classes of medications in psychiatry and an example of each.
3. What is Cognitive Behavioral Therapy (CBT), and for which disorders is it most effective?
4. How does Electroconvulsive Therapy (ECT) work, and when is it typically used?
5. What are the main side effects of antipsychotic medications? Name at least two.

Answer to Critical Thinking Questions

1. (c); 2. (c); 3. (c); 4. (c); 5. (a)

REFERENCES

1. Sun, H., Jiang, R., Qi, S., Narr, K. L., Wade, B. S., Upston, J., Espinoza, R., Jones, T., Calhoun, V. D., Abbott, C. C., & Sui, J. (2020). Preliminary prediction of individual response to electroconvulsive therapy using whole-brain functional magnetic resonance imaging data. *NeuroImage. Clinical*, *26*, 102080. https://doi.org/10.1016/j.nicl.2019.102080 (accessed on 28th July 2025).
2. Abedinzadeh, M., Mozafari, S., & Noorian, K. (2013). Effect of lidocaine on duration of seizure and hemodynamic alterations in electroconvulsive therapy. 5 / Journal of Gorgan University of Medical Sciences Spring 2013 / vol 15 / no 1. https://core.ac.uk/download/143845654.pdf (accessed on 28th July 2025).
3. Adinoff, B., Fiore, V. G., Gu, X., et al. (2018). A multilevel computational characterization of endophenotypes in addiction. https://core.ac.uk/download/160809873.pdf (accessed on 28th July 2025).
4. Ahmed, F., Khalil, M., Yoga, B., et al. (2014). Neurostimulation for refractory primary chronic headache disorders: A review. https://core.ac.uk/download/47263646.pdf (accessed on 28th July 2025).
5. Meling D, Ehrenkranz R, Nayak SM, Aicher HD, Funk X, van Elk M, Graziosi M, Bauer PR, Scheidegger M, Yaden DB. Mind the Psychedelic Hype: Characterizing the Risks and Benefits of Psychedelics for Depression. *Psychoactives*. 2024; 3(2):215-234. https://doi.org/10.3390/psychoactives3020014(accessed on 28th July 2025).
6. Albert, U., Arumugham, S. S., Bailey, B. E., et al. (2019). Treatments used for obsessive-compulsive disorder—An international perspective. https://core.ac.uk/download/287581917.pdf (accessed on 28th July 2025).
7. Verdejo-Garcia, A., Lorenzetti, V., Manning, V., Piercy, H., Bruno, R., Hester, R., Pennington, D., Tolomeo, S., Arunogiri, S., Bates, M. E., Bowden-Jones, H., Campanella, S., Daughters, S. B., Kouimtsidis, C., Lubman, D. I., Meyerhoff, D. J., Ralph, A., Rezapour, T., Tavakoli, H., Zare-Bidoky, M., ... Ekhtiari, H. (2019). A Roadmap for Integrating Neuroscience Into Addiction Treatment: A Consensus of the Neuroscience Interest Group of the International Society of Addiction Medicine. *Frontiers in psychiatry*, *10*, 877. https://doi.org/10.3389/fpsyt.2019.00877(accessed on 28th July 2025).
8. Assogna, F., Baugh, L. A., Bhattacharya, A. K., et al. (2020). The ENIGMA Stroke Recovery Working Group: Big data neuroimaging to study brain–behavior relationships after stroke. https://core.ac.uk/download/322929945.pdf (accessed on 28th July 2025).
9. Avdibegović, E., Brkić, M., & Hasanović, M. (2021). Integrating the concept of creative psychopharmacotherapy and group psychotherapy in clinical practice. https://core.ac.uk/download/512507772.pdf (accessed on 28th July 2025).
10. Costa, M. B., & Melnik, T. (2016). Effectiveness of psychosocial interventions in eating disorders: an overview of Cochrane systematic reviews. *Einstein (Sao Paulo, Brazil)*, *14*(2), 235–277. https://doi.org/10.1590/S1679-45082016RW3120(accessed on 28th July 2025).
11. Barry-Walsh, J., Pathé, M., & Every-Palmer, S. (2015). Harassment, stalking, threats and attacks targeting New Zealand politicians: A mental health issue. https://core.ac.uk/download/pdf/30672120.pdf (accessed on 28th July 2025).

12. Bauer, C. C., Himle, M. B., Ran, D., et al. (2016). Pilot open case series of Voice over Internet Protocol-delivered assessment and behavior therapy for chronic tic disorders. https://core.ac.uk/download/213085582.pdf (accessed on 28th July 2025).

13. Beck, F., Chin, P., Gorman, F., et al. (2024). A systematic review of brief respiratory, embodiment, cognitive, and mindfulness interventions to reduce state anxiety. https://core.ac.uk/download/636776767.pdf (accessed on 28th July 2025).

14. Morland, L. A., Macdonald, A., Grubbs, K. M., Mackintosh, M. A., Monson, C. M., Glassman, L. H., Becker, J., Sautter, F., Buzzella, B., Wrape, E., Wells, S. Y., Rooney, B. M., & Glynn, S. (2019). Design of a randomized superiority trial of a brief couple treatment for PTSD. *Contemporary clinical trials communications*, *15*, 100369. https://doi.org/10.1016/j.conctc.2019.100369(accessed on 28th July 2025).

15. Bir, A., Berndt, E. R., Frank, R. G., Normand, S. L. T., & Busch, S. H. (2025). The medical treatment of depression, 1991–1996: Productive inefficiency, expected outcome variations, and price indexes. https://core.ac.uk/download/pdf/6863980.pdf (accessed on 28th July 2025).

16. Borrione, L., Brunoni, A. R., Passos, I. C., et al. (2020). Precision non-implantable neuromodulation therapies: A perspective for the depressed brain. https://core.ac.uk/download/479501287.pdf (accessed on 28th July 2025).

17. Campbell, A., McTiernan, A., McTiernan, A., Silvestri, A., Visser, A., Kornblith, A. B., Utter, A. C., et al. (2006). Study protocol to investigate the effect of a lifestyle intervention on body weight, psychological health status and risk factors associated with disease recurrence in women recovering from breast cancer treatment. https://core.ac.uk/download/57819.pdf (accessed on 28th July 2025).

18. Caponigro, J. M., Elis, O., & Kring, A. M. (2013). Psychosocial treatments for negative symptoms in schizophrenia: Current practices and future directions. https://core.ac.uk/download/323311087.pdf (accessed on 28th July 2025).

19. Carbajal, J. (2018). Trauma focused interventions: A clinical practice analysis. The Practitioner Scholar: Journal of Counseling and Professional Psychology, 7, 19-33.(accessed on 28th July 2025).

20. Carcione, A., Riccardi, I., Bilotta, E., Leone, L., Pedone, R., Conti, L., Colle, L., Fiore, D., Nicolò, G., Pellecchia, G., Procacci, M., & Semerari, A. (2019). Metacognition as a Predictor of Improvements in Personality Disorders. *Frontiers in psychology*, *10*, 170. https://doi.org/10.3389/fpsyg.2019.00170 (accessed on 28th July 2025).

21. Carli, D., Parolin, &, Santona, D., et al. (2016). Implicit attitude toward caregiving: The moderating role of adult attachment styles. https://core.ac.uk/download/168404853.pdf (accessed on 28th July 2025).

22. Marzilli, E., Cerniglia, L., & Cimino, S. (2018). A narrative review of binge eating disorder in adolescence: prevalence, impact, and psychological treatment strategies. *Adolescent health, medicine and therapeutics*, *9*, 17–30. https://doi.org/10.2147/AHMT.S148050(accessed on 28th July 2025).

23. Certa, K., Huege, S., Kenning, T., et al. (2012). Electroconvulsive therapy: A review of its current status. https://core.ac.uk/download/46968142.pdf (accessed on 28th July 2025).

24. Chang, P., Cosley, D., Frank, E., et al. (2016). Self-monitoring practices, attitudes, and needs of individuals with bipolar disorder: Implications for the design of technologies to manage

mental health. https://core.ac.uk/download/213087764.pdf (accessed on 28th July 2025).

25. Chiesa, M., Sharp, R., & Fonagy, P. (2011). Clinical associations of deliberate self-injury and its impact on the outcome of community-based and long-term inpatient treatment for personality disorder. *Psychotherapy and psychosomatics*, *80*(2), 100–109. https://doi.org/10.1159/000320975(accessed on 28th July 2025).

26. Elliott, R., & Zucconi, A. (2006). Doing research on the effectiveness of psychotherapy and psychotherapy training: A person-centered/experiential perspective. https://core.ac.uk/download/9029991.pdf (accessed on 28th July 2025).

27. O'Neill, J., & Feusner, J. D. (2015). Cognitive-behavioral therapy for obsessive-compulsive disorder: access to treatment, prediction of long-term outcome with neuroimaging. *Psychology research and behavior management*, *8*, 211–223. https://doi.org/10.2147/PRBM.S75106(accessed on 28th July 2025).

28. Guggenmos, M., Schmack, K., Veer, I.M. *et al.* A multimodal neuroimaging classifier for alcohol dependence. *Sci Rep* **10**, 298 (2020). https://doi.org/10.1038/s41598-019-56923-9(accessed on 28th July 2025).

29. Gazdag, G., Marić, N. P., Samardzic, R., Milovanović, S., Spiric, Z., & Stojanovic, Z. (2014). Electroconvulsive therapy practice in Serbia today. https://core.ac.uk/download/81388296.pdf (accessed on 28th July 2025).

30. Ramirez-Zamora, A., Giordano, J., Boyden, E. S., Gradinaru, V., Gunduz, A., Starr, P. A., Sheth, S. A., McIntyre, C. C., Fox, M. D., Vitek, J., Vedam-Mai, V., Akbar, U., Almeida, L., Bronte-Stewart, H. M., Mayberg, H. S., Pouratian, N., Gittis, A. H., Singer, A. C., Creed, M. C., Lazaro-Munoz, G., ... Okun, M. S. (2019). Proceedings of the Sixth Deep Brain Stimulation Think Tank Modulation of Brain Networks and Application of Advanced Neuroimaging, Neurophysiology, and Optogenetics. *Frontiers in neuroscience*, *13*, 936. https://doi.org/10.3389/fnins.2019.00936(accessed on 28th July 2025).

31. Griffiths, M. D., Shonin, E., & Van Gordon, W. (2015). Mindfulness in mental health: A critical reflection. https://core.ac.uk/download/30649717.pdf (accessed on 28th July 2025).

32. Hoque, S. (2016). Care team education on the use of sensory resources in inpatient psychiatry. https://core.ac.uk/download/79664899.pdf (accessed on 28th July 2025).

33. Ng, F., Charles, A., Pollock, K., Rennick-Egglestone, S., Cuijpers, P., Gillard, S., van der Krieke, L., Bongaardt, R., Pomberth, S., Repper, J., Roe, J., Llewellyn-Beardsley, J., Yeo, C., Hui, A., Hare-Duke, L., Manley, D., & Slade, M. (2019). The mechanisms and processes of connection: developing a causal chain model capturing impacts of receiving recorded mental health recovery narratives. *BMC psychiatry*, *19*(1), 413. https://doi.org/10.1186/s12888-019-2405-z (accessed on 28th July 2025).

34. Kerick, S. E., Lance, B. J., McDowell, K., et al. (2012). Brain computer interface technologies in the coming decades. http://arxiv.org/abs/1211.0886 (accessed on 28th July 2025).

35. Kusumaningrum, A. E., & Sucinta, A. (2024). Exploring legal frameworks for the clinical use of psychedelic substances in mental health treatment. https://core.ac.uk/download/617930797.pdf (accessed on 28th July 2025).

36. Lim, C. R., Lai, C. Y. Y., Ho, C. S. H., & Ho, R. C. M. (2017). Functional near-infrared spectroscopy in psychiatry. https://www.cambridge.org/core/services/aop-cambridge-core/content/view/DEBC97B8F3B5424CB84F3718DF778C88/S2056467800002760a.pdf/div-class-title-

functional-near-infrared-spectroscopy-in-psychiatry-div.pdf (accessed on 28th July 2025).

37. Masiriri, T. (2008). The effects of managed care on social work mental health practice. https://core.ac.uk/download/10685663.pdf (accessed on 28th July 2025).

38. Micallef-Trigona B. (2014). Comparing the effects of repetitive transcranial magnetic stimulation and electroconvulsive therapy in the treatment of depression: a systematic review and meta-analysis. *Depression research and treatment, 2014*, 135049. https://doi.org/10.1155/2014/135049(accessed on 28th July 2025).

39. Noel, C. (2017). Evidence for the use of "medical marijuana" in psychiatric and neurologic disorders. https://core.ac.uk/download/213033329.pdf (accessed on 28th July 2025).

40. Pace, R., Roscoe, S., & University of San Diego. (2023). Exercise As a Prescription for Patients with Depressive Disorders: A Quality Improvement Project. *UC San Diego*. Retrieved from https://escholarship.org/uc/item/42n2p0qz(accessed on 28th July 2025).

41. Snyder AD, Venkatachalam V, Pandurangi AK. Electroconvulsive therapy in geriatric patients: A literature review and program report from Virginia Commonwealth University, Richmond, Virginia, USA. J Geriatr Ment Health 2017;4:115-22.f (accessed on 28th July 2025).

42. Rhoda, D. (2014). Ayurvedic psychology: Ancient wisdom meets modern science. https://core.ac.uk/download/217367428.pdf (accessed on 28th July 2025).

INDEX

L

M

N

O

P